A Lange Medical Book

INTERNAL MEDICINE ON CALL

Fourth Edition

Edited by

Steven A. Haist, MD, MS, FACP
Professor of Medicine and Residency Program Director
Department of Internal Medicine
University of Kentucky Medical Center
Lexington, Kentucky

John B. Robbins, MD
General Internist
Private Practice
Internal Medicine Associates
Bozeman, Montana
Series Editor

Leonard G. Gomella, MD
The Bernard W. Godwin, Jr. Professor and Chair
Department of Urology
Jefferson Medical College
Thomas Jefferson University Medical Center
Philadelphia, Pennsylvania

Lange Medical Books/McGraw-Hill
Medical Publishing Division

New York Chicago San Francisco Lisbon London
Madrid Mexico City Milan New Delhi San Juan
Seoul Singapore Sydney Toronto

The McGraw·Hill Companies

Internal Medicine On Call, Fourth Edition

Copyright © 2005 by the **McGraw-Hill Companies, Inc.** All rights reserved. Printed in the United States of America. Except as permitted under the United States Copyright Act of 1976, no part of this publication may be reproduced or distributed in any form or by any means, or stored in a data base or retrieval system, without the prior written permission of the publisher.

Previous editions copyright © 2002 by The McGraw-Hill Companies, Inc.; copyright © 1997 and 1991 by Appleton & Lange

67890 DOC/DOC 0

ISSN:1052-6854
ISBN: 0-07-143902-1

The book was set in Helvetica by Pine Tree Composition, Inc.
The editors were Janet Foltin, Harriet Lebowitz, and Regina Y. Brown.
The production supervisor was Catherine H. Saggese.
The index was prepared by Katherine Pitcoff.
The art manager was Charissa Baker.

R.R. Donnelley was the printer and binder.

This book was printed on acid-free paper.

INTERNATIONAL EDITION ISBN 0-07-110493-3
Copyright © 2005. Exclusive rights by the McGraw-Hill Companies, Inc., for manufacture and export. This book cannot be re-exported from the country to which it is consigned by McGraw-Hill. The international Edition in not available in North America.

Dedicated to Meg, Sarah and Will, and Mary. Our inspiration for everything we do. We also want to thank all of our former teachers who instilled in us the importance of knowledge and scholarship and our former, current, and future students who inspire our continued learning.

Contents

Associate Editors

Aimee G. Adams, PharmD
Ambulatory Care Specialist
Assistant Professor
College of Pharmacy
University of Kentucky
Lexington, Kentucky

James A. Barker, MD
Professor and Chief,
Pulmonary and Critical Care Medicine
University of South Carolina School of Medicine
Columbia, South Carolina

David P. Haynie, MD, MBA, FACC
Cardiovascular Specialists, PA
Lewisville, Texas

Dianna S. Howard, MD
Assistant Professor
Division of Hematology and Oncology
Department of Internal Medicine
University of Kentucky
Lexington, Kentucky

Lisbeth Ann Selby, MD
Assistant Professor
Division of Gastroenterology
Department of Internal Medicine
University of Kentucky
Lexington, Kentucky

Kelly M. Smith, PharmD
Drug Information Specialist
Clinical Associate Professor
College of Pharmacy
University of Kentucky
Lexington, Kentucky

Benjamin J. Stahr, MD, FCAP
Chief of Dermatopathology
Greensboro Pathology Associates
Greensboro, North Carolina

Contributors

Aimee G. Adams, PharmD
Ambulatory Care Specialist
Assistant Professor
College of Pharmacy
University of Kentucky
Lexington, Kentucky

Jerri Alley Alexiou, MD
Dermatologist
Private Practice
Harrisonburg Dermatology
Harrisonburg, Virginia

James A. Barker, MD
Professor and Chief,
Pulmonary and Critical Care Medicine
University of South Carolina School of Medicine
Columbia, South Carolina

Donald R. Barnett, MD
Service Line Manager for Primary Care
Veterans Administration Eastern Kansas Health Care System
Topeka, Kansas

P. Ricky Bass, MD
Assistant Professor
Department of Internal Medicine and
Department of Pediatrics
Louisiana State University—Shreveport
Shreveport, Louisiana

David J. Bensema, MD
General Internist
Private Practice
Lexington, Kentucky

Rolando Berger, MD
Professor of Medicine
Division of Pulmonary and Critical Care Medicine
Department of Internal Medicine
University of Kentucky
Lexington, Kentucky

Eric W. Byrd, MD
General Internist
Private Practice
Carolina Mountain Internal Medicine
Hendersonville, North Carolina

William Coble, MD
Fellow
Division of Cardiology
Department of Internal Medicine
Medical College of Virginia
Richmond, Virginia

Thadis C. Cox, MD
Fellow
Division of Gastroenterology
Department of Internal Medicine
University of Kentucky
Lexington, Kentucky

Robert T. Davis, MD
Associate Professor of Medicine
Division of General Internal Medicine
Department of Internal Medicine
University of Kentucky
Lexington, Kentucky

David W. Dozer, MD
Gastroenterologist
Private Practice
Milwaukee Digestive Diseases Consultants, SP
Milwaukee, Wisconsin

Rita M. Egan, MD, PhD
Rheumatologist
Private Practice
Bluegrass Rheumatology Associates
Lexington, Kentucky

G. Paul Eleazer, MD
Professor of Medicine and Director
Division of Geriatrics
University of South Carolina School of Medicine
Columbia, South Carolina

Kim R. Emmett, MD
Assistant Professor
Department of Medicine
University of Tennessee Graduate School of Medicine
Knoxville, Tennessee

Christopher Feddock, MD, MS
Assistant Professor
Division of General Internal Medicine
Department of Internal Medicine
University of Kentucky
Lexington, Kentucky

Joan B. Fowler, PharmD, BCPP, CGP
President, Creative Educational Concepts Foundation
Lexington, Kentucky

David K. Goebel, MD
Hematologist/Oncologist
Private Practice
Tri-State Regional Cancer Center
Ashland, Kentucky

John J. Gohmann, MD
Medical Oncologist
Private Practice
Central Baptist Hospital
Lexington, Kentucky

Leonard G. Gomella, MD
The Bernard W. Godwin, Jr. Professor and
Chair
Department of Urology
Jefferson Medical College
Thomas Jefferson University Medical Center
Philadelphia, Pennsylvania

Tricia L. Gomella, MD
Assistant Professor, Part-time
Division of Neonatology
Department of Pediatrics
Johns Hopkins University
Baltimore, Maryland

Steven A. Haist, MD, MS, FACP
Professor of Medicine and
Residency Program Director
Department of Internal Medicine
University of Kentucky
Lexington, Kentucky

David P. Haynie, MD, MBA, FACC
Cardiovascular Specialists, PA
Lewisville, Texas

David M. Hiestand, MD
Fellow
Division of Pulmonary and Critical Care Medicine
Department of Internal Medicine
University of Kentucky Lexington, Kentucky

Alan T. Lefor, MD
Director, Surgical Education and Academic Affairs
Director, Division of Surgical Oncology
Cedars-Sinai Medical Center
Professor of Clinical Surgery
Department of Surgery
University of California, Los Angeles
Los Angeles, California

Jerry J. Lierl, MD
Associate Professor of Medicine
Director, Cardiac Cath Lab
Director of Interventional Cardiology Fellowship
University of Cincinnati
Cincinnati, Ohio

Shantae L. Lucas, MD
Hematologist/Oncologist
Private Practice
Cancer Care of Western North Carolina
Asheville, North Carolina

Ralph A. Manchester, MD, FACP
Director
University Health Service
Associate Professor of Medicine
General Medicine Unit
Department of Medicine
University of Rochester School of Medicine and Dentistry
Rochester, New York

Andrew D. Massey, MD
Associate Professor of Medicine
Department of Internal Medicine
Department of Psychiatry
Department of Neurology—Kansas City
University of Kansas School of Medicine–Wichita
Wichita, Kansas

Rick R. McClure, MD, FACC
Associate Professor
Division of Cardiovascular Medicine
Department of Internal Medicine
University of Kentucky
Lexington, Kentucky

Thomas B. Montgomery, MD
Professor of Medicine
Division of Medical Education
Department of Internal Medicine
University of South Alabama
Mobile, Alabama

William C. Moore, MD
General Internist
Private Practice
Ferrell Duncan Clinic, Inc.
Springfield, Missouri

Rita M. Kramer, MD
Associate Professor
The Breast Center
Baylor College of Medicine
Houston, Texas

Brain Murphy, MD
Fellow
Division of Infectious Diseases
Department of Internal Medicine
University of Kentucky
Lexington, Kentucky

John C. Parker, MD
Endocrinologist
Hanover Medical Specialists, PA
Wilmington, North Carolina
Consulting Associate in Medicine
Duke University
Durham, North Carolina

Carol B. Peddicord, MD
General Internist
Private Practice
Albany, Kentucky

Holly G. Pursely, MD, MSPH
General Internist
Mobile, Alabama

John B. Robbins, MD
General Internist
Private Practice
Internal Medicine Associates
Bozeman, Montana

David W. Rudy, MD
Associate Professor of Medicine
Division of General Internal Medicine
Department of Internal Medicine
University of Kentucky Lexington, Kentucky

Steven I. Shedlofsky, MD
Marcos Lins Andrade Professor of Medicine
Division of Digestive Diseases and Nutrition
Department of Internal Medicine
University of Kentucky Medical Center and Veteran's Administration Hospital
Lexington, Kentucky

Michael H. Sifford, MD
Fellow
Division of Gastroenterology
Department of Internal Medicine
University of Kentucky
Lexington, Kentucky

Kelly M. Smith, PharmD
Drug Information Specialist
Clinical Associate Professor
College of Pharmacy
University of Kentucky
Lexington, Kentucky

Benjamin J. Stahr, MD, FCAP
Chief of Dermatopathology
Greensboro Pathology Associates
Greensboro, North Carolina

R. Douglas Strickland, MD
Gastroenterologist
Private Practice
Holston Valley Hospital
Gastroenterology Associates
Kingsport, Tennessee

Gregg M. Talente, MD, MS
Assistant Professor of Medicine and Pediatrics
Brody School of Medicine
East Carolina University
Greenville, North Carolina

Timothy A. Winchester, MD
General Internist
Private Practice
Lexington, Kentucky

Preface

The fourth edition of *Internal Medicine On Call* is a user-friendly reference that will assist in the initial evaluation and treatment of the most frequently encountered problems in internal medicine. It will serve as an aid to house officers and medical students when they are called about medical problems, whether common or potentially life-threatening. *Internal Medicine On Call* provides a concise and practical approach to these problems and serves to bridge the gap between textbooks and patient care. Unlike many books or manuals, *Internal Medicine On Call* is organized by the presenting problem or complaint rather than the diagnosis. We have not attempted to provide a comprehensive discussion, but rather the essential elements in the initial assessment and management of each problem. This will aid the house officer or student when called to evaluate a patient with a specific problem.

Each on-call problem is introduced with a case scenario. This is followed by the questions the clinician should initially ask. A differential diagnosis is given with key points to help one arrive at the final diagnosis. A database section includes key points on the physical examination, laboratory tests, and other tests that are important in making the diagnosis. A plan for the treatment of specific diagnoses is also included. Recommendations for treatment are specific with regard to dosage and dosing intervals, but it is emphasized that hepatic and renal disease as well as other factors (eg, age) can greatly affect the metabolism of drugs. In addition, variations in institutional practices exist. For these reasons, treatment may need to be individualized from patient to patient or from institution to institution.

House officers and medical students often have questions regarding frequently used medications, laboratory tests, and procedures including step-by-step instruction, as well as indications and contraindications. These areas, as well as ventilator management and transfusion therapy, have been included to provide house officers and medical students a manual to answer many of the questions that arise in the day-to-day management of their patients. The fourth edition of *Internal Medicine On Call* includes significant changes from the second edition. Each problem has been updated to include the latest diagnostic tests and treatment. The Laboratory Diagnosis, Procedures, Blood Component Therapy and Ventilator Management sections have been up-dated to reflect the current state of mecical parcatice. Section VII, Therapeutics, includes sections on minerals, natural products (herbals), and vitamins, as well as over 50 new medications.

We are grateful to Tricia Gomella, MD, for providing the "on-call" concept originally used in her book *Neonatology: Basic Management, On Call Problems, Diseases, and Drugs*, first published in 1988. We thank McGraw-Hill for providing us the forum to present a unique approach for medical student and house officer education. In particular, we want to thank our copy editor, Alison T. Kelley, whose diligence and keen eye for detail has helped us improve the quality of the fourth edition of *Internal Medicine On Call*. We also want to thank Janet Foltin, our editor at McGraw-Hill, whose support and guidance has been invaluable through the third and fourth editions of this book.

Finally, we want to thank Lindsey Sutton and Mary Robbins, RN, for their efforts in the completion of this book. Without their assistance, hard work and support, the completion of this manual would not have been possible.

We sincerely hope that this manual will enhance your training and help you to provide the best care for your patients.

Steven A. Haist, MD, MS, FACP
Lexington, Kentucky

John B. Robbins, MD
Bozeman, Montana

June 2005

I. On-Call Problems

1. ABDOMINAL PAIN, ACUTE

I. **Problem.** A 34-year-old woman admitted for control of diabetes develops acute abdominal pain that increases in severity over several hours.

II. Immediate Questions

A. **What are the patient's vital signs?** Acute abdominal pain may signify a condition as benign as gastroenteritis or as catastrophic as an infarcted bowel or perforated viscus. The significant morbidity and mortality of the acute surgical abdomen can be obviated by early diagnosis. *Tachycardia* and *hypotension* suggest circulatory or septic shock from perforation, hemorrhage, or fluid loss into the intestinal lumen or peritoneal cavity. Orthostatic blood pressure and pulse changes would also be helpful in ascertaining the presence of volume loss. *Fever* occurs in inflammatory conditions such as cholecystitis and appendicitis. When the temperature exceeds 102 °F, gangrene or perforation of a viscus should be suspected. Fever may not be present in elderly patients, patients on corticosteroids, or those who are immunocompromised.

B. **Where is the pain located?** Abdominal pain is produced by three mechanisms: (1) *tension* within the walls of the alimentary tract (biliary or intestinal obstruction) or the capsules of solid organs; (2) *ischemia* (strangulated bowel, mesenteric vascular occlusion); and (3) *peritoneal irritation*. The first two causes result in visceral pain, a dull pain perceived in the midline and *poorly localized*. Generally, *pain arising from the GI tract* is perceived in the midline because of the symmetric and bilateral innervation of these organs. *Unilateral pain* should prompt consideration of a disorder of organs with unilateral innervation such as the kidney, ureter, or ovary, although unilateral pain can also be seen in disorders arising from the gut. Generally, *midepigastric pain* is caused by disorders of the stomach, duodenum, pancreas, liver, and biliary tract. Disease of the small intestine, appendix, upper ureters, testes, and ovaries results in *periumbilical pain*. *Lower abdominal pain* is caused by processes in the colon, bladder, lower ureters, and uterus. Inflammation of the parietal peritoneum results in more severe pain that is *well localized* to the area of inflammation. It is also important to realize that *referred pain* (pain originating from a site more central than where it is perceived) occurs because the cutaneous dermatomes and visceral organs share the same spinal cord level. In addition, perceived abdominal pain may arise outside of the abdomen. For example, zoster involving the thoracic dermatomes may present as severe right upper quadrant pain.

C. Does the pain radiate? Pain that becomes rapidly generalized implies perforation and leakage of fluid into the peritoneal cavity. Biliary pain can radiate from the right upper quadrant to the right inferior scapula. Pancreatic and abdominal aneurysmal pain may radiate to the back. Ureteral colic classically is referred to the groin and thigh.

D. When did the pain begin? Sudden onset suggests perforated ulcer, mesenteric occlusion, ruptured aneurysm, or ruptured ectopic pregnancy. A more gradual onset (> 1 hour) implies an inflammatory condition such as appendicitis, cholecystitis, diverticulitis, or an obstructed viscus such as bowel obstruction.

E. What is the quality of the pain? Intestinal colic occurs as cramping abdominal pain interspersed with pain-free intervals. Biliary colic is not a true colicky pain in that it usually presents as sustained persistent pain. Unfortunately, the terms *sharp, dull, burning,* and *tearing,* although used by patients to describe pain, seldom assist in determining the cause.

F. What relieves the pain or makes it worse? Pain with deep inspiration is associated with diaphragmatic irritation, such as with pleurisy or upper abdominal inflammation. Patients with intestinal or ureteral colic tend to be restless and active, whereas patients with peritonitis attempt to avoid all motion. Coughing frequently exacerbates abdominal pain from peritonitis.

G. Are there any associated symptoms? *Vomiting* may result from intestinal obstruction or may result from a visceral reflex caused by pain. In conditions causing an acute surgical abdomen, the vomiting usually follows rather than precedes the onset of pain. *Hematemesis* suggests gastritis or peptic ulcer disease. *Diarrhea* may result from gastroenteritis, but may also result from ischemic colitis or inflammatory bowel disease. *Obstipation* (absence of passage of stool or flatus) suggests mechanical bowel obstruction. *Hematuria* indicates genitourinary disease such as nephrolithiasis. *Cough* and *sputum production* might occur if lower lobe pneumonia is present.

H. For women, what is the patient's menstrual history? A missed period in a sexually active woman suggests ectopic pregnancy. A foul vaginal discharge may indicate pelvic inflammatory disease.

I. What is the patient's medical history? Is there a history of peptic ulcer disease, gallstones, diverticulosis, alcohol abuse, abdominal operations suggesting adhesions, or an abdominal aortic aneurysm? Is there any known history of cardiac arrhythmias or other cardiac disease that could result in embolization to a mesenteric artery? Is there a history of a hypercoagulable state?

J. What medications is the patient taking? Is the patient already on chronic pain medications or steroids that mask the clinical picture? Does the patient use nonsteroidal anti-inflammatory agents or other medications that might lead to abdominal pain? Is the patient taking a medication associated with acute pancreatitis?

III. **Differential Diagnosis.** The list of causes of acute abdominal pain is extensive; some of these are listed in Table I-1. Many of these diseases can be managed medically; others require urgent surgery. Abdominal pain can result from extra-abdominal processes as well as intra-abdominal disease.

   A. **Intra-abdominal disease**

      1. **Hollow viscera.** Perforation of a hollow viscus represents a surgical emergency.

         a. **Upper abdomen.** Esophagitis, gastritis, peptic ulcer disease, cholecystitis, cholelithiasis, and biliary colic.

TABLE I–1. COMMON CAUSES OF ACUTE ABDOMEN: CONDITIONS IN ITALIC TYPE OFTEN REQUIRE SURGERY.

■ **Gastrointestinal tract disorders** Nonspecific abdominal pain *Appendicitis* *Small and large bowel obstruction* *Incarcerated hernia* *Perforated peptic ulcer* *Bowel perforation* *Meckel's diverticulitis* *Boerhaave's syndrome* Diverticulitis Inflammatory bowel disorders Mallory-Weiss syndrome Gastroenteritis Acute gastritis Mesenteric adenitis Parasitic infections	■ **Urinary tract disorders** Ureteral or renal colic Acute pyelonephritis Acute cystitis Renal infarct ■ **Gynecologic disorders** *Ruptured ectopic pregnancy* *Twisted ovarian tumor* *Ruptured ovarian follicle cyst* Acute salpingitis Dysmenorrhea Endometriosis ■ **Vascular disorders** *Ruptured aortic and visceral aneurysms* *Acute ischemic colitis* *Mesenteric thrombosis*
■ **Liver, spleen, and biliary tract disorders** *Acute cholecystitis* *Acute cholangitis* *Hepatic abscess* *Ruptured hepatic tumor* *Spontaneous rupture of the spleen* Splenic infarct Biliary colic Acute hepatits	■ **Peritoneal disorders** *Intra-abdominal abscesses* Primary peritonitis Tuberculous peritonitis ■ **Retroperitoneal disorders** Retroperitoneal hemorrhage
■ **Pancreatic disorders** Acute pancreatitis	

Doherty GM, Boey JH: The Acute Abdomen. In Way LW, Doherty GM, eds. Current Surgical Diagnosis and Treatment. 11th ed. McGraw-Hill; 2003.

   b. **Midgut.** Small bowel obstruction or infarction.
   c. **Lower abdomen.** Inflammatory bowel disease, appendicitis, large bowel obstruction, diverticulitis.
2. **Solid organ**
   a. **Hepatitis**
   b. **Budd-Chiari syndrome**
   c. **Pancreatitis**
   d. **Splenic infarction or abscess**
   e. **Pyelonephritis/urolithiasis/renal infarction**
3. **Pelvis**
   a. **Pelvic inflammatory disease**
   b. **Ruptured ectopic pregnancy**
4. **Vascular system**
   a. **Ruptured aneurysm**
   b. **Dissecting aneurysm**
   c. **Mesenteric thrombosis or embolism**
5. **Spontaneous bacterial peritonitis**

B. **Extra-abdominal disease.** To prevent unnecessary surgery, the following causes of acute abdominal pain should be considered.
   1. **Diabetic ketoacidosis**
   2. **Acute adrenal insufficiency**
   3. **Acute porphyria**
   4. **Pneumonia involving lower lobes**
   5. **Pulmonary embolism involving lower lobes**
   6. **Pneumothorax**
   7. **Sickle cell crisis**
   8. **Herpes zoster of thoracoabdominal dermatomes**
   9. **Myocardial infarction**
   10. **Lead toxicity**

C. **Special populations.** In these patients, pain is secondary to unusual causes or unusual presentation of common problems.
   1. **Elderly patients.** Pain is often present without signs and symptoms commonly seen in younger patients.
   2. **Patients with HIV.** See Section I, Chapter 23, Fever in the HIV-Positive Patient, p 141.
   3. **Patients with coagulopathies including hemophilia and patients taking warfarin. Hematoma of bowel wall.**

D. **Rare causes**
   1. **Celiac axis compression syndrome**
   2. **Painful rib syndrome**
   3. **Wandering spleen syndrome**
   4. **Abdominal migraine**
   5. **Fitz-Hugh-Curtis syndrome.** Perihepatitis secondary to gonococcal or chlamydia salpingitis.
   6. **Mesenteric vasculitis**

TABLE I–2. PHYSICAL FINDINGS WITH VARIOUS CAUSES OF ACUTE ABDOMEN.

Condition	Signs
Perforated viscus	Scaphoid, tense abdomen; diminished bowel sounds (late); loss of liver dullness; guarding or rigidity
Peritonitis	Motionless, absent bowel sounds (late); cough and rebound tenderness; guarding or rigidity
Inflamed mass or abscess	Tender mass (abdominal, rectal, or pelvic); punch tenderness; special signs (Murphy's, psoas, or obturator)
Intestinal obstruction	Distention; visible peristalsis (late); hyperperistalsis (early) or quiet abdomen (late); diffuse pain without rebound tenderness; hernia or rectal mass (some)
Paralytic ileus	Distention; minimal bowel sounds; no localized tenderness
Ischemic or strangulated bowel	Not distended (until late); bowel sounds variable; severe pain but little tenderness; rectal bleeding (some)
Bleeding	Pallor, shock; distention; pulsatile (aneurysm) or tender (eg, ectopic pregnancy) mass; rectal bleeding (some)

Reproduced with permission from Doherty GM, Boey JH: The Acute Abdomen. In Way LW, Doherty GM, eds. Current Surgical Diagnosis and Treatment. 11th ed. McGraw-Hill; 2003.

IV. Database

A. Physical examination key points. See Table I-2.

1. **Vital signs and general appearance.** Does the patient appear uncomfortable? (See Section II.A.) Is the patient jaundiced? Is there a position that provides some relief of the pain? Patients with peritonitis resist movement, whereas patients with colic writhe in pain.

2. **Lungs.** Percuss for dullness at the bases, which suggests a pleural effusion or consolidation. In addition to dullness, crackles or bronchial breath sounds suggest a pneumonia, infarction, or atelectasis associated with decreased inspiratory effort because of pain. A friction rub suggests pleuritis as a cause of upper abdominal pain.

3. **Heart.** Look for jugular venous distention, S_3 gallop, or a displaced apical impulse indicative of congestive heart failure that might predispose to passive congestion of the liver or mesenteric ischemia. An irregular pulse could indicate atrial fibrillation, which might result in mesenteric artery embolism. Pericarditis is suggested by a friction rub and could be associated with upper abdominal discomfort.

4. **Abdomen**
   a. **Inspection.** Examine for distention (obstruction, ileus, ascites), ecchymoses (hemorrhagic pancreatitis), caput medusae (portal hypertension), and surgical scars (adhesions).

        b. Auscultation. Listen for bowel sounds (absent or an occasional tinkle with ileus, hyperperistaltic with gastroenteritis, high-pitched rushes with small bowel obstruction).

        c. Percussion. Tympany is associated with distended loops of bowel. Shifting dullness and a fluid wave suggest ascites with peritonitis.

        d. Other signs. Pain with active hip flexion or with extension of the patient's right thigh while lying on the left side (*psoas sign*) could result from an inflamed appendix. *Obturator sign* (pain on internal rotation of the flexed thigh) can occur with appendicitis.

    5. Rectum. Evaluation of acute abdominal pain is not complete until a rectal exam has been performed. A mass suggests the presence of rectal carcinoma. Lateral rectal tenderness occurs with appendicitis, a condition in which examination of the abdomen may not reveal localized findings. If stool is present, evaluate for occult blood.

    6. Female genitalia. Examine for pain with cervical motion and cervical discharge that may suggest pelvic inflammatory disease. Also, palpate for adnexal masses that would indicate an ectopic pregnancy, ovarian abscess, cyst, or neoplasm.

B. Laboratory data. The decision to operate is seldom made solely on the basis of laboratory data. This information serves mainly (1) as an adjunct in cases in which the cause of the pain is unclear or (2) for assistance in preoperative assessment in individuals for whom the diagnosis is certain and the decision to operate has already been made.

    1. Hematology. An increased hematocrit suggests hemoconcentration from volume loss (pancreatitis). A low hematocrit may suggest a process that has resulted in chronic blood loss or possibly acute intra-abdominal hemorrhage or an acute gastrointestinal (GI) hemorrhage. With acute blood loss, however, the hematocrit may not decrease for several hours. An elevated white blood cell count suggests an inflammatory process such as appendicitis or cholecystitis.

    2. Electrolytes, blood urea nitrogen (BUN), creatinine. Bowel obstruction with vomiting can result in hypokalemia, azotemia, and volume contraction alkalosis. A strangulated bowel or sepsis may result in a metabolic gap acidosis. An elevated BUN/creatinine ratio is seen with volume depletion and GI bleeding.

    3. Liver function tests including bilirubin, transaminases, and alkaline phosphatase. Results are elevated in acute hepatitis, cholecystitis, and other biliary tract disease.

    4. Amylase/lipase. Markedly elevated levels are associated with pancreatitis. However, in up to 30% of patients with acute pancreatitis, amylase may be initially normal, especially in patients with lipemic serum. Conversely, amylase can also be elevated in conditions other than pancreatitis, such as acute cholecystitis, perforated ulcer, small bowel obstruction with strangulation, and ruptured ectopic pregnancy. Serum lipase helps to differentiate pancreatitis from other causes of hyperamylasemia.

5. **Arterial blood gases.** Hypoxemia is often an early sign of sepsis and may occur with pancreatitis. As mentioned, metabolic acidosis may result from ischemic bowel or sepsis.

6. **Pregnancy test.** All premenopausal women with acute right or left lower abdominal pain should be tested for human chorionic gonadotropin levels to rule out ectopic pregnancy, regardless of whether or not they missed their last period.

7. **Urinalysis.** Hematuria may indicate nephrolithiasis; pyuria and hematuria can be present in urinary tract infections. In addition, pyuria is occasionally present with appendicitis.

8. **Cervical culture.** Obtain a cervical culture for chlamydia and gonorrhea when pelvic inflammatory disease is suspected.

C. Radiology and other studies

1. **Flat and upright abdominal films.** These films can be readily obtained and may provide important information. Watch for the following indicators: gas pattern; evidence of bowel dilation; air—fluid levels; presence or absence of air in the rectum; pancreatic calcifications; biliary and renal calcifications; aortic calcifications; loss of psoas margin (suggesting retroperitoneal bleeding); and presence or absence of air in the biliary tract.

2. **Chest film.** A chest x-ray may reveal lower lobe pneumonia, pleural effusion, or elevation of a hemidiaphragm indicating a subdiaphragmatic inflammatory process. Free air under the diaphragm suggests a perforated viscus and is most often seen on the upright chest film. The sensitivity of this test has been reported as low as 38%.

3. **Ultrasound (US).** This readily obtainable and noninvasive test is the preferred modality for right upper quadrant pain or gynecologic disease. US may reveal the presence or absence of gallstones, biliary tract dilation, or ectopic pregnancy.

4. **Computed tomography (CT).** The most sensitive test when considering many possible diagnoses. CT has a sensitivity of 96% and a specificity of 83—89% for appendicitis compared with 75—90% and 86—100%, respectively, for ultrasound. The American College of Radiology, Expert Panel on Gastrointestinal Imaging, states that if the patient has fever or is HIV-positive, CT imaging is the preferred modality.

5. **Electrocardiogram (ECG).** An ECG is needed to rule out an acute myocardial infarction or pericarditis, which may present with acute upper abdominal pain.

    6. Arteriography. This may be necessary in patients in whom mesenteric artery ischemia is suspected

    7. Paracentesis. See Section III, Chapter 11, Paracentesis, p 447. With known ascites and acute abdominal pain, this test is required to rule out the possibility of spontaneous bacterial peritonitis. If ascites is suspected but has not been documented, an ultrasound should be performed before an attempted paracentesis.

    8. Other studies may be necessary to determine the nature of the pain, provided that the patient does not appear to have acute abdominal pain that requires surgery. These tests can include the following:

       a. Intravenous pyelogram

       b. Hepato-iminodiacetic acid (HIDA) scan, to rule out acute cholecystitis

       c. Contrast bowel studies, such as an upper GI and small bowel series, to look for evidence of occult perforation or mechanical obstruction. A barium enema may be helpful in evaluation for sigmoid or cecal volvulus.

       d. Endoscopic studies, such as esophagogastroduodenoscopy, colonoscopy, or endoscopic retrograde cholangiopancreatography.

V. Plan. As mentioned previously, the initial goal in evaluating acute abdominal pain is to determine whether or not surgical treatment is indicated to prevent further morbidity. When pain has been present 6 or more hours and has not improved, there is an increased likelihood that the patient will require surgical exploration to determine the cause. Often, the specific cause of the patient's abdominal pain is not determined until laparotomy. The use of analgesics remains controversial, but many surgeons now favor the use of moderate doses of pain medication to make the patient more comfortable and facilitate further examination (See Section I, Chapter 54, Pain Management, V, p 306.)

    A. Observation. With the exception of conditions requiring urgent surgical exploration (Table I-3), most cases of abdominal pain can be initially managed with close observation, correction of any fluid or electrolyte disturbances, and judicious use of analgesics.

       1. Surgery consultation. Any patient developing acute abdominal pain should be evaluated by a general surgeon.

       2. Gastric decompression. When mechanical obstruction is suspected or vomiting is present, a nasogastric tube should be placed for decompression. (See Section III, Chapter 8, Gastrointestinal Tubes, p 436.)

       3. Intravenous fluids. Septic or circulatory shock should be treated with vigorous intravenous volume replacement. If hypotension persists, vasopressors such as dopamine may be needed (See Section I, Chapter 42, Hypotension, V, p 237.)

TABLE I–3. INDICATIONS FOR URGENT OPERATION IN PATIENTS WITH ACUTE ABDOMEN.

■ **Physical findings**
Involuntary guarding or rigidity, especially if spreading
Increasing or severe localized tenderness
Tense or progressive distention
Tender abdominal or rectal mass with high fever or hypotension
Rectal bleeding with shock or acidosis
Equivocal abdominal findings along with
    Septicemia (high fever, marked or rising leukocytosis, mental changes, or increasing
        glucose intolerance in a diabetic patient)
    Bleeding (unexplained shock or acidosis, falling hematocrit)
    Suspected ischemia (acidosis, fever, tachycardia)
    Deterioration on conservative treatment

■ **Radiologic findings**
Pneumoperitoneum
Gross or progressive bowel distension
Free extravasation of contrast material
Space-occupying lesion on CT scan with fever
Mesenteric occlusion on angiography

■ **Endoscopic findings**
Perforated or uncontrollably bleeding lesion

■ **Paracentesis findings**
Blood, bile, pus, bowel contents, or urine

[1]*Reproduced with permission from Doherty GM, Boey JH: The Acute Abdomen. In Way LW, Doherty GM, eds. Current Surgical Diagnosis and Treatment. 11th ed. McGraw-Hill; 2003.*

    4. Serial physical examinations. Periodic examinations by the same clinician are helpful in determining a change in the patient's condition and establishing a diagnosis or need for surgery.

  B. Surgery. Indications for an urgent operation without a period of observation or establishment of a specific preoperative diagnosis are outlined in Table I-3.

REFERENCES

Balthazar EJ, Birnbaum BA, Yee J et al: Acute appendicitis: CT and ultrasound correlation in one hundred patients. Radiology 1997;202:137.

Fishman MB, Aronson MD: Approach to the patient with abdominal pain. In: Fletcher SW, Fletcher RH, Aronson MD, eds. UpToDate [CD-ROM]. Version 8.2. Wellesley, MA;2000. www.uptodate.com

Jung PJ, Merrell PC: Acute abdomen. Gastroenterol Clin North Am 1988;17:227.

Ray BS, Neill CL: Abdominal visceral pain in man. Ann Surg 1947;126:709.

Silen W: *Cope's Early Diagnosis of the Acute Abdomen.* 20th ed. Oxford University Press;2000.

Wagner JM, McKinney P, Carpentar JL: Does this patient have appendicitis? JAMA 1996;276:1589.

2. ACIDOSIS

I. **Problem.** A 30-year-old man is brought into the emergency room uncon-scious. A friend found him at home. No other history is available. Physi-cal examination is unremarkable except for rapid, shallow breathing. Arterial blood gas (ABG) reading reveals a pH of 7.10.

II. **Immediate Questions**

A. **Is the acidemia from a metabolic, respiratory, or mixed acido-sis?** A quick look at the pCO_2 on the ABG slip will reveal whether the disturbance is a primary metabolic or respiratory acidosis. If the pCO_2 is less than 40 mm Hg, then the primary disturbance is a metabolic acidosis. If the pCO_2 is greater than 40 mm Hg, the disturbance may be a primary respiratory acidosis or may be a mixed disturbance. Many ABG slips list the base excess (BE). The BE may help determine the cause of the acidosis. If the BE is posi-tive, the acidosis is respiratory; if the BE is negative, the acidosis is at least partially metabolic. Remember that the BE is calculated from the pH; the calculation assumes that both the pH and pCO_2 are cor-rect.

B. **What are the patient's vital signs?** Metabolic acidosis is often the result of lactic acid production from hypoperfusion and hypoxia. If the patient has hypotension or is orthostatic, immediate fluid resuscita-tion is indicated. Vasopressor agents may also be needed after vol-ume resuscitation. (See Section I, Chapter 42, Hypotension, p 237.) Bradypnea may suggest a narcotics overdose. Tachypnea may arise from hyperventilation as respiratory compensation for a metabolic acidosis or from increased respiratory effort with hypoventilation (eg, pulmonary edema), resulting in a respiratory acidosis.

C. **Are there any arrhythmias or ectopy?** With a profound acidemia from any cause, there may be an associated cardiac arrhythmia (ventricular ectopy common). Obtain an electrocardiogram and moni-tor the patient.

D. **What is the serum bicarbonate?** To fully understand an acid–base problem, it is imperative to obtain the serum bicarbonate from an electrolyte panel. A high serum bicarbonate is evidence of a primary respiratory acidosis. A low serum bicarbonate is evidence of either a primary metabolic acidosis or a mixed metabolic and respiratory aci-dosis.

E. **Do the values for serum bicarbonate, pH, and pCO_2 fit?** Once you have the serum bicarbonate, you should make sure the pH, pCO_2, and HCO_3^- fit:

$$pH = pK_a + \log \frac{HCO_3^-}{H_2CO_3}$$

which can be simplified to:

$$H^+ = 24 \times \frac{pCO_2}{HCO_3^-}$$

In this patient with a pH of 7.10, if the pCO_2 is 20 mm Hg and the serum bicarbonate is 6 mmol/L, then:

$$H^+ = 24 \times \frac{20}{6}$$

$$H^+ = 80$$

Does a pH of 7.10 equal a $[H^+]$ of 80 nmol/L? There are some simple rules to help convert pH to $[H^+]$. At a pH of 7.40, the $[H^+]$ = 40 nmol/L. pH is a log scale, and for every 0.3 change in pH, the $[H^+]$ doubles or is halved. For instance, if pH = 7.70, $[H^+]$ = 20 nmol/L, and at pH = 8.00, $[H^+]$ = 10 nmol/L. In this patient, if pH = 7.10, then $[H^+$ = 80 nmol/L. Also, around a pH of 7.40 (7.25–7.48), the $[H^+]$ changes 1 nmol/L for every 0.01 change in pH. Lastly, on the back of many ABG slips, there may be a scale showing the relation between pH and $[H^+]$. If the numbers do not fit reasonably well (± 10%) into the equation

$$[H^+] = 24 \times \frac{pCO_2}{HCO_3^-}$$

then it is difficult to determine the acid–base disturbance, and the blood gas and serum bicarbonate should be repeated. For instance, if pH = 7.30, pCO_2 = 45 mm Hg, and HCO_3^- = 30 mmol/L, a superficial interpretation might be respiratory acidosis; however, closer scrutiny is necessary.

A pH of 7.30 corresponds to H^+ of 50 nmol/L

$$50 = 24 \times \frac{45}{30}$$
$$50 \neq 36$$

The pH, the pCO_2, or the HCO_2^- is in error. For instance, if the blood was not transported on ice to the laboratory, the pH would be falsely low.

F. Is the compensation appropriate? Checking to see whether the compensation is appropriate may unmask mixed disturbances.

1. For **respiratory acidosis,** immediate compensation is through buffers. In the short term, one expects the HCO_3^- to increase by 1 mmol/L for every 10 mm Hg increase in pCO_2 over normal (40

mm Hg). Renal compensation is not present for up to 24 hours. For chronic respiratory acidosis, expect an increase in the HCO_3^- of 3.5–4.0 mmol/L for every 10 mm Hg increase in pCO_2. It takes several days (3–5 days) for maximal renal compensation for a respiratory acidosis. For instance, in a 25-year-old with an acute episode of asthma, the ABG revealed a pCO_2 of 90. One would expect the bicarbonate to increase by 5 mmol/L from the calculation 1 mmol/L $\times$ (90 mm Hg – 40 mm Hg)/10 mm Hg. One would expect the HCO_3^- to be 31 mmol/L from the calculation 26 mmol/L (normal bicarbonate range 23–29) + 5 mmol/L. If the bicarbonate were 25 mmol/L, then a relative metabolic acidosis would be present along with the primary respiratory acidosis. If the bicarbonate were 36 mmol/L, then a metabolic alkalosis would also be present along with the primary respiratory acidosis.

2. For **metabolic acidosis,** compensation begins immediately through buffers and hyperventilation; however, steady state may not be reached for up to 24 hours. The expected change in pCO_2 = (1.5 $\times$ HCO_3^-) + 8 $\pm$ 2. For instance, in a 40-year-old with renal failure, the serum bicarbonate was found to be 14 mmol/L. The expected change in pCO_2 would be (1.5 $\times$ 14) + 8 $\pm$ 2, or 29 $\pm$ 2. One would expect the pCO_2 to be between 27 and 31 mm Hg. If the actual pCO_2 were 19 mm Hg, then a respiratory alkalosis would also be present along with the primary metabolic acidosis. If the actual pCO_2 were 36 mm Hg, then a relative respiratory acidosis would be present along with the primary metabolic acidosis.

III. **Differential Diagnosis.** An acidemia is from either a metabolic or respiratory acidosis. There are many causes of both, and sometimes a patient may have more than one cause.

A. **Respiratory acidosis.** By definition, respiratory acidosis occurs secondary to hypoventilation. Hypoventilation can be caused by lung, chest, or central nervous system (CNS) disorders.

1. **Lungs**
   a. **Asthma.** May progress from a respiratory alkalosis to respiratory acidosis. A normal or elevated pCO_2 indicates impending respiratory failure and may indicate the need for prompt intubation.
   b. **Pulmonary edema.** Mild pulmonary edema usually causes a respiratory alkalosis. Severe pulmonary edema may cause a respiratory acidosis, and intubation will probably be required.
   c. **Pneumonia.** Again, pneumonia usually causes respiratory alkalosis. But if more than one lobe is involved, or if there is underlying chronic obstructive disease, pneumonia may cause a respiratory acidosis.
   d. **Upper airway obstruction.** Causes of obstruction may include foreign bodies, tumors, or a laryngospasm.

    e. **Pneumothorax.** Usually causes respiratory alkalosis; can cause a respiratory acidosis.

    f. **Large pleural effusion.** Usually causes a respiratory alkalosis; can cause a respiratory acidosis.

  2. **Chest abnormalities**

    a. **Kyphoscoliosis.** Results in a restrictive defect.

    b. **Scleroderma.** Results in a restrictive defect.

    c. **Marked obesity (pickwickian syndrome)**

    d. **Muscular disorders.** These include muscular dystrophy, severe hypophosphatemia, and myasthenia gravis.

    e. **Peripheral neurologic disorders, such as Guillain-Barré syndrome.**

  3. **CNS disorders**

    a. **Drugs or toxins.** Cause respiratory drive depression.

      i. **Ethanol intoxication at levels of 400–500 mg%**

      ii. **Barbiturates, especially overdoses**

      iii. **Narcotics**

      iv. **Benzodiazepines.** Especially when taken with alcohol.

    b. **Cerebrovascular accident**

    c. **Brain stem bleed or cervical spinal cord injuries**

B. Pseudorespiratory alkalosis. Arterial hypocapnia is present; however, there is an increase in the mixed venous pCO_2. It is seen in severe cardiac dysfunction and associated pulmonary hypoperfusion with normal pulmonary function. Total body carbon dioxide is increased, resulting in an increase in H^+ and an acidosis.

C. Metabolic acidosis. This can be divided into high anion gap and normal anion gap acidosis. The anion gap can be calculated as follows:

$$\text{Anion gap} = [Na^+] - ([Cl^-] + [HCO_3^-])$$

The normal anion gap is 8–12 mmol/L. An increase in anion gap may result from an increase in an unmeasured anion. Other causes of an elevated anion gap include dehydration; alkalosis; use of penicillin antibiotics that contain large amounts of sodium, such as carbenicillin; and therapy with sodium salts or organic acids such as sodium lactate, acetate, and citrate. Sodium citrate is used in whole blood and packed red cells as an anticoagulant. However, only a metabolic acidosis causes an appreciable increase in the anion gap.

  1. **Normal anion gap (metabolic nongap acidosis)**

    a. **Loss of bicarbonate through the GI tract**

      i. **Diarrhea**

      ii. **Small bowel fistula**

      iii. **Pancreatocutaneous fistula**

      iv. **Ureterosigmoidostomy**

      v. **Chloride-containing exchange resins,** such as cholestyramine; or with calcium chloride or magnesium chloride

   b. **Loss of bicarbonate through the kidneys**
      i. **Renal tubular acidosis.** If the history does not reveal an obvious cause such as diarrhea, then you need to consider renal tubular acidosis.
         (a.) Distal renal tubular acidosis. Impaired net acid excretion; causes include hypercalcemia, amphotericin B, and medullary sponge kidney.
         (b.) Proximal renal tubular acidosis. Impaired proximal tubular reabsorption of HCO_3^-. Causes include lead, cadmium and mercury toxicity, and amyloidosis.
      ii. **Carbonic anhydrase inhibitors**
   c. **Other causes not from gastrointestinal or renal loss of HCO_3^-**
      i. **Early renal failure**
      ii. **Hydrochloric acid**
      iii. **Hyperalimentation**
      iv. **Dilutional**
2. **Elevated anion gap (metabolic gap acidosis)**
   a. **Lactic acidosis.** Results from overproduction or impairment of lactate utilization by the liver, often from tissue hypoperfusion and hypoxia.
      i. **Shock. Cardiogenic, hypovolemic, septic shock.**
      ii. **Severe anemia**
      iii. **Hypoxia**
      iv. **Malignancy**
      v. **Seizures**
      vi. **Ethanol**
      vii. **Crush injury**
   b. **Renal failure.** Loss of acid secretion and failure to filter anions.
   c. **Ketoacidosis**
      i. **Diabetic ketoacidosis**
      ii. **Alcoholic ketoacidosis**
      iii. **Starvation ketoacidosis**
   d. **Toxins**
      i. **Salicylates.** These compounds cause an isolated metabolic gap acidosis (10%), an isolated respiratory alkalosis (30%), but most commonly a mixed metabolic gap acidosis and respiratory alkalosis (57%).
      ii. **Methanol.** Metabolized to formic acid and formaldehyde; may cause blindness, abdominal pain, and headache.
      iii. **Ethylene glycol.** Metabolized to oxalate, glycolaldehyde, and hippurate. Renal failure, neurologic disturbances, hypertension, and cardiovascular collapse may occur.
      iv. **Toluene.** Seen in glue sniffing or huffing. Toluene can cause metabolic gap acidosis (hippurate anion) or metabolic nongap acidosis.

      v. **Note:** Isopropyl alcohol ingestion does not cause an acidosis because isopropyl alcohol is metabolized to acetone. It may therefore cause a positive nitroprusside test for ketones. It may cause gastritis.

  e. The anion gap is also helpful in differentiating a pure metabolic acidosis, a mixed metabolic gap acidosis and metabolic nongap acidosis, and a mixed metabolic gap acidosis and metabolic alkalosis. For instance, if the HCO_3^- were 14 with a gap of 23, this would most likely represent a pure metabolic gap acidosis as calculated by:

        23 mmol/L   Actual gap
  −<u>10</u> mmol/L   Normal gap
        13 mmol/L   Expected change in HCO_3^- from normal

        26 mmol/L   Normal HCO_3^- (range 23–29)
  −<u>13</u> mmol/L   Expected change in HCO_3^-
        13 mmol/L   Expected HCO_3^-

Actual HCO_3^- 14 mmol/L = expected gap of 13 mmol/L

An HCO_2^- of 19 with a gap of 25 would most likely represent a *mixed metabolic acidosis and metabolic alkalosis* as calculated by:

        25 mmol/L   Actual gap
  −<u>10</u> mmol/L   Normal gap
        15 mmol/L   Expected change in HCO_3^- from normal

        26 mmol/L   Normal HCO_3^- (range 23 – 29)
  −<u>15</u> mmol/L   Expected change in HCO_3^-
        11 mmol/L   Expected HCO_3^-

The actual HCO_3^-, however, is 19 mmol/L, 8 mmol/L higher than expected. Thus, there must also be a metabolic alkalosis in addition to the metabolic gap acidosis.

  An HCO_3^- of 8 mmol/L with a gap of 22 mmol/L would most likely represent a *mixed metabolic gap acidosis and metabolic nongap acidosis* as calculated by:

        22 mmol/L   Actual gap
  −<u>10</u> mmol/L   Normal gap
        12 mmol/L   Expected change in HCO_3^-

26 mmol/L Normal HCO_3^- (range 23 – 29)
$\underline{-12}$ mmol/L Expected change in HCO_3^-
14 mmol/L Expected HCO_3^-

The actual HCO_3^-, however, is 8 mmol/L, or 6 mmol/L lower than expected. Thus, there must also be a metabolic nongap acidosis in addition to the metabolic gap acidosis.

IV. Database

A. Physical examination key points

1. **Vital signs.** A low respiratory rate suggests hypoventilation; a high rate points toward respiratory failure or compensation for a metabolic acidosis. Hypotension suggests hypoperfusion.
2. **Skin.** Changes, which characterize scleroderma, indicate a restrictive defect. Cool, clammy, and mottled skin on the extremities suggests shock.
3. **HEENT.** Ketosis or fruity odor on breath suggests diabetic ketoacidosis. Look for tracheal shift from a space-occupying lesion or venous distention (congestive heart failure or tension pneumothorax). Pinpoint pupils are consistent with drug overdose.
4. **Lungs.** Evaluate for absent or decreased breath sounds, stridor in upper airway obstruction, wheezes, and rales.
5. **Abdomen.** Peritoneal signs indicate an acute abdomen; marked distention may inhibit respiration.
6. **Neuromuscular examination.** Generalized weakness or focal neurologic signs, depressed level of consciousness, obtundation, and coma should be noted.

B. Laboratory data

1. **Hemograms.** Anemia may be associated with renal failure. Anemia may cause ischemia resulting in lactic acidosis. Leukocytosis with a left shift may suggest sepsis.
2. **Electrolytes.** Serum chloride is usually elevated in metabolic nongap acidosis. Serum potassium is usually increased with acidosis, but may be low in diabetic ketoacidosis or renal tubular acidosis. The serum potassium may be especially helpful in predicting the acid–base status before the ABG analysis. For instance, a serum bicarbonate of 34 mmol/L could indicate a primary metabolic alkalosis, or compensation for a chronic respiratory acidosis. If the potassium were 5.6 mmol/L, this would argue that the bicarbonate of 34 mmol/L was from compensation for a chronic respiratory acidosis. If the potassium were 3.1 mmol/L, this would argue that the bicarbonate of 34 mmol/L was from a metabolic alkalosis. The potassium, blood urea nitrogen (BUN), and creatinine may be elevated with renal failure. The creatinine may be falsely elevated with ketoacidosis.

3. **Metabolic gap acidosis.** The following tests *must be* ordered:
   a. **Glucose.** If elevated, may indicate diabetic ketoacidosis.
   b. **Ketone levels.** May indicate alcoholism, starvation, or diabetic ketoacidosis.
   c. **Lactate.** Lactic acidosis may be seen with alcohol use, severe anemia, sepsis, hypoperfusion (either generalized or local), hypoxemia, end-stage liver disease, and postictally.
   d. **Salicylate level**
   e. **Ethanol**
   f. **Methanol**
   g. **Ethylene glycol**
   h. **Paraldehyde.** Very rare cause of metabolic acidosis.
   i. **BUN and creatinine**
4. **Metabolic nongap acidosis.** If the history does not reveal an obvious cause such as diarrhea, then consider renal tubular acidosis.
   a. **Distal renal tubular acidosis.** Inability to lower urine pH below 5.5 with NH_4Cl (ammonium chloride).
   b. **Proximal renal tubular acidosis.** Urine pH will decrease to < 5.5; however, the excretion of HCO_3^- is increased to > 15% when serum HCO_3^- is raised to the normal range.
5. **Respiratory acidosis.** Order a serum and urine drug screen. If there is hypoventilation with decreased respirations, you need to rule out a drug overdose. Also, with an intentional salicylate overdose, ingestion of other substances must be ruled out, because intentional overdoses often involve multiple substances.

C. **Radiologic and other studies.** If there is respiratory acidosis, radiologic studies may be needed.
   1. **Chest x-ray.** Rule out pneumothorax, pulmonary edema, pleural effusion, and infiltrative processes.
   2. **CT scan of head.** Consider with hypoventilation and altered mental status or with focal neurologic exam.
   3. **Electromyography.** May be helpful in assessment of neuromuscular disorders.

V. **Plan.** In general, for both respiratory and metabolic acidosis, treatment of the underlying cause of the acidemia is the primary goal. In emergent situations, the two methods for short-term reversal of metabolic and respiratory acidosis are (1) to administer IV sodium bicarbonate and (2) to hyperventilate the patient. Be sure to check serial pH values to monitor the progress of therapy.

A. **Severe acidosis (pH < 7.20).** Use continuous cardiac monitoring for potential arrhythmias.

B. **Metabolic acidosis.** Sodium bicarbonate is the mainstay for therapy. Sodium acetate, citrate, and lactate can be used, but all three must be metabolized to bicarbonate. If hypoperfusion is a problem,

the metabolism of one of the precursors to bicarbonate may be delayed.
1. **Bicarbonate therapy.** Although controversial, the present recommendation is to administer IV bicarbonate if the pH < 7.10. The goal is to raise the HCO_3^- to 10–12 mmol, which should be sufficient to attain a serum pH > 7.20.
    a. Calculate the amount of sodium bicarbonate needed to raise the HCO_2^- to a given level.

    $$NaHCO_3 \text{ needed} = wt \text{ (in kg)} \times 0.80\,^*$$
    $$\times \text{ (desired } HCO_3^- - \text{measured } HCO_3^-).$$

    b. Give 50% of this amount over the first 12 hours as a mixture of bicarbonate with D5W. A normal bicarbonate drip is made by adding 3 ampules of $NaHCO_3$ (50 mEq/ampule) to 1 L of D5W. Discontinue the bicarbonate infusion when the pH is > 7.20.
    c. Complications of bicarbonate therapy include:
        i. **Hypernatremia**
        ii. **Volume overload**
        iii. **Hypokalemia.** Caused by intracellular shifts of potassium as the pH increases.
        iv. **Overshoot metabolic alkalosis.** From overaggressive therapy.
2. **THAM (0.3 *N* tromethamine).** Is a commercial carbon dioxide–consuming alkalinizing solution. It is not clinically proven to be more beneficial than sodium bicarbonate. Side effects include hyperkalemia, hyperglycemia, and respiratory depression.
3. **Treatment of underlying causes**
    a. **Sepsis and hemorrhagic shock.** Volume resuscitation with normal saline is indicated. Vasopressors may be needed. See Section I, Chapter 42, Hypotension, Section V, p 241.
    b. **Renal failure.** Dialysis as needed.
    c. **Diabetic ketoacidosis.** Normal saline and insulin for diabetic ketoacidosis. See Section I, Chapter 32, Hyperglycemia, Section V, p 193.
    d. **Alcoholic ketoacidosis.** Normal saline and dextrose for alcoholic ketoacidosis, along with replacement of other electrolytes and vitamins such as thiamine and folate as needed.
    e. **Starvation ketosis.** Normal saline and dextrose.
    f. **Salicylate intoxication.** Treated with alkalinization of urine. Intravenous fluids containing $NaHCO_3$ (3 ampules 50 mEq in 1 L of D5W or 2 ampules $NaHCO_3$ in 1 L D5 1/4NS) are administered at 100–250 mL/hr. Check urine pH every 1–2 hours. Urine pH should be maintained at or above 7.5–8.0. ABG and serum bicarbonate should be followed closely, and severe alkalemia (pH > 7.55) avoided. Hemodialysis may be required.

g. **Methanol and ethylene glycol ingestion.** Treated with ethanol infusion (desired serum concentration of ethanol is 100–120 mg/dL), which decreases the accumulation of toxic metabolites. More recently fomepizole (4-methylpyrazole) has been shown to be a safe and effective treatment alternative to ethanol. Hemodialysis may be required.

C. **Respiratory acidosis.** The main goal is to treat the underlying cause.

1. If indicated, intubate the patient and treat with mechanical ventilation. If a patient is already intubated and has a significant respiratory acidosis, then increase alveolar ventilation by increasing tidal volume (up to 8–10 mL/kg), while following peak inspiratory pressures, or by increasing the respiratory rate. See Section I, Chapter 19; Dyspnea, V, p 121; and Section VI, Ventilator Management, Chapter 3C, p 482.

2. In an emergent situation, disconnect the patient from the ventilator and hyperventilate by hand. The importance of good pulmonary toilet (ie, suctioning of secretions) cannot be overemphasized. Sedation is often a necessary adjunct to mechanical ventilation. See Section VI, Ventilator Management, Chapters 3A (p 476) and 3C (p 482).

REFERENCES

Adrogue HJ, Madias NE: Management of life-threatening acid-base disorders. N Engl J Med 1998;338:26.

Brent J, McMartin K, Phillips S, Aaron C, Kulig K: Fomepizole for the treatment of methanol poisoning. N Engl J Med 2001;344:424.

Kaehny WD: Pathogenesis and management of respiratory and mixed acid-base disorders. In: Schrier RW, ed. *Renal and Electrolyte Disorders.* 6th ed. Lippincott Williams & Wilkins;2003:154.

Narins RG, Emmett A: Simple and mixed acid-base disorders: A practical approach. Medicine 1980;59:161.

Shapiro JI, Kaehny WD: Pathogenesis and management of metabolic acidosis and alkalosis. In: Schrier RW, ed. *Renal and Electrolyte Disorders.* 6th ed. Lippincott Williams & Wilkins;2003:115.

3. ALKALOSIS

I. **Problem.** You are consulted to see a 60-year-old man with a pH of 7.65, who is 3 days status postcholecystectomy.

II. **Immediate Questions**

A. **Is the alkalemia from a metabolic, respiratory, or mixed alkalosis?** A quick look at the pCO_2 on the arterial blood gas (ABG) slip will reveal whether the disturbance is a primary metabolic or respiratory alkalosis. If the pCO_2 is > 40 mm Hg, the primary disturbance is a metabolic alkalosis with at least partial respiratory compensation. If the pCO_2 is < 40 mm Hg, the disturbance may be a primary respiratory alkalosis or a mixed disturbance. Many arterial blood gas slips list the base excess (BE), which may help determine the cause of the alkalosis. If the BE is negative, the alkalosis is respiratory; if the BE is positive, the alkalosis is at least partially metabolic. Remember that the BE is calculated from the pH and assumes that both the pH and pCO_2 are correct.

B. What are the patient's vital signs? An elevated respiratory rate, fever, hypotension, or all three may indicate sepsis. Respiratory alkalosis is associated with sepsis. Tachypnea may also indicate anxiety, CNS disease, or pulmonary disease.

C. What medications is the patient taking? Diuretics can cause a contraction alkalosis. Acetate in hyperalimentation solutions, antacids, exogenous steroids, or large doses of penicillin or carbenicillin may cause an alkalosis. Salicylate overdose and progesterone can cause a respiratory alkalosis.

D. Is a nasogastric tube in place? Is the patient vomiting? Loss of HCl from the stomach is a common cause of metabolic alkalosis.

E. Is there any history of mental status changes, seizures, paresthesias, or tetany? Alkalemia may cause the latter; if so, prompt action is indicated.

F. Is there any ventricular ectopy? Severe alkalemia may cause ventricular arrhythmias unresponsive to the usual pharmacologic treatments.

   Caution: Mortality in critically ill surgical patients is associated with a high serum pH. One study indicated that mortality was 69% in patients with a pH > 7.60, but fell to 44% in patients with a pH between 7.55 and 7.59.

G. Is there any associated chest pain? Severe alkalemia causes arteriolar constriction, resulting in a decrease in coronary blood flow. The anginal threshold may be reduced.

H. What is the serum bicarbonate? To fully understand an acid–base problem, you must obtain the serum bicarbonate from an electrolyte panel. A low serum bicarbonate is evidence of a primary respiratory alkalosis with at least partial metabolic compensation. A high serum bicarbonate is evidence of either a primary metabolic alkalosis or a mixed metabolic and respiratory alkalosis.

I. Does the serum bicarbonate fit the pH and pCO_2? See Section I, Chapter 2, Acidosis, Section II.E, p 10.

J. Is the compensation appropriate? Checking to see whether the compensation is appropriate may unmask mixed disturbances.

   1. For respiratory alkalosis, immediate compensation takes place through buffers. The compensation for acute respiratory alkalosis

is a decrease of 2 mmol of HCO_3^- (range 1–3 mmol) for each 10 mm Hg decrease in pCO_2. Renal compensation is complete between 2 and 4 days. The compensation for chronic respiratory alkalosis is a decrease of about 5 mmol of HCO_3^- for each 10 mm Hg decrease in pCO_2. For instance, in a 35-year-old woman who is 36 weeks pregnant, the ABG revealed a pCO_2 of 25. One would expect the HCO_3^- to decrease by 7.5 mmol from the calculation 5 mmol/L × (40 mm Hg – 25 mm mg)/10 mm Hg. One would expect the HCO_3^- to be 18.5 or 26 mmol/L (normal HCO_3^- – 7.5 mmol (expected change in HCO_3^-). If the HCO_3^- were 25 mmol, a relative metabolic alkalosis would be present along with the primary respiratory alkalosis, since the serum bicarbonate is higher than expected. If the HCO_3^- were 13 mmol, a metabolic acidosis would be present along with the primary respiratory alkalosis, since the serum bicarbonate is lower than expected.

2. For metabolic alkalosis, compensation begins immediately through buffers and hypoventilation. Hypoventilation as a means of compensation is limited by resulting hypoxemia. Seldom is the $pCO_2 > 55$ mm Hg secondary to compensation. The expected increase in pCO_2 is 0.6 mm Hg (range 0.25–1.0 mm Hg) for each 1-mmol increase in HCO_3^-. For instance, in a 60-year-old status postcholecystectomy, the HCO_3^- was 36 mmol/L. The expected pCO_2 is 46 mm Hg (36 mmol/L – 26 mmol/L) × 0.6 mm Hg per 1 mmol/L change in HCO_3^-. If the pCO_2 were 40 mm Hg, a relative respiratory alkalosis would be present along with the primary metabolic alkalosis. If the pCO_2 were 55 mm Hg, there would be a respiratory acidosis along with a primary metabolic alkalosis.

III. **Differential Diagnosis.** Alkalemia results either from a metabolic or respiratory alkalosis. There may be many causes for both, and sometimes a patient may have more than one cause.

A. **Respiratory alkalosis.** By definition, respiratory alkalosis occurs secondary to hyperventilation. Hyperventilation can result from either central or peripheral stimulation of respiration. Common causes include medications, CNS disease, pulmonary disease, anxiety, and systemic disorders.

1. **Medications**
   a. **Salicylate overdose.** Causes an isolated respiratory alkalosis (30%), isolated metabolic gap acidosis (10%), and most commonly a mixed metabolic gap acidosis and respiratory alkalosis (57%).
   b. **Progesterone**
2. **CNS disease.** See Section I, Chapter 13, Coma, Acute Mental Status Changes, p 76.
   a. **Cerebrovascular accident**
   b. **Infection**

      c. **Tumor.** Primary or metastatic.

      d. **Trauma**

  3. **Pulmonary disease.** See Section I, Chapter 19, Dyspnea, p 116.

      a. **Interstitial lung disease**

      b. **Pneumonia.** Usually causes respiratory alkalosis; if multiple lobes or underlying lung disease is present, it may cause respiratory acidosis.

      c. **Asthma.** If mild to moderate, asthma causes a respiratory alkalosis; if severe, respiratory acidosis may result.

      d. **Pulmonary emboli**

      e. **Pneumothorax**

  4. **Anxiety**

  5. **Pulmonary edema.** If mild, pulmonary edema causes a respiratory alkalosis; if severe, it may cause a respiratory acidosis.

  6. **Pain**

  7. **Pregnancy.** Secondary to progesterone.

  8. **Liver disease.** Cirrhosis.

  9. **Fever**

 10. **Early sepsis**

 11. **Hyperthyroidism**

 12. **Iatrogenic**

 13. **Hypoxemia**

 14. **Residence at high altitude**

B. **Pseudorespiratory alkalosis.** Arterial hypocapnia is present; however, there is an increase in the mixed venous pCO_2. Pseudorespiratory alkalosis is seen in severe cardiac dysfunction and associated pulmonary hypoperfusion with normal pulmonary function. Total body carbon dioxide is decreased, resulting in an increase in H^+ and an acidosis.

C. **Metabolic alkalosis.** Can be divided into chloride-responsive and chloride-unresponsive. The urine Cl^- is < 10–20 mmol/L with the chloride-responsive causes, and > 20–30 mmol/L with the chloride-unresponsive causes (provided no diuretic has been given). Severe metabolic alkalosis is usually the chloride-responsive type.

  1. **Chloride-responsive causes**

      a. **Gastric losses.** Vomiting or nasogastric tube.

      b. **Diarrhea.** Chloride wasting.

      c. **Diuretics**

      d. **Correction of chronic hypercapnia**

      e. **Sulfates, phosphates, or high-dose penicillins**

      f. **Massive blood transfusion.** Citrate is used as an anticoagulant and is metabolized to HCO_3^-. One unit of whole blood and 1 unit of packed red cells contain 17 and 5 mEq of citrate, respectively.

  2. **Chloride-unresponsive causes**

a. **Cushing's syndrome.** Elevated glucocorticoids from a variety of causes including pituitary adenoma, adrenal adenoma, and ectopic production. Cushing's syndrome also causes hypertension, glucose intolerance, fluid retention, and osteoporosis.
b. **Hyperaldosteronism.** Rare cause of hypertension; also associated with hypokalemia and hypernatremia.
c. **Exogenous steroid ingestion**
d. **Bartter's syndrome.** Also causes hypokalemia. Hyperreninemia and hyperaldosteronemia secondary to hyperplasia of the juxtaglomerular apparatus. Patients are normotensive.
e. **Potassium or magnesium deficiency**
f. **Calcium carbonate–containing antacids**
g. **Milk-alkali syndrome**
h. **Refeeding with glucose after starvation**

IV. Database
A. Physical examination key points
1. **Vital signs.** Tachypnea may indicate pulmonary disease, pulmonary edema, or CNS respiratory stimulation. Bradypnea suggests a metabolic alkalosis. An elevated temperature may indicate an infection or sepsis.
2. **Chest.** Examination must be thorough; look for evidence of pneumothorax, pleural effusion, pneumonia, bronchospastic disease, and pulmonary edema.
3. **Abdomen.** Look for evidence of chronic liver disease such as ascites and caput medusae.
4. **Skin.** Check for evidence of chronic liver disease such as palmar erythema, Dupuytren's contractures, and spider angiomas. Also, look for changes associated with Cushing's syndrome, such as buffalo hump, purple striae, and easy bruisability.
5. **Neurologic exam.** Check for focal abnormalities as evidence for tumor, cerebrovascular accident, and infection. Tremor and hyperreflexia may suggest hyperthyroidism.

B. Laboratory data
1. **Anion gap.** May unmask a mixed metabolic gap acidosis and metabolic alkalosis. See Section I, Chapter 2, Acidosis, III.B, p 13.
2. **Serum electrolytes.** Hypokalemia and hypomagnesemia may cause a metabolic alkalosis. Hypokalemia, hypomagnesemia, hypocalcemia, and hypophosphatemia may result from alkalosis.
3. **Respiratory alkalosis**
   a. **Salicylate level.** If elevated, check serum and urine drug screen for other ingested substances.
   b. **Liver function tests**
   c. **Thyroid function studies**
   d. **Blood cultures**

    4. Metabolic alkalosis. You will need a spot urine for chloride. A urine chloride below 10–20 mmol/L represents a **chloride-responsive** alkalosis. A urine chloride above 20 mmol/L represents a **chloride-unresponsive** alkalosis.

    5. Chloride-unresponsive metabolic alkalosis. You may need to rule out Cushing's syndrome and primary aldosteronism.

C. Radiologic and other studies. If respiratory alkalosis, consider the following:

    1. Chest x-ray. To look for pulmonary disease and pulmonary edema.

    2. CT scan of head. Rule out CNS disease.

V. Plan. It is essential to identify the cause of the alkalemia and treat it.

A. Respiratory alkalosis

    1. If hypoxic, give supplemental oxygen.

    2. If anxious, give sedative. Diazepam 1–5 mg PO or 1–2 mg IV; or lorazepam 1–2 mg PO or 0.5 mg IV.

    3. If nonintubated, increase $FiCO_2$ (fraction of inspired carbon dioxide). Use a rebreathing mask (or a paper bag). Would consider for pH > 7.55.

    4. If the patient is intubated, decrease minute ventilation. Decrease the rate or tidal volume. Be sure the tidal volume is set for 8–10 mL/kg. The respirator may need to be changed from assist control to intermittent ventilation. Increasing the amount of dead space would also increase the pCO_2.

    5. Salicylate overdose. Consider alkalinization of urine. Alkalinization of urine should be done cautiously in a patient who is already alkalotic. Follow serum pH and serum bicarbonate closely. See Section I, Chapter 2, Acidosis, Section V, p 17, for instructions on alkalinization of urine. Hemodialysis may be required.

B. Metabolic alkalosis

    1. In the presence of severe alkalemia with seizures or ventricular arrhythmias, prompt, immediate action is needed. Treatment includes increasing the pCO_2, or administering an acid such as hydrochloric acid. HCl 0.1–0.2 N solution (100–200 mmol of H^+ per liter) is administered slowly through a central line. The amount of required HCl to be administered can be calculated by taking the desired change in HCO_3^- and multiplying by the weight in kg and by 0.50 (bicarbonate space). For instance, in a 80-kg man with a pH of 7.68, if the actual bicarbonate is 52 mmol/L and the desired bicarbonate is 40 mmol/L, the required amount of HCl would be (52 mmol/L – 40 mmol/L) × 80 kg × 0.5 = 480 mmol, or about 2.5 liters of 0.2 N solution.

    2. Ammonium chloride and arginine hydrochloride. Both are precursors to HCl; however, there is significant risk (an increase in ammonia with ammonium chloride in patients with liver failure and hyperkalemia with arginine hydrochloride with renal failure).

 3. **Bicarbonate precursors.** Acetate salts (amino acids) found in hyperalimentation solutions or solutions containing lactate should be eliminated.
 4. **If chloride-responsive,** give normal saline.
 5. **If chloride-unresponsive,** treat underlying disorder.
    a. Potassium or magnesium deficiency often requires massive replacement.
    b. Evaluation and specific treatment of endogenous mineralocorticoid disorders.

REFERENCES

Adrogue HJ, Madias NE: Management of life-threatening acid-base disorders. N Engl J Med 1998;338:107.

Kaehny WD: Pathogenesis and management of respiratory and mixed acid-base disorders. In: Schrier RW, ed. *Renal and Electrolyte Disorders.* 6th ed. Lippincott Williams & Wilkins;2003:154.

Narins RG, Emmett A: Simple and mixed acid–base disorders: A practical approach. Medicine 1980;59:161.

Shapiro JI, Kaehny WD: Pathogenesis and management of metabolic acidosis and alkalosis. In: Schrier RW, ed. *Renal and Electrolyte Disorders.* 6th ed. Lippincott Williams & Wilkins;2003:115.

Wilson RF, Gibson D, Percinel AK et al: Severe alkalosis in critically ill surgical patients. Arch Surg 1972;105:197.

4. ANAPHYLACTIC REACTION

 I. **Problem.** Within 10 minutes of receiving an intramuscular injection, a patient develops diffuse pruritus, wheezing, and shortness of breath.

 II. **Immediate Questions.** Anaphylaxis can be a life-threatening situation and requires immediate evaluation and treatment.

 A. **What are the patient's vital signs?** Tachycardia is a common finding. It results from sympathetic response or vasodilatory hypotension. Hypotensive shock, which can occur with or without other symptoms, poses the greatest danger from anaphylaxis and must be recognized and treated promptly.

 B. **Can the patient still communicate?** The ability to provide appropriate answers to simple questions implies adequate cerebral perfusion. Inability to speak, dysphonia, hoarseness, or stridor probably indicates an upper airway obstruction from laryngospasm or laryngeal edema.

 C. **What medication(s) did the patient receive?** Anaphylaxis can result from a variety of agents, including medications, foods (especially shellfish and nuts), latex, blood products, venoms, and pollens. The most common medications causing anaphylaxis are penicillins, cephalosporins, sulfonamides, angiotensin-converting enzyme (ACE) inhibitors, chemotherapeutic agents, and local anesthetics. Nonimmunologically mediated anaphylactoid reactions result from opiates, aspirin (and other nonsteroidal anti-inflammatory drugs), and radiocontrast material. Any medicines suspected of causing an anaphylactic reaction must be stopped immediately. Similarly, transfusion can result in an anaphylactoid reaction.

III. **Differential Diagnosis.** Signs and symptoms of anaphylaxis are produced by the release of biologically active mediators such as histamine from basophils and mast cells. This release either can be mediated immunologically through the interaction of antigen with IgE residing on the basophils and mast cells or can occur as the result of a nonimmunologic release of mediators. These mediators affect several organ systems, including the skin, upper and lower airways, cardiovascular system, and gastrointestinal tract. Anaphylaxis may involve only one or all of the preceding organ systems and thus must be distinguished from other disease processes occurring at these sites.

A. **Upper airway obstruction.** This could result from epiglottitis, aspiration of a foreign body, vocal cord dysfunction syndrome, globus hystericus, or other causes of laryngeal edema such as hereditary angioedema. Angioedema involving the tongue and lips may occur secondary to ACE inhibitor therapy.

B. **Lower airway obstruction.** Think of status asthmaticus, bolus aspiration, cardiogenic pulmonary edema, and lung cancer.

C. **Syncope.** See Section I, Chapter 59, Syncope, p 337.

D. **Flushing syndromes.** Think of carcinoid syndrome; postmenopausal state; "red man" syndrome, which may be seen with too rapid infusion of vancomycin; and autonomic epilepsy. Pheochromocytoma usually causes pallor; however, 10–15% of the cases of pheochromocytoma have flushing.

E. **Urticaria.** This condition can be produced by a wide variety of causes other than anaphylaxis.

F. **Excess histamine states.** These states are found in systemic mastocytosis, basophilic leukemia, and acute promyelocytic leukemia.

G. **Serum sickness.** Usually occurs 5–7 days after exposure to an agent compared with anaphylaxis, which occurs in 5–60 minutes. This may be seen with beta-lactams (especially oral cefaclor) and horse serum–based snake antivenom.

IV. **Database.** Knowledge of the patient's history of allergies and current medications is essential. The temporal relationship between administration of medication and the onset of symptoms is also important, because anaphylaxis usually occurs within 1 hour of administration.

A. **Physical examination key points**
1. **Vital signs.** Hypotension must be recognized immediately.
2. **HEENT.** Evaluate for swelling of lips, tongue, and oropharynx.

3. **Lungs.** Listen for stridor (suggests upper airway obstruction) and wheezing (suggests bronchospasm).
4. **Skin.** Generalized flushing, urticaria, and angioedema may occur.
5. **Extremities.** Look for cyanosis.
6. **Mental status.** Impaired mentation may indicate significant respiratory compromise or hypotension and suggests the need for immediate respiratory and/or blood pressure support.

B. **Laboratory data**
   1. **Serum tryptase.** A protease specific to mast cells, reaches a peak 1 hour after an anaphylactic reaction occurs and remains elevated for approximately 6 hours. A serum tryptase during this period would help confirm the diagnosis.
   2. **N-methylhistamine.** A histamine metabolite, remains elevated in the urine for several hours after an anaphylactic reaction and can be measured by a 24-hour urine sample for N-methylhistamine.

C. **Radiologic and other studies**
   1. **Chest x-ray.** Can be obtained after the patient is stabilized to exclude other causes of respiratory distress, such as pneumonia and congestive heart failure.
   2. **Electrocardiogram.** Acute myocardial infarction can present with severe dyspnea. Anaphylaxis can also cause myocardial ischemia and arrhythmias (mainly in the elderly population).

V. **Plan.** Treatment should be initiated quickly—without waiting for the results of laboratory testing. Any medicines or transfusions suspected of causing an anaphylactic reaction must be stopped immediately. Initial therapy consists of epinephrine, oxygen, nebulized beta$_2$-agonist, and antihistamines.
   1. **Epinephrine.** Give epinephrine 0.3–0.5 mL of 1:1000 dilution intramuscularly immediately for laryngeal edema, bronchospasm, or urticaria. This may be repeated every 10–15 minutes to a total of three doses. Patients with severe hypotension, severe bronchospasm, severe upper airway edema may be administered intravenous epinephrine given as 0.5–1.0 mL of 1:10,000 dilution in bolus fashion (can be given in intervals of 5–10 minutes). If no improvement is seen, a continuous infusion of epinephrine (1–4 μg/min) titrated to effect may be administered. If IV access cannot be obtained immediately, deliver twice the above IV dose down the endotracheal tube.
   2. **Oxygen.** Oxygen by face mask should be instituted if the patient appears dyspneic. Intubation may be required if the patient is severely somnolent or hypoxemic. Tracheostomy may be necessary if upper airway edema precludes intubation. The goal is to maintain a pulse oximetry > 90% (pO$_2$ > 60 mm Hg).
   3. **Bronchodilators.** Albuterol (0.5 mL of 0.5% solution in 2.5 mL of saline) can be administered by nebulizer for persistent bronchospasm.

4. **Antihistamines.** Diphenhydramine (Benadryl) 25–50 mg IV/IM/PO Q 4–6 hr and ranitidine 50 mg IV or 150 mg PO Q 8 hr (or other H_2 blockers) should follow epinephrine to reduce the effects of histamine release. This may alleviate hypotension as well as lessen the symptoms associated with mild urticaria.

5. **Glucocorticoids.** Methylprednisolone 120 mg IV × 1 dose then 60 mg IV Q 6 hr should be given in patients with anaphylactic bronchospasm. This may also help the late-phase response that sometimes occurs 6–12 hours after the initial presentation.

6. **Glucagon.** Patients on beta-blockers may be resistant to treatment with epinephrine and can develop refractory hypotension and bradycardia. Glucagon 1 mg IV/IM/SC bolus × 1 dose is administered for inotropic and chronotropic effects not mediated through beta-receptors.

7. **Blood pressure support.** Hypotension usually responds to epinephrine; however, normal saline may be necessary for patients who fail to respond, as well as glucagon, as noted above. Vasopressor medications such as continuous norepinephrine or epinephrine should be used for persistent hypotension despite aggressive fluid administration.

8. **Monitoring.** Telemetry or intensive care unit admission is mandatory for anaphylaxis requiring epinephrine therapy. Relapse of anaphylaxis (late-phase response) can occur hours after the initial presentation. Close monitoring through the first 24 hours is essential. Even with rapid and appropriate treatment, patients may fail to respond. Always be prepared for the possible need for emergent intubation or tracheostomy.

VI. **Prevention.** Patients who have experienced anaphylaxis should be evaluated by an allergist.

A. **EpiPen.** Patients should be provided with, and instructed regarding the use of, a self-administered epinephrine injection device.

B. **Medic Alert bracelet.** Patients at risk for anaphylaxis should wear a Medic Alert bracelet at all times to expedite diagnosis and appropriate treatment in the event of subsequent anaphylaxis.

REFERENCES

Bochner BS, Lichtenstein LM: Anaphylaxis. N Engl J Med 1991;324:1785.
Ellis A, Day J: Diagnosis and management of anaphylaxis. CMAJ 2003;169:4.
Freeman TM: Anaphylaxis: Diagnosis and treatment. Primary Care 1998;25:809.
Ring J, Behrendt H: Anaphylaxis and anaphylactoid reactions. Clin Rev Allergy Immunol 1999;28:723.
Winbery SL, Lieberman PL: Anaphylaxis. Immunol Allergy Clin North Am 1995;15:447.

5. ANEMIA

I. **Problem.** A 50-year-old man is admitted for pneumonia. Laboratory testing reveals a hemoglobin of 11.2 g/dL (7.0 mmol/L).

II. Immediate Questions

A. What are the patient's vital signs? If the patient is not hypotensive or severely tachycardic, transfusion therapy is not emergently indicated.

B. Is the patient symptomatic? In the absence of angina, congestive heart failure, syncope, pre-syncope, or hemodynamic compromise, transfusion therapy is not emergently indicated.

C. Is there evidence of acute or recent blood loss such as hematemesis, melena, or hematochezia? Gastrointestinal (GI) blood loss can be divided into acute or chronic, upper GI (see Section I, Chapter 27, Hematemesis, Melena, p 166) and lower GI (see Section I, Chapter 28, Hematochezia, p 171). Patients more frequently succumb from acute upper GI blood loss than from lower GI blood loss.

D. Is there a history of hematuria or menorrhagia? Longstanding hematuria or menorrhagia can cause iron deficiency anemia.

E. What medications does the patient take? Aspirin and nonsteroidal anti-inflammatory drugs may lead to GI blood loss. Alkylating agents (cyclophosphamide, chlorambucil, melphalan, *cis*-platinum), antimetabolites (methotrexate), folate antagonists (trimethoprim-sulfamethoxazole, pentamidine), anticonvulsants (phenytoin), some antibiotics (chloramphenicol) and anti-inflammatory drugs (phenylbutazone) may cause marrow suppression or aplasia. Penicillin, sulfonamides, cyclosporine, tacrolimus, and methyldopa (Aldomet) may cause hemolysis. Alcohol, isoniazid, and trimethoprim may cause maturation defects.

F. Is significant organ dysfunction or a current inflammatory disease present? Severe liver, kidney, adrenal, and thyroid dysfunction may lead to anemia. Chronic inflammatory diseases such as rheumatoid arthritis, systemic lupus erythematosus (SLE), and other vasculitides, as well as chronic suppurative infections such as subacute bacterial endocarditis, chronic osteomyelitis and, more recently, patients with AIDS are associated with anemia of chronic disease.

G. Does the patient have other medical problems associated with excess total body water that may lead to a pseudoanemia, such as congestive heart failure, cirrhosis, and pregnancy? In the setting of increased plasma volume relative to the red blood cell (RBC) mass, an apparent anemia may be manifest or an existing anemia may be made more apparent.

H. Does the patient have a personal or family history of anemia, thalassemia, sickle cell anemia, or red cell membrane metabolism disorders such as glucose-6-phosphatase deficiency? Hereditary disorders of hemoglobin usually present nonacutely, and a family history may be suggestive of an inherited cause of the anemia.

    I. Does the patient have an autoimmune disease? Pernicious ane-
mia, the most common cause of vitamin B_{12} deficiency, may be associated with other autoimmune endocrinopathies such as Hashimoto's
thyroiditis, insulin-dependent diabetes mellitus, and Addison's disease.

    J. Does the patient have a malignancy? Anemia of cancer can be
found in patients with any malignancy.

III. Differential Diagnosis. There are over 100 causes of anemia. Visualiz-
ing the peripheral smear and paying careful attention to the RBC indices
(mean corpuscular volume [MCV], mean corpuscular hemoglobin, mean
corpuscular hemoglobin concentration) are essential when evaluating an
anemia. Anemia may result from decreased production of RBCs, blood
loss, or increased destruction of RBCs.

    A. Pancytopenia. The platelet and white blood cell (WBC) counts are
decreased along with the hemoglobin and hematocrit. Pancytopenia
is usually caused by marrow invasion, failure, or suppression; it is
most commonly caused by drugs, carcinoma, hematologic malignancies, autoimmune conditions and inflammatory diseases. It may be
idiopathic.

    B. Anemia with a low mean corpuscular volume. Associated with mi-
crocytic RBCs on the peripheral smear. Iron deficiency is the most
common cause of anemia and is seen in approximately 20% of men-
struating females. Hypochromic, microcytic RBCs, target cells, basophilic stippling, marked anisocytosis, and poikilocytosis are seen
with thalassemias. Sideroblastic anemia and anemia of chronic disease may also be associated with low MCV. The MCV should never
be < 70 if it is due to chronic disease. Microcytic anemias can easily
be differentiated by looking at the peripheral smear and various laboratory studies. Serum iron, total iron binding capacity or transferrin,
ferritin, and hemoglobin electrophoresis may be helpful (Table I–4).
Blockade of heme synthesis induced by such chemicals as lead and
isoniazid can create a microcytic anemia that may be confused with
iron deficiency.

TABLE I–4. CAUSES OF MICROCYTIC ANEMIA.

	Iron Deficiency	β-Thalassemia	Chronic Disease	Sideroblastic Anemia
Iron	Low	Normal/increased	Low	Increased
TIBC	Increased	Normal	Low	Normal
Ferritin	Low	Normal/increased	Normal/increased	Increased
Hemoglobin A_2[1]	Normal	Increased	Normal	Normal

[1]A type of hemoglobin detected by hemoglobin electrophoresis.
TIBC, total iron binding capacity.

C. **Normal-MCV anemias.** Many anemias are associated with a normal MCV. Anemia of chronic disease is probably the most common normocytic anemia. Chronic infections (tuberculosis, osteomyelitis), collagen vascular diseases, and malignancies may produce an anemia with a normal MCV. Kidney, liver, thyroid, and adrenal dysfunction may also lead to a normal-MCV anemia. Correction of the underlying disorder should correct the anemia. Acute GI blood loss results in a normal-MCV anemia

D. **High-MCV anemias.** Many anemias are macrocytic, but only a few are megaloblastic. Folate and vitamin B_{12} deficiencies are the most common megaloblastic anemias. Vitamin B_{12} deficiency can be secondary to pernicious anemia (lack of intrinsic factor), bacterial overgrowth, ileal disease, and, rarely, dietary deficiency. Vitamin B_{12} stores last 3–4 years. Folate deficiency is often caused by dietary deficiency but may be secondary to increased needs such as with pregnancy or hyperthyroidism. If there is no obvious cause of folate deficiency, then the possibility of malabsorption must be considered. Along with macrocytic RBCs, the peripheral smear of folate or vitamin B_{12} deficiency may demonstrate hypersegmented neutrophils and nucleated RBCs. Other anemias that may be associated with macrocytes are myelodysplasias, aplastic anemias, acquired sideroblastic anemias, anemias induced by chemotherapy (antimetabolites), and anemia associated with hypothyroidism and chronic liver disease. An increased MCV may be seen in the presence of a markedly increased reticulocyte count, because reticulocytes are large cells that increase the mean RBC size.

E. **Anemias with increased reticulocytosis.** Many anemias listed above are associated with an increased reticulocyte count. A *reticulocyte* is a very young RBC ~ 1 day old. Because the RBC life span is 120 days, the normal reticulocyte count is 1/120, or ~ 1%. An increased reticulocyte count indicates that the bone marrow is producing RBCs faster than normal. This is usually due to red cells having a shortened life span or to acute blood loss. The peripheral smear may reveal large polychromatophilic RBCs that are reticulocytes; however, a reticulocyte stain is needed to perform a definitive reticulocyte count. Examples of anemias with an increased reticulocyte count include acquired or autoimmune hemolytic anemias and congenital hemolytic anemias (sickle cell anemia, thalassemias). Correction of a particular deficit such as B_{12} deficiency by the administration of vitamin B_{12} also leads to a reticulocytosis.

IV. **Database**

A. **Physical examination key points**
1. **Vital signs.** Make sure the patient is not hypotensive. The patient may be *orthostatic*. Look for a decrease in systolic blood pressure of 10 mm Hg and/or an increase in heart rate of 20 bpm on move-

ment from a supine to a standing position after 1 minute. Orthostatic changes suggest acute blood loss or symptomatic anemia.

2. **Skin.** Telangiectasia, palmar erythema, and jaundice may indicate liver disease. Isolated jaundice may point toward hemolysis.
Excessive bruising and the presence of cytopenias are suggestive
of hematologic malignancy.

3. **Oropharynx.** Glossitis is commonly seen in iron and B_{12} deficiency.

4. **Heart.** Murmurs indicate either hemolysis from valvular disease or
a flow murmur resulting from the anemia.

5. **Abdomen.** Check for splenomegaly, which is associated with hemolysis, thalassemias, chronic leukemias, lymphomas, and occasionally acute leukemias. It could also indicate portal hypertension
secondary to cirrhosis. Also look for ascites and hepatomegaly.

6. **Rectum.** Test for stool Hemoccult to look for acute or chronic GI
blood loss.

7. **Neurologic examination.** Loss of vibration and position sense as
well as dementia are associated with B_{12} deficiency but may also
represent effects of alcohol.

B. **Laboratory data**

1. **Peripheral smear.** Review of the peripheral smear is essential.
Note the size and shape of the RBCs and the presence or absence of platelets. Nucleated RBCs, reticulocytes, schistocytes,
sickle cells, and target cells may aid in the diagnosis. Examine
WBC morphology for hypersegmented neutrophils, presence of
Pelger-Huët anomaly (monolobed or bilobed appearance of neutrophils, inherited disorder, or seen in acute myelogenous
leukemia), or immature blasts.

2. **Reticulocyte count.** The most important laboratory test after reviewing the peripheral smear. An increased reticulocyte count indicates either an appropriate response to anemia or shortened
RBC survival through blood loss or hemolysis. A low reticulocyte
count indicates that the marrow is responding inappropriately to
the anemia either secondary to a nutritional deficiency or marrow
failure from immune-mediated suppression, toxin exposure, fibrosis or replacement (lymphoma, leukemia, carcinoma).

3. **Iron and total iron-binding capacity (TIBC) or transferrin.** Occasionally, a ferritin value should also be obtained if the anemia is
microcytic. This aids in the diagnosis of iron deficiency anemia.
Iron deficiency anemia results in low iron and normal or elevated
TIBC or transferrin; ferritin is also low. If the patient has a very low
MCV (< 70) and a normal iron and TIBC, the likelihood of thalassemia is high. It is important to realize that many acute and
chronic illnesses can dramatically affect the iron and TIBC, com-
promising their usefulness as measures in the diagnosis of anemia. If the question of iron deficiency requires a definite answer, a
bone marrow exam with iron stains is indicated.

4. **B₁₂ and folate.** Order these tests for any patient suspected of having B_{12} and folate deficiency before transfusion. If folate deficiency is secondary to malnutrition, a serum folate may be normal after one or two well-balanced meals. If folate deficiency is suspected and the patient has recently eaten, then consider checking an RBC folate.

5. **Haptoglobin and urine hemosiderin.** A low haptoglobin and a positive urine hemosiderin are indicative of hemolysis. When haptoglobin is low, free hemoglobin in the serum or urine and/or increased lactate dehydrogenase are also suggestive of hemolysis.

6. **Direct and indirect Coombs' test.** These tests may indicate that the hemolysis is immunologic. A direct Coombs' test measures the presence of antibody or complement on the RBC; an indirect Coombs' test detects antibody in the plasma that has dissociated from the RBC but is directed at the RBC. Direct Coombs' is the more valuable test in evaluating the possibility of immunohemolytic disease, whereas indirect Coombs' is primarily of value as a blood banking procedure. Detection of an antibody in the plasma but not on the RBC indicates that it is an alloantibody rather than an autoantibody. Most immunohemolytic anemias are due to warm-reacting antibodies, usually IgG. These are manifest by a direct Coombs' test result that is positive for IgG with or without complement. Cold-reacting antibodies may be induced by infections such as mycoplasma.

7. **Platelet count.** May be elevated in early iron deficiency. Decreased in folate and vitamin B_{12} deficiency as well as with marrow replacement.

C. **Radiologic studies.** Not usually needed unless GI blood loss is suspected; then order as clinically indicated.

D. **Pathologic evaluations.** A bone marrow aspirate and biopsy are generally indicated in all but the very straightforward explanations for anemia. Even when iron deficiency anemia is suspected, absence of iron stores in the marrow supports the diagnosis.

V. **Plan**

A. **Anemia with hemodynamic compromise or complications**
   1. If the patient is hemodynamically unstable or is having angina, a transfusion is urgently indicated. In such cases, the source of blood loss is usually obvious. For specific information on transfusion, consult Section V, Blood Component Therapy, p 465.
   2. Be sure the patient has adequate intravenous access if there is evidence of acute bleeding.

B. **Anemia without hemodynamic compromise or complications.** If the patient is not hemodynamically compromised, proceed with the workup in an orderly fashion. In many cases, the cause of the anemia is not obvious. Furthermore, laboratory testing is not always diagnostic. If the patient has an unremarkable history and physical, ambivalent laboratory testing, and no obvious underlying infectious, malignant, or inflammatory disease, a bone marrow biopsy is indicated.

C. **Iron deficiency anemia.** Iron deficiency occurs as a result of chronic blood loss, inadequate dietary iron intake, malabsorption of iron, hemolysis, or a combination of these factors. The plan of care must address these potential causes. The source of blood loss must first be found. This usually entails an endoscopy of the upper GI tract and a flexible sigmoidoscopy and air-contrast barium enema, or a colonoscopy of the lower GI tract. Keep in mind that heavy menstrual losses are the most common cause of iron deficiency anemia in young women. After the source of blood loss is determined, the iron stores need to be repleted. Most patients tolerate oral iron as ferrous sulfate 325 mg PO tid between meals. Treatment must be continued for 3–6 months after normalization of the CBC to ensure adequate repletion of iron stores. Gradually increasing the dose over several days from every day to bid to tid improves tolerance to oral iron. Vitamin C 500–1000 units with each dose of iron may improve absorption. Rarely, patients require parenteral iron replacement, which raises the suspicion of GI malablsorption of iron. These conditions are uncommon but may be frequently seen in patients who have undergone subtotal gastric resection.

D. **Folate deficiency.** This condition is usually due to dietary deficiency (chronic alcoholism), impaired absorption, or increased requirements such as that seen in pregnancy. In this setting, daily folate supplementation at 1 mg PO is indicated.

E. **Vitamin B_{12} deficiency.** Inadequate dietary intake is a rare cause of B_{12} deficiency. It is most often a result of defective absorption—most commonly pernicious anemia, an autoimmune condition in which intrinsic factor production fails. True pernicious anemia can be diagnosed by serum tests that detect anti–parietal cell and/or intrinsic factor antibodies or by a Schilling test. A Schilling test involves giving a loading dose of 1000-mg vitamin B_{12} to saturate receptor sites. This dose is followed by the administration of radiolabeled B_{12} and measurement of the radioactivity in a 24-hour urine sample. If the amount of radioactive B_{12} in the urine is small, oral intrinsic factor can be given along with a second dose of radioactive B_{12}, and a 24-hour urine can be re-collected. An abnormal first step and a normal second step help differentiate between pernicious anemia and other causes of vitamin B_{12} deficiency (eg, bacterial overgrowth and ileal diseases). The history may also provide an obvious cause of B_{12} deficiency (status post gastrectomy or ileal resection). Vitamin B_{12} is replaced by administration of 30–100 µg IM daily for 2–3 weeks, then 100–200 µg IM every 2–4 weeks for life.

F. **Hemolytic anemia.** In the face of an elevated reticulocyte count with no obvious source of blood loss, a destructive process must be considered. Immune-mediated processes can be diagnosed by use of the Coombs' test. In the setting of Coombs'-negative hemolytic anemia, other disease processes must be considered, such as hemolysis due to chemical or physical agents (arsenic, postcardiac bypass), disseminated intravascular coagulation, paroxysmal nocturnal hemoglobinuria, or microangiopathic hemolytic anemia (thrombotic thrombocytopenic purpura, hemolytic uremic syndrome). A review of the peripheral smear is helpful. A concomitant low platelet count, low fibrinogen, and elevated prothrombin time, partial thromboplastin time, and D-dimer or fibrin degradation products as well as schistocytes on the peripheral smear point toward disseminated intravascular coagulation (see Section I, Chapter 12, Coagulopathy, V, p 70). The presence of spherocytes, however, is suggestive of extravascular hemolysis such as that seen with immune-complex deposition and subsequent destruction of the red cell via the reticuloendothelial system of the spleen. The possibility of an inherited disorder such as thalassemia, sickle cell anemia, or an enzymopathy must be ruled out. Hemoglobin electrophoresis and review of the peripheral smear are indicated. If an enzymopathy is considered, specific assays are indicated (such as glucose-6-phosphate dehydrogenase, pyruvate kinase). The possibility of paroxysmal nocturnal hemoglobinuria must be considered in cases in which the cause is unclear. Ham's test and sucrose lysis test have historically been used to suggest this diagnosis. Currently, flow cytometric analysis of the peripheral blood for absence of phosphoinositol-anchored proteins from the surfaces of the red cell or white blood cell populations or genetic analysis for a mutation in the *PIG-A* gene is diagnostic for this condition. Discussion of specific treatments for hemolytic anemias is beyond the scope of this book.

G. **Anemia of chronic disease.** This is usually a diagnosis of exclusion. However, if the patient has end-stage renal disease, endogenous erythropoietin levels may be low, and the patient may respond to replacement therapy with one of the currently available erythropoietin products approved for use in anemia of chronic disease and chemotherapy-induced anemia. In other cases, the cause may be obvious, as with advanced malignancy. There is no specific diagnostic test for anemia of chronic disease; treatment is of the underlying disease. It is generally manifest by a low reticulocyte count, a low iron and a low TIBC or transferrin, and normal bone marrow morphology. These are not specific findings, however.

REFERENCES

Beutler E, Lichtman MA, Coller RS et al, eds. *Williams Hematology.* 6th ed. McGraw-Hill;2001.

Bolinger A: Anemias. In: Koda-Kimbel MA, Young LY, eds. *Applied Therapeutics: The Clinical Use of Drugs.* 7th ed. Lippincott Williams & Wilkins;2001.

Izaks GJ, Westendorp RGJ, Knook DL: The definition of anemia in older persons. JAMA 1999;281:1714.

Lux SE: Introduction to anemia. In: Handin RI, Lux SE, Stossel TP, eds. *Blood: Principles and Practice of Hematology.* Lippincott;1995:1383.

Toh B-H, van Driel IR, Gleeson PA: Pernicious anemia. N Engl J Med 1997;337:1441.

6. ARTERIAL LINE PROBLEMS

See also Section III, Chapter 1, Arterial Line Placement, p 416.

I. **Problem.** You are called to the intensive care unit to see a patient in whom a low, dampened arterial line pressure is being obtained.

II. **Immediate Questions**

   A. **Does the pressure accurately reflect the patient's status?** Mental status changes (see Section I, Chapter 13, Coma, Acute Mental Status Changes, p 36), tachycardia, and a decreased urine output would be expected with hypotension.

   B. **Is the problem with the catheter itself or with the monitoring apparatus (tubing, transducer, electronic equipment)?** If the patient's clinical status does not reflect the low blood pressure obtained by the arterial line, the problem may lie in the equipment.

   C. **Is an extremity at risk?** Thrombosis secondary to the arterial line can cause ischemia and tissue loss.

   D. **Has the quality of the tracing changed recently?** Find out whether the tracing was satisfactory earlier. A good tracing followed by a poor one suggests either deterioration in clinical status or a new problem with the catheter.

III. **Differential Diagnosis.** A low or dampened blood pressure may result from problems with the monitoring equipment, problems with the arterial line catheter, or actual hemodynamic deterioration of the patient.

   A. **Patient status.** If the patient's hemodynamic status has deteriorated, the decrease in blood pressure or dampening of the waveform is actually indicative of the patient's status. Often, other clinical indicators of the patient's status such as mental status changes, tachycardia, decreased urine output, and electrocardiographic changes suggest that the patient is genuinely hypotensive.

   B. **Monitoring apparatus problems**
      1. Air is present in the tubing/transducer.
      2. The tubing is kinked.
      3. Electrical equipment is faulty.

   C. **Catheter problems**
      1. There are kinks in the catheter.
      2. A thrombus is present in the catheter or in the vessel.
      3. The catheter tip is resting against the wall of the artery because of the way the catheter was anchored (by suture or taping).

   4. The catheter has punctured the arterial wall, causing bleeding and compression of the catheter.

IV. Database

A. Physical examination key points

1. **Blood pressure.** If the arterial line pressure is low, perform a brachial artery cuff pressure. If the reading confirms hypotension, prompt action is indicated. The manual blood pressure is usually within 10–20 mm Hg of the arterial line pressure, unless severe vasoconstriction is present; in which case indirect measurement may underestimate direct measurement by 20–30 mm Hg.

2. **Pulses.** Check at once for distal pulses and for swelling or tenderness in the area of the catheter insertion. Failure to find a pulse or finding a decrease in the pulse, with significant swelling at the catheter site, represents a potentially serious vascular compromise.

3. **Inspection of the equipment**
   a. Check for air in the lines or the transducer. The search must be thorough and almost certainly requires the assistance of the nursing staff.
   b. Have nursing staff confirm that the electrical equipment is working properly.
   c. Attempt to withdraw blood through the catheter. Inability to do so suggests either that the catheter tip is poorly positioned or that there is a kink or a thrombus in the catheter, at the catheter tip, or in the artery. *Caution:* Do not attempt to flush a catheter through which blood cannot be drawn!

V. Plan

A. Maintaining perfusion to the extremity.
A limb may be susceptible to ischemic injury as the result of systemic hypotension, a large catheter-to-vessel ratio, bleeding into surrounding tissues, inadequate flushing techniques, or prolonged catheter indwelling time.

1. Failure of the pulse to return will probably necessitate a surgical attempt at thrombus removal or repair of the artery. Consult a vascular surgeon immediately.

2. If bleeding from the artery into the surrounding tissue seems likely, watch carefully for compartmental syndrome (pain, pain with extension of the digits, pallor, hypesthesia, and loss of motor function). Surgical evacuation of the blood may be necessary. Consult a vascular surgeon at once if compartmental syndrome is suspected.

3. Search for evidence of infection. If infection is present, culture and treat appropriately, and remove the catheter.

B. Monitoring apparatus problems

1. Flush the transducer and tubing thoroughly.

2. Retape the tubing to eliminate kinks.
3. Replace faulty electrical equipment.
4. An armboard may prevent the catheter or tubing from extra-arterial kinking.

C. **Catheter problems**
1. Loosen sutures or tape to reposition the catheter tip away from the wall.
2. If a thrombus or kink in the intra-arterial catheter is suspected, the line will probably have to be removed and relocated.
3. In general, do not attempt to place a new arterial line over a guidewire. Remove the old catheter and replace it with a new one, preferably at a different site. Perforation of the catheter with the guidewire may cause a foreign body embolus, damage to the arterial wall, or dislodgement of a thrombus in or at the tip of the catheter. All these potentially serious complications make the risk of using a catheter guidewire to assess a dampened waveform unwise.

7. ASPIRATION

I. **Problem.** After a generalized seizure, a patient is observed to vomit and subsequently develops acute respiratory distress.

II. **Immediate Questions**

A. **What are the vital signs?** On the basis of the history, it must be assumed that the patient has aspirated gastric contents. This can result in acute respiratory compromise from lodging of particulate matter in the larynx or trachea, by induction of laryngospasm, or through the rapid onset of pulmonary edema. Both *tachycardia* and *tachypnea* are often present. In severe episodes of respiratory compromise, *respiratory arrest* or *shock* may also occur.

B. **Is the patient able to communicate?** Aphonia may result from lodging of particulate matter in the larynx or trachea; it requires immediate intervention to dislodge the bolus by either the Heimlich maneuver or forceful coughing.

C. **Is the patient cyanotic?** Cyanosis would indicate severe respiratory compromise and probable need for emergent intubation.

D. **Does the patient need to be repositioned?** To prevent further aspiration of gastric contents, the patient should be placed in a lateral decubitus position with the head down.

III. **Differential Diagnosis.** *Aspiration* is defined as the entry of oropharyngeal contents into the larynx below the vocal cords. Three distinct aspiration syndromes are recognized: (1) acidic gastric contents; (2) nonacidic and/or particulate material; and (3) oropharyngeal bacterial pathogens. These syndromes should be distinguished from one another as well as from other causes of acute respiratory distress, because the complications and treatment differ for each.

A. **Acid aspiration.** Aspiration of gastric contents with a pH < 2.5 and a volume of at least 25 mL results in immediate alveolar injury and chemical pneumonitis. Acute respiratory distress syndrome and shock may occur. Clinically, there is abrupt onset of dyspnea, fever, wheezing, rales, and hypoxemia.

B. **Particulate aspiration.** This can result in mechanical obstruction and bronchospasm. Pneumonia can ensue if particulate material remains lodged in peripheral airways.

C. **Oropharyngeal bacteria.** Saliva contains 10^8 organisms per milliliter. Aspiration of saliva into the lower airway can cause an early pneumonitis followed by necrotizing pneumonia or abscess in 3–14 days.

D. **Asthma.** See Section I, Chapter 63, Wheezing, p 364.

E. **Pneumonia (community-acquired or nosocomial).** Pneumonia can be difficult to distinguish from acute aspiration of gastric contents, since both can result in sputum production, tachycardia, tachypnea, fever, rales, and radiographic infiltrates.

F. **Pulmonary embolism.** This diagnosis must be considered in the differential of any patient developing acute respiratory distress.

G. **Foreign body aspiration.** This occurs mainly in younger children and occasionally in debilitated elderly people who aspirate a food bolus.

H. **Upper airway obstruction.** Acute edema of the vocal cords or glottis may follow aspiration. A high-pitched wheeze is heard over the larynx (stridor).

IV. **Database.** Attempt to identify conditions that predispose to aspiration, including reduced consciousness, impaired swallowing, and esophageal dysfunction. Disorders resulting in *reduced consciousness* include anesthesia, alcohol abuse, seizure disorder, acute cerebrovascular accident, cardiopulmonary arrest, and drug overdose. *Esophageal dysfunction* predisposes to aspiration and includes esophageal neoplasm or stricture, hiatal hernia, and nasogastric intubation. *Impaired swallowing* may result from a cerebrovascular accident, polymyositis, myasthenia gravis, Parkinson's disease, an artificial airway, advanced age with impaired esophageal motility, or cancer involving the head and neck. Other causes include protracted emesis, gastric outlet obstruction, and large-volume nasogastric tube feedings. Be aware that deficits in the pharyngeal phase of swallowing may persist for 2–3 days after extubation of a patient with an artificial airway.

A. **Physical examination key points**
   1. **Vital signs.** See Section II.A.

2. **HEENT.** Check dentition for loose or missing teeth and evidence of gingivitis.

3. **Neck.** Examine for evidence of tumor involving the oropharynx. Also, look for any evidence of prior surgical procedures or radiation of the head and neck.

4. **Lungs.** Wheezing and crackles can occur after aspiration of gastric contents. Wheezing and diminished breath sounds may result from aspiration of particulate material. Listen for stridor (laryngeal wheeze).

5. **Skin.** Examine for presence of cyanosis.

6. **Neurologic examination.** Determine the degree of consciousness and the presence or absence of a gag reflex. Note, however, that even with an intact gag reflex dysphagia and aspiration may still occur.

B. **Laboratory data**

1. **Arterial blood gases.** Hypoxemia and hypercapnia may occur, and, if present, intubation may be required.

2. **Hemogram.** Aspiration of acid contents and pneumonia can cause a leukocytosis and left shift.

3. **Sputum Gram's stain and culture.** If the patient manifests fever, leukocytosis, and sputum production 2–3 days after aspiration, a sputum Gram's stain and culture may be helpful in confirming pneumonia and directing subsequent antibiotic therapy. However, aspiration pneumonia is often anaerobic and may be polymicrobial.

C. **Radiologic and other studies**

1. **Chest x-ray** may show:

   a. Hyperaeration from air trapping on the side of foreign body aspiration.

   b. Infiltrate in dependent segments of the lungs: the lower lobes if aspiration occurs while upright; the superior segments of the lower lobes or posterior segments of the upper lobes when recumbent. Infiltrates may not be seen immediately after aspiration; therefore, if the initial chest x-ray is normal but there is a strong clinical suspicion of aspiration, repeat the chest x-ray in 4–5 hours. Bilateral alveolar infiltrates may appear within 2 hours with acute acid aspiration.

   c. A wedge-shaped, pleural-based density suggests pulmonary infarction from pulmonary embolism.

   d. Clear fields and hyperinflation are common in uncomplicated asthma.

   e. Lung abscess formation does not generally occur until 7–14 days after aspiration and is not observed on initial films.

2. **Other studies.** Ventilation/perfusion ($\dot{V}/\dot{Q}$) scan or CT pulmonary angiogram if a pulmonary embolism is suspected.

V. **Plan.** Aspiration should be suspected in any patient with a predisposing factor who develops sudden respiratory distress. Early treatment is important because death from respiratory failure can occur if the condition is not recognized early. Ideally, the best treatment is prevention.

A. Prevention
1. For patients being administered tube feedings, gastric emptying should be confirmed and the head of the bed elevated to 45 degrees. Flexible, small-bore feeding tubes are preferable to stiffer large-bore tubes. Duodenal placement of the tube may confer a reduction in risk of aspiration compared to gastric feeding.
2. Unconscious patients should be placed in a lateral, slightly head-down position whenever possible.
3. When not being used for enteral feedings, nasogastric tubes should be placed only when continuous suction is required.
4. Up to one-third to one-half of patients presenting with acute cerebrovascular accidents will experience aspiration. Consider ordering videofluoroscopy in these patients to determine aspiration risk and appropriate feeding.

B. Oxygenation. Supplemental oxygen should be given in an amount sufficient to ensure oxygen saturation greater than 90%.

C. Intubation and positive pressure breathing. This is required in the patient for whom supplemental oxygen therapy is not sufficient to maintain adequate oxygenation, or in the patient who is obtunded and unable to protect her or his airway.

D. Medications
1. Bronchodilators such as albuterol 0.5 mL with 3 mL normal saline may relieve bronchospasm.
2. Prophylactic corticosteroids have not been shown to decrease subsequent morbidity and mortality from aspiration and are not indicated.
3. Prophylactic antibiotics likewise have not been shown to diminish morbidity and mortality. Antibiotics should be administered only if the patient continues to manifest fever, leukocytosis, purulent sputum, and infiltrates 2–3 days after the initial aspiration. For patients with in-hospital aspiration, a regimen that provides coverage for gram-negative aerobes and *Staphylococcus aureus* is more important than anaerobic coverage.

E. Fiberoptic bronchoscopy. This procedure is indicated when lobar or segmental collapse is present, when foreign body aspiration is suspected, or when abscess drainage is required.

REFERENCES

Bartlett JG: Aspiration pneumonia. In: Rose BD, ed. UpToDate, Wellesley, MA,2003.
Elpern E: Pulmonary aspiration in hospitalized adults. Nutr Clin Pract 1997;12:5.
Marik PE: Aspiration pneumonitis and aspiration pneumonia. N Engl J Med 2001;344:665.

Marom E, McAdams HP, Erasmus JJ et al: The many faces of pulmonary aspiration. Am J Radiol 1999;172:121.

Teofilo L: Pulmonary aspiration. Comp Ther 1997;23:371.

Tietjen PA, Kaner RD, Quin CE: Aspiration emergencies. Clin Chest Med 1994;15:117.

8. BRADYCARDIA

I. **Problem.** A nurse on the telemetry unit notifies you that a 66-year-old woman has a heart rate of 40 beats per minute (bpm). She was admitted earlier in the day with syncope.

II. **Immediate Questions**

   A. **What are the patient's other vital signs?** Heart rate must always be considered in relation to the blood pressure (BP) and other signs of the patient's condition. A patient with a BP below 90 mm Hg and bradycardia requires more immediate attention than a patient with bradycardia, a normal BP, and no other associated symptoms.

   B. **What has the patient's heart rate been since admission?** The range of normal heart rates is wide and is influenced by many factors, such as activity, age, medications, presence of pain or fever, and type of illness. Bradycardia can be seen in both healthy and ill patients.

   C. **Does the patient have any symptoms possibly related to the bradycardia?** Such may be fatigue, dizziness, syncope, nausea, dyspnea, chest pain, decreased urinary output, or altered mental status.

III. **Differential Diagnosis**

   A. **Sinus bradycardia.** Defined as a sinus node rhythm below 60 bpm. Changes in sinus rate are modulated primarily by parasympathetic nervous system tone. Causes of sinus bradycardia include the following:

   1. **Increased parasympathetic tone.** Sinus bradycardia can be precipitated many times by sudden stressful or painful events. An example is a vasovagal syncopal episode related to nervousness or to fear from venipuncture.

   2. **Sinoatrial node dysfunction.** Characterized by the presence of bradycardia at inappropriate times. Sinus node dysfunction can also be manifested by periods of sinoatrial node arrest, or sinoatrial exit block, or by alternating sinus bradycardia and atrial tachyarrhythmias, commonly referred to as *sick sinus syndrome.*

   3. **Myocardial infarction.** Sinus bradycardia is seen frequently with inferior wall infarctions, involving the proximal portion of the right coronary artery and its branch to the sinoatrial node. The presence of sinus bradycardia during the early phases of an acute myocardial infarction is, in general, a good prognostic sign. It does not require therapy, as long as left ventricular cardiac output is

adequate and hypotension or congestive heart failure is absent. In fact, raising the heart rate in this instance may raise cardiac demand and cause further ischemia or infarction.

4. **Cushing's reflex.** Sinus bradycardia in combination with hypertension is associated with an increase in intracranial pressure (hemorrhagic stroke, meningitis, intracranial tumor, or trauma).

5. **Other medical disorders.** Sinus bradycardia can occur in patients with hypothyroidism, hypothermia, obstructive sleep apnea, advancing age, carotid sinus hypersensitivity, and certain infiltrative diseases of the myocardium, such as amyloidosis and sarcoidosis.

6. **Drug effect.** Sinus bradycardia is a common secondary effect of several classes of medications, including beta-blockers, digoxin, calcium channel blockers, clonidine (Catapres), lithium carbonate, and certain antiarrhythmic drugs such as amiodarone (Cordarone) and sotalol (Betapace).

B. **Atrioventricular (AV) node blocks**

1. **Mobitz type I second-degree AV block (Wenckebach).** Characterized by progressive, cyclical prolongation of the PR interval with each cardiac cycle until a ventricular beat is dropped. This results in intermittent AV block in a repeated cycle.

   a. **Acute myocardial infarction.** Most commonly seen early in inferior wall infarctions related to ischemia affecting the AV nodal branch of the right coronary artery.

   b. **Drug effect.** Excessive serum levels of certain cardiac medications can result in Wenckebach-type second-degree AV block (digoxin, beta-blockers, calcium channel blockers, and amiodarone).

   c. **Infections.** A Wenckebach rhythm is occasionally seen during the acute phases of rheumatic fever and Lyme disease, when the inflammatory process affects the cardiac conduction system.

   d. **Other.** Wenckebach rhythms can occasionally be seen in asymptomatic, otherwise normal adults; they are related to the level of parasympathetic nervous system tone, such as in highly trained aerobic athletes, particularly during sleep.

2. **Mobitz type II second-degree AV block.** Cyclical AV block without the progressive prolongation of the PR interval. The QRS complex of conducted beats may be prolonged because of disease involvement of the bundle of His.

   a. **Acute myocardial infarction.** Large anterior wall infarctions are a more common cause than inferior infarctions.

   b. **Degenerative fibrosing diseases.** Involving the bundle of His.

   c. **Infectious diseases.** Examples are viral myocarditis, acute rheumatic fever, and Lyme disease.

3. **Third-degree AV block.** This rhythm is associated with the same conditions as Mobitz type II second-degree heart block. Third-degree AV block occurs when there is no conduction of the P waves from the sinoatrial node through the AV node to the ventricle. This results in the P waves and QRS complexes being independent of one another. Usually, the ventricular rate and rhythm are controlled by a secondary intraventricular pacemaker, which is normally suppressed when AV conduction is intact.

4. **Malfunctioning pacemaker.** See Section I, Chapter 53, Pacemaker Troubleshooting, p 301.

IV. Database

A. Physical examination key points

1. **Vital signs.** Obtain the patient's BP during the bradycardic rhythm, and assess the patient's level of consciousness.

2. **Neck veins.** Intermittent cannon "A" waves in the jugular venous pulsations are observed in the presence of complete AV dissociation. A *cannon A wave* is an exaggerated A wave in the jugular venous pulse that results from right atrial contraction on an already closed tricuspid valve, caused by simultaneous atrial and ventricular contraction. This results in backward ejection of right atrial blood into the superior vena cava and jugular veins.

3. **Lungs.** Rales during periods of bradycardia suggest congestive heart failure from inadequate left ventricular cardiac output.

4. **Heart.** Listen for murmurs and gallops. An S_4 gallop may be present during an acute myocardial infarction. A new cardiac murmur may be seen in myocardial infarction, acute rheumatic fever, and myocarditis. See Section I, Chapter 26, Heart Murmur, p 159.

5. **Skin.** Cool, pale extremities suggest an inadequate cardiac output.

6. **Mental status.** Inadequate cerebral perfusion may result in an altered level of consciousness.

B. Laboratory data

1. **Electrolytes.** Exclude hypokalemia if the patient is on digoxin.

2. **Digoxin level.** Bradycardia can be a sign of digitalis intoxication.

3. **Thyroid hormone levels.** Rule out hypothyroidism as a cause.

C. Electrocardiogram and rhythm strip

1. Identify P waves and their timing and relation to the QRS complexes. Leads I, II, aVR, aVF, and V_1 demonstrate the morphology of the P waves best. The absence of P waves suggests an AV nodal rhythm, or atrial fibrillation with a slow ventricular response, as the cause of the bradycardia.

2. An increasing PR interval with a dropped QRS complex, recurring in a cyclical pattern, indicates Mobitz type I second-degree heart block.

3. P waves that occur intermittently without an associated QRS complex, but with an otherwise constant PR interval, suggest Mobitz

type II second-degree heart block. The QRS duration is usually prolonged.
4. Third-degree heart block is present when the P waves and QRS complexes demonstrate no relationship to each other.
5. Look for evidence of myocardial ischemia or infarction. ST-segment elevation or depression, T-wave inversion, and the presence of new Q waves are common findings.
6. Look for the presence and timing of pacemaker spikes, if appropriate. See Section I, Chapter 53, Pacemaker Troubleshooting, p 301.

V. Plan. Therapy is dictated by the most likely cause of the bradycardia and the presence of symptoms. Some bradycardic rhythms do not require treatment.

A. Drugs
1. Consider stopping or holding doses of medications associated with bradycardic rhythms. If the patient is asymptomatic, and otherwise fine, discontinuing a medication such as propranolol is all that needs to be done.
2. **Atropine.** 0.5–1.0 mg IV push, up to a total dose of 2.0 mg, is the initial treatment of symptomatic sinus bradycardia. Remember to be careful in raising the heart rate of a patient with a recent myocardial infarction, because myocardial demand could increase the likelihood of precipitating further myocardial injury.
3. Since atropine is only a temporary measure, its effects are not likely to last beyond an hour or so. Transcutaneous cardiac pacing if available, dopamine 5–20 µg/kg/min, or epinephrine 2–10 µg/min can be used after atropine if the heart rate is not adequate to maintain hemodynamic stability.
4. If digitalis overdose or intoxication is responsible for a potentially life-threatening, hemodynamically unstable arrhythmia and rapid treatment is necessary, consider giving the patient intravenous digoxin immune Fab fragments (**Digibind**). The dose is based on the amount of digoxin acutely ingested or the serum digoxin concentration and body weight. See dosing charts provided with the drug.

B. Treatment of bradycardia secondary to a CNS event. Initial steps to decrease intracranial pressure include hyperventilation, furosemide, and dexamethasone if there is an increase in intracranial pressure resulting in bradycardia. See Section I, Chapter 13, Coma, Acute Mental Status Changes, V, p 85.

C. Temporary pacemakers. Temporary pacemakers include external and transvenous devices. External pacemakers can be applied quickly in an emergent situation such as cardiac arrest. A transvenous pacemaker should be placed using central venous cannulation and fluoroscopy when the patient is more hemodynamically stable.

1. **Indications for temporary pacing**
   a. Mobitz type II second-degree or third-degree AV block associated with an acute myocardial infarction.
   b. Symptomatic AV block associated with drug toxicity that is likely to be prolonged (amiodarone toxicity).
   c. Sinus bradycardia with severe congestive heart failure.
   d. Prolonged sinus pauses (> 3.5 seconds) associated with syncope.
2. **Indications for permanent pacing**
   a. Sick sinus syndrome **with** symptoms as a result of bradycardia or sinus pauses.
   b. Mobitz type II second-degree or third-degree AV block.
   c. Occasionally, patients with cardiomyopathies and class III congestive heart failure may benefit from placement of a dual-chambered permanent pacemaker to raise heart rate and cardiac output.

REFERENCES

Mangrum JM, DiMarco JP: The evaluation and management of bradycardia. Primary Care 2000;342:703.

Miller JM, Zipes DP: Management of patient with cardiac arrhythmias. In: Braunwald E, Zipes DP, Libby P, eds. *Heart Disease: A Textbook of Cardiovascular Medicine.* 6th ed. Saunders;2001:700.

Wagner GS, ed: *Marriott's Practical Electrocardiography.* 9th ed. Williams & Wilkins;1994.

9. CARDIOPULMONARY ARREST

I. **Problem.** You are the first member of a code team to arrive at the bedside of a patient found unresponsive by the nurse.

II. **Immediate Questions**

A. **Is the patient unresponsive?** Cardiopulmonary resuscitation (CPR) begins with an attempt to arouse the patient. Call the patient by name and gently shake him or her by the shoulders. If the patient is unresponsive, send someone to call a code and begin CPR.

B. **Is the patient in optimal position for CPR?** The patient must be supine and lying on a firm and flat surface to provide effective external chest compression. The head must be at the same level as the thorax for optimal cerebral perfusion.

C. **Is the airway obstructed?** In an unconscious patient, the tongue and epiglottis may fall posteriorly and occlude the airway. A head tilt/chin lift maneuver will lift these structures and open the airway. Vomitus or foreign material should be removed from the mouth by either a finger sweep or suction.

D. **After establishment of airway patency, note whether the patient is breathing?** Respiration can be assessed for no more than 10 seconds by looking for chest movement, listening for air movement, and feeling for breath on the rescuer's face (rescuer's face is turned to face the patient's chest; rescuer's cheek is above the patient's mouth). If the patient is not breathing, institute rescue breathing with two slow full breaths, preferably via either a pocket mask or Ambu bag, if available.

E. **Is there evidence of adequate circulation?** Establish the presence of a carotid pulse. If no pulse is felt after 10 seconds of palpation, begin external chest compressions. After basic and then advanced cardiac life support has been instituted, asking other questions may help elucidate the cause of the patient's arrest.

F. **What medications has the patient been taking?** Cardiac medications are particularly important. Drugs that prolong the QT interval, such as quinidine and procainamide, amiodarone, and sotalol, may predispose to *torsades de pointes,* characterized by recurrent ventricular tachycardia and ventricular fibrillation. Phenothiazines and tricyclic antidepressants may also cause this condition. Digoxin (Lanoxin) is a common cause of a variety of cardiac arrhythmias.

G. **Has the patient received any administered medications that could have resulted in an anaphylactic reaction?** See Section I, Chapter 4, Anaphylactic Reaction, p 25.

H. **Is there any history of electrolyte disturbance or conditions that could predispose to electrolyte disturbance?** Hypokalemia and hypomagnesemia can predispose to arrhythmias. Hyperkalemia can cause complete heart block and cardiac arrest.

I. **What are the patient's medical problems?** Inquire specifically regarding a history of cardiac disease. Is there a recent history to suggest an acute stroke or any conditions that predispose to acute pulmonary embolism, such as recent surgery? The aggressiveness of CPR can be directed by knowing whether the patient has any terminal medical problems such as advanced cancer.

III. **Differential Diagnosis.** Cardiopulmonary arrest can result either from a primary cardiac disturbance or from primary respiratory arrest. There are many causes of cardiopulmonary arrest; some of the more common are listed here:

A. **Cardiac**
 1. **Acute myocardial infarction**
 2. **Acute pulmonary edema**
 3. **Ventricular arrhythmias**
 4. **Third-degree heart block**
 5. **Cardiac tamponade**

B. **Pulmonary**
  1. **Acute pulmonary embolism (usually massive)**
  2. **Acute respiratory failure**
  3. **Aspiration**
  4. **Tension pneumothorax (large)**

C. **Hemorrhagic.** Acute severe hemorrhage such as from a ruptured aortic aneurysm or rapid gastrointestinal bleeding.

D. **Metabolic**
  1. **Electrolyte disturbances.** Hypokalemia, hyperkalemia, and hypomagnesemia can induce arrhythmias. Hypophosphatemia can induce respiratory failure.
  2. **Acidosis and alkalosis**
  3. **Hypothermia and rewarming.** During the treatment of acute hypothermia, rewarming may induce ventricular fibrillation or other arrhythmias as body temperature increases.

E. **Drug overdoses.** Especially tricyclic antidepressants, digitalis, and beta and calcium channel blockers.

IV. **Database**
  A. **Physical examination key points.** The initial assessment of airway, breathing, and circulation is described in Section II, p 369. Resuscitation should be initiated before a detailed physical examination is performed. Other signs to watch for are:
  1. **Tracheal deviation.** This indicates the possibility of tension pneumothorax.
  2. **Distended neck veins.** May indicate a tension pneumothorax or a hemodynamically significant pericardial effusion.
  3. **Cannon A waves on jugular venous pulsations**. May indicate third-degree heart block.

  B. **Laboratory data.** These should be obtained early in resuscitation efforts but should not delay initiation of specific therapy.
  1. **Arterial blood gases.** Acidosis could be the cause of an arrhythmia or result from prolonged hypoperfusion. A low pO_2 can result from a variety of causes, including pulmonary edema and pulmonary embolus, or it may be the result of prolonged hypoperfusion.
  2. **Serum electrolytes.** Particularly potassium, magnesium, and ionized calcium.
  3. **Complete blood count.** Keep in mind that with massive hemorrhage the hematocrit may not have had sufficient time to equilibrate and therefore may not be an accurate indicator of the severity of blood loss.

  C. **Radiologic and other studies**
  1. **Continuous cardiac monitoring.** Three-lead monitoring is acceptable; however, a 12-lead electrocardiogram (ECG) should be obtained as early as possible.

2. Chest x-ray. A chest x-ray should be obtained to determine the position of the endotracheal tube or any central venous line. This should be performed after the patient is stabilized.

V. Plan. A full description of definitive therapy for each of the causes of cardiopulmonary arrest is beyond the scope of this text. The reader is referred to the excellent reference at the end of this chapter. In general, the best success in performing CPR has been achieved in patients in whom basic life support has been initiated *within 4 minutes* of the time of arrest and advanced cardiac life support *within 8 minutes.* Fairly early recognition of unresponsiveness and initiation of CPR is crucial. Once basic life support has been instituted, the next goal should be to determine the cardiac rhythm. Ventricular fibrillation is treated with immediate defibrillation. The next priority is endotracheal intubation followed by establishment of venous access via an antecubital vein or other large, visible superficial vein. Once a 12-lead ECG has been obtained, the physician may be able to establish a specific cause of the arrest and direct treatment accordingly. Listed here are brief summaries of the management of the major cardiac causes of arrest.

A. Ventricular fibrillation (Figure I–1). Immediate defibrillation is the most important step in the treatment of ventricular fibrillation. In fact, defibrillation should be attempted before attempts to intubate the patient or establish intravenous access. Defibrillation is facilitated by the use of quick-look paddles now available on most defibrillators.

1. The first attempt at ventricular fibrillation should be with 200 joules. If the patient remains in ventricular fibrillation, the second attempt should use 200–300 joules, administered immediately. If fibrillation still persists, a third countershock with 360 joules should be delivered.

2. If the patient remains in ventricular fibrillation after three countershocks, CPR should be resumed. The patient should be intubated, intravenous access should be established, and the patient should be connected to a 12-lead ECG. Epinephrine (1 mg of a 1:10,000 solution) should be administered every 3–5 minutes or a one-time dose of vasopressin (40 U IV) given followed by epinephrine every 5 minutes (if needed). Epinephrine is probably the most important pharmacologic agent used during CPR.

3. Within 30–60 seconds, defibrillation should be attempted again with 360 joules. If the patient remains in ventricular fibrillation, a 300-mg bolus of amiodarone should be administered.

4. After administration of amiodarone, defibrillation should again be attempted. If fibrillation persists, a second bolus of 150 mg of amiodarone or a 1.5 mg/kg bolus of lidocaine can be administered, followed by another attempt at defibrillation.

5. Upon return to spontaneous circulation after either step 3 or 4, a constant infusion of 1 mg/min of amiodarone or 2–4 mg/min of lidocaine should be started.

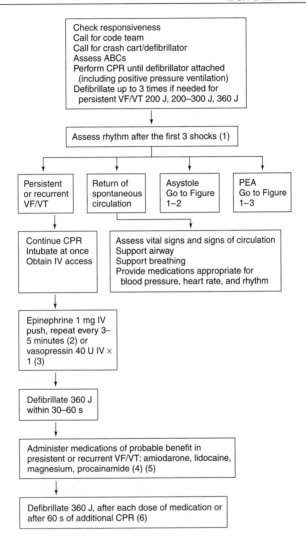

Figure I–1. Algorithm for ventricular fibrillation and pulseless ventricular tachycardia (VF/VT). *(Reproduced with permission from American Heart Association: Guidelines 2000 for cardiopulmonary resuscitation and emergency cardiovascular care. Circulation 2000[August 22]:102.)*

Footnotes to Figure I–1

(1) Hypothermic cardiac arrest is treated differently after this point. See Section I, Chapter 43, Hypothermia, p. 243.

(2) The recommended dose of epinephrine is 1 mg IV push every 3–5 min. If this approach fails, consider high-dose epinephrine 0.2 mg/kg IV push, every 3–5 min; however, there is evidence this may be harmful.

(3) No evidence to support use of vasopressin for asystole or PEA or to support using more than one dose. If no response in 5–10 minutes after vasopressin, start or restart epinephrine administration.

(4) Amiodarone 300 mg IV push, consider additional dose of 150 mg IV. No more than 2.2 g should be given in a 24-hr period.
   Lidocaine 1.0–1.5 mg/kg IV push. Consider repeat dose in 3–5 min to total loading dose of 3 mg/kg.
   Magnesium sulfate 1–2 g IV (if hypomagnesemia present, or polymorphic VT [torsades de pointes])
   Procainamide 30 mg/min in refractory VF (maximum total 17 mg/kg)

(5) Sodium bicarbonate (1 mEq/kg IV), for conditions known to provoke cardiac arrest:
   If preexisting hyperkalemic,
   If preexisting bicarbonate-responsive acidosis,
   If overdose with tricyclic antidepressants,
   To alkalinize the urine in drug overdoses (aspirin),
   If intubated and continued long arrest interval,
   Upon return of spontaneous circulation after long arrest interval.
   Note: May be harmful in respiratory acidosis.

(6) Follow either CPR-drug-shock-repeat sequence or CPR-drug-shock-shock-repeat sequence.

6. If ventricular fibrillation still persists, procainamide at a rate of 30 mg/min for a total dose of 17 mg/kg can be given followed by defibrillation.

B. Sustained ventricular tachycardia with no palpable pulse. This arrhythmia should be managed like ventricular fibrillation.

C. Ventricular tachycardia with a palpable pulse

1. **Stable monomorphic ventricular tachycardia (with decreased ejection fraction).**

   a. Amiodarone is the drug of choice, especially in patients with decreased ejection fractions. An initial loading dose of 150 mg over 10 minutes should be given followed by infusion of 1 mg/min. An additional 150-mg bolus over 10 minutes can be used 15 minutes after the first dose if needed. Lidocaine can be used as well with initial 0.5–0.75 mg/kg IV bolus, and this can be administered every 5–10 minutes as necessary until a total loading dose of 3 mg/kg has been given.

   b. If amiodarone or lidocaine fails to convert the patient, synchronized cardioversion with an initial energy level of 100 joules may be attempted, followed by 200 joules, 300 joules, and 360 joules if necessary. Premedicate the patient with a sedative and analgesic whenever possible.

2. **Stable monomorphic ventricular tachycardia (with normal ejection fraction).** Use one agent, if possible, to avoid adverse side effects (ie, proarrhythmic effects of dual drugs). Procainamide and sotalol are the top choices. Procainamide can be ad-

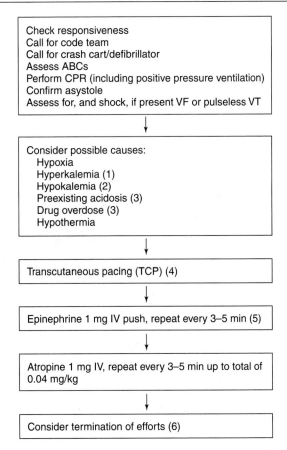

Check responsiveness
Call for code team
Call for crash cart/defibrillator
Assess ABCs
Perform CPR (including positive pressure ventilation)
Confirm asystole
Assess for, and shock, if present VF or pulseless VT

↓

Consider possible causes:
  Hypoxia
  Hyperkalemia (1)
  Hypokalemia (2)
  Preexisting acidosis (3)
  Drug overdose (3)
  Hypothermia

↓

Transcutaneous pacing (TCP) (4)

↓

Epinephrine 1 mg IV push, repeat every 3–5 min (5)

↓

Atropine 1 mg IV, repeat every 3–5 min up to total of
0.04 mg/kg

↓

Consider termination of efforts (6)

Figure I–2. Asystole treatment algorithm. *(Reproduced with permission from American Heart Association: Guidelines 2000 for cardiopulmonary resuscitation and emergency cardiovascular care. Circulation 2000[August 22]:102.)*

ministered IV in 100-mg increments Q 5 minutes until the arrhythmia is suppressed, the QRS complex widens more than 50%, or a loading dose of 17 mg/kg has been given. Other acceptable drugs are amiodarone and lidocaine dosed as above.

3. **Stable polymorphic ventricular tachycardia.** Identification of ischemia and correction of electrolytes are first priority. If baseline

ECG has a normal QT interval, refer to treatment of stable monomorphic ventricular tachycardia with decreased ejection fraction (amiodarone or lidocaine followed by cardioversion). If baseline ECG has a prolonged QT interval, consider torsades de pointes. In this case magnesium, lidocaine, or isoproterenol is effective as well as overdrive pacing.

   4. Unstable ventricular tachycardia
   a. If the patient has a pulse but is hemodynamically unstable (hypotension, unconsciousness, pulmonary edema), antiarrhythmic therapy should be deferred; instead, immediate *synchronized* cardioversion with 100 joules should be administered.
   b. If an unstable ventricular tachycardia does not convert with 100 joules, administer 200–300 joules; if still unsuccessful, 360 joules.
   c. After cardioversion, an amiodarone bolus followed by continuous infusion should be administered. Alternatively, a continuous infusion of lidocaine can be administered to prevent recurrence of the arrhythmia.

D. Asystole (Figure I–2). This rhythm has an extremely poor prognosis.
   1. Epinephrine 1 mg should be administered IV and repeated Q 3–5 minutes. (At the time this edition was under review, an original article appeared in the *New England Journal of Medicine* regarding vasopressin versus epinephrine for out-of-hospital cardiac arrest. The preliminary results indicated that vasopressin 40 units IV given twice [3 minutes apart], followed by epinephrine was more effective than epinephrine alone for treatment of asystolic cardiac arrest.)

Check responsiveness
Call for code team
Call for crash cart/defibrillator
Assess ABCs
Perform CPR until defibrillator attached
  (including positive pressure ventilation)
Defibrillate up to 3 times if needed for persistent VF/VT 200 J,
  200–300 J, 360 J

↓

Continue CPR
Intubate at once
Obtain IV access
Identify rhythm
Administer appropriate drugs
Identify and treat underlying cause

↓

Consider possible causes (and immediate treatment):
  Hypovolemia (volume infusion)
  Hypoxia (ventilation)
  Cardiac tamponade (pericardiocentesis)
  Tension pneumothorax (needle decompression)
  Hypothermia (see Section I, Chapter 43,
    Hypothermia, V, p. 243)
  Massive pulmonary embolism (surgery, thrombolytics)
  Hyperkalemia (1) or Hypokalemia (2)
  Acidosis (3)
  Drug overdoses (tricyclics, digitalis, β-blockers, calcium
    channel blockers) (3)
  Massive acute myocardial infarction (thrombolytics,
    intra-aortic balloon pump, angiography with intervention)

↓

Epinephrine 1 mg IV push, repeat every 3–5 min (4)

↓

If bradycardia is absolute or relative, give atropine 1 mg IV.
Repeat every 3–5 min to a total of 0.04 mg/kg

Figure I–3. Algorithm or pulseless activity. PEA, rhythm on monitor without detectable pulse. *(Reproduced with permission from American Heart Association: Guidelines 2000 for cardiopulmonary resuscitation and emergency cardiovascular care. Circulation 2000[August 22]:102.)*

Footnotes to Figure I–3

(1) Sodium bicarbonate 1 mEq/kg if patient has known preexisting hyperkalemia.

(2) KCl 40–60 mmol/hr IV, if > 40 mmol/hr must be administered through a central line; for rates > 15 mmol/hr cardiac monitoring is mandatory; be sure concomitant hypomagnesemia is not present.

(3) Sodium bicarbonate 1 mEq/kg:

   If known preexisting bicarbonate-responsive acidosis,

   If intubated and continued long arrest interval,

   Upon return of spontaneous circulation after long arrest interval,

   Hypoxic lactic acidosis,

   To alkalinize the urine in drug overdose (eg, aspirin),

   If overdose with tricyclic antidepressants.

   Note: May be harmful in respiratory acidosis.

(4) The recommended dose of epinephrine is 1 mg IV push every 3–5 min. If this approach fails, consider high-dose epinephrine 0.2 mg/kg every 3–5 min. Vasopressin is not recommended for PEA.

   2. Because massive parasympathetic discharge can occasionally result in asystole, an initial dose of atropine 1 mg may be administered if there is no response to the epinephrine. This dose may be repeated after 3–5 minutes if there is no response to a total dose of 0.04 mg/kg.

   3. Sodium bicarbonate and calcium chloride are no longer recommended for management of asystole.

   4. In general, pacemaker therapy will not be successful if the heart fails to respond to either of the preceding measures.

   5. Keep in mind that fine ventricular fibrillation occasionally may be mistaken as asystole. This problem can be avoided by evaluating the ECG in several leads.

E. Pulseless electrical activity (PEA) (Figure I-3). This condition is characterized by the presence of electrical activity on the ECG but no detectable pulse. It is important to recall that some causes of this condition can be reversed if they are recognized and treated appropriately.

   1. PEA is caused by a variety of conditions including hypoxemia, severe acidosis, pericardial tamponade, tension pneumothorax, hypovolemia, and pulmonary embolus. It is therefore important to evaluate for potentially reversible causes such as pericardial tamponade and pneumothorax.

   2. If tamponade is suspected, pericardiocentesis should be performed.

   3. If tension pneumothorax is suspected, insertion of a catheter-over-needle device in the second intercostal space in the midclavicular line should be attempted.

   4. Otherwise, treatment consists of epinephrine 1 mg IV along with CPR. If the heart rate is slow, atropine 1 mg IV should be given with repeated doses after 3–5 minutes to a total dose of 0.04 mg/kg.

   5. A fluid challenge should also be administered. Give 500 mL of normal saline over 15 minutes.

6. The administration of calcium chloride for this condition is no longer recommended.

7. Coronary or pulmonary thrombosis should also be considered as a possible cause of PEA.

REFERENCES

American Heart Association: Guidelines 2000 for cardiopulmonary resuscitation and emergency cardiovascular care. Circulation 2000;August 22:102.

Wenzel V, Krismer AC, Arntz HR et al: A comparison of vasopression and epinephrine for out-of-hospital cardiopulmonary resuscitation. N Engl J Med 2004;350:105.

10. CENTRAL VENOUS LINE PROBLEMS

See also Section I, Chapter 57, Pulmonary Artery Catheter Problems, p 324.

I. Problem. The nursing staff calls to report that a subclavian line has stopped functioning.

II. Immediate Questions

A. If the central line is used for central venous pressure (CVP) monitoring, what does the waveform look like? The CVP waveform drops on inspiration, rises with expiration, and should show monophasic to triphasic fluctuations with each cardiac cycle. If there is no waveform, the catheter may not be patent, or a thrombus may be in the vein or catheter.

B. Do intravenous fluids flow easily into the catheter, or does fluid leak from the insertion site? Again, these developments might indicate a thrombosed central vein or a kinked catheter.

C. Is the patient febrile? A fever in conjunction with a malfunctioning catheter suggests a central line infection, deep venous thrombosis, or both. If there is any suspicion of associated infection or thrombosis, malfunctioning lines should be removed immediately and cultured.

D. Are there any arrhythmias? A central line catheter that extends into the right atrium or right ventricle can cause atrial or ventricular ectopy and arrhythmias.

E. What is the line's purpose? What is its relative necessity? If drugs are being administered centrally that should not be given peripherally (vincristine or doxorubicin [Adriamycin] as a continuous infusion), the situation is different from one in which the central line could be replaced by a peripheral line.

III. Differential Diagnosis

A. Clotted catheter. This can occur when central lines are allowed to run dry or are running very slowly. Blood backs up into the catheter lumen and thrombosis occurs.

B. Misdirected catheter. Subclavian catheters from either the right or the left side may be inadvertently placed retrograde into the ipsilateral internal jugular vein. This results in a line that cannot be used to measure CVP. Much more rarely, subclavian or internal jugular attempts end up in the long thoracic vein, again failing to function properly. The catheter may also extend into the right atrium or right ventricle rather than the proximal venous circulation.

C. Kinked catheter. Catheters can kink at the skin or more deeply. From the right subclavian insertion site, it is not uncommon for catheters within relatively stiff sheaths to kink at the turn from the subclavian vein to the brachiocephalic vein as it joins the superior vena cava. Kinking at this bend is uncommon for single-lumen catheters or triple-lumen catheters not inside a sheath. Internal jugular lines and left subclavian lines are not generally subject to this problem. It should be stressed that any line can be misdirected and kink. The catheters are easily seen fluoroscopically and radiographically; a chest x-ray usually allows you to diagnose this problem.

D. Infected catheter. Central line sepsis usually does not result in any apparent malfunction of the catheter. Fever, sepsis, and positive blood cultures all may result from the spread of skin flora to the intravascular segment of the catheter.

E. Thrombosis of the vein of insertion. Any deep vein accessed for central line insertion can thrombose as a result of the trauma associated with the procedure, as well as the presence of a foreign body within the vein. Clinically, these events resemble natural deep venous thrombosis and can result in associated bland or septic pulmonary emboli.

IV. Database

A. Physical examination key points

1. **Vital signs.** An elevated temperature suggests an infection. If the catheter has been in place more than 3 days, you must assume the central venous catheter is the source of the fever.
2. **Extremities.** Look for evidence of deep venous thrombosis, such as unilateral edema and venous engorgement.
3. **Skin.** Examine the insertion site for evidence of tissue infiltration, bleeding, catheter kinking, or leakage. Also, erythema around the insertion site may result from a localized infection.

B. Laboratory data

1. **Complete blood count with differential.** An elevated white blood count with an increase in banded neutrophils is often present with catheter-related sepsis.
2. **Prothrombin time (PT), partial thromboplastin time (PTT), platelet count.** These values should be obtained if a central line

needs to be changed and a coagulopathy is suspected, such as in patients with severe liver disease or malnutrition.

3. **Blood cultures.** These should be obtained as part of routine evaluation of a fever. Remember, if a central venous catheter has been in place for more than 3 days, there is a significant risk of catheter-related sepsis.

C. Radiologic and other studies

1. **Chest x-ray.** Useful in determining whether a catheter is in the correct position or is kinked.

2. **Culture of catheter tip.** If catheter-related sepsis or infection is suspected, the catheter must be removed and the tip sent for culture.

3. **Impedance plethysmography and Doppler ultrasound.** Noninvasive tests for suspected extremity venous thrombosis.

4. **Venography.** This is the gold standard for diagnosing venous thrombosis. If there is a history of allergy to contrast media, venography should be preceded by treatment with corticosteroids and diphenhydramine.

5. **Nuclear venogram.** Can diagnose venous thrombosis and pulmonary embolism simultaneously with lower extremity injection.

V. Plan. For replacement of central venous catheters, see Section III, Chapter 6, Central Venous Catheterization, p 426.

A. Clotted catheter. A line can sometimes be salvaged by aspirating the catheter while it is slowly pulled out. Sterile technique and a small syringe are necessary. Use of a guidewire or manual flushing, or injection of urokinase 5000 U (5000 U/mL) or tissue plasminogen activator (10 mg) may result in embolization. However, these measures seldom cause any significant problem, probably because of the small volume of the embolus. The only completely safe approach, however, is aspiration. The risk of replacement of the line has to be weighed against the risk of using any of the other techniques besides aspiration. Other factors must be considered, such as the length of time the catheter has been in place, the necessity of a central rather than peripheral placement, and the presence of fever or local evidence of infection.

B. Misdirected catheter. This situation usually requires removal and replacement. With fluoroscopic guidance, a guidewire might be manipulated into the superior vena cava, which then can guide the catheter correctly. If fluoroscopy is not an option, a new puncture may be unavoidable. If the catheter is in the right atrium or right ventricle and does not have to be removed for other reasons, it can be partially withdrawn using sterile technique, so that it is in the superior or inferior vena cava.

C. Kinked catheter. A new line that is kinked at the site of insertion can sometimes be salvaged by repositioning the line with new skin sutures. More proximal kinks can sometimes be fixed by replacing the catheter over a guidewire. If the kink is within a sheath or is located where the catheter emerges from the sheath, the sheath can sometimes be withdrawn, leaving the catheter in the same place, provided there is enough catheter left onto which the sheath can be withdrawn. The best way to deal with this problem is to prevent it by avoiding the right subclavian approach in patients who have shallow chests in the lateral dimension. In these patients, the lines must negotiate a sharp angle from the subclavian to the superior vena cava.

D. **Infected catheter.** An infected or possible infected central line *must be removed.* This almost always requires replacement elsewhere if central venous access is still desired. Intravenous line–associated sepsis is caused in large part by skin contamination. The practice of removing the line over a guidewire and traversing the same insertion site with the replacement line is **not** recommended. A new site is a better idea. It is important to draw two sets of blood cultures from the suspect line as well as two sets from the peripheral veins before the line is removed and to culture the tip of the catheter after it is removed. Antibiotics are indicated for 10–14 days in the event that a blood culture was positive, matching a tip culture or catheter culture, and antibiotics should be tailored to the sensitivity of the organism. The use of antibiotic- or antiseptic-impregnated catheters is associated with reduction in catheter infection. The clinical application of this research is not yet evident in catheters available for routine use.

E. **Thrombosis of the vein of insertion.** This also requires line removal and replacement at a site distant from the thrombosed vein. Heparin 80 U/kg IV bolus followed by 18 U/kg continuous infusion is recommended unless contraindicated for other reasons. The PTT should be checked 6 hours after the infusion is begun; the heparin dose should be adjusted so that the PTT is one and one-half to two times the control. If sepsis is also suspected, antibiotics are necessary, as is a surgical consultation for possible removal of the infected vein. Vancomycin 1000 mg Q 12 hours is the preferred antibiotic if normal renal function is present. Vancomycin covers *Staphylococcus epidermidis* as well as *Staphylococcus aureus*. Be sure to decrease the dose if renal insufficiency is present.

REFERENCES

Fares LG, Block PH, Feldman SD: Improved house staff results with subclavian cannulation. Am Surg 1986;52:108.

Gil RT, Kruse JA, Thill-Baharozian MC et al: Triple- vs. single-lumen central venous catheters. Arch Intern Med 1989;149:1139.

Maki DG, Stolz SM, Wheeler S et al: Prevention of central venous catheter-related bloodstream infection by use of an antiseptic-impregnated catheter. Ann Intern Med 1997;127:257.

Mansfield PF, Hohn DC, Fornage BD et al: Complications and failures of subclavian-vein catheterization. N Engl J Med 1994;331:1735.

McGee DC, Gould MK: Preventing complications of central venous catheterization. N Engl J Med 2003;348:1123.

Raad I, Darouiche R, Dupuis J et al: Central venous catheters coated with minocycline and rifampin for the prevention of catheter-related colonization and bloodstream infections. Ann Intern Med 1997;127:267.

11. CHEST PAIN

I. **Problem.** A 48-year-old man with a history of tobacco abuse is admitted for elective bronchoscopy. On the evening of his admission, he develops substernal chest pain lasting 15 minutes.

II. **Immediate Questions.** Because of potentially serious conditions, patients complaining of chest pain should be evaluated urgently. By far, the most important tool in identifying the cause of chest pain is a meticulous history.

A. **Does the patient have a history of coronary artery disease, and if so, does the current pain resemble previous episodes of angina pectoris?** If the patient has a documented history of coronary artery disease, particularly if the current episode resembles previously known anginal pain, assume that the pain represents myocardial ischemia and treat accordingly.

B. **What is the location, quality, and severity of the pain?** Location (substernal, epigastric); radiation (jaw, arms, back); quality (burning, crushing, tearing, stabbing, sharp); and severity of pain are features that may suggest a particular diagnosis. Because the same spinal cord segments innervate several intrathoracic and extrathoracic structures, the location and quality of different causes of chest pain may overlap.

C. **Are there any factors that are known to precipitate or relieve the pain?** Sharp pain worsened by coughing or deep inspiration suggests pleuritis, pericarditis, or pneumothorax. Although classic angina is brought on by exertion, acute myocardial infarction (MI) may produce chest pain at rest, especially in the early morning. Movement of the arms or trunk that reproduces pain would indicate a musculoskeletal origin; however, pericarditis can also cause chest pain worsened by movement of the trunk. The pain of esophagitis is frequently exacerbated by recumbency. Relief of chest pain with sublingual nitroglycerin implies myocardial ischemia, although chest pain resulting from esophageal spasm and gallbladder colic may also be relieved. Myocardial ischemia is relieved in 3–5 minutes, whereas esophageal spasm is relieved in 10 minutes by sublingual nitroglycerin.

D. **Has there been any recent trauma, fall, or thoracic procedure?** Fractured ribs, chest wall contusions, or other musculoskeletal conditions such as recent excessive physical activity can result in chest pain.

III. Differential Diagnosis. The differential diagnosis includes a variety of conditions, ranging from musculoskeletal chest wall pain to life-threatening conditions such as acute MI and dissecting aneurysm. The clinician's initial goal is to exclude potentially catastrophic conditions; if such conditions are identified, institute immediate therapy.

A. Cardiac causes of chest pain

1. **Acute MI.** The pain of MI is characterized as a severe, crushing, retrosternal pain that may radiate into the arms and neck. This pain is generally described as the worst ever experienced and generally persists 30 minutes or longer. One seldom relieves it with 1 or 2 nitroglycerin tablets, and frequently morphine sulfate is required for relief. The pain of MI may begin at rest or even during sleep and is only infrequently preceded by strenuous physical activity. Associated symptoms include nausea, diaphoresis, dyspnea, and palpitations. Because more than 50% of deaths caused by acute MI occur within the initial 2 hours, the physician must maintain a high index of suspicion for MI when evaluating any patient with acute chest pain.

2. **Angina pectoris.** The pain of angina is similar to that of MI, although it generally lasts less than 20 minutes and is not nearly as severe. Relief can generally be obtained with sublingual nitroglycerin. The pain is usually exacerbated by exertion, but can also occur at rest or with emotional stress. Any recent change in a stable pattern of angina, such as occurrence with rest or increased frequency or severity, should imply an unstable pattern that mandates close monitoring and aggressive medical therapy. Although coronary artery disease is the most common cause of angina pectoris, other potential causes include coronary artery spasm, aortic stenosis, and angina precipitated by thyrotoxicosis, anemia, and a low diastolic blood pressure.

3. **Acute pericarditis.** Pain is usually described as sharp, but may be dull, and is frequently pleuritic. The pain may be worsened by recumbency and relieved by sitting and leaning forward. Rotation of the trunk may precipitate pain. Possible causes include the following:

   a. **Infection.** Most commonly viral, but may also be bacterial, fungal, or tuberculous.

   b. **Myocardial infarction.** Pericarditis may occur in the first 2–3 days after infarction or may not occur until 1–4 weeks after MI (Dressler's syndrome).

   c. **Uremia**

   d. **Malignancy.** Most often breast cancer, lung carcinoma, or lymphoma.

   e. **Connective tissue diseases.** Including rheumatoid arthritis, scleroderma, systemic lupus erythematosus, or acute rheumatic fever.

B. Vascular causes of chest pain
   1. Acute aortic dissection. Usually described as an excruciatingly severe pain that is tearing in nature and may radiate to the back (especially if the descending aorta is involved). The pain is most severe at its onset. A history of hypertension, chest trauma, or connective tissue disorders such as Marfan's syndrome is usually present. On presentation, however, the blood pressure may be normal or even low. Aortic dissection is a potentially life-threatening condition that must be recognized and treated early.
   2. Primary pulmonary hypertension. The pain is frequently similar to angina. It is usually mild, may be associated with syncope or dyspnea, and may occur with exertion.

C. Pulmonary causes of chest pain
   1. Pulmonary embolism (PE) with infarction. Infarction results in inflammation of the overlying pleura and thus causes pleuritic chest pain. Embolism without infarction may cause a more vague, nondescript chest pain. Dyspnea is often present. Hemoptysis may be present if there is underlying pulmonary infarction. Several conditions predispose to deep venous thrombosis or PE; they include pregnancy; postoperative state; prolonged immobilization; malignancy (especially adenocarcinoma); obesity; exogenous estrogen use; paraplegia; cerebral vascular accident with resultant hemiplegia; congestive heart failure; and hypercoagulable states such as protein C, protein S, factor V Leiden, or antithrombin III deficiency; or the presence of a lupus anticoagulant or anticardiolipin antibody. PE is a potentially fatal condition that is too often underdiagnosed. It should be suspected in any hospitalized patient who develops acute shortness of breath or chest pain, especially with any of the above risk factors and a clear lung examination.
   2. Pneumothorax. This is characterized by the acute onset of pleuritic chest pain associated with dyspnea. *Tension pneumothorax* is a potentially life-threatening condition that is characterized by hypotension, tracheal deviation, venous distention, and severe respiratory distress. There are three broad categories of causes of pneumothorax:
      a. Spontaneous. This most often occurs in 20- to 30-year-old men and in older patients with bullous emphysema.
      b. Iatrogenic. Pneumothorax may be a complication of subclavian vein catheterization or thoracentesis. Barotrauma from mechanical ventilation, especially in patients requiring high inspiratory pressures, may also cause pneumothorax.
      c. Traumatic. Any patient with a penetrating chest injury, as well as patients with rib fractures, may sustain a pneumothorax.
   3. Pleurodynia. This is frequently associated with Coxsackie virus.
   4. Pneumonia/pleuritis. The pain is typically pleuritic and associated with fever, productive cough, and rigors.

D. **Gastrointestinal causes of chest pain**
1. **Gastroesophageal reflux.** This condition is usually described as a burning pain that is made worse with recumbency and relieved by antacids.
2. **Esophageal spasm.** This condition is easily confused with angina pectoris. It may cause substernal chest pain or tightness that is relieved by nitrates. Intermittent dysphagia, if it occurs, suggests esophageal disease; however, it may be difficult by history alone to distinguish esophageal spasm from angina. Remember that both conditions may occur together.
3. **Gastritis.** Alcohol use, stress associated with severe burns, trauma, major surgery, or intensive care unit admission, as well as use of nonsteroidal anti-inflammatory drugs (NSAIDs) all may induce inflammation of the gastric mucosa, resulting in epigastric and lower chest pain.
4. **Peptic ulcer disease.** This is typically described as an epigastric discomfort that may be burning or gnawing and frequently radiates to the back. Pain may be either relieved or exacerbated by eating. Antacids frequently relieve it.
5. **Biliary colic.** This condition is characterized by postprandial pain that occurs 1–2 hours after eating and may last several hours. In contrast to the term *colic,* the pain is actually constant and intense and may last several hours. The pain is usually located in the right upper quadrant and radiates to the right scapula; however, the pain may also be perceived largely in the epigastrium and lower chest and therefore may be confused with angina.
6. **Pancreatitis.** The patient usually has a history of gallstones or alcohol ingestion. Pain is generally midepigastric with radiation to the back. Similar to pericarditis, the pain of pancreatitis may be exacerbated by recumbency and relieved by sitting upright and leaning forward. Often nausea and vomiting accompany it.
E. **Musculoskeletal chest pain.** Pain is usually reproduced by palpation over the costochondral or sternochondral junctions. Pain is fairly well localized.
1. **Costochondritis.** Point tenderness is elicited over the costochondral junction.
2. **Muscle strain/spasm.** Most typically, there is a preceding history of exercise or overexertion.
3. **Rib fractures after trauma**

IV. **Database**
A. **Physical examination key points**
1. **Vital signs**
a. **Hypotension.** An ominous sign that may result from any one of several potentially catastrophic causes, including massive MI, cardiac tamponade, tension pneumothorax, acute massive

PE, rupture of a dissecting aneurysm, or gastritis or peptic ulcer disease with hemorrhage.

   b. Hypertension. May result from any painful condition, but must be particularly looked for in the setting of acute MI or aortic dissection in which emergent therapy to reduce the pressure is essential.

   c. Fever. May result from PE, MI, pneumonia, or pericarditis.

   d. Tachycardia. Can be from sinus tachycardia associated with pain, but could also indicate ventricular tachycardia that has developed because of myocardial ischemia. If untreated, ventricular tachycardia may progress into ventricular fibrillation. (See Section I, Chapter 60, Tachycardia, p 345). PE frequently causes sinus tachycardia or acute atrial fibrillation.

   e. Bradycardia. A common occurrence with inferior MI, this may result from either sinus node dysfunction or atrioventricular heart block (second- or third-degree). (See Section I, Chapter 8, Bradycardia, p 42.)

2. **HEENT.** Evidence of oral thrush, especially in an immunosuppressed patient, could indicate *Candida* esophagitis.

3. **Neck.** Significant venous distention may occur with either acute tension pneumothorax or cardiac tamponade. Pain with hyperextension of the neck may indicate a cervical nerve or disk problem as a cause of referred shoulder and chest pain. Tracheal deviation suggests tension pneumothorax.

4. **Chest.** Localized chest wall tenderness may result from a contusion, costochondritis, or rib fracture.

5. **Lungs**

   a. Absent breath sounds and hyperresonance to percussion indicate a pneumothorax.

   b. Crackles and signs of pneumonic consolidation such as increased tactile fremitus or egophony may occur with pneumonia.

   c. A pleural friction rub may result from pneumonia, pulmonary infarction, or any process resulting in pleuritis.

   d. Bibasilar crackles and/or wheezes may occur with decompensated congestive heart failure resulting from myocardial ischemia or infarction.

   e. Lung examination may be normal in a patient with acute PE.

6. **Heart**

   a. The point of maximal impulse may not be palpable in a patient with a pericardial effusion. Heart sounds may likewise be distant. In a patient with acute pericarditis, a friction rub may be present, but this is an evanescent finding and therefore the patient must be reexamined periodically.

   b. Most often, the cardiac exam is normal in a patient with acute MI or angina pectoris. If there is significant associated left ventricular dysfunction, an S_3 gallop may be heard. An S_4 gallop may also be present. A harsh systolic ejection murmur over the aortic outflow area may indicate aortic stenosis, which can cause angina pectoris even in the presence of normal coronary arteries. In the setting of a recent MI, a new holosystolic murmur at the apex suggests papillary muscle dysfunction or rupture. If dissection is suspected, listen for a decrescendo diastolic murmur of aortic regurgitation at the left lower sternal border, which may develop if the dissection spreads to involve the aortic ring.

7. **Abdomen.** For a discussion of abdominal conditions that can also produce epigastric and lower chest pain, see Section I, Chapter 1, Abdominal Pain, p 1.

8. **Neurologic exam.** A careful and detailed exam is important in any patient in whom aortic dissection is suspected. The dissection may occlude cerebral or spinal arteries and thereby cause a variety of neurologic deficits.

9. **Extremities**
   a. In a patient with suspected PE, examine for evidence of deep venous thrombosis; however, the physical exam is notoriously inaccurate in this condition and may be entirely normal despite the presence of significant venous thrombosis. Be sure to examine the upper extremities.
   b. In patients with suspected dissection, it is important to examine the pulses bilaterally in both upper and lower extremities for symmetry.

B. **Laboratory data**
   1. **Hemogram.** Leukocytosis may result from any form of inflammation such as pulmonary infarction or MI. If there is an increase in banded neutrophils, suspect a bacterial infection such as pneumonia.
   2. **Arterial blood gases (ABGs).** These values should be obtained if a pulmonary process is suspected, such as embolism, pneumothorax, or pneumonia. It should also be ordered with decompensated cardiac function resulting in pulmonary edema.
   3. **Cardiac enzymes.** Serial measurements of cardiac enzymes such as creatine phosphokinase (CK) with isoenzymes and the cardiac-specific troponin I may initially be normal, but they should be followed every 4–6 hours over the first 24–48 hours watching for elevation to help exclude or confirm an acute MI. Troponin I is usually elevated within the first 4–6 hours after an acute cardiac injury and may remain elevated for 5–9 days. Serial measurements of CK with isoenzymes every 8–12 hours over the first 24–48 hours may help to confirm or exclude an MI. Note that CK may not become elevated until several hours after the beginning of infarction. Therefore, a single measurement of CK cannot be used to exclude the diagnosis of MI. Troponin I is cardiac specific, is elevated in the first 4–6 hours after an acute MI, and remains elevated for 5–9 days.

C. Radiologic and other studies

1. **Electrocardiogram (ECG).** An ECG should be obtained in any patient with a new complaint of chest pain. If available for comparison, an old ECG is helpful. New T-wave changes, ST-segment depression or elevation, or the presence of new Q waves are helpful in identifying the cause of the chest pain as myocardial ischemia/infarction. Patients presenting with MI may initially have an entirely normal ECG, and the diagnosis of MI cannot be excluded on the basis of a normal ECG. With a pulmonary embolism, sinus tachycardia, nonspecific ST-T wave changes, right axis deviation, right bundle branch block, P pulmonale, right ventricular hypertrophy, or the classic S_I, Q_{III}, T_{III}, (S wave in I and Q wave and inverted T wave in III) may be present.

2. **Chest x-ray.** Request a chest x-ray in any patient in whom the cause of the chest pain is unclear. Chest films may be helpful in diagnosing pneumothorax, pneumonia, and pleural and pericardial effusions. A widened mediastinum suggests dissection of the thoracic aorta.

3. **Echocardiogram.** This can be performed on an emergent basis if cardiac tamponade is suspected. It is also helpful in diagnosing thoracic aortic dissection and assessing regional wall abnormalities in acute MI.

4. **Contrast CT scan.** This should be obtained in any patient in whom aortic dissection is suspected.

5. **Spiral CT of the chest.** Helpful for ruling in PE. A negative test does not rule out the diagnosis.

6. **Ventilation/perfusion (V̇/Q̇) lung scan.** A lung scan may be helpful if pulmonary emboli are suspected. Impedance plethysmography and Doppler ultrasound of the lower extremities may also be obtained if there is a strong suspicion of acute deep venous thrombosis.

V. Plan. In assessing any patient with acute chest pain, the overriding goal is to exclude the presence of the previously mentioned life-threatening conditions. In the acute setting, it is better to maintain a high index of suspicion for these conditions.

A. Emergency management (for all patients with chest pain)

1. **Oxygen.** Administer oxygen therapy with 2–4 μL/min by nasal cannula. If the patient has a history of chronic obstructive airway disease, it is preferable to administer 24% O_2 by Venturi face mask initially.

2. **Intravenous access.** Establish at least one intravenous line for administration of medications if the patient's condition deteriorates.

3. **Nitroglycerin.** If chest pain is still present and the systolic blood pressure is above 90 mm Hg, 0.4 mg nitroglycerin may be administered sublingually.

   4. 12-lead ECG
   5. Stat portable chest x-ray and ABGs. Obtain if your initial assessment suggests any evidence of a pneumothorax, pneumonia, or heart failure.

B. **Myocardial ischemia.** If your initial assessment suggests the possibility of acute MI, the following are brief guidelines offered for the initial treatment. A full discussion of acute MI is beyond the scope of this section.

   1. **Aspirin.** Administer two chewable 81-mg aspirin (consider ticlopidine [Ticlid] if there is a history of aspirin hypersensitivity).

   2. **Nitrates**
      a. Nitroglycerin in a dose of 0.4–0.6 mg may be administered sublingually every 5 minutes, provided that the systolic blood pressure remains above 90 mm Hg. It is preferable to administer the nitroglycerin while the patient is recumbent. This may provide relief for angina pectoris and possibly unstable angina pectoris.
      b. The pain of acute MI is seldom relieved by sublingual nitroglycerin and requires treatment with either intravenous nitroglycerin or morphine. If the nitroglycerin is effective but pain recurs, begin a nitroglycerin infusion initially at 10 µg/min and increase by 10 µg/min every 10 minutes until relief of pain or to a maximum dose of 200 µg/min. The systolic blood pressure must be maintained above 90 mm Hg during the administration of nitroglycerin. Hemodynamic monitoring with a pulmonary artery catheter (see Section III, Chapter 12, Pulmonary Artery Catheterization p 449) is often necessary if hypotension develops.

   3. **Morphine sulfate.** If pain is not relieved by nitroglycerin sublingually or intravenously, 3–5 mg of morphine IV every 5–10 minutes can be administered for relief. Close monitoring of the patient's blood pressure and respirations is necessary, because hypotension and respiratory suppression may occur. These adverse effects may be reversed with naloxone (Narcan) 0.4 mg IV.

   4. **Beta-blockers.** Administration should strongly be considered. Metoprolol 5 mg every 2–5 minutes for 3 doses intravenously; or atenolol 5 mg every 5 minutes for 2 doses intravenously. Watch for bradycardia and acute heart block (second- or third-degree), especially in a patient with suspected right ventricular infarction.

   5. **Heparin.** Unfractionated heparin 70 U/kg bolus, followed by 15 U/kg/hr continuous infusion. Dose is titrated to a partial thromboplastin time (PTT) 1.5–2 times the control value (usually 50–60 seconds); some cardiologists prefer the PTT to be 2–2.5 times the control value. Low molecular weight heparins may also be used. Dalteparin (Fragmin) 120 U/kg SC Q 12 hr, to a maximum of 10,000 units per dose, or enoxaparin (Lovenox) 1 mg/kg SC Q 12

hr can be used. Treatment is usually continued for 2–8 days after the patient has stabilized.

6. **Transfer to a coronary care unit or intensive care.** This is especially important in the first 24 hours of MI, when arrhythmia monitoring and ready access to a defibrillator are essential.

7. **Platelet glycoprotein IIb/IIIa inhibitors.** Should be considered in the setting of chest pain with ST depression in two contiguous leads or typical chest pain with a history of coronary artery disease. In patients undergoing percutaneous coronary intervention, abciximab (ReoPro) 0.25 mg/kg IV bolus, followed by infusion of 0.125 µg/kg/min (maximum of 10 µg/min) for 18–24 hours. Infusion should be discontinued 1 hour after percutaneous coronary intervention. Eptifibatide (Integrilin) 180 µg/kg IV bolus, followed by infusion of 2 µg/kg/min. Eptifibatide may be administered for up to 96 hours. Tirofiban (Aggrastat) 0.4 µg/kg/min initial infusion for 30 minutes, followed by 0.1 µg/kg/min continuous infusion. Tirofiban may be given for up to 108 hours after presentation. Aspirin and heparin should be used along with the platelet glycoprotein IIb/IIIa inhibitors.

8. **Thrombolytic therapy.** Discussion of thrombolytic agents is beyond the scope of this section, but *should always be considered* in any patient presenting with chest pain that is consistent with MI; at least 1 mm ST-segment elevation in two contiguous leads and no contraindication to thrombolytics. See the discussions of alteplase, anistreplase, and streptokinase in Section VII, Therapeutics.

C. **Aortic dissection.** The initial treatment goal is to reduce pain and to reduce blood pressure if elevated. Surgical correction is indicated for all ascending thoracic aneurysms.

1. **Transfer to a coronary or intensive care unit.** Make arrangements for immediate transfer where hemodynamic monitoring can be instituted.

2. **Immediate vascular surgical consult**

3. **Intravenous esmolol or labetalol.** Esmolol is given as a 30-mg bolus followed by 3 mg/min and titrated to 12 mg/min. Labetalol is given as 10 mg over 2 minutes followed by 20- to 80-mg doses every 10–15 minutes to a total dose of 300 mg, and then a maintenance dose of 2 mg/min, titrating to 5–20 mg/min. If there is a contraindication to using beta-blockers, then IV verapamil or diltiazem can be used.

4. **Relieve pain.** Morphine sulfate 3–5 mg may be administered intravenously every 10 minutes. Again, close monitoring of the blood pressure and respirations is necessary.

D. **PE**

1. **Oxygen.** Ensure adequate oxygenation.

2. **Heparin.** After checking a baseline prothrombin time and PTT, administer a bolus of heparin 80 U/kg IV and follow it with a con-

tinuous IV infusion of 18 U/kg/hr. Repeat the PTT in 4–6 hours and adjust the heparin to maintain a PTT approximately 1.5–2.5 times the control value (50–70 seconds).
3. **Surgical or radiologic consultation.** For placement of a venocaval filter if systemic anticoagulation is contraindicated.
4. **Thrombolytic therapy or surgical consultation for embolectomy.** Should be considered for massive PE with hypotension. *Caution:* Thrombolytics are contraindicated postoperatively.

E. **Acute pneumothorax**
   1. **Decompression.** An acute tension pneumothorax should be treated by immediate placement of a 16-gauge needle into the second intercostal space in the midclavicular line. This potentially life-saving measure can be instituted while the patient awaits placement of a chest tube.
   2. **Oxygen.** A spontaneous pneumothorax occurring in an otherwise healthy person and involving 20% or less of the lung can usually be treated with oxygen and observation. Chest tube insertion or pneumothorax catheter placement with aspiration should be used to treat all other pneumothoraces.

F. **Pericarditis**
   1. **Ketorolac** (Toradol) 30 mg IM or IV initially or indomethacin (Indocin) 25–50 mg PO tid.
   2. **Emergent echocardiogram.** If tamponade is suspected and confirmed, a cardiology consultation for pericardiocentesis should be requested.

G. **Gastritis/esophagitis**
   1. **Antacids.** Mylanta-II 30 mL Q 4–6 hr may provide immediate relief.
   2. **H_2 antagonists.** Cimetidine (Tagamet), ranitidine (Zantac), famotidine (Pepcid), or nizatidine (Axid) may also relieve symptoms. Hydrogen proton pump inhibitors such as omeprazole (Prilosec) are also effective.
   3. **Elevating head of the bed.** Elevation by 6 inches on blocks may help to reduce the reflux that occurs with recumbency.
   4. ***H pylori* antibody.** May be helpful in making a diagnosis of peptic ulcer disease.

H. **Costochondritis.** Treat with NSAIDs such as ibuprofen 800 mg Q 8 hr.

REFERENCES

Raschke RA, Reilly BM, Guidry JR et al: The weight-based heparin dosing nomogram compared with a "standard care" nomogram. Ann Intern Med 1993;119:874.

Silverman ME: *Examination of the Heart: The Clinical History.* 3rd ed. American Heart Association;1990.

12. COAGULOPATHY

I. Problem. After cardiac catheterization, a patient has oozing from the femoral arterial puncture site.

II. Immediate Questions

A. What is the patient's blood pressure? Determine immediately if the bleeding is extensive enough to cause hypovolemia and shock (Refer to Section I, Chapter 42, Hypotension (Shock), p 237.) If central lines need to be placed, determine the extent of the coagulopathy before inserting needles into major noncompressible vessels. Hypotension and coagulopathy can also be seen with sepsis.

B. How much external bleeding is there? Look at wounds or needle puncture sites to see if there is active bleeding.

C. Do factors exist that increase the likelihood of generalized bleeding? In critically ill patients, disseminated intravascular coagulation (DIC) should be considered. In general, when you have a bleeding patient, inquire about liver disease; nutritional status; family history of bleeding disorders; any bleeding with prior surgical procedures (including dental extractions); and use of medications such as aspirin, nonsteroidal anti-inflammatory drugs (NSAIDs), antiplatelet drugs, and anticoagulants.

III. Differential Diagnosis

A. Inadequate hemostasis. This is the most common cause of localized bleeding in the postoperative patient. The bleeding is usually minimal.

B. Platelet disorders

1. Thrombocytopenia. See Section I, Chapter 61, Thrombocytopenia, p 355.

a. Decreased platelet production. This is often secondary to chemotherapy, fibrosis, neoplasia, or infection (tuberculosis, histoplasmosis) involving the bone marrow. Ethanol, thiazides, estrogens, and other drugs can impair platelet production. Vitamin B_{12}, folic acid, and iron deficiencies may result in decreased production.

b. Sequestration. Caused by splenic enlargement resulting from portal hypertension, neoplasia, infection, or storage diseases.

c. Destruction. Idiopathic thrombocytopenic purpura (ITP), thrombotic thrombocytopenic purpura (TTP), hemolytic-uremic syndrome (HUS), collagen vascular diseases, and reactions to drugs (penicillins, sulfa drugs, quinidine, thiazides, heparin, and others) can cause platelet destruction.

d. Dilution. May occur with a large volume of blood transfused over a short interval.

      2. Qualitative platelet disorders
        a. Inherited disorders
          i. **von Willebrand's disease (vWD).** Autosomal dominant adhesion defect with many variants; prevalence as high as 1%.
          ii. **Bernard-Soulier syndrome.** Inherited adhesion defect characterized by giant platelets and absence/dysfunction of glycoprotein Ib/IX.
          iii. **Glanzmann's thrombasthenia.** Inherited aggregation defect with absence/dysfunction of glycoprotein IIb/IIIa.
        b. Acquired disorders
          i. **Drugs.** Aspirin and NSAIDs affect cyclooxygenase metabolism (aspirin for the life of the platelet, NSAIDs in the presence of the drug). Glycoprotein IIb/IIIa inhibitors and other antiplatelet agents affect platelet aggregation only in the presence of the drug.
          ii. **Uremia.** Abnormal platelet aggregation caused by an unknown mechanism.

C. Coagulation defects
  1. Congenital
    a. Hemophilia A. Factor VIII deficiency, X-linked recessive. Incidence of 1/10,000 male births.
    b. Hemophilia B. Factor IX deficiency, X-linked recessive. Incidence of 1/100,000 male births.
    c. Congenital deficiencies of other coagulation factors. These are much less common than factor VIII and IX deficiencies.
  2. Acquired
    a. DIC. Associated with sepsis, trauma, burns, and malignancy. DIC may be a complication of pregnancy and delivery, liver disease, or heat stroke.
    b. Vitamin K deficiency. Vitamin K is required for synthesis of factors II, VII, IX, and X. The most common setting for deficiency is the malnourished patient receiving antibiotics.
    c. Severe liver disease. Cirrhosis, hepatitis, hemochromatosis, biliary cirrhosis, or cancer. Coagulopathy is caused by decreased production of coagulation factors, production of abnormal coagulation factors, or a failure to clear activated coagulation factors.
    d. Autoantibodies. Circulating anticoagulant antibodies occur in postpartum women and in autoimmune diseases such as systemic lupus erythematosus (SLE).

IV. Database. The most important factor in diagnosing a coagulopathy is understanding and utilizing appropriate laboratory tests. It is imperative to draw blood for needed tests before instituting therapy or transfusions.

  A. History and physical examination key points
    1. Vital signs. *Orthostatic hypotension* (a decrease in systolic blood pressure of 10 mm Hg, and/or an increase in heart rate of 20 bpm

1 minute after changing from a supine to a standing position) signifies a major loss of blood. Also, look for resting or supine tachycardia or hypotension. Fever or hypothermia suggests DIC as the
cause.

2. **Skin and incisions.** Petechiae, purpura, easy bruising, and oozing from intravenous sites suggest a systemic rather than a local
cause. Examine any incision for hematoma or for active bleeding.

3. **Abdomen.** Splenomegaly, hepatomegaly, or ascites provide
clues to the diagnosis.

4. **Extremities.** Hemarthrosis may be seen with hemophilia or other
causes of coagulopathy.

5. **Neurologic exam.** To assess for CNS bleeding.

B. **Laboratory data**

1. **Complete blood count.** Follow serial hematocrits with ongoing
bleeding. Patients with acute hemorrhage may have normal
hematocrits initally. An adequate platelet count does not imply adequate function of platelets. Generally, platelet counts of
50,000–100,000 are adequate to maintain hemostasis if function
is normal. Large platelets suggest shortened survival and rapid
platelet turnover.

2. **Prothrombin time (PT) and partial thromboplastin time (PTT).**
PTT assesses all coagulation proteins except factors VII and XIII.
PT is elevated if there is a deficiency of factor I, II, V, VII, or X
(Table I–5). Factor VII has the shortest half-life; a deficiency in
factor VII is the usual cause in generalized problems such as liver
disease. In SLE, there may be a circulating anticoagulant, which
usually prolongs PTT and less frequently PT. This condition generally does not cause a bleeding diathesis but may predispose to
thrombosis. To determine whether a prolonged PT or PTT is at-
tributable to factor deficiency or an inhibitor, a mixing study can

**TABLE I–5. COMMON CAUSES OF COAGULOPATHY DIFFERENTIATED BY ALTERATIONS IN
PROTHROMBIN TIME, PARTIAL THROMBOPLASTIN TIME, AND PLATELET COUNT**

PT	PTT	Platelets	Most Common Causes
↑	–	–	Deficiency or inhibitor of factor VII (early liver disease, vitamin K deficiency, warfarin therapy, dysfibrinogenemia, some cases of DIC)
–	↑	–	Deficiency or inhibitor of factors VIII, IX, or XI; vWD; heparin
↑	↑	↓	DIC, liver disease, heparin therapy associated with thrombocytopenia
–	–	↓	Increased platelet destruction, decreased platelet production, hypersplenism, hemodilution
–	–	↑	Myeloproliferative disorders
–	–	–	Mild vWD, acquired qualitative platelet disorders (eg, uremia)

DIC, disseminated intravascular coagulation; vWD, von Willebrand's disease.

be performed. Correction after addition of pooled normal plasma suggests a factor deficiency, whereas lack of correction suggests the presence of an inhibitor.

3. **Peripheral blood smear.** May reveal fragments and helmet cells seen in DIC and TTP. It may suggest other causes of thrombocytopenia such as vitamin B_{12} (or folate deficiency (marcocytic anemia and hypersegemted neutrophils). The presence of nucleated red blood cells suggests the presence of marrow infiltrative disorders (eg, prostate cancer) as the cause.

4. **Renal function.** Uremia inhibits platelet function.

5. **Thrombin time (TT).** TT assays functional fibrinogen; it can also assay for heparin effect and presence of fibrinogen degradation products.

6. **Fibrinogen, fibrin split products, and D-dimer assay.** In DIC, fibrinogen may be decreased and fibrin split products are increased. Fibrinogen is an acute-phase reactant. The absolute fibrinogen level may be normal, but a downward trend is helpful. D-dimer increase may suggest ongoing DIC.

7. **Bleeding time.** This test evaluates platelet function. Uremia, liver disease, and aspirin therapy within the last week may adversely affect function. Thrombocytopenia (platelets < 50,000 per microliter) can increase the bleeding time. Bleeding time is also prolonged by rare disorders of collagen that may impair the integrity of the vessel wall. Bleeding time may be prolonged in vWD, but normal bleeding time should not preclude testing.

8. **Blood replacement.** Type and cross-match if needed.

9. **Future studies.** Save one or two tubes of blood prior to transfusion therapy to assay for any coagulation factors or other studies that may be ordered later.

C. **Radiologic and other studies**

1. **X-ray/CT.** Obtain a chest x-ray if there is concern about intrathoracic bleeding; obtain a CT scan of the head if intracranial bleeding is suspected.

2. **Bone marrow aspiration and biopsy.** Might be performed to assess platelet production in the presence of unexplained thrombocytopenia or if leukemia or another infiltrative marrow disorder is suspected.

V. **Plan.** Assess the rate of bleeding and differentiate between mechanical bleeding and true coagulopathy. Almost all external bleeding that is mechanical can be controlled by applying direct pressure and elevation. Treatment of coagulopathy requires appropriate laboratory tests to make the diagnosis and then institution of the correct treatment. In the acute setting, assess the amount of blood loss and the volume status, and treat with IV fluids if hypovolemia is present. For further information regarding transfusion of blood products, refer to Section V, Blood Component Therapy, p 465.

A. Thrombocytopenia

1. Use random donor platelet transfusion, usually 5–10 U at a time (often a "six-pack" is ordered), for a platelet count below 20,000 or with higher platelet counts if there is ongoing bleeding. Platelet transfusions are generally not indicated in immune thrombocytopenias unless there is active bleeding. Patients receiving multiple platelet transfusions may develop HLA antibodies, and they will have better incremental increases in the platelet count with HLA-matched single-donor platelets. Immunocompromised patients should receive irradiated single-donor platelets that are leuko-filtered to avoid a transfusion-induced graft-versus-host reaction and to avoid sensitivity to alloantigens. Such patients include bone marrow transplant patients and possibly patients with acute leukemia or lymphoma who are undergoing aggressive therapy.

2. For a drug reaction, discontinue the drug and transfuse platelets if necessary.

3. In the presence of ITP, no treatment is usually needed until the platelet count is below 10,000 unless there is bleeding. For counts below 10,000, IV immunoglobulin (for Rh-negative patients) or WinRho (for Rh-positive patients) with or without prednisone may be used. Chronic ITP is treated with prednisone, cyclophosphamide, azathioprine, or danazol. The best long-term results are obtained with splenectomy. Platelet transfusions before splenectomy are very short-lived in ITP.

4. Document functional defect with bleeding time and treat the underlying condition, such as uremia. Deamino-8-D-arginine vasopressin (DDAVP; desmopressin), a vasopressin analogue, may be useful in uremic patients whose bleeding time is prolonged. The usual dose is 0.3 µg/kg IV. Discontinue drugs adversely affecting function.

5. TTP and HUS are treated with plasmapheresis.

B. von Willebrand's disease (vWD)

1. Cryoprecipitate or fresh-frozen plasma is the plasma product of choice. (See Section V, Blood Component Therapy, p 465.)

2. DDAVP increases von Willebrand factor (vWF) levels by releasing stores from endothelium. DDAVP can be effective for certain types of vWD with mild bleeding, but is contraindicated in type IIb because it may exacerbate thrombocytopenia.

C. Hemophilia A. Specific recommendations for factor replacement depend on site of bleeding and severity of factor deficiency and are beyond the scope of this book. The reader is referred to a standard hematology text for this information. The half-life of factor VIII is about 8–12 hours. Because many factor VIII concentrates are now available, treatment of choice should be only with genetically engineered products that minimize risk of transmission of viral hepatitis and human immunodeficiency virus (HIV). For individuals with inhibitor antibodies to factor VIII, treatment with recombinant factor VIIa may be indicated. The usual dose for this indication is 90 μg/kg every 2 hours.

D. Hemophilia B. As with hemophilia A, the reader is referred to a standard hematology text for specific recommendations for factor replacement. Factor IX concentrate has a half-life of approximately 24 hours. Several factor IX preparations are available. There is concern about some preparations containing activated coagulation factors that may induce thrombosis or DIC. New preparations probably avoid this risk. Recombinant factor VIIa is also used in patients with severe factor IX inhibitor antibodies.

E. DIC. Treat the underlying cause. Support the bleeding patient with fresh-frozen plasma, platelet transfusions, and blood transfusions. Heparin therapy in chronic DIC decreases the bleeding severity and incidence of thromboembolic events. Results of studies using heparin to treat acute DIC (especially from sepsis) have been less encouraging. The dose of heparin used varies from 5 to 140 U/kg intravenously every 4 hours to 15–20 U/kg/hr by continuous infusion. Lower doses (< 50 U/kg Q 4 hours) are recommended if marked thrombocytopenia is present.

F. Vitamin K deficiency/liver disease. If immediate treatment is needed, transfuse with 2–4 units of fresh-frozen plasma and follow the PT/PTT. Because factor VII, which has a half-life of 6 hours, is metabolized quickly, repeated infusions may be needed in 6–12 hours. In all cases, begin treatment with vitamin K 10 mg SC every day for 3 consecutive days. Vitamin K may be given intravenously, but because of rare anaphylactic reactions, it must be given slowly— the rate should not exceed 1 mg/min. IV vitamin K has a faster onset and shorter time to maximal effect than SC vitamin K. If the coagulopathy is secondary to vitamin K deficiency, a response to vitamin K should be evident after 24 hours. If there is no response to vitamin K, the coagulopathy is not due to vitamin K deficiency.

G. Severe hemorrhage of any cause. Therapy with activated recombinant factor VIIa appears to be useful in uncontrollable bleeding due to any cause. Indications, efficacy, and dose remain under investigation.

REFERENCES

Rodgers GM: Acquired coagulation disorders. In: Greer JP, Foerster J, Lukens J et al, eds. *Wintrobe's Clinical Hematology.* 11th ed. Lippincott Williams & Wilkins; 2004:1668.
Rodgers GM: Diagnostic approach to the bleeding disorders. In: Greer JP, Foerster J, Lukens J et al, eds. *Wintrobe's Clinical Hematology.* 11th ed. Lippincott Williams & Wilkins;2004:1511.

13. COMA, ACUTE MENTAL STATUS CHANGES

I. **Problem.** You are called to the emergency room to evaluate a 63-year-old man with confusion and lethargy.

II. **Immediate Questions**

A. **What are the patient's vital signs?** Hypotension from any cause can decrease cerebral perfusion and lower the level of consciousness. Fever might implicate an infectious process such as pneumonia or urinary tract infection as the cause. This is particularly true in the elderly patient. Meningitis should be suspected in any patient presenting with acute mental status changes and fever. Respiratory rate and pattern are also important diagnostic clues.

B. **What is the time course of the mental status alteration?** When possible, it is important to question the patient's family or friends while obtaining the history. If the alteration is longstanding or recurrent, the patient may have dementia or psychiatric illness.

C. **What medications is the patient taking?** Medications, especially in the elderly, may alter mental status. If the patient is hospitalized, review the medication orders and then check the medication administration record to define the actual quantity of analgesic or sedative given.

D. **Is there a history of trauma?** Recent head trauma may result in a subdural or epidural hematoma. The elderly, alcoholics, and patients receiving oral anticoagulation are particularly susceptible.

E. **Is there evidence of central nervous system pathology such as headache, hemiparesis, ataxia, or vomiting?** Increased intracranial pressure from tumor, subdural hematoma, or cerebral hemorrhage may lead to delirium, lethargy, or coma.

F. **Does the patient drink ethanol or use any recreational medications?** Exposure to drugs or toxins is the most common cause of coma. Intoxication with ethanol or other substances, as well as alcohol withdrawal (see Section I, Chapter 16, Delirium Tremens: Major Alcohol Withdrawal, p 94), can cause alterations in the level and content of consciousness.

G. **What is the pertinent past medical history?** Hyperglycemia from diabetes mellitus (see Section I, Chapter 32, Hyperglycemia, p 190) or hypoglycemia (see Section I, Chapter 37, Hypoglycemia, p 213) from its treatment can cause altered mental status. Severe liver disease, renal failure, or hypothyroidism can depress the level of consciousness or cause delirium. Respiratory failure with hypoxemia causes agitation followed by lethargy. Ventilatory failure with hypercapnia causes somnolence. A seizure disorder might present as stupor in the postictal state. Non–tonic-clonic seizures should always be considered in a patient with unexplained mental status changes.

H. Is there a history of psychiatric illness? Patients with depression may present with confusion and disorientation. Patients with catatonic schizophrenia may not be responsive to verbal or other cues.

I. Are there occupational or environmental exposures? Consider carbon monoxide, cyanide, organic solvents, lead, or arsenic as possible causes.

J. Is the patient in the perioperative period? Perioperative delirium is common. Potential causes include intraoperative hypotension or anoxia; infection, myocardial ischemia or infarction; and medications such as anticholinergics, sedatives, and narcotics.

III. Differential Diagnosis

A. Trauma

1. **Subdural hematoma.** The most common intracranial mass lesion resulting from head injury.
2. **Epidural hematoma.** Usually associated with a skull fracture resulting in a lacerated meningeal vessel, particularly the middle meningeal artery.
3. **Concussion.** Cerebral dysfunction that clears within 24 hours, a clinical diagnosis.
4. **Contusion.** Usually associated with neurologic deficits that persist longer than 24 hours. Small hemorrhages are present in the cerebral parenchyma on CT scan or MRI.

B. Metabolic causes

1. **Exogenous**
   a. **Medications.** The following are a few of the many medications that can alter the content or level of consciousness: narcotics, benzodiazepines, barbiturates, amphetamines, tricyclic antidepressants, H_1 and H_2 antagonists, antiparkinsonian agents, antiepileptics (phenytoin and carbamazepine), digoxin, corticosteroids, lithium, psychotropics, and salicylates.
   b. **Toxins**
      i. **Environmental/occupational.** These include carbon monoxide, cyanide, organic solvents, and heavy metals such as lead and arsenic.
      ii. **Drugs of abuse.** Intoxication with ethanol, amphetamines, methanol, or ethylene glycol, or withdrawal from ethanol, barbiturates, benzodiazepines, or opiates (see Section I, Chapter 16, Delirium Tremens: Major Alcohol Withdrawal, p 94).
2. **Endogenous**
   a. **Fluids/electrolytes**
      i. **Sodium.** Hyponatremia (see Section I, Chapter 40, Hyponatremia, p 226) and hypernatremia (see Section I, Chapter 34, Hypernatremia, p 201) may cause confusion. With hyponatremia, the severity of the mental status alteration is related to the level and rate of sodium decrease.

ii. **Potassium.** Hypokalemia (see Section I, Chapter 38, Hypokalemia, p 217) or hyperkalemia (see Section I, Chapter 33, Hyperkalemia, p 197). Potassium abnormalities infrequently cause mental status changes. Hypokalemia may precipitate hepatic encephalopathy in the cirrhotic patient.

iii. **Calcium.** Hypocalcemia (see Section I, Chapter 36, Hypocalcemia, p 210) or hypercalcemia (see Section I, Chapter 31, Hypercalcemia, p 185).

iv. **Magnesium.** Hypomagnesemia (see Section I, Chapter 39, Hypomagnesemia, p 222). Often there is associated hypokalemia and hypocalcemia. The patient may be anxious, delirious, or psychotic. Hypermagnesemia is a rare cause of coma.

v. **Acid–base alterations.** Mental status changes often result from underlying acidemia or alkalemia. Acute, and to a lesser extent, chronic hypercapnia can cause confusion, hallucinations, and coma. See Section I, Chapter 2, Acidosis, p 10 and Chapter 3, Alkalosis, p 19.

vi. **Osmolarity disturbances.** Common causes are hypernatremia and marked hyperglycemia.

b. **Organ failure**

i. **Renal failure.** Usually with markedly elevated blood urea nitrogen.

ii. **Hepatic encephalopathy.** Seen in fulminant hepatitis and cirrhosis. Often precipitated by worsening hepatic function, gastrointestinal bleeding, spontaneous bacterial peritonitis, dehydration, azotemia, hypokalemia, alkalosis, constipation, and medications such as sedatives.

iii. **Respiratory failure.** Hypoxia and/or hypercapnia.

c. **Endocrine**

i. **Pancreas.** Hypoglycemia (most often secondary to treatment of diabetes) or marked hyperglycemia resulting in a hyperosmolar state.

ii. **Pituitary.** Hypopituitarism secondary to tumor or apoplexy can lead to adrenal insufficiency and hypothyroidism.

iii. **Thyroid.** Thyrotoxicosis and hypothyroidism. Both may have associated mental status changes. Thyrotoxicosis is associated with agitation and nervousness. Hypothyroidism is associated with lethargy. A high index of suspicion is required for diagnosis in the elderly because mental status changes may be the only sign.

iv. **Parathyroid.** Either hyperparathyroidism resulting in hypercalcemia or hypoparathyroidism resulting in hypocalcemia can cause mental status alteration.

v. **Adrenal.** Cushing's syndrome can cause irritability, emotional lability, profound depression, confusion, and overt psychosis. Addisonian crisis can present with stupor or coma.

d. Vitamin deficiencies

i. Thiamine (vitamin B₁). Wernicke's encephalopathy is often seen in alcoholics but also occurs in patients with hyperemesis gravidarum, AIDS, peritoneal dialysis, malnutrition, and eating disorders. Mental status changes range from mild confusion to coma. Patients presenting in coma with Wernicke's encephalopathy are often not diagnosed until autopsy. Ataxia, bilateral horizontal nystagmus, or other ophthalmoplegias are frequently present. Korsakoff's psychosis is a part of Wernicke's encephalopathy and is characterized by anterograde amnesia, impaired ability to learn, and confabulation. Recovery from Korsakoff's psychosis can be expected in only 50% of cases.

ii. Cobalamin (vitamin B₁₂). Symptoms include forgetfulness, dementia, irritability, and psychosis. Neurologic manifestations can precede macrocytic anemia.

iii. Niacin (vitamin B₃). In pellagra, fatigue and insomnia often precede an encephalopathic syndrome of memory loss, confusion, and psychosis. Other symptoms include dermatitis and diarrhea.

e. Alteration in body temperature

i. Hypothermia. Occurs most commonly from exposure and is frequently observed in patients with alcohol or barbiturate intoxication, extracellular fluid deficit, sepsis, adrenal insufficiency, and myxedema. See Section I, Chapter 43, Hypothermia, p 243.

ii. Hyperthermia. Most commonly seen from heat stroke. Hyperthermia also occurs with neuroleptic malignant syndrome in patients taking phenothiazines and as malignant hyperthermia secondary to inhaled anesthetics or succinylcholine. It may be seen in hyperthyroidism (thyroid storm). See Section I, Chapter 22, Fever, p 133.

f. Miscellaneous

i. Porphyria. Anxiety, depression, disorientation, and hallucinations can occur in attacks of acute intermittent porphyria.

ii. Reye's encephalopathy. This rare syndrome can follow influenza or varicella upper respiratory infections in children less than 15 years old. It is classically associated with salicylate use (salicylate use not necessary).

C. Infection

1. Central nervous system infections. Consider meningitis, encephalitis, tertiary syphilis, and stage 3 Lyme disease.

2. Sepsis

3. Infections in the elderly. Especially urinary or respiratory.

D. Tumors
   1. **Primary or metastatic to CNS**
   2. **Hypercalcemia from metastatic disease**
   3. **Paraneoplastic syndromes.**
      a. **Parathyroid hormone–related peptide.** Secretion by squamous cell bronchogenic carcinoma causes hypercalcemia.
      b. **Syndrome of inappropriate antidiuretic hormone.** Inappropriate secretion of antidiuretic hormone by small cell lung cancer can cause symptomatic hyponatremia.
      c. **Cushing's syndrome.** This can be due to ectopic adrenocorticotropic hormone (ACTH) production by small cell lung cancer or carcinoid.
      d. **Paraneoplastic neurologic syndromes.** These include paraneoplastic encephalomyelitis and limbic encephalitis, both associated with small cell lung cancer.

E. Psychiatric causes
   1. **Psychogenic coma.** In pseudocoma, patients appear unarousable and unresponsive but have no structural, metabolic, or toxic disorder.
   2. **Catatonia.** State of muteness characterized by drastically decreased motor activity with preserved ability to sit, stand, and maintain body posture. Catatonia is usually psychiatric in etiology (schizophrenia), but frontal lobe dysfunction and drug effects can mimic.
   3. **Depression.** May mimic dementia or cause vegetative state, especially in the elderly.
   4. **ICU psychosis.** This form of delirium classically occurs in the ICU but can occur with any hospitalization, particularly in the elderly patient.

F. Miscellaneous
   1. **Hypotension.** See Section I, Chapter 42, Hypotension, p 237.
   2. **Hypertensive encephalopathy.** Blood pressure is markedly elevated. Funduscopic exam is notable for exudates, hemorrhages, and papilledema.
   3. **Seizures.** Non–tonic-clonic seizures as well as postictal confusion.
   4. **Cerebrovascular accident**
      a. **Ischemic infarction.** The most common causes include atherosclerosis with thromboembolism and cardiogenic embolism from mural thrombus or endocarditis. Also, consider vasculitis and vasospasm.
      b. **Intracranial hemorrhage.** Causes include hypertension, trauma, ruptured aneurysm, arteriovenous malformation, coagulopathy, tumor, and cocaine.
   5. **Locked-in syndrome.** In this de-efferented state, bilateral pontine lesions cause quadriplegia and lower cranial nerve palsies. Patients are alert and awake but mute.

6. **Anoxic encephalopathy.** Can occur after resuscitation of sudden cardiac death.
7. **Syncope.** See Section I, Chapter 59, Syncope, p 337.
8. **Dementia.** Common causes include Alzheimer's disease, multi-infarct dementia, alcoholism, and Parkinson's disease. Also consider normal pressure hydrocephalus if ataxia and incontinence are present.
9. **Hyperviscosity syndrome.** This uncommon syndrome is associated with Waldenstrom's macroglobulinemia, multiple myeloma, leukemia, and polycythemia vera (see Section I, Chapter 55, Polycythemia, p 312). Somnolence, stupor, coma, and psychiatric illness can occur within a triad of bleeding, visual abnormalities, and neurologic deficits.

IV. Database

A. Physical examination key points

1. **Vital signs**

   a. **Blood pressure.** Hypotension can cause decreased cerebral perfusion and is a common finding in acute mental status changes due to ethanol or barbiturate intoxication, GI hemorrhage, myocardial infarction, dissecting aortic aneurysm, Addison's disease, and gram-negative sepsis. Hypertension occurs with hypertensive encephalopathy, cerebral or brain stem infarction, subarachnoid hemorrhage, or increased intracranial pressure.

   b. **Heart rate.** Tachycardia may be secondary to many causes of mental status alteration such as sepsis, pulmonary embolus, hypoglycemia, and myocardial infarction. Bradycardia in association with hypertension and respiratory irregularity may indicate increased intracranial pressure (Cushing's reflex).

   c. **Respiratory rate and pattern.** Bradypnea may indicate ethanol, narcotic, or barbiturate intoxication. Tachypnea may indicate significant hypoxia or sepsis. Hyperpnea causing hyperventilation can be compensation for metabolic acidosis (*Kussmaul respiration*). A normal breathing pattern suggests the absence of brain stem damage. *Cheyne-Stokes respiration,* characterized by periods of waxing and waning hyperpnea alternating with shorter periods of apnea, implies an intact brain stem and may be present in bilateral hemispheric lesions or metabolic disturbance. Apneustic or ataxic breathing strongly suggests brain stem damage.

   d. **Temperature.** In the comatose patient, temperature should be measured with a rectal probe. A fever suggests infection, thyroid storm, anticholinergic toxicity, heat stroke, malignant hyperthermia, or neurogenic hyperthermia due to subarachnoid hemorrhage or hypothalamic pathology. The elderly may not have a fever in response to an infection. Hypothermia suggests myxedema, adrenal insufficiency, exposure, intoxication with ethanol or barbiturates, or a posterior hypothalamic lesion.

2. **General.** An unkempt patient might be an alcoholic or schizophrenic. Cachexia points to malnutrition or malignancy. Emesis can indicate increased intracranial pressure. Decerebrate posturing occurs in bilateral midbrain or pontine lesions, bilateral supratentorial motor pathway lesions, and metabolic disturbances. Decorticate posturing can occur with any lesion above the brain stem.

3. **HEENT**
   a. **Head.** Look for evidence of trauma that may point to a subdural or epidural bleed or a cerebral contusion.
   b. **Eyes**
      i. **Pupils.** Pinpoint pupils (< 1 mm) may indicate narcotic use or a pontine lesion. A unilateral, fixed, and dilated pupil suggests ipsilateral temporal lobe herniation. Bilateral, fixed, and dilated pupils suggest anticholinergic poisoning, anoxia, or brain death. Pupils may be dilated or sluggish to direct and indirect light in hypothermia or hyperthermia.
      ii. **Fundus.** Conjunctival or fundal petechiae suggest fat embolism or endocarditis. Papilledema suggests a mass, intracranial bleed, or hypertensive encephalopathy. Subhyaloid hemorrhages may be seen trapped behind the vitreous humor at the edge of the optic disc, suggesting a sudden rise in intracranial pressure.
      iii. **Ocular movements.** Assessment of unprovoked eye movements can be valuable. Smooth, fully conjugate, spontaneous eye movements (roving) in a comatose patient suggest an intact brain stem and a bihemispheric cause of coma. Nystagmus is seen with Wernicke's encephalopathy.
   c. **Ears.** Blood behind the tympanic membrane suggests a traumatic basilar skull fracture. Otitis media could be a source of meningitis or brain abscess.
   d. **Nasopharynx.** A fruity odor suggests diabetic ketoacidosis. A uriniferous smell implicates uremia. Fetor hepaticus points to hepatic encephalopathy. A burnt-almond odor is found with cyanide toxicity. A garlic scent may be found in arsenic poisoning.
   e. **Neck.** Resistance to passive flexion of the neck without resistance to other neck movements is evidence for meningitis or subarachnoid bleed. Positive Kernig's and Brudzinski's signs indicate meningeal irritation. Thyroid enlargement points to hypothyroidism or hyperthyroidism. A bruit over an enlarged thyroid gland is pathognomonic of Graves' disease.

4. **Chest.** Findings of consolidation implicate pneumonia. A prolonged expiratory phase with rhonchi and wheezing suggests underlying obstructive airways disease and possible hypoxia and/or hypercapnia.

5. **Heart.** An irregularly irregular apical pulse (*atrial fibrillation*) points to embolization from a mural thrombus. A new murmur with fever and/or leukocytosis suggests endocarditis.

6. **Abdomen.** Splenomegaly, ascites, and stigmata of chronic liver disease suggest hepatic encephalopathy.

7. **Skin.** Jaundice, spider angiomata, and palmar erythema point to hepatic encephalopathy. Petechiae and ecchymoses may suggest a coagulation abnormality or thrombocytopenia. A maculohemorrhagic rash suggests meningococcal infection, staphylococcal endocarditis, or other infection. In carbon monoxide poisoning, the skin may be cherry-red. Needle marks on extremities indicate possible drug abuse.

8. **Neurologic exam.** A thorough neurologic exam, including mental status evaluation, is essential. To avoid missing the locked-in syndrome, all patients should be asked to open their eyes and look up and down. Focal findings suggest an intracranial process. Hyperreflexia may be seen with upper motor neuron lesions or thyrotoxicosis. Clonus is absent with thyrotoxicosis and present in upper motor neuron lesions. Absent or sluggish reflexes are seen in hypothyroidism and hypothermia. The relaxation phase of the reflex is delayed in hypothyroidism and increased in thyrotoxicosis. An extensor plantar reflex can be present in coma from any cause. The Glasgow Coma Scale is helpful in evaluating and following the comatose patient (see Appendix, Table A–3, p 636). Testing the oculocephalic reflex (after clearance of the cervical spine if clinically indicated) is also beneficial: Hold the eyes open and turn the patient's head quickly to one side. The eyes should move toward the midline as if staring at a fixed point (*positive* or *intact doll's eyes*). Movement of the eyes in the direction the head is turned (*absent doll's eyes*) suggests a brain stem lesion, bilateral labyrinth dysfunction, or drugs such as sedatives or anticonvulsants. Doll's eyes are not present in normal, alert persons.

B. **Laboratory data**

1. **Complete blood count with differential.** To evaluate for infection and anemia.

2. **Complete blood chemistry.** Includes electrolytes, glucose, blood urea nitrogen, creatinine, bilirubin, alkaline phosphatase, transaminases, calcium, and magnesium. This rules out many organ-failure or metabolic causes. Serum glucose can be rapidly checked with a glucometer via a "finger stick."

3. **Arterial blood gases.** Along with serum bicarbonate, these measurements uncover a metabolic or respiratory acid–base

disturbance, which may point to the underlying cause. Arterial blood gas measurements are also helpful to rule out hypoxemia, hypercapnia, and carbon monoxide poisoning.

4. **Osmolal gap.** This helpful diagnostic clue refers to the difference between measured and calculated serum osmolality (see Section II, Laboratory Diagnosis, p 369). A gap greater than 10 implies the presence of a low molecular weight solute such as ethanol, methanol, isopropyl alcohol, ethylene glycol, ketones, or lactate.

5. **Platelet count and coagulation studies.** Especially useful if trauma is known or suspected and the diagnosis of an intracranial hemorrhage is entertained.

6. **Thyroid-stimulating hormone (TSH) and thyroxine ($T_4$4) levels.** To rule out suspected hypothyroidism or hyperthyroidism. Occasionally, T_4 is normal with hyperthyroidism, and only tri-iodothyronine (T_3) is elevated along with a low TSH.

7. **Urine and serum toxicology screening.** This is mandatory if the cause of the mental status alteration is uncertain or if there are medicolegal issues. The screening is also important in the presence of an anion or osmolal gap.

8. **Blood and urine cultures.** If infection is suspected.

9. **Drug levels.** When appropriate, consider obtaining digoxin and phenytoin (Dilantin) levels.

10. **Miscellaneous labs.** Hyperammonemia is indicative of hepatic failure; however, not all patients with hepatic encephalopathy have an elevation in ammonia. Creatine kinase levels should be assessed serially for several days because of the high risk of rhabdomyolysis in the coma patient. When addisonian crisis is suspected, an ACTH stimulation test should be performed and presumptive steroid therapy initiated even before the results of the ACTH stimulation test are returned.

C. **Radiologic and other studies**

1. **Chest x-ray.** Especially if an infectious or pulmonary source is suspected.

2. **CT scan of the head.** If there are any indications of a CNS etiology, especially in the presence of headache, vomiting, focal neurologic signs, or papilledema, or in the absence of any other etiology.

3. **Lumbar puncture.** This should be performed in any patient with unexplained fever and mental status alteration. If focal neurologic deficits exist or if the patient's mental status alteration precludes thorough neurologic exam, perform a STAT head CT before lumbar puncture. See Section III, Chapter 10, Lumbar Puncture, p 440.

4. **Electrocardiogram.** Look for myocardial infarction or atrial fibrillation. Myocardial infarction, especially in the elderly, may present with acute mental status changes.

     5. Electroencephalogram. Diffuse theta and delta changes may be present with most metabolic causes. This test is often not diagnostic except for herpes encephalitis.

V. Plan

A. General. Although the therapy of altered mental status must be directed at the underlying cause, certain steps should be taken immediately: Ensure adequate airway, breathing, and circulation (the ABCs of basic life support). In the comatose patient with normal respiration, an oropharyngeal airway is usually adequate. However, intubation may be necessary to protect the airway. If trauma is known or suspected, stabilize the neck until radiographic clearance is obtained.

B. Metabolic causes. Treat the underlying defect. Refer to the specific abnormality in the index. Any patient in coma should receive thiamine 100 mg slow IV push. Empiric dextrose administration is controversial. Because the administration of D50 has been associated with a poorer outcome in patients with anoxic or ischemic coma, some experts recommend intravenous dextrose only if an immediate finger-stick glucose is low. If dextrose is given, it should be in conjunction with thiamine to avoid precipitation of acute Wernicke's syndrome.

C. Exogenous causes. Any suspicion of narcotic-induced somnolence can be safely treated with naloxone 0.4–0.8 mg IV push. A repeat dose may be necessary (up to 4–5 ampules are commonly given in this situation). Consider gastric aspiration and lavage if toxic ingestion is suspected. If indicated, administer the appropriate antidote (see Section I, Chapter 52, Overdoses, p 292) such as ethanol for methanol or ethylene glycol ingestion, 100% FiO_2 for carbon monoxide poisoning, amyl nitrite and sodium nitrite followed by sodium thiosulfate for cyanide poisoning, and digitalis antibody for "digitalis delirium."

D. Tumor. Altered mental status in the presence of metastatic or primary CNS tumors can require emergent radiation therapy. Intracranial pressure should be acutely decreased with steroids, hyperventilation, and osmotic diuresis. Give dexamethasone 0.1–0.2 mg/kg IV bolus. The patient should be intubated to protect the airway and can be hyperventilated by increasing the ventilator rate to achieve a pCO_2 of 20–25 mm Hg. Osmotic diuresis with mannitol 50 g in a 20% solution over 20 minutes is also beneficial if cerebral edema is associated.

E. Infection. Treat with appropriate antibiotics. Gram's stain may help direct initial antibiotic therapy prior to culture results.

F. Cardiac syncope or low cardiac output. Treat the underlying cardiac problem.

G. Intracranial hemorrhage. Consult neurosurgery immediately. Increased intracranial pressure should be emergently treated as outlined above.

REFERENCES

Berger JR: Clinical approach to stupor and coma. In: Bradley WG, ed: *Neurology in Clinical Practice*. 3rd ed. Butterworth-Heinemann;2000:37.

Mendez Ashla MF: Delirium. In Bradley WG, ed: *Neurology in Clinical Practice*. 3rd ed. Butterworth-Heinemann;2000:25.

Victor M, Ropper AH: Coma and related disorders of consciousness. In: *Adams and Victor's Principles of Neurology*. 7th ed. McGraw-Hill;2001:366

Victor M, Ropper AH: Delirium and other acute confusional states. In: *Adams and Victor's Principles of Neurology*. 7th ed. McGraw-Hill;2001:431.

14. CONSTIPATION

I. **Problem.** A 75-year-old bedridden woman from a nursing home was admitted with dehydration and a urinary tract infection. She has not had a bowel movement in 7 days.

II. **Immediate Questions**

A. **What are the patient's normal bowel habits?** Normal bowel habits vary from three stools per day to three stools per week. Constipation can be defined as infrequent defecation, but one also needs to include excessive straining, passage of hard stools, and a sensation of incomplete evacuation.

B. **What medications is the patient taking?** Constipation is a side effect of many drugs. A careful medication history including use of vitamins and herbal products is necessary.

C. **Is the abdomen distended, tender, or tense?** Is the patient passing flatus or vomiting? Intestinal obstruction (obstipation) from sigmoid volvulus, intussusception, and hernia can lead to constipation. Mechanical obstruction often has other symptoms. Flatus signifies an intact, functioning gastrointestinal tract. Obstipation can result in tremendous abdominal distention.

D. **Does the patient have a history of hemorrhoids or rectal bleeding?** Rectal lesions, including hemorrhoids, proctitis, and fissures, may induce constipation. The patient suppresses bowel movements to avoid discomfort.

E. **Has the patient undergone any recent radiographic or surgical procedures?** Barium from radiologic studies can cause constipation. Many postoperative patients have an ileus resulting in constipation.

F. **What is the patient's fluid status?** Decrease in fluid intake or increase in diuretic use, especially in the elderly patient, can cause constipation.

III. **Differential Diagnosis**

A. **Systemic disorders**

1. **Drugs.** Constipation is a side effect of many medications, including analgesics (inhibitors of prostaglandin synthesis, opiates);

anticholinergics; antihistamines, antiparkinsonism agents, phenothiazines, tricyclic antidepressants; antacids containing aluminum hydroxide or calcium carbonate; barium sulfate; clonidine; diuretics (non–potassium sparing); calcium channel blockers (especially verapamil); ganglionic blockers; iron preparations; polystyrene sodium sulfonate, and 5-HT$_3$-receptor antagonists.

2. **Endocrine disorders.** Hypothyroidism, diabetes mellitus, and hyperparathyroidism are associated with constipation secondary to metabolic changes.

3. **Metabolic disorders.** Hypercalcemia, hypokalemia, and hypomagnesemia.

4. **Volume status.** Dehydrated patients, especially the elderly, can become constipated.

B. **Gastrointestinal disorders**

1. **Tumors.** Benign or malignant tumors can lead to constipation through obstruction by mass effect. This is of greater concern in the elderly.

2. **Inflammatory lesions.** With development of pain, the patient suppresses the urge to defecate, resulting in constipation. Common inflammatory disorders include diverticulitis, proctitis, hemorrhoids, fistula-in-ano, and inflammatory bowel diseases (IBD), in particular Crohn's disease. Diarrhea is a much more common symptom with IBD.

3. **Mechanical obstruction.** Constipation can be secondary to physical blockage from adhesions, incarcerated hernias, volvulus, ischemic strictures, or intussusception.

C. **Neurologic conditions**

1. **Spinal or pelvic trauma.** Results in colonic dysmotility or anal sphincter dysfunction.

2. **Autonomic neuropathy.** Results in colonic dysmotility and can even cause pseudo-obstruction.

3. **Cerebral vascular accident.** Constipation may develop via an associated decrease in activity level.

D. **Functional disorders—irritable bowel syndrome, constipation predominant.** This is a common cause of long-term constipation, which is often associated with abdominal bloating, lower abdominal pain, passage of small hard stools, and a sense of incomplete evacuation.

IV. Database

A. **Physical examination key points**

1. **Vital signs.** Fever suggests an inflammatory source such as diverticulitis. Orthostasis suggests dehydration.

2. **Abdomen.** Distention may result from obstruction. Evidence of prior surgery suggests adhesions. Listen for bowel sounds and quality to assess for ileus or obstruction. Absence of bowel

sounds is consistent with any cause of complete obstruction. While palpating, assess for tenderness or rebound. Rebound suggests peritoneal inflammation. Feel for stool-filled colon.

3. **Rectum.** Rule out external lesions (hemorrhoids or fissures) as the cause; this requires anoscopy. Be sure the anal sphincter is not stenotic. Check the quality of sphincter tone. Absence of sphincter tone suggests a spinal cord lesion. Presence of blood suggests an inflammatory cause or a tumor.

4. **Neurologic exam.** Look for evidence of prior cerebrovascular accident or spinal injury, such as decreased motor function or asymmetric reflexes. A delay in the relaxation phase of the reflexes suggests hypothyroidism.

B. **Laboratory data**
   1. **Electrolytes and calcium.** Check calcium level to rule out hypercalcemia. Hypokalemia or uremia can cause constipation.
   2. **Complete blood count.** Elevated white blood cell count may indicate an inflammatory disorder. A low hemoglobin accompanies blood loss and can result from a variety of causes, such as tumors, diverticulitis, or IBD.
   3. **Sedimentation rate or C-reactive protein (CRP).** With active inflammation, the sedimentation rate or CRP is elevated, but an elevated sed rate or CRP is not specific.
   4. **Stool for occult blood.** Inflammatory disorders and tumors can result in blood loss.
   5. **Thyroid function studies.** If history and physical examination are consistent with hypothyroidism, thyroid function studies (thyroid-stimulating hormone [TSH], T_4) should be obtained.

C. **Radiologic and other studies**
   1. **Acute abdominal series.** Obtain these x-rays if acute obstruction is considered. This assesses the area of obstruction, the degree of intestinal distention, and the amount of stool in the colon.
   2. **Proctosigmoidoscopy.** To further assess the colon for obstructing or inflammatory lesions.
   3. **Barium enema.** This demonstrates partial obstruction, or mass lesion, diverticulosis, or ischemic strictures.
   4. **Colonoscopy.** The procedure of choice if colon carcinoma or colonic polyps are suspected.
   5. **CT scan of abdomen.** To further evaluate for partial obstruction, inflammation, and lesions extrinsic to the colon.

V. **Plan.** Once the cause is determined, the underlying cause should be corrected. Medicines inducing constipation should be discontinued whenever possible. Electrolyte abnormalities should be corrected or obstruction relieved.

A. **Prevention.** Patients taking narcotics should receive stool softeners and bowel stimulants. Bedridden patients should also be given stool softeners. Place patients on high-fiber diets; encourage activity and adequate fluid intake.

B. Laxatives and enemas. There are several modalities from which to choose, depending on preference and etiology (Table I–6). Use bulk laxatives (psyllium) and high-fiber diets for control and prevention of constipation.

Although bulk laxatives and high-fiber diets are commonly recommended for the maintenance of normal defecation, many chronically constipated patients derive little benefit from these agents and require daily use of another agent. Osmotic agents such as magnesium hydroxide (Milk of Magnesia) are widely available and useful in doses from 1.2–3.6 g/day. Newer flavorless polyethylene glycol compounds (eg, MiraLax) are good for the severely constipated patients who require large volumes of daily laxatives. Oral mineral oil should be discouraged because of the risk of lipoid pneumonia if aspirated.

5-HT$_4$-receptor agonist tegaserod can improve colonic transit and improve constipation related to irritable bowel syndrome.

Surfactants or wetting agents, osmotic laxatives, and colonic stimulants for rapid action can also be used to relieve constipation. Sup-

TABLE I–6. LAXATIVES.

Type	Name	Dosage
Bulk—daily use	Citrucel (methylcellulose)	1 teaspoon (6–7 g) in fluid 1 or 2 × daily
	Metamucil (psyllium)	1 teaspoon (6–7 g) in fluid 1 or 2 × daily
Softeners/wetting agents—daily use	Docusate sodium (Colace)	50–200 mg 1 or 2 × daily Available: Capsules 50–100 mg Solution 10 mg/mL Syrup 25 mg/mL
	Docusate calcium (Surfak)	240 mg 1 or 2 × daily
	Lactulose (Chronuluc)	15–30 mL 1 or 2 × daily
	Sorbitol	15–30 mL 1 or 2 × daily
	Mineral oil	14–45 mL; one-time dose
Stimulants—prn	Bisacodyl (Dulcolax)	Oral 5–15 mg, 5-mg tablets Rectal 10 mg, 10-mg suppository
	Senna (Senokot)	1 tablet 1 or 2 × daily
	Glycerin suppository	3 g; 1 rectally
Osmotic—prn	Milk of Magnesia	15–30 mL 1 or 2 × daily
	Magnesium citrate	200 mL; one-time dose
	Polyethylene glycol (PEG) (MiraLax)	17 g in fluid 1 or 2 × daily
Enema—prn	Fleet Enema	120 mL rectally
	Oil retention enema	
Prokinetics	Tegaserod (Zelnorm)	6 mg 2 × daily

positories or enemas, such as gentle tap-water or oil retention enemas, and glycerin suppositories are useful for rapid action.

C. **Disimpaction.** Digital disimpaction is occasionally required when hard stool will not pass through the rectum. This is more common in the elderly. After disimpaction, the patient should receive laxatives or preferably enemas to relieve the constipation. Use stool softeners or bulk laxatives to prevent recurrence.

D. **Other.** If obstructing or inflammatory lesions are demonstrated, they should be treated with surgery, anti-inflammatory medicines, or antibiotics.

REFERENCES

Arce DA: Evaluation of constipation. Am Fam Physician 2002;65:2283.

Camilleri M, Thompson WG, Fleshman JW et al: Clinical management of intractable constipation. Ann Intern Med 1994;121:520.

Harari D, Gurwitz JH, Minaker KL: Constipation in the elderly. J Am Geriatr Soc 1993;41:1130.

Lange RL, DiPiro JT: Diarrhea and constipation. In: DiPiro JT, Talbert RL, Hayes PE et al, eds. *Pharmacotherapy: A Pathophysiologic Approach.* 2nd ed. Appleton & Lange;1993:566.

Lennard-Jones JE: Constipation. In: Feldman M, Friedman LS, Sleisenger MH, eds. *Gastrointestinal and Liver Diseases: Pathophysiology/Diagnosis/Management.* 7th ed. Saunders;2002:181.

Locke GR III, Pemberton JH, Phillips SF: AGA technical review on constipation. Gastroenterology 2000;119:1161.

Rao S: Constipation: Evaluation and treatment. Gastroenterol Clin North Am 2003;32(2):659.

Wald A: Constipation in elderly patients. Drugs Aging 1993;3:220.

15. COUGH

I. **Problem.** A nurse notifies you that one of your patients is unable to sleep because of a persistent cough.

II. **Immediate Questions**

A. **Is the cough acute or chronic?** Acute onset of cough most often results from infections such as the common cold, but can result from urgent conditions such as acute bronchospasm (see Section I, Chapter 63, Wheezing, p 364), pulmonary embolism (see Section I, Chapter 11, Chest Pain, p 60), aspiration (see Section I, Chapter 7, Aspiration, p 38), or decompensated congestive heart failure. A chronic cough is unlikely to represent a condition that is an immediate danger to the patient. Chronic cough is most often due to postnasal drip, postviral infection, asthma, chronic bronchitis from smoking, or gastroesophageal reflux.

B. **Is the cough productive of sputum?** If so, what does the sputum look like? A productive cough implies an inflammatory condition such as bronchitis, bronchiectasis, or pneumonia. Blood in the sputum leads to consideration of several other causes. (See Section I, Chapter 30, Hemoptysis, p 180.)

C. Is the patient tachypneic or dyspneic? Either of these suggests a significant underlying respiratory disease such as pulmonary embolism or pneumonia.

D. Is the patient on an angiotensin-converting enzyme (ACE) inhibitor? Cough is a side effect in 1–19% of patients on ACE inhibitors. The cough is nonproductive and persistent. It can begin 3–12 months after therapy initiation and remits 1–7 days after the drug is discontinued. There is a female predominance.

III. Differential Diagnosis. Cough reflex receptors are present throughout the respiratory tract and ear. Stimulation of these receptors can come from many possible sources.

A. Ear. Impacted cerumen, foreign body, or hair in the ear can produce cough.

B. Oropharynx/nasopharynx. Postnasal drip from allergic and nonallergic rhinitis or sinusitis is a common cause of cough. The common cold is a very frequent cause of cough.

C. Larynx. Acute viral laryngitis can produce cough.

D. Tracheobronchial tree. Any process irritating the mucosal receptors or preventing clearance of secretions can result in cough.

1. **Bronchospasm.** Asthma is a common cause of cough, especially nocturnal cough. Wheezing may be absent.

2. **Bronchitis.** Both acute and chronic bronchitis can cause irritation of mucosal receptors and result in cough.

3. **Pneumonia.** Viral, bacterial, tuberculous, and fungal causes all should be considered, especially in a patient with any immunocompromised condition such as AIDS, immunosuppressive therapy, or lymphoproliferative or hematologic malignancy.

4. **Gastroesophageal reflux.** Aspiration of oropharyngeal and gastric contents can produce cough. Symptoms typically worsen at night or after meals.

5. **Inhaled irritants.** Tobacco smoke, strong perfumes, and other irritants may initiate cough.

6. **Bronchogenic carcinoma.** Produces mechanical irritation of mucosal receptors. Chronic cough is common with bronchogenic carcinoma at some point in the illness.

E. Others. There are many other causes of cough; a few are listed here.

1. **Congestive heart failure.** A nocturnal cough may be the only manifestation of early congestive heart failure.

2. **Interstitial lung disease.** Includes usual interstitial pneumonitis, collagen vascular disease–related fibrosis, and granulomatous diseases such as sarcoidosis.

      3. Thoracic aneurysm. Produces bronchial or tracheal compression.

IV. Database

A. Physical examination key points

1. **Vital signs.** Fever occurs with infection and pulmonary infarction. Tachypnea and use of accessory respiratory muscles suggest significant underlying pulmonary disease.
2. **Ears.** Examine for impacted cerumen, foreign body, or hair in the external auditory canal.
3. **Mouth.** Examine posterior pharynx for evidence of sinusitis or rhinitis (postnasal drip or cobblestoning resulting from lymphoid hyperplasia). Look for evidence of head and neck cancer.
4. **Sinuses.** Check for tenderness or opacification.
5. **Lungs**
   a. **Stridor.** This is a manifestation of upper airway obstruction resulting from conditions such as laryngeal edema or epiglottitis. Stridor also frequently occurs after extubation or after an aspiration event.
   b. **Rhonchi.** Occur with bronchitis and inhalation injuries.
   c. **Signs of consolidation.** Peripheral bronchial breath sounds, egophony, and increased tactile fremitus occur with pneumonia.
   d. **Crackles.** Occur in congestive heart failure, pneumonia, and interstitial lung disease.
   e. **Wheezing.** Occurs in asthma. If localized, wheezing may signify a foreign body or obstructing neoplasm.
6. **Heart.** Jugular venous distention, laterally displaced point of maximal impulse, and left third heart sound (S_3) gallop indicate congestive heart failure.
7. **Lymph nodes.** Lymphadenopathy suggests metastatic carcinoma, a lymphoproliferative disorder, or a granulomatous disease such as sarcoidosis or tuberculosis.
8. **Extremities.** Clubbing occurs in patients with bronchiectasis, bronchogenic carcinoma, or usual interstitial pneumonitis.

B. Laboratory data

1. **Hemogram.** Leukocytosis with left shift occurs with infectious diseases. Thrombocytosis may result from underlying malignancy.
2. **Arterial blood gases.** Important to evaluate in patients who appear tachypneic or cyanotic.

C. Radiologic and other studies

1. **Chest x-ray.** Look for congestive heart failure, neoplasm, pneumonia, interstitial lung disease, hilar adenopathy, and thoracic aortic aneurysm.
2. **Sputum.** Examine for color, viscosity, odor, and amount. A good quality Gram's stain with PMNs and few epithelial cells may guide antibiotic therapy for pneumonia.

3. **Purified protein derivative (PPD) skin test.** Should be performed if tuberculosis is considered.
4. **Pulmonary function tests.** A restrictive pattern occurs in interstitial lung disease and a *restrictive pattern* is characterized by a decrease in all lung volumes: forced expiratory volume at 1 second (FEV_1), forced vital capacity (FVC), total lung capacity, and other lung volumes. The FEV_1/FVC ratio is maintained near normal or may be high. A *reversible obstructive defect* (a decrease in the FEV_1 and FEV_4/FVC ratio) suggests underlying asthma. Bronchial provocation with methacholine may be necessary to diagnose occult asthma if baseline pulmonary function tests are normal.
5. **Bronchoscopy.** This is of value only when there is an abnormality on chest x-ray, or a localized wheeze.

V. **Plan.** The treatment of cough is dependent on identifying the cause and then directing treatment toward that cause. Symptomatic cough suppression often helps the patient rest at night.

A. **Infectious conditions.** See Section VII for drug dosages.
   1. **Community-acquired pneumonia.** Hospitalized patients should receive a third-generation cephalosporin such as ceftriaxone or cefipime plus a macrolide or a fluoroquinolone such as moxifloxacin. If *Pseudomonas aeruginosa* infection is suspected, coverage with an antipseudomonal penicillin and an aminoglycoside is recommended.
   2. **Acute bronchitis.** Most often, acute bronchitis has a viral etiology; however, when mycoplasma or bacteria are suspected, trimethoprim-sulfamethoxazole, doxycycline, amoxicillin, or a macrolide antibiotic can be given.
   3. **Chronic bronchitis.** Most often occurs in smokers; cough improves with cessation of smoking. Ipatroprium bromide metered dose inhaler may provide relief as well.

B. **Rhinitis/sinusitis.** In these instances, cough is best managed by treatment with a first-generation antihistamine such as chlorpheniramine. Nasal ipratropium bromide may also have efficacy. Antibiotics are indicated if bacterial sinusitis is suspected.

C. **Asthma.** Inhaled bronchodilators such as albuterol represent the best treatment for those whose cough is due to asthma. A long-acting beta drug such as formoterol (Foradil) or salmeterol (Serevent) will provide excellent night-time coverage for the patient. Initially, oral steroids may be required to eliminate the cough.

D. **Gastroesophageal reflux.** These patients should have the head of their beds elevated and should not eat before going to bed. Antacids, histamine H_2 antagonists such as famotidine (Pepcid), or proton pump blockers such as omeprazole (Prilosec) may also be required.

E. General measures. In patients with a nonproductive cough in whom infection is not a concern, cough suppression can provide much-needed symptomatic relief.

   1. Cough suppression

   a. Codeine phosphate is the most effective cough suppressant. The usual dose is 10–30 mg Q 4–6 hr (maximum dose is 120 mg/day). Other narcotics such as oxycodone may be likewise effective in those patients who are codeine intolerant.

   b. Dextromethorphan, a codeine derivative, acts centrally and is the best nonnarcotic for cough suppression. The dose is 10–30 mg Q 4–8 hr or 60 mg Q 12 hr for sustained-action liquid (maximum dose 120 mg/day).

   c. Diphenhydramine HCl acts centrally to suppress cough; the dose is 25 mg Q 4–6 hr (maximum 150 mg/day).

   2. Expectorants. Have been shown to be of no value and should not be used.

REFERENCES

Bryant BG, Lombardi TP: Cold, cough, and allergy products. In: Covington TR, Lawson LC, Young LL et al, eds. *The Handbook of Non-Prescription Drugs.* 10th ed. American Pharmaceutical Association;1993:89.

Infectious Diseases Society of America: Update of practice guidelines for the management of community-acquired pneumonia in immunocompetent adults. Clin Infect Dis 2003;37:1405.

Irwin RS, Corrao WM, Pratter MR: Chronic persistent cough in the adult: Spectrum and frequency of causes and successful outcome of specific therapy. Am Rev Respir Dis 1981;123:413.

Irwin RS, Madison JM: The diagnosis and treatment of cough. N Engl J Med 2000;343:1715.

Poe RH, Harder RV, Israel RH et al: Chronic persistent cough: Experience in diagnosis and outcome using an anatomic diagnostic protocol. Chest 1989;95:723.

16. DELIRIUM TREMENS (DTS): MAJOR ALCOHOL WITHDRAWAL

I. Problem. A 55-year-old intoxicated man is admitted with abdominal pain and elevated amylase. On the third hospital day, he is found talking incoherently and is markedly diaphoretic and very tremulous.

II. Immediate Questions

   A. What are the patient's vital signs? Hypertension, tachycardia, and fever may represent signs of autonomic overactivity, common in DTs and minor alcohol withdrawal. A fever may also point to an infection as the cause of the delirium.

   B. What is the patient's mental status? Altered levels of consciousness and impaired cognitive function define delirium. Hallucinations and confusion are common in major alcohol withdrawal. These, combined with autonomic hyperactivity, are typical of DTs. DTs can also present as unresponsiveness. Most (80%) of the hallucinations occur after ethanol cessation and occur 12–24 hours after the last drink. The hallucinations may be visual (most common), auditory, olfactory, or tactile.

C. **What is the patient's airway status?** With an altered level of consciousness, there is an increased risk of aspiration.

D. **What medications or illicit drugs is the patient taking?** Medications may cause disorientation. Likely offenders include narcotics (morphine, codeine, meperidine), phencyclidine (PCP), cocaine, barbiturates, amphetamines, atropine, scopolamine, H_2 blockers (cimetidine, ranitidine, famotidine, nizatidine) or aspirin; and especially in the elderly, digitalis, sedatives (benzodiazepines), tricyclic antidepressants, and steroids. Individuals who abuse one substance are more likely to abuse others. Ask specifically regarding the use of narcotics, sedatives, barbiturates, and atropine-like substances.

E. **Is there a history of alcohol abuse?** This is central to the diagnosis. Historical information may need to be obtained from family or friends because of the delirium.

F. **Is there a history of DTs?** Alcohol withdrawal is often more severe in individuals who have experienced previous episodes of withdrawal. The absence of such a history does not exclude DTs.

G. **Is there a history of alcohol withdrawal seizures?** One-third of patients with a history of alcohol withdrawal seizures develop DTs, whereas only 5% of patients with minor alcohol withdrawal develop DTs. The seizures are tonic-clonic and occur 12–24 hours after ethanol cessation. Usually, there is a single seizure, but there can be multiple seizures in a short period of time.

H. **When was the patient's last drink?** Knowing the length of time since the last drink will assist in the diagnosis of DTs. Minor alcohol withdrawal usually begins 6–8 hours after cessation of drinking, peaks at about 24 hours, and usually resolves within 48 hours. The onset of DTs varies between 2 and 14 days after ethanol cessation, but usually occurs during the first 4 days.

III. **Differential Diagnosis.** DTs is a manifestation of diffuse cerebral dysfunction. Focal neurologic deficits point to a structural abnormality (stroke or brain tumor). The differential diagnosis of delirium is more extensive than given here and includes any cause of diffuse cerebral dysfunction. (See Section I, Chapter 13, Coma, Acute Mental Status Changes, p 76). Patients presenting with DTs may have a wide range of concomitant problems, any of which could cause delirium.

A. **Withdrawal syndromes**
   1. **Minor alcohol withdrawal.** A less severe form of alcohol withdrawal, which occurs between 8 and 48 hours after the last drink. The disorientation is usually mild. It is characterized by autonomic

hyperactivity: tachycardia, diaphoresis, insomnia, irritability, and tremor. Seizures and hallucinations may also occur.

2. **Barbiturate withdrawal.** Indistinguishable from DTs clinically.

3. **Opioid withdrawal.** Symptoms usually begin within 48 hours after cessation of the agent (most rapid with heroin). Symptoms include restlessness, rhinorrhea, lacrimation, nausea, diarrhea, and hypertension.

B. **Metabolic abnormalities.** Multiple metabolic abnormalities can cause altered levels of consciousness and impaired cognitive function similar to DTs (see Section I, Chapter 13, Coma, Acute Mental Status Changes, p 76).

1. **Wernicke's encephalopathy.** Results from nutritional deficiency of thiamine. Characterized by a triad of symptoms: (1) mental status changes (confusion to coma), (2) ataxia, and (3) ocular dysfunction (nystagmus or ophthalmoplegia).

C. **Endocrine abnormalities**

1. **Hypoglycemia.** Hypoglycemia results either from an insulin-secreting tumor or from intentional or accidental insulin overdose. See Section I, Chapter 37, Hypoglycemia, p 213.

2. **Hyperglycemia.** Extreme hyperglycemia, especially in the elderly, can result in delirium. See Section I, Chapter 32, Hyperglycemia, p 190.

3. **Hyperthyroidism.** The signs and symptoms of hyperthyroidism may mimic alcohol withdrawal syndrome; mental status changes, diaphoresis, tachycardia, tremor, and agitation may be seen. There is often a history of weight loss, heat intolerance, and hyperdefecation. The thyroid gland is often enlarged. The T_3 or T_4 is elevated and the TSH level suppressed. The signs and symptoms of hyperthyroidism are usually more subacute or chronic; however, thyroid storm is manifested by thermoderegulation (hyperthermia) and mental status changes. There is usually an identifiable precipitating event such as an operation or infection).

D. **Hypertensive encephalopathy.** Encephalopathy induced by poorly controlled hypertension. Headache is common. Exudates, hemorrhages and papilledema may be present on funduscopic examination.

E. **Central nervous system (CNS) infections.** In anyone with disorientation, consider CNS infection, including meningitis, brain abscess, and encephalitis. With bacterial causes, fever, meningismus, and leukocytosis with an increase in banded neutrophils are often present. If focal findings or papilledema are present, a CT scan should be performed prior to lumbar puncture.

F. **Intracranial hemorrhage.** Symptoms and level of consciousness vary depending on the location and size of the hemorrhage.

G. **Psychiatric disturbances: "sundowning."** Night-time agitation and confusion are common problems, especially in the elderly and those with dementia. Symptoms improve with reorientation and a quiet environment and always resolve by morning.

H. Sepsis. Sepsis can cause mental status changes. A fever and elevated white blood cell count with an increase in banded neutrophils are common.

I. Low cardiac output states. From either ischemia or cardiomyopathy. Low cardiac output states can cause confusion secondary to decreased cerebral perfusion and may cause agitation. Inquire about chest pain and congestive heart failure symptoms (orthopnea, paroxysmal nocturnal dyspnea, and dyspnea on exertion).

J. Intoxications
   1. **Cocaine**
   2. **Amphetamines**
   3. **Anticholinergic toxicity**

IV. Database

A. Physical examination key points

1. **Vital signs.** Tachycardia, hypertension, and fever are common. With severe hypertension and delirium, consider hypertensive encephalopathy. Fever may also be a manifestation of a localized infection or sepsis. Hypothermia could be associated with sepsis or could be the cause of the delirium. Carpal spasm with inflation of the blood pressure cuff between the diastolic and systolic blood pressure for 3 minutes (*Trousseau's sign*) is seen with hypocalcemia.

2. **Eyes.** Nystagmus suggests Wernicke's encephalopathy. Lid lag or proptosis suggests hyperthyroidism. Papilledema may occur with meningitis, hypertensive encephalopathy, CNS hemorrhage, or a space-occupying lesion.

3. **Nose.** Rhinophyma (hypertrophy and follicular dilation) is a late complication of rosacea, which is exacerbated by alcohol intake.

4. **Neck.** Thyromegaly suggests hyperthyroidism as a cause of the delirium. Jugular venous distention points toward congestive heart failure.

5. **Chest.** Signs of congestive heart failure and other causes of pulmonary edema and hypoxia should be sought.

6. **Abdomen.** Check for bladder distention, a common cause of agitation in the elderly.

7. **Skin.** Profuse sweating is typical of DTs. Telangiectasias and gynecomastia are associated with chronic ethanol use and chronic liver disease.

8. **Neurologic exam.** Hallucinations, confusion, and disorientation are typical. Tremulousness is a common sign of alcohol withdrawal. Reflexes are exaggerated but symmetric. Hyperreflexia is also seen in hyperthyroidism. Twitching at the corner of the mouth with tapping over the facial nerve (*Chvostek's sign*) is seen in

hypocalcemia. Any focal findings on motor, sensory, deep tendon, or cranial nerve examination point to a structural abnormality.

B. Laboratory data. Multiple electrolyte abnormalities may cause delirium or may be associated with heavy ethanol use.

1. **Sodium.** Hyponatremia could be the cause of the delirium.
2. **Glucose.** Both hypoglycemia and hyperglycemia may be associated with heavy ethanol ingestion and may cause delirium.
3. **Calcium.** May reveal hypocalcemia or hypercalcemia as the cause.
4. **Potassium.** Hypokalemia often complicates heavy ethanol ingestion and may also cause delirium.
5. **Blood urea nitrogen and creatinine.** May point to uremia/renal failure as the cause of the delirium.
6. **Liver function tests.** Transaminases (alanine aminotransferase [AST] and aspartate aminotransferase [ALT]), total bilirubin, and alkaline phosphatase to rule out hepatic failure as a cause. Liver dysfunction is common with chronic alcohol use.
7. **Arterial blood gases.** To eliminate hypoxemia or hypercapnia as a cause.
8. **Complete blood count with differential.** An elevated white blood cell count with an increase in banded neutrophils suggests a bacterial etiology. An elevated mean corpuscular volume may be from associated folate or vitamin B_{12} deficiency. Long-standing vitamin B_{12} deficiency can cause mental status changes. Anemia from a variety of causes is commonly seen in heavy ethanol use.
9. **Thyroid function tests.** Thyroid-stimulating hormone (TSH) is suppressed and thyroxine is usually elevated with hyperthyroidism. Hypothyroidism may cause changes in mental status and result in an elevated TSH and a decrease in the thyroxine.
10. **Phosphorus.** Hypophosphatemia is associated with heavy ethanol use and results from poor nutritional intake, malabsorption, or refeeding after prolonged starvation. Severe hypophosphatemia can cause an encephalopathy.
11. **Magnesium.** Hypomagnesemia is commonly seen with heavy ethanol use. Hypomagnesemia may result from poor intake, diarrhea, renal losses, and excessive sweating.

C. Radiologic and other studies

1. **Chest x-ray.** May reveal cardiomegaly, pulmonary edema, or pneumonia.
2. **Electrocardiogram.** To rule out myocardial ischemia as a cause of delirium. Also tachyarrhythmias are associated with alcohol withdrawal (major or minor).
3. **CT scan of head.** May be indicated if there are focal findings on examination, or seizures associated with DTs. Alcohol withdrawal seizures should occur before the onset of DTs.

4. **Lumbar puncture.** Indicated in any patient with mental status changes and fever. It may be difficult to rule out meningitis in a patient with DTs without performing a lumbar puncture.
5. **Electroencephalogram.** Rarely is an electoencephalogram necessary, but it may help diagnose encephalitis. It usually shows increased nonfocal activity with DTs.

V. Plan

A. **Strategies.** There are four treatment strategies for minor or moderate alcohol withdrawal:

1. **Supportive care.** A calm environment with frequent assessment and nursing care is all that is required for many patients with *mild* alcohol withdrawal. Individuals with a history of alcohol withdrawal seizures or DTs, or a coexisting acute illness, require medical management in addition to supportive care.

2. **Front-load dosing.** A long-acting benzodiazepine is given every 1–2 hours until symptoms abate; for example, diazepam (Valium) 10–20 mg PO every 1–2 hours (or 5 mg IV every 5 minutes) until symptoms subside or lorazepam (Ativan) 2 mg PO every 2 hours can be used. Symptoms are alleviated faster, and the total dose of benzodiazepines required is less than the conventional scheduled dosing method.

3. **Symptom-triggered dosing.** The benzodiazepines are administered according to the patient's symptoms. This method requires frequent assessment using a validated withdrawal symptom scale (a common example is the Clinical Institute Withdrawal Assessment for Alcohol). Symptom-triggered therapy has been shown to require less medication and to require a shorter duration of treatment compared with scheduled dosing regimens. Initially, diazepam (Valium) 10–20 mg PO or chlordiazepoxide (Librium) 50–100 mg PO is given; or lorazepam (Ativan) 2–4 mg PO initially with additional doses every 1–2 hours if assessment indicates a need for more medication.

4. **Scheduled dosing.** A fixed dose of a benzodiazepine is given on a regular schedule and tapered over several days, for example, diazepam (Valium) 10–20 mg every 4–6 hours for 1–3 days, decreasing the dose by half every day. An as-needed dose of 5–10 mg every 2–4 hours is made available. Chlordiazepoxide (Librium) 50–100 mg every 6 hours can be given for 1–3 days, decreasing the dose by half every day with an additional 25–50 mg every 2–4 hours as needed. Lorazepam (Ativan) or oxazepam (Serax) PO or IM should be considered with moderate to severe hepatic dysfunction.

B. **Delirium tremens**

1. **ICU setting**

2. **Thiamine replacement.** Thiamine 100 mg IV or IM should be given before the administration of any IV fluids containing glu-

cose. Glucose can precipitate Wernicke's encephalopathy in a patient with marginal thiamine stores. Thiamine should be given for at least 3 days.

3. **IV fluids.** May require 3–6 L per day; use D5 NS.
4. **Correction of electrolyte disorders**
   a. **Hypokalemia.** Replacement with potassium supplements either PO or IV. A total replacement dose of 100 mEq of potassium is required to raise a potassium level of 3.0 mEq/L to 4.0 mEq/L. IV replacement is generally 10–15 mEq per hour. Oral replacement is 20–60 mEq per dose and can be repeated in 2–4 hours.
   b. **Hypophosphatemia.** IV replacement is reserved for severe, life-threatening hypophosphatemia (levels < 1 mg/dL). IV replacement is with 5–10 mmol over 4–6 hours. PO replacement can be with Neutra-Phos capsules (250 mg per capsule) or skim milk (1 quart contains 1 g of phosphorus, or about 30 mmol).
   c. **Hypomagnesemia.** Replacement is generally either IV or IM. The oral route often causes diarrhea. Magnesium sulfate can be given 1 g IM in each hip or 1 g IV per hour for 4 hours. The magnesium level should be checked 1–2 hours after the fourth gram has been infused. This regimen may need to be repeated. Magnesium is mostly an intracellular cation. With extremely low levels of magnesium, often 10–15 g are required.
5. **Other vitamins.** Multivitamins and folate should be given daily either orally or intravenously.
6. **Restraints.** Often needed to prevent injury.
7. **Benzodiazepines.** Diazepam (Valium) 5–10 mg IV every 5–10 minutes until sedated, or lorazepam (Ativan) 1–2 mg IV every 5–10 minutes. The dose of diazepam should not exceed 100 mg/hr or 250 mg over 8 hours.
8. **Other treatments.** Phenobarbital 100–200 mg IM or IV every 1–2 hours can be used if benzodiazepines cannot be used. Carbamazepine (800 mg/day, taper over 7 days) has been used for mild and moderate withdrawal as a single agent. Advantages are that it is nonaddictive and nonsedating, and metabolism is not affected by liver dysfunction.
9. **Adjunct therapy.** These agents are useful to treat some symptoms of withdrawal, but are ineffective at preventing delirium or seizures
   a. A beta-blocker, atenolol (Tenormin 50–100 mg/d) has been shown to be beneficial for mild to moderate withdrawal, in both outpatient and inpatient settings.
   b. Clonidine (Catapres) 0.1–0.2 mg PO bid can also be used for autonomic symptoms.
   c. **Haloperidol (Haldol).** 2–10 mg PO, IV, or IM, can be used for hallucinations or for agitation not responding to benzodi-

azepines. Neuroleptics decrease the seizure threshold, however, and may precipitate alcohol withdrawal seizures. Butyrophenones are a better choice than phenothiazines.

10. Antipyretics. Acetaminophen 650–1000 mg or aspirin 650 mg and a cooling blanket may be required because of fever associated with DTs.

REFERENCES

Chang PH, Steinberg MB: Alcohol withdrawal. Med Clin North Am 2001;85:1191.

Hall W, Zador D: The alcohol withdrawal syndrome. Lancet 1997;349:1897.

Kosten TR, O'Connor PG: Management of drug and alcohol withdrawal. N Engl J Med 2003;348:1786.

Kraus ML, Gottlieb LD, Horwitz RI et al: Randomized clinical trial of atenolol in patients with alcohol withdrawal. N Engl J Med 1985;313:905.

Mayo-Smith MF: Pharmacological management of alcohol withdrawal: A meta-analysis and evidence based practice guideline. JAMA 1997;278:144.

Saitz R, O'Malley SS: Pharmacotherapies for alcohol abuse: Withdrawal and treatment. Med Clin North Am 1997;81:881.

Turner RC, Lichstein PR, Peden JG et al: Alcohol withdrawal symptoms: A review of pathophysiology, clinical presentations, and treatment. J Gen Intern Med 1989;4:432.

Williams D, McBride AJ: The drug treatment of alcohol withdrawal symptoms: A systematic review. Alcohol Alcohol 1998;33:103.

17. DIARRHEA

I. Problem. A 50-year-old woman is admitted after having 36 hours of diarrhea.

II. Immediate Questions

A. What are the patient's vital signs? Hypotension suggests volume depletion or possible septic shock. Fever implies an infectious etiology. Diarrhea with associated hypotension or fever should be evaluated immediately.

B. Is the diarrhea grossly bloody? This usually is seen with ischemic bowel or infarction, invasive infections, neoplasms, or inflammatory bowel disease (IBD). Bloody diarrhea requires more active and immediate intervention.

C. Is this an acute or chronic problem? *Acute diarrhea* is usually a self-limited disease and can often be treated symptomatically. Acute diarrhea in the outpatient setting is commonly due to infection. In the inpatient setting, *Clostridium difficile* diarrhea and drugs are the most likely causes. *Chronic diarrhea* is defined as diarrhea that has been present 4–6 weeks or longer. Common causes include lactose intolerance, irritable bowel syndrome, IBD, postsurgical procedures, malabsorptive syndromes, drugs, and various infections. The intial presentation of a chronic diarrheal disorder may be sudden and therefore easily mistaken for an acute diarrhea.

D. Are there risk factors that suggest a specific cause? This is a critical step in the evaluation, which is often undervalued. Risk factors include drug-induced diarrhea; travel; sexual activities that involve the anus, especially oral-anal contact; abdominal surgery; abdominal/pelvic radiation; vascular disease; and various endocrine disorders such as diabetes mellitus and Addison's disease. Any recent contacts with ill persons should be elicited. Family history may be positive for diarrhea, especially in IBS, IBD, and celiac sprue. Dietary habits may predispose to infectious diarrheas (eg, rare meats, unpasteurized milk, fresh cheeses, sushi, raw oysters).

E. Is there associated abdominal pain? Absence of pain makes inflammatory causes such as ischemic bowel disease or ulcerative colitis (UC) less likely.

F. What is the volume of the stool? Does the patient have diarrhea (> 300 g stool per day) or just loose stools? Large volumes suggest small bowel or right colon; small volumes suggest left colon.

G. Has the patient participated in any recreational water activities? Many outbreaks of gastroenteritis have been associated with recreational water activities (swimming pools, interactive water fountains at water parks, lakes, rivers, hot tubs). Offending agents include *Shigella sonnei* and *Cryptosporidium parvum*.

H. Is there any reason to suspect laxative abuse (eg, a young woman with a history of bulimia)? Testing the stool for laxatives may secure the diagnosis without an extensive workup.

I. Does the diarrhea stop if the patient is not eating? If the answer is yes, the cause of diarrhea is likely osmotic rather than secretory, in which the diarrhea does not vary with the oral intake.

III. Differential Diagnosis

A. Infection

1. **Viruses.** Viral syndromes usually resolve in a few days and can be treated symptomatically. Rotavirus and Norwalk virus are the most common viruses causing diarrhea.

2. **Bacteria.** *Shigella dysenteriae, S sonnei, Salmonella typhimurium, Campylobacter jejuni, Yersinia* species, *Staphylococcus aureus, Vibrio cholerae, Vibrio parahaemolyticus, Escherichia coli, Bacillus cereus, Clostridium perfringens,* and *Clostridium difficile* all cause diarrhea by producing enterotoxins or by enteroinvasion. The spectrum of illness may range from asymptomatic to life threatening. *S aureus, B cereus,* and *C perfringens* are often associated with food poisoning. *C jejuni* and enterohemorrhagic *E coli* often cause a bloody diarrhea and may be associated with hemolytic-uremic syndrome in adults. *V cholerae* can cause severe life-threatening diarrhea and is associated with contaminated

food or water. Other non–*Cholera/Vibrio* species are halophilic and therefore often cause diarrhea in the setting of consumption of raw or improperly handled seafood.

3. **Parasites.** *Giardia lamblia, Entamoeba histolytica,* and *Cryptosporidium. G lamblia* is often contracted by drinking contaminated water. *E histolytica* is seen in travelers to developing countries and in institutionalized patients. *Cryptosporidium* can cause a self-limited diarrhea in immunocompetent individuals working with livestock. *G lamblia, E histolytica,* and *Cryptosporidium* are common etiologic agents causing diarrhea in homosexual men. *Cryptosporidium* results in a severe, unremitting diarrhea in patients infected with human immunodeficiency virus (HIV).

B. **Inflammatory diseases**
1. **Ischemic bowel** secondary to thrombosis, embolism, or vasculitis such as polyarteritis nodosa or systemic lupus erythematosus can result in bloody or guaiac-positive diarrhea. Atrial fibrillation is a common source of embolism.
2. **Inflammatory bowel disease (IBD).** Ulcerative colitis begins in the rectum and spreads proximally in a continuous manner. Presenting complaints may begin abruptly and usually include rectal bleeding and diarrhea. Patients with Crohn's disease (CD) usually present with diarrhea as well; however, the diarrhea is less often bloody.

C. **Tumor**
1. **Malignant carcinoid syndrome.** Flushing is also common.
2. **Colon carcinoma.** Rarely presents with diarrhea. Bright red blood per rectum as well as occult blood loss or anemia is common.
3. **Medullary thyroid carcinoma**
4. **Lymphoma involving the bowel**
5. **Villous adenomas**
6. **Gastrinomas.** Usually a history of peptic ulcer disease or gastroesophageal reflux.

D. **Endocrinopathies**
1. **Hyperthyroidism.** Hyperdefecation (loose, frequent stools) rather than diarrhea. Diarrhea may be present with thyroid storm.
2. **Diabetes.** Associated with longstanding diabetes with neuropathy.
3. **Hypoparathyroidism**
4. **Addison's disease.** Nausea, vomiting, abdominal pain, weight loss, and lethargy along with diarrhea.

E. **Drugs**
1. **Laxatives.** Chronic laxative abuse causes chronic diarrhea.
2. **Antacids.** Magnesium-containing antacids can cause osmotic diarrhea.
3. **Lactulose.** Used to treat hepatic encephalopathy; should be titrated to two to three loose stools per day but can result in se-

vere, life-threatening hypernatremia secondary to an osmotic diarrhea if not dosed properly.

4. **Cardiac agents.** Diarrhea is a common reason for discontinuation of quinidine. Digoxin may cause diarrhea.

5. **Colchicine.** In treatment of acute gout, diarrhea can occur with increasing doses.

6. **Antibiotics.** Antibiotics can produce diarrhea by altering gut flora. This leads to malabsorption or induction of *C difficile* overgrowth and toxin production, resulting in pseudomembranous colitis. Pseudomembranous colitis is most often secondary to antibiotics, especially broad-spectrum antibiotics such as clindamycin and the cephalosporins, and it can occur up to 4 months after antibiotic use.

7. **Antihypertensives.** Reserpine, guanethidine, methyldopa, guanabenz, and guanadrel all can cause diarrhea.

8. **Metformin.** Many patients develop diarrhea, especially at higher doses.

9. **Other agents.** Bethanechol, metoclopramide, and neostigmine all may cause diarrhea.

F. **Abdominal surgery.** Can cause chronic diarrhea.

    1. **Gastric surgery.** Vagotomy, resection, or bypass procedures.

    2. **Cholecystectomy**

    3. **Bowel resection**

G. **Malabsorption.** A common cause of chronic diarrhea that may result in deficiencies of fat-soluble vitamins A, D, E, and K; weight loss; and hypoalbuminemia.

    1. **Chronic pancreatitis**

    2. **Bowel resection**

    3. **Bacterial overgrowth**

    4. **Celiac or tropical sprue**

    5. **Whipple's disease**

    6. **Eosinophilic gastroenteritis**

H. **Lactose intolerance.** A common cause of chronic diarrhea resulting from lactase deficiency. It is often associated with flatulence. Milk or milk products exacerbate the diarrhea.

I. **Irritable bowel syndrome.** Intermittent diarrhea may alternate with constipation. Symptoms are aggravated by stress. Abdominal pain may be present. Physical examination and routine laboratory tests are normal.

J. **Fecal impaction.** Can present with diarrhea. Fecal impaction often occurs in an older age group.

K. **Human immunodeficiency virus (HIV) infection.** Diarrhea is common in patients positive for HIV or with acquired immunodeficiency syndrome (AIDS). Parasitic infections mentioned in III.A.3. are common in men who have sex with men with or without HIV infection. *Isospora belli, Microsporidia,* and *Cyclospora* are three other parasites that can cause diarrhea in HIV patients. Other nonparasitic etiologies associated with HIV infection include *S typhimurium,* which often results in bacteremia; *C jejuni, Mycobacterium avium-intracellulare,* and cytomegalovirus. Often the diarrhea is idiopathic and associated with fever and weight loss.

IV. Database

A. Physical examination key points

1. **General.** Cachexia suggests a chronic process such as carcinoma, AIDS, IBD, or malabsorption.
2. **Vital signs.** Hypotension or postural changes suggest sepsis or significant volume depletion. Tachycardia implies volume depletion or infection, or could be secondary to pain. Tachypnea may indicate fever, anxiety, pain, or sepsis or may represent compensation for a metabolic acidosis from a variety of causes including sepsis and bowel infarction.
3. **HEENT.** Aphthous ulcers are associated with IBD. Glossitis, cheilitis, or stomatitis can be seen with vitamin deficiencies secondary to malabsorption, especially the B vitamins. An enlarged thyroid suggests hyperthyroidism or medullary carcinoma.
4. **Abdomen.** Look for surgical scars. Distention may be from carbohydrate malabsorption. Absent bowel sounds suggest bowel infarction or associated peritoneal inflammation. Metastatic cancer can result in hepatomegaly.
5. **Rectum.** Rule out rectal carcinoma. Look for fissures suggesting CD. Patients with fecal impaction can present with diarrhea. Sphincter tone should be evaluated, since many patients with fecal incontinence associated with poor tone actually report "diarrhea" because of embarrassment.
6. **Musculoskeletal exam.** Arthritis is associated with IBD, Whipple's disease, and infection by *Yersinia enterocolitica.*
7. **Skin.** Hyperpigmentation can be seen with Addison's disease. Erythema nodosum and pyoderma gangrenosum point to IBD. Dermatitis herpetiformis suggests celiac sprue, a relatively common cause of chronic diarrhea.

B. Laboratory data:
The laboratory evalaution is more commonly required in chronic diarrheas. The number of studies that can be done is extensive. It is useful to categorize the diarrhea as completely as possible with history and physical examinations before proceeding with diagnostic tests. If history and physical do not suggest a specific cause, then lab tests aimed at placing a diarrhea into one of three categories—watery, fatty, or inflammatory—are helpful in narrowing the evaluation.

C. Blood tests

1. **Electrolytes.** With severe diarrhea, various electrolyte abnormalities can occur, including hypokalemia, metabolic acidosis, hypernatremia, and hyponatremia.

2. **Complete blood count with differential.** An elevated hematocrit suggests volume depletion. An anemia (see Section I, Chapter 5, Anemia, p 28) may be associated with IBD, carcinoma, or HIV infection. A microcytic anemia suggests chronic gastrointestinal blood loss or malabsorption of iron. Macrocytic anemia may be secondary to vitamin B_{12} deficiency after gastric surgery, or may result from malabsorption or folate deficiency.

3. **Sedimentation rate, C-reactive protein (CRP).** Expect sedimentation rate to be increased in patients with IBD, metastatic carcinoma, bowel ischemia, and systemic infections.

4. **Prothrombin time (PT) and partial thromboplastin time (PTT).** An elevated PT and PTT could be secondary to vitamin K deficiency from malabsorption or associated liver disease.

5. **Albumin.** Expect a low albumin in diarrhea secondary to malabsorption, IBD, and metastatic carcinoma.

6. **Calcium.** To rule out hypoparathyroidism as a cause. Hypocalcemia associated with vitamin D deficiency secondary to steatorrhea may also be seen.

7. **Endocrine tests.** Helpful as clinically indicated; these include thyroid tests (thyroxine, thyroid-stimulating hormone), parathyroid hormone, Cortrosyn stimulation test, and gastrin.

D. **Stool studies**

1. **Twenty-four- to 72-hour collection of stool for fecal fat.** Useful to categorize steatorrhea, which is often associated with malabsorption. The patient should be on a 100-g fat diet before and during the stool collection.

2. **Stool for leukocytes.** Presence of fecal leukocytes suggests an inflammatory cause such as infection, ischemia, or IBD. In the absence of fecal leukocytes, viruses, enterotoxic food poisoning, or parasites can be suspected, as can drugs, causes of malabsorption or endocrinopathies, cancer, irritable bowel, lactose intolerance, and abdominal surgery. The sensitivity and specificity of fecal leukocyte testing to distinguish inflammatory from noninflammatory causes are noted to be 70% and 50%, respectively. As a result, a fecal lactoferrin latex agglutination assay, which is noted to have a sensitivity and specificity between 90% and 100%, is being used in some institutions.

3. **Stool electrolytes.** Measurement of the stool osmotic gap is useful to separate osmotic and secretory diarrheas. The osmotic gap is calculated as follows: the stool sodium and potassium are measured directly and then the sum is multiplied by 2. This number is subtracted from the estimated plasma osmolality of 290 mOsm/kg.

stool osmotic gap = 290 mOsm/kg–2(stool Na + stool K)

Stool osmotic gaps that are (< 50 mOsm/kg) are consistent with secretory diarrhea. Large stool osmotic gaps (> 100 mOsm/kg) are consistent with osmotic diarrheas. A negative stool osmotic gap suggests ingestion of a multivalent poorly absorbed anion such as phosphate or sulfate.

Stool osmolality is useful only for detecting the contamination of the stool, such as with urine or water. The osmolality in such cases is less than 290 mOsm/kg if measured on a fresh specimen (the stool osmolality tends to rise after passage from the body owing to ongoing bacterial fermentation).

4. **Stool for occult blood.** Follow with serial exams to increase sensitivity. Occult blood suggests UC, neoplasm, ischemic bowel, or various infections such as *C jejuni*.

5. **Stool cultures.** Indicated for clinical dysentery (fever, abdominal cramps, fecal leukocytes), inflammatory causes, prolonged diarrhea (longer than 7–14 days), immunocompromised (including HIV), symptoms suggestive of acute proctitis, or a prolonged illness. Contact lab regarding special procedures to identify *Yersinia, Vibrio,* or *E coli* O157:H7 if clinically indicated.

6. **Stool for ova and parasites (O&P). Routinely three specimens are needed, with each specimen collection separated over 24 hours because of the intermittent nature of parasite excretion.**
   a. Parasitic infections often require a "fresh" specimen within several hours of collection.
   b. Amebic dysentery is diagnosed with presence of trophozoites. Cysts suggest the carrier state in the absence of trophozoites. Serology may help in the diagnosis.
   c. Identification of *Giardia* cysts is diagnostic of active infection. A small bowel aspirate may be required to recover *Giardia*.

7. *Clostridium difficile* toxin. If antibiotics have been given in the last 4 months (usually 4–14 days). The presence of *C difficile* without the toxin should not cause diarrhea. Toxin-negative pseudomembranous colitis must also be considered.

8. **Stool *Giardia* antigen.** The preferred stool exam with a sensitivity of about 90% with at least two specimens tested.

C. **Radiologic studies**
   1. **Barium enema.** May reveal carcinoma or IBD.
   2. **Upper GI series with small bowel follow-through.** May suggest CD, celiac sprue, Whipple's disease, or lymphoma.

D. **Endoscopy**. Useful for detecting and defining mucosal diseases such as IBD and pseudomembranous colitis. UC is distinguished from CD largely on the basis of the endoscopic distribution of the mucosal lesions. *Microscopic colitis* is a term that encompasses diarrheal disorders with mucosal abnormalities that are detectable only on histopathology.

E. **Other tests**
   1. **D-Xylose test.** Abnormal in diseases involving the small bowel mucosa such as CD, celiac sprue, Whipple's disease, and lymphoma.

V. Plan. Symptomatic treatment with fluids, electrolytes, and antidiarrheal agents is usually all that is required for acute diarrhea. The initial use of antibiotic therapy should be avoided and implemented only in specific situations and guided by stool culture results. Many cases of diarrhea resolve by addressing the underlying cause (eg, discontinuation of a drug).

   A. Fluid replacement. Essential in the early treatment.
      1. Oral. Helpful if given as hyperosmolar solution and with glucose to facilitate uptake of sodium and water.
      2. Intravenous. Necessary if the patient is markedly volume depleted or has accompanying nausea and vomiting. Patient may need potassium replacement.

   B. Diet. Place the patient on a lactose-free diet to prevent diarrhea secondary to lactase deficiency, which may be transient as a result of acute gastroenteritis. Diarrhea can also be secondary to lactose intolerance. Administer a clear liquid diet for 24–48 hours, and then advance diet slowly.

   C. Antidiarrheal agents. Often helpful but should not be used if invasive diarrhea is clinically suspected. Antimotility drugs are contraindicated in patients with pseudomembranous colitis or IBD because of the risk of precipitating toxic megacolon. Commonly used agents include bismuth subsalicylate (Pepto-Bismol) 30 mL or 2 tablets Q 30 minutes to 1 hour as needed up to 8 doses/day; diphenoxylate with atropine (Lomotil 2.5 mg) 1–2 tablets qid, not to exceed 20 mg/day; and loperamide (Imodium) 4 mg initially, then 2 mg after each loose stool, not to exceed 16 mg/day. Both diphenoxylate and loperamide may facilitate development of hemolytic-uremic syndrome in patients with enterohemorrhagic *E coli.* Paregoric is an extremely effective agent (5 mL after each loose stool, up to 40 mL/day).

   D. Antibiotics. Antibiotic treatment often does not shorten the duration of illness. It may select out resistant strains of organisms and may lead to pseudomembranous colitis.
      1. *Salmonella.* Does not usually require antibiotics unless the patient remains ill or is predisposed to developing complications (osteomyelitis, bacteremia), such as a patient with sickle cell disease. Treatment is chloramphenicol, ampicillin, trimethoprim-sulfamethoxazole (Bactrim or Septra), or ciprofloxacin.
      2. Shigellosis. Antibiotics are recommended to decrease duration of illness and fecal shedding. Antibiotic sensitivity is crucial because resistance, especially to trimethoprim-sulfamethoxazole and ampicillin, is common. Treatment is an oral quinolone bid for 5 days, with trimethoprim-sulfamethoxazole or ampicillin used as a second-line therapy.
      3. *Clostridium difficile.* Recommended treatment is metronidazole (Flagyl) 250–500 mg PO Q 6 hours for 10 days. If symptoms per-

sist or recur, re-treatment with metronidazole is recommended. If a third course of treatment is needed, give vancomycin 125 mg PO Q 6 hours. Metronidazole is less expensive and is equally effective. Addition of cholestyramine (Questran) qid may help control diarrhea if given with antibiotics. If the patient cannot take medications orally or through a nasogastric tube, intravenous metronidazole can be used.

4. ***Campylobacter.*** Often self-limiting illness. With severe or persistent diarrhea, erythromycin or ciprofloxacin for 5–7 days is effective. Fluoroquinolone resistance has been reported.

REFERENCES

Aranda-Michel J, Giannella RA: Acute diarrhea: A practical review. Am J Med 1999;106:670.

Centers for Disease Control and Prevention: Outbreak of gastroenteritis associated with an interactive water fountain at a beachside park—Florida, 1999. MMWR 2000; 49:565.

Cimolai N, Carter JE, Morrison BJ, Anderson JD: Risk factors for the progression of *Escherichia coli* O157:H7 enteritis to hemolytic-uremic syndrome. J Pediatr 1990; 116:589.

Fine KD: Diarrhea. In: Feldman M, Scharschmidt BF, Sleisenger MH, eds. *Gastrointestinal and Liver Diseases: Pathophysiology/Diagnosis/Management.* 6th ed. Saunders;1998:128.

Guerrant RL, Araujo V, Soares E et al: Measurement of fecal lactoferrin as a marker of fecal leukocytes. J Clin Microbiol 1992;30:1238.

Lebwohl B, Deckelbaum RJ, Green PHR: Giardiasis. Gastrointest Endosc 2003; 57:906.

Schiller LR, Sellin, JH: Diarrhea. In: Feldman M, Friedman LS, Sleisenger MH, eds. *Gastrointestinal and Liver Diseases: Pathophysiology/Diagnosis/Management.* 7th ed. Saunders;2004:131.

18. DIZZINESS

I. **Problem.** You are called by the nurse to evaluate a 65-year-old woman complaining of dizziness.

II. **Immediate Questions**

A. **What is the patient's description of the dizziness?** Obtaining a detailed description of the patient's symptoms enables you to classify dizziness into one of four specific categories (vertigo, pre-syncope, disequilibrium, or lightheadedness).

B. **What are the patient's vital signs?** Blood pressure and heart rate should be obtained lying and standing after 1 minute in all patients with dizziness. Orthostatic hypotension (a decrease of 10 mm Hg systolic blood pressure) can often be attributed to drugs, volume depletion, or autonomic insufficiency. The heart rate increases by 20 bpm (16 bpm in the elderly) in volume depletion, whereas with autonomic insufficiency the heart rate does not change. Consider an arrhythmia if the patient is tachycardic or bradycardic or has an irregular rhythm. Blood pressure and heart rate should be checked in both arms. A significant difference in systolic blood pressure (> 20 mm Hg) between the two arms may be suggestive of subclavian steal. Tachypnea may suggest hyperventilation or anxiety. Fever could represent an infectious cause such as meningitis or otitis media.

C. **What are the patient's medications?** Medications are a common cause of dizziness. Vasodilators, antihypertensives, and tricyclic antidepressants often cause orthostatic hypotension. Digoxin, beta-blockers, and calcium channel blockers (non–dihydropyridine calcium antagonists) can result in bradycardia and varying degrees of heart block. Antiarrhythmics such as quinidine, procainamide, and sotalol can induce ventricular arrhythmias. Aminoglycoside antibiotics (amikacin, gentamicin, streptomycin, tobramycin) and loop diuretics have been associated with ototoxicity and vertigo.

D. **What are the onset and duration of the dizziness?** Sudden onset of vertigo is suggestive of a peripheral vestibular disorder, whereas central vestibular disorders are associated with vertigo that is gradual in onset. In general, episodic symptoms occur with peripheral vestibular disorders and constant symptoms with central vestibular disorders. Knowing the duration of episodes can be helpful in differentiating benign positional vertigo (seconds), transient ischemic attack (minutes to hours), Ménière's disease (hours), and vestibular neuronitis/labyrinthitis (days). Common nonvestibular disorders (postural hypotension, vasovagal reactions, and cardiac arrhythmias) cause episodic dizziness usually lasting a few minutes. Chronic continuous dizziness is commonly caused by psychogenic factors and hyperventilation syndrome.

E. **Are there precipitating factors of the dizziness?** Dizziness related to position change can be attributed to vestibular and nonvestibular disorders. Positional vertigo is precipitated by changes in head position (turning/tilting head or rolling over in bed) or middle ear pressure (coughing, sneezing, or Valsalva maneuver). Postural hypotension is typically associated with a change in position (lying to standing). Generally, dizziness associated with exercise or stress is suggestive of a nonvestibular disorder.

F. **Are there other associated symptoms?** Hearing loss and tinnitus indicate a vestibular disorder, usually a peripheral disorder (eg, Ménière's disease). Nausea and vomiting are nonspecific findings often associated with vestibular disorders. Focal neurologic deficits usually represent a central nervous system disorder. Dyspnea, palpitations, and sweating occur with nonvestibular disorders, such as hyperventilation or cardiac disease.

III. Differential Diagnosis. Dizziness is a common complaint with an extensive differential diagnosis. A common approach is to categorize dizziness as vertigo, pre-syncope, disequilibrium, or lightheadedness. In general, the most common causes of dizziness are peripheral vestibular disorders, psychiatric disorders, and pre-syncope.

A. Vertigo. Vertigo is a symptom of vestibular dysfunction. It is a sensation of motion either of one's surroundings or of one's body, commonly described as a spinning or tilting sensation. If dizziness is attributed to vertigo, you must determine whether it is due to a peripheral or to a central vestibular disorder.

    1. Peripheral vestibular disorders. Due to disease of the inner ear or vestibular nerve (CN VIII).

        a. Benign positional vertigo. The most common cause of vertigo. Characterized by brief episodes of severe vertigo that are associated with changes of head position, it often occurs after ear trauma or infection.

        b. Vestibular neuronitis. Sudden onset of severe vertigo associated with nausea and vomiting. Symptoms may persist for hours to days. It usually follows a viral upper respiratory infection.

        c. Labyrinthitis. Similar to vestibular neuronitis except associated with hearing loss.

        d. Ménière's disease. Characterized by episodic vertigo, tinnitus, aural fullness, and progressive sensorineural hearing loss.

        e. Ototoxic medications. Aminoglycoside antibiotics, loop diuretics, aspirin, *cis*-platinum, alcohol.

        f. Other peripheral disorders. Post-traumatic vertigo, acute or chronic otitis media, cholesteatoma, perilymphatic fistula, and acoustic neuroma.

    2. Central vestibular disorders. Due to disease of brain stem or cerebellum. Usually, vertigo is not the dominant manifestation of these disorders.

        a. Cerebrovascular disease. Ischemia involving the vertebrobasilar circulation often causes vertigo. Other signs of brain stem involvement such as diplopia, dysarthria, dysphagia, weakness, or numbness usually accompany vertigo due to brain stem ischemia. Cerebellar ischemia typically presents with vertigo and cerebellar signs; however, it may present with only vertigo. Altered mental status may indicate cerebellar infarction or hemorrhage with potential for herniation and progression to coma.

        b. Tumors. Brain stem, cerebellar, and cerebellopontine-angle tumors. *Acoustic neuromas,* which are benign tumors of the vestibular nerve, are the most common cerebellopontine-angle tumors. Tinnitus and hearing loss are common complaints, whereas vertigo is usually mild or absent.

   c. **Multiple sclerosis.** Vertigo is the presenting symptom in ~
      10% of patients. Up to one-third of patients with multiple scle-
      rosis experience vertigo.
   d. **Subclavian steal syndrome.** Vertigo and other signs of verte-
      brobasilar insufficiency occur during arm exercise.
   e. **Other central disorders.** Temporal lobe seizures, basilar
      artery migraines, meningitis, Friedreich's ataxia and related
      heredofamilial disorders, vasculitis.
B. **Pre-syncope.** A sensation of an impending faint, often described as
   "nearly fainting." Unlike syncope, there is no loss of consciousness.
   Pre-syncope typically lasts less than 1 minute. (See Section I, Chapter 59, Syncope, p 337.)
   1. **Vasovagal reaction.** Common in young patients and usually pre-
      ceded by diaphoresis, pallor, and nausea. Frequently provoked by
      stressful, painful, or other noxious stimuli (ie, venipuncture).
   2. **Orthostatic hypotension.** Hypovolemia, medications, or auto-
      nomic insufficiency.
   3. **Cardiac disease.** Arrhythmias, valvular disease, atrial myxoma,
      cardiac ischemia, tamponade.
   4. **Carotid sinus hypersensitivity.** Associated with head turning,
      tight collars, and shaving.
   5. **Metabolic.** Hypoxia, hypoglycemia, hyponatremia, hypokalemia,
      hypocalcemia.
C. **Disequilibrium.** A sense of imbalance with ambulation, typically not
   occurring at rest.
   1. **Multisensory deficit disorder.** The most common cause of dise-
      quilibrium in the elderly. It is due to any combination of peripheral
      neuropathy, visual impairment, vestibular disorder, or muscu-
      loskeletal disorder (ie, arthritis, cervical spondylosis). Multisensory
      deficit disorder is often worsened by the patient's fear of falling.
   2. **Altered visual input.** The elderly with vision loss and cataracts
      are prone to gait disturbances, particularly at night or in unfamiliar
      surroundings.
   3. **Cerebellar disease**
   4. **Parkinson's disease**
   5. **Medications.** Psychotropics, benzodiazepines, anticonvulsants.
D. **Lightheadedness.** Dizziness that is difficult to define and not otherwise classifiable. The description given by the patient is often vague.
   1. **Psychiatric.** Frequently nonspecific dizziness is a symptom of an
      underlying psychiatric disorder, including anxiety, depression, and
      panic disorder. The dizziness associated with anxiety is frequently
      associated with hyperventilation.
   2. **Hyperventilation.** Dizziness is the most common symptom with
      hyperventilation syndrome. Dyspnea, palpitations, and paresthe-
      sias are associated symptoms. An abnormal pattern of breathing
      is often not recognized by the patient.

IV. Database

A. Physical examination key points

1. **Vital signs.** See above Section II.B.
2. **Ears.** The external auditory canal should be evaluated for cerumen impaction or foreign body. The tympanic membrane should be examined for evidence of fluid, infection, or perforation. Do a simple assessment for hearing loss through whispered voice or finger rub. If hearing loss is suspected, then distinguish between sensorineural and conductive hearing loss (Weber and Rinne tests). Sensorineural hearing loss is suggestive of Ménière's disease or an acoustic neuroma, whereas conductive hearing loss is often due to middle ear disease interfering with conduction, such as otitis media.
3. **Eyes.** Eyes should be examined for nystagmus, which is commonly associated with vertigo. Assess pupils and extraocular muscles for cranial nerve dysfunction, which may be due to a CNS lesion. Do a funduscopic exam to evaluate for papilledema (increased intracranial pressure). A quick check of visual acuity should also be done.
4. **Neck.** Auscultate for carotid/vertebral bruits, which may suggest possible cerebrovascular disease. Determine whether head and neck movement precipitates dizziness.
5. **Cardiac.** Assess cardiac rate and rhythm to determine presence of arrhythmia. Auscultate for heart murmurs suggestive of aortic stenosis or idiopathic hypertrophic subaortic stenosis.
6. **Neurologic exam.** A careful neurologic exam is essential.
   a. **Mental status exam.** May give evidence of underlying psychiatric disorder. Altered mental status associated with non-vestibular dizziness may be attributed to drug toxicity, metabolic abnormalities, or CNS infection, whereas altered mental status with vertigo is often associated with life-threatening CNS disorders such as cerebellar hemorrhage or infarction.
   b. **Cranial nerves.** Cranial nerve abnormalities suggest a CNS disorder. Sensory: peripheral neuropathy, especially of lower extremities, contributes to disequilibrium.
   c. **Cerebellar.** Observe gait. Evaluate for limb ataxia and gait ataxia.

B. Diagnostic physical tests

1. **Nystagmus.** The presence of nystagmus suggests that dizziness is caused by vertigo. It may be the only objective finding in the examination of a patient with vertigo. Nystagmus associated with a peripheral lesion is different from that seen with a central lesion. Peripheral lesions cause only horizontal or rotary nystagmus; central lesions may cause nystagmus in any direction. Vertical nystagmus is seen only with central lesions. Visual fixation tends to suppress nystagmus that is due to peripheral but not central le-

sions. Changing the direction of gaze does not change the direction of nystagmus with peripheral lesions, but it may change the direction of nystagmus with central lesions.

2. **Nylen-Barany (Hallpike-Dix) maneuver.** Indicated with a history of vertigo. This maneuver helps to differentiate peripheral positional vertigo from central vertigo. The physician moves the patient from a sitting to a supine position, with the head rotated 45 degrees to one side and hanging off the table at 45 degrees. The patient is then observed for vertigo and nystagmus. The maneuver is repeated with the head turned to the other side. With peripheral positional vertigo (benign positional vertigo), the maneuver produces vertigo and rotary nystagmus after a latency of 2–20 seconds, which diminishes in intensity within 30 seconds and fatigues with repetitive testing. Variation of these features often indicates a central disorder.

3. **Romberg test.** The patient stands with feet together, without support from the arms. Monitor the patient with his eyes open and then closed. Pronounced imbalance with eyes closed compared with eyes open suggests proprioceptive impairment. A *positive* Romberg test is common with disequilibrium.

4. **Hyperventilation maneuver.** The patient hyperventilates for 2–3 minutes. Monitor for reproduction of dizziness.

C. **Laboratory data**
   1. **Complete blood count.** To rule out anemia or infection.
   2. **Glucose.** To rule out hypoglycemia.
   3. **Serum electrolytes.** To rule out electrolyte abnormalities such as hypokalemia or hypocalcemia.
   4. **Thyroid function tests.** If hypothyroidism is suspected.
   5. **Urine drug screen/drug levels.** If illicit drug use or drug toxicity is suspected.
   6. **Serologic test for syphilis (RPR/VDRL).** If tertiary syphilis is suspected.

D. **Special tests**
   1. **Brain imaging.** Not all patients with dizziness need neuroimaging. If a patient's findings on exam are suggestive of a CNS disorder, neuroimaging is indicated. MRI is more sensitive than CT in diagnosing posterior fossa lesions and acoustic neuromas.
   2. **Electronystagmogram.** Testing of vestibular function by evaluating nystagmus. This test is able to confirm nystagmus when the physical examination is equivocal. It detects peripheral and central vestibular disorders and should be considered when the cause of vertigo is uncertain.
   3. **Audiometry.** Should be considered with hearing complaints or with hearing loss on examination. It may help with the diagnosis of peripheral vertigo (ie, Ménèire's disease or acoustic neuroma).
   4. **Brain stem–evoked audiometry.** Very sensitive in the detection of acoustic neuromas.

5. **Electroencephalogram.** If seizures are suspected.
6. **Lumbar puncture.** If meningitis or multiple sclerosis is suspected.
7. **Electrocardiogram.** To rule out arrhythmia.
8. **Telemetry/Holter monitor/event recorder.** Useful in the evaluation of suspected arrhythmias.
9. **Echocardiogram.** If valvular heart disease or atrial myxoma is suspected.

V. Plan. Effective management of dizziness requires establishing the cause.

A. **Vertigo.** The management of central vertigo usually requires treatment of the underlying cause. The therapeutic goal of peripheral vertigo is to provide symptomatic relief from the vertigo as well as the nausea and vomiting. Most of the causes of peripheral vertigo are not life threatening, and most episodes subside with conservative therapy (drug therapy and physical therapy).

1. **Drug therapy.** Antihistamines and anticholinergics are the drugs of choice. Phenothiazines and benzodiazepines are more sedating and usually reserved for patients with severe vomiting.
   a. **Antihistamines.** Meclizine (Antivert), 12.5–25 mg PO Q 6 hr; dimenhydrinate (Dramamine), 50 mg PO Q 6 hr; diphenhydramine (Benadryl), 25–50 mg PO/IM/IV Q 6 hr.
   b. **Anticholinergics.** Scopolamine (Transderm Scop), 0.5 mg/patch Q 3 days.
   c. **Phenothiazines.** Prochlorperazine (Compazine), 5–10 mg PO/IM/IV Q 6 hr; promethazine (Phenergan), 25–50 mg PO/IM/IV Q 6 hr.
   d. **Benzodiazepines.** Diazepam (Valium), 2–10 mg PO/IM/IV Q 6 hr.
2. **Physical therapy.** Vestibular rehabilitation often promotes recovery in patients with peripheral vertigo. Patients with vertigo tend to avoid head motion, which actually prolongs symptoms. Physical therapy forces them to perform exercises that may decrease the duration and severity of vertigo.
3. **Surgery.** Surgical intervention is reserved for refractory cases of vertigo. Endolymphatic shunts and labyrinthectomies have been performed for disabling cases of Ménière's disease.

B. **Pre-syncope.** See Section I, Chapter 59, Syncope, V, p 344.

C. **Disequilibrium**
1. **Treat any underlying treatable disorders.**
2. **Correct vision** if indicated.
3. **Advise to use cane or walker** when indicated.
4. **Consider physical therapy.**
5. **Assess environmental risks.** Prevent falls by eliminating hazards in environment.
6. **Avoid sedating medications.**

  D. Lightheadedness
    1. **Treat any underlying psychiatric disorder** (ie, give anxiolytics or antidepressants).
    2. **Supportive psychotherapy.**
    3. **Teach relaxation techniques.**
    4. **Teach breathing techniques to relieve symptoms.**

REFERENCES

Branch WT: Approach to the patient with dizziness. In: Fletcher SW, Fletcher RH, Aronson MD, eds. UpToDate [CD-ROM]. Version 8.2. Wellesley, MA;2000. www.uptodate.com

Hoffman RM, Einstadter D, Kroenke K: Evaluating dizziness. Am J Med 1999;107:468.

Warner EA, Wallach PM, Adelman HM et al: Dizziness in primary care patients. J Gen Intern Med 1992;7:454.

19. DYSPNEA

  I. Problem. A patient admitted to the coronary care unit to rule out a myocardial infarction (MI) complains of difficulty breathing.

  II. Immediate Questions

    A. Was the onset of dyspnea acute or gradual? The differential diagnosis for acute dyspnea differs from subacute or chronic dyspnea. Causes of acute dyspnea include bronchospasm, pulmonary embolism (PE), pneumothorax, pulmonary infection, acute respiratory distress syndrome, diaphragmatic paralysis, myocardial ischemia, acute cardiogenic pulmonary edema, and anxiety. Chronic dyspnea can present with an acute exacerbation.

    B. Are there other associated symptoms? The patient may focus on the shortness of breath and fail to disclose chest pain, pressure, or discomfort unless specifically asked. Qualify the chest pain; for example, chest pain of a pleuritic nature characterizes pneumothorax or PE with infarction. Bear in mind that dyspnea rather than angina may be the primary or the only symptom of acute myocardial ischemia. Determination of the effect of positional changes on dyspnea is important. *Orthopnea* (difficulty breathing when lying flat) suggests congestive heart failure, or diaphragmatic dysfunction. *Platypnea* (difficulty breathing when sitting upright) invokes intrapulmonary or intracardiac shunting. *Trepopnea* (an inability to lie on one's side) implies pleural effusion or congestive heart failure. Assessment for precipitants, including exertion, exposure to chemicals, and other irritants is also helpful.

    C. Is the patient cyanotic? Hypoxemia is a potentially lethal condition. If cyanosis (or evidence of hypoxia, such as by pulse oximetry) is noted, immediate oxygen therapy is indicated.

III. Differential Diagnosis. *Dyspnea* is the subjective sensation of difficult, labored, uncomfortable breathing. It may occur through increased respiratory muscle work, stimulation of neuroreceptors throughout the respiratory tract, or stimulation of peripheral and central chemoreceptors. Although many diseases produce dyspnea, two-thirds are caused by pulmonary or cardiac disorders.

A. Pulmonary

1. **Pulmonary embolism.** This diagnosis must be considered in any patient presenting with acute dyspnea. Also, recurrent pulmonary emboli can cause intermittent dyspnea at rest. This diagnosis should be considered especially in the presence of risk factors such as prolonged immobilization, recent operative procedure, obesity, malignancy (especially adenocarcinomas), venous trauma, known venous thrombosis, hypercoagulable risk factor (such as factor V Leiden mutation, prothrombin gene mutation, antithrombin, protein C or S deficiency) or state (such as antiphospholipid antibody syndrome), or high-dose estrogen therapy, especially in women over 35 years of age who take birth control pills and smoke.

2. **Pneumothorax.** This can occur after trauma, spontaneously in patients with bullous emphysema, or in young people—especially males with a tall, thin body habitus. Patients on ventilators are at increased risk. Iatrogenic pneumothoraces may occur after central line insertion, bronchoscopy, or thoracentesis.

3. **Asthma/chronic obstructive airway disease (COPD).** Sometimes patients with asthma have primarily chest hyperinflation and increased work of breathing before actual wheezing occurs. A careful examination and review of history are important. However, anaphylaxis can also produce wheezing. (See Section I, Chapter 4, Anaphylactic Reaction, p 25). In addition to bronchospasm, these patients often demonstrate other evidence of anaphylaxis, such as stridor, wheezing, pruritus, hypotension, and urticaria.

4. **Aspiration.** An altered mental status or advanced age is often present (eg, from intoxication, psychosis, delirium); also ask about dysphagia and muscle weakness suggesting an acute cerebral vascular accident. See Section I, Chapter 7, Aspiration, III.H. Upper Airway Obstruction, p 39.

5. **Pneumonia.** It is characterized by fever, productive cough, radiographic infiltrates, and leukocytosis or leukopenia.

6. **Interstitial lung disease.** This usually produces progressive dyspnea and is caused by diseases such as sarcoidosis, idiopathic pulmonary fibrosis, collagen vascular disease, and occupational lung disease.

7. **Pleural effusion.** This is more likely to cause chronic or subchronic dyspnea rather than acute dyspnea, except in the setting of significant parapneumonic effusion or in association with congestive heart failure, renal failure, or pulmonary hemorrhage.

8. **Acute respiratory distress syndrome.** This is defined as acute bilateral lung injury with severe hypoxemia and is commonly associated with pneumonia, aspiration, sepsis, trauma, pancreatitis, or receiving multiple transfusions.

B. **Cardiac**
   1. **Acute MI.** Myocardial ischemia can present primarily with dyspnea rather than chest pain. In addition, patients with acute MI can develop acute PE or congestive heart failure with pulmonary edema.
   2. **Congestive heart failure.** Accumulation of fluid in the interstitial spaces of the lung stimulates neuroreceptors, which produce a sensation of dyspnea often causing orthopnea and paroxysmal nocturnal dyspnea. Common causes include myocardial ischemia, hypertension, dilated cardiomyopathy, and valvular disease.
   3. **Pericarditis/pericardial tamponade.** Dyspnea and fatigue, as well as chest discomfort, are frequently significant complaints. Suspect pericardial effusion in a patient with a pulmonary malignancy.
   4. **Arrhythmias.** Dyspnea may accompany tachyarrhythmias (eg, atrial fibrillation, supraventricular tachycardia, ventricular tachycardia) or bradyarrhythmias (eg, complete atrioventricular block, sinus bradycardia).
   5. **Valvular and other cardiac diseases.** Aortic stenosis, aortic insufficiency, mitral stenosis, and mitral insufficiency, as well as intracardiac shunt and atrial myxoma, can cause dyspnea.

C. **Neuromuscular diseases.** Dyspnea can be caused by central nervous system disorders, myopathies, neuropathies, phrenic nerve and diaphragmatic disorders, spinal cord disorders, or systemic neuromuscular disorders.

D. **Other organic causes.** Anemia, gastroesophageal reflux, thyrotoxicosis, hypothyroidism, metabolic acidosis (particularly diabetic ketoacidosis), renal failure (with concomitant pulmonary edema and/or uremic pericarditis), carbon monoxide poisoning, massive ascites (effectively resulting in restrictive lung disease), and deconditioning all can cause dyspnea.

E. **Psychogenic breathlessness.** Dyspnea associated with hyperventilation can be difficult to separate from dyspnea due to organic causes. Typically, anxiety, acral paresthesias, and lightheadedness are present. The dyspnea is often worse at rest and improves during exercise. Psychogenic breathlessness as a diagnosis should not be made until organic causes have been excluded. These patients often have an increased frequency of sighing.

IV. **Database**

A. **Physical examination key points**
   1. **Vital signs.** Fever may signify infection, but also occurs with PE and MI. Tachypnea occurs in most cases of dyspnea; however,

dyspnea can occur with a normal respiratory rate. Hypotension may result from a tension pneumothorax, anaphylaxis, pericardial tamponade, acute MI, or anemia from hemorrhage. Tachycardia is also seen in the above conditions. *Pulsus paradoxus* (inspiratory diminution in systolic pressure exceeding 10 mm Hg) may occur with acute exacerbation of asthma, COPD, constrictive pericarditis, or pericardial tamponade, and its significance is established only during normal cardiac rhythm and with respirations of normal rhythm and depth (*tidal breathing*). Bedside pulse oximetry is a valuable measurement.

2. **Lungs.** Observe the patient for accessory muscle use. Paradoxical abdominal movement during respiration suggests diaphragmatic and respiratory muscle fatigue. Palpate for tracheal deviation, which may be encountered in pneumothorax, large pleural effusion, or pulmonary mass. Percuss the lung fields to survey for asymmetry of resonance, as found in pneumothorax. Listen for wheezes, stridor, crackles, friction rubs, and absent breath sounds.

3. **Heart.** Elevated jugular venous pressure, a displaced point of maximal impulse, or an S_3 gallop suggests decompensated heart failure. Jugular venous distention on inspiration, a nonpalpable apical impulse, and muffled heart tones occur with pericardial tamponade. Irregular heart beat and murmurs are also important signs.

4. **Extremities.** Examine for swelling or other evidence of deep venous thrombosis, which predisposes to pulmonary embolus. Also, evaluate for pallor and peripheral cyanosis. Clubbing may be seen in the dyspneic patient with chronic suppurative lung disease, bronchial carcinoma, cyanotic heart disease, bacterial endocarditis, cirrhosis, or Graves' hyperthyroidism.

5. **Neurologic exam.** Confusion and impaired mentation may signify severe hypoxemia or may elucidate the cause of dyspnea, such as infection.

B. **Laboratory data**

1. **Hemogram.** Leukocytosis with an increase in banded neutrophils occurs with pneumonia. Anemia can cause dyspnea on exertion and may precipitate myocardial ischemia in patients with established coronary heart disease.

2. **Arterial blood gases (ABGs).** These values should be obtained in any patient with significant dyspnea or when hypoxemia is suspected based on a decreased percentage of oxygen saturation as measured by pulse oximetry. Assess for elevation of the alveolar-arterial (A-a) PO_2 gradient.

3. **Sputum Gram's stain and culture.** Obtain if pneumonia is suspected.

4. **Electrolytes and renal function tests.** Metabolic acidosis or renal failure may be discovered. Potential causes of cardiac ar-

rhythmias (eg, hypocalcemia, hypokalemia, hypomagnesemia) or diaphragmatic dysfunction (hypophosphatemia) can be uncovered.

5. **Thyroid function tests.** Obtain if thyroid disease is considered.
6. **Markers of cardiac disease.** Elevations in creatinine kinase (particularly MB fraction) and troponin are supportive of myocardial ischemia or infarction. Brain natriuretic peptide increases in acute ventricular dysfunction, but also may be elevated in chronic heart failure, PE, and cor pulmonale.

C. **Radiologic and other studies**

1. **Chest x-ray.** Obtain a stat portable upright chest x-ray if there is obvious distress. If the patient is unable to sit for an adequate film, obtain lateral decubitus films to rule out the possibility of a basilar pneumothorax. A clear chest x-ray raises the possibility of airway obstruction or PE. An increased cardiac silhouette (implies either cardiomegaly from heart disease or pericardial effusion), pulmonary vascular congestion, infiltrates, pleural effusion, elevated diaphragm (seen in neuromuscular disorders), or pneumothorax may be discovered.

2. **Electrocardiogram (ECG).** Should always be obtained in evaluating acute dyspnea to rule out myocardial ischemia or infarction (ST depression; ST elevation–convex upward; T-wave inversion; new Q waves); arrhythmia; pericarditis (PR depression; ST elevation–diffuse and concave upward; T-wave inversion); pericardial effusion (low QRS amplitude, electrical alternans); or PE ($S_1Q_3T_3$; right-axis deviation; right bundle branch block; T-wave inversion).

3. **Pulmonary function tests.** These are not applicable to the acute situation, but can assist in the evaluation of patients with obstructive or restrictive lung disease. Bronchial provocation testing may help increase yield of pulmonary function testing when looking for causes of chronic dyspnea or cough. (See Section I, Chapter 15, Cough; Section IV.C.4., Pulmonary Function Tests, p 93).

4. **Ventilation/perfusion (V̇/Q̇) scan.** To evaluate for PE. With underlying cardiopulmonary disease, spiral computed tomography (CT) of the chest may be the preferred test because of the higher rate of ventilation defects, thus lowering the number of high-probability scans. Remember that spiral CT is an excellent rule-in test, but a negative test does not rule out pulmonary embolus. For CT, reader expertise is essential.

5. **Pulmonary angiogram.** In patients with a low or moderate probability V̇/Q̇ scan or negative spiral CT in whom there still exists a suspicion for PE, this test is the gold standard for diagnosing PE. A venogram or impedance plethysmography and Doppler ultrasound of lower extremities may be helpful, potentially obviating the need for pulmonary angiogram if results demonstrate thrombosis.

6. **Echocardiogram.** Should be obtained emergently if there is a strong clinical suspicion for cardiac tamponade. Otherwise, an echocardiogram can be useful for assessing left ventricular function and valvular function and whether or not cardiac disease is responsible for the dyspnea.

7. **Cardiopulmonary exercise testing.** Useful if the diagnosis is unclear. It can help to determine whether a cardiac or pulmonary abnormality exists.

V. Plan

A. Emergent therapy

1. **Oxygen supplementation.** The initial goal of treatment for acute dyspnea should be to ensure adequate oxygenation; thus, most patients should be treated with 100% oxygen therapy. In patients with a history of COPD in whom one is concerned about the possibility of suppression of their hypoxic ventilatory drive, therapy should be initiated with 24–28% oxygen by Venturi mask. In either case, ABG values should be obtained to direct subsequent adjustments of the oxygen. Continuous oxygen saturation monitoring by pulse oximetry can be helpful.

2. **Stat portable chest x-ray, ECG, and ABG.** Indicated in any patient who complains of acute dyspnea.

B. Asthma/acute exacerbation of chronic bronchitis

1. **Albuterol.** Request a stat nebulizer treatment with albuterol 0.5 mL in 23 mL normal saline or give 4 puffs albuterol by metered-dose inhaler via a spacer device.

2. **Epinephrine.** For anaphylaxis or in young patients with acute asthma, epinephrine 0.250.4 mL of a 1:1000 concentration can be given SC.

3. **Methylprednisolone (Solu-Medrol).** 125 mg stat IV will provide relief of bronchospasm in 36 hours as the effectiveness of the albuterol dissipates.

C. Anaphylaxis. (See Section I, Chapter 4, Anaphylactic Reaction, V, p 27.)

D. Myocardial ischemia. If initial assessment suggests myocardial ischemia, administer aspirin 325 mg (chewable) and nitroglycerin 0.4 mg SL, provided the systolic blood pressure is > 100. (See Section I, Chapter 11, Chest Pain, V, p 66.)

E. Acute congestive heart failure. Furosemide (Lasix) 40–80 mg IV may be given, provided the patient is not hypotensive. Morphine sulfate 25 mg IV may also be helpful initially for acute pulmonary edema. Invasive monitoring via pulmonary artery catheter, IV inotropes, and angiotensin-converting enzyme inhibitor therapy may be warranted.

F. **Pneumonia.** Treat with pulmonary toilet (bronchodilators, incentive spirometry, percussion and postural drainage) and antibiotics as directed by results of the sputum Gram's stain. Be mindful of nosocomial pathogens when beginning empiric antibiotic treatment.

G. **Pleural effusion.** Removal of pleural fluid by thoracentesis can often produce a significant improvement in a patient's dyspnea, particularly in the setting of an exudative process such as malignancy. (See Section III, Chapter 14, Thoracentesis, p 459.)

H. **Aspiration.** (See Section I, Chapter 7, Aspiration, V, p 40.)

REFERENCES

Burki NK: Acute dyspnea: Is the cause cardiac or pulmonary—or both? Consultant 2000;40:542.

DeGowin RL, Brown DD: *DeGowin's Diagnostic Examination.* 7th ed. McGraw-Hill;2000:247.

Gillespie DJ, Staats BA: Concise review for primary-care physicians: Unexplained dyspnea. Mayo Clin Proc 1994;69:657.

Gulsun M, Goodman LR: CT for the diagnosis of venous thromboembolic disease. Curr Opin Pulm Med 2003;9:367.

Mahler DA: Acute dyspnea. In: Mahler DA, ed. *Dyspnea.* Futura Publishing Co.;1990:127.

Maisel AS, Krishnaswamy P, Nowak RM et al: Rapid measurement of B-type natriuretic peptide in the emergency diagnosis of heart failure. N Engl J Med 2002;347:161.

Manning HL, Schwartzstein RM: Pathophysiology of dyspnea. N Engl J Med 1995;327:1547.

Salzman GA: Evaluation of dyspnea. Hosp Pract 1997;195.

Task Force on Pulmonary Embolism, European Society of Cardiology: Guidelines on diagnosis and management of acute pulmonary embolism. Eur Heart J 2000;21:1301.

Ware LB, Matthay MA: Medical progress: The acute respiratory distress syndrome. N Engl J Med 2000;342:1334.

20. DYSURIA

I. **Problem.** A 36-year-old sexually active woman complains of pain with urination.

II. **Immediate Questions**

A. **How long have the symptoms been present?** Acute onset of symptoms of dysuria, frequency, and urgency within 1–2 days indicates lower urinary tract infection (UTI). Patients with symptoms for more than 1 week are more likely to have a more serious infection (upper tract involvement). A gradual onset of several days' duration suggests a chlamydial or gonorrheal infection. Prostatitis can also present with several days of symptoms.

B. **Are there any associated symptoms?** Fever, chills, nausea, vomiting, and back pain are often signs of upper UTIs such as pyelonephritis. Dysuria, frequency, urgency, and suprapubic pain are lower UTI signs and symptoms and can occur with cystitis, prostatitis, and urethritis. A vaginal discharge suggests a vaginitis, such as that caused by *Gardnerella vaginalis* in bacterial vaginosis, *Candida albicans,* or *Trichomonas vaginalis,* as a cause of dysuria. Also, remember that other sexually transmitted diseases such as chlamydia and gonorrhea can cause urethritis. In men, ask about a recent penile discharge.

C. Does the patient have a history of UTIs or urologic abnormality?
Women and patients with a urinary tract abnormality are predisposed to recurrent UTIs. Patients with recurrent UTIs (> 2 UTIs per year) are managed with longer courses of antibiotics and possibly prophylactic antibiotics. Bladder cancer can sometimes present with dysuria.

D. Has the patient recently had a Foley catheter removed? Catheter placement may result in an infection or transient urethral irritation.

E. What types of contraception or sexual protection are used by the patient? Use of diaphragm and spermicide enhance UTI susceptibility in women. In men, unprotected anal intercourse, intercourse with an infected partner, and an uncircumcised penis all are risk factors for UTIs.

III. Differential Diagnosis. The principal causes of dysuria differ for men and women.

A. Women. Women presenting with acute dysuria are likely to have one of seven conditions, each of which may require different management.

1. **Acute pyelonephritis.** Suggested by fever, rigors, flank pain, nausea, and vomiting with or without lower UTI symptoms.
2. **Complicated UTI.** Seen in patients with diabetes, immunosuppression, pregnancy, abnormal genitourinary tracts, resistant organisms, and history of relapsing infections. These patients can present only with signs of lower UTI but can have an upper UTI as well (subclinical pyelonephritis).
3. **Lower UTI.** These patients have either cystitis or urethritis, with bacteria confined to either the bladder or urethra.
4. **Chlamydial urethritis.** This is characterized by a gradual onset over several days. The patient often reports intercourse with a partner with similar symptoms. An associated mucopurulent endocervical secretion may be noted on pelvic exam.
5. **Other urethral infections.** Urethritis may also be caused by *Neisseria gonorrhoeae* and *T vaginalis.*
6. **Vaginitis.** In contrast to the internal sensations of dull pain associated with dysuria caused by cystitis, vaginitis causes external burning pain as the urine stream flows over the inflamed labia. The most common causes include bacterial vaginosis, candida vulvovaginitis, and trichomoniasis.

7. **No recognized pathogen.** These patients have no pyuria and no evidence of infection. The most common cause is atrophic vaginitis. Consider bladder or urethral carcinoma. "Urethral syndrome" is seen in some women who may be exquisitely sensitive to pH changes in the urine.

B. **Men**

1. **Acute pyelonephritis.** Presents with the same symptoms and signs as in women. Patients require further anatomic workup after infection is resolved.

2. **Lower UTI.** Presents with the same signs and symptoms as in women. If an isolated event, no further workup is needed, presuming that the patient is cured with treatment. Recurrent UTIs require workup.

3. **Urethritis.** Always keep in mind that chlamydia and gonorrhea often coexist.

   a. **Nongonococcal.** The most common etiologic agent is *Chlamydia trachomatis*. Discharge occurs 8–21 days after exposure and is typically thin and clear.

   b. **Gonococcal.** In contrast to nongonococcal urethritis, the discharge associated with this condition is heavy and purulent. Symptoms occur 2–6 days after exposure.

4. **Prostatitis.** Symptoms include dysuria, frequency, hesitancy, and vague groin and/or back pain. Associated fever, chills, and malaise suggest acute prostatitis. Chronic bacterial prostatitis is less common and associated with recurrent UTIs in men. Nonbacterial prostatitis is the most common and is sometimes referred to as "prostatodynia."

5. **Cancer.** Think of bladder, prostate, and urethral cancer.

6. **Benign conditions.** Urethral stricture, meatal stenosis, and benign prostatic hypertrophy.

IV. **Database**

A. **Physical examination key points**

1. **Vital signs.** Check for fever, tachycardia, and hypotension, which suggest upper tract involvement and, in the case of hypotension, urosepsis.

2. **Abdomen/back.** Examine for evidence of suprapubic tenderness or costovertebral angle tenderness.

3. **Genitalia.** In women who present with acute dysuria and also complain of a vaginal discharge, pelvic exam is mandatory to rule out vaginitis, cervicitis, and pelvic inflammatory disease. In men with a history of urethral discharge, penile stripping may be necessary to produce a discharge. Examine for evidence of epididymitis or orchitis.

4. **Prostate.** In acute prostatitis, the gland is swollen, tender, and boggy. In patients presenting with acute prostatitis, digital exam of

the prostate can result in bacteremia, so vigorous massage of the prostate is contraindicated. In patients with chronic prostatitis, examination of the prostate may be unremarkable.

B. Laboratory data

1. **Urinalysis.** Pyuria, which can be quickly detected by testing the urine for the presence of leukocyte esterase, is present in almost all cases of UTI (sensitivity 90%, specificity 95%). Bacteriuria, which can be detected using the nitrite test (except for the following uropathogens: *Enterococcus, Staphylococcus saprophyticus,* and *Acinetobacter* species that do not split nitrates to nitrites), confirms a bacterial cause. Remember that false-negative nitrite results may occur in patients who consume a low-nitrate diet or who take diuretics. Also, examine for white blood cell casts with microscopy, which indicates pyelonephritis. Hematuria occurs with cystitis and pyelonephritis but is seldom seen with urethritis. Gram's stain of uncentrifuged urine is also helpful in assessing the presence of bacteria and may help direct therapy, especially if gram-positive bacteria are seen.

2. **Urine culture.** Although useful in determining a bacterial cause of dysuria, a urine culture is usually indicated only in women if acute pyelonephritis or complicated UTI is suspected or if the patient is presenting with a relapse from a UTI. In men, a urine culture should always be obtained to confirm and direct subsequent treatment.

3. **Blood cultures.** Should be ordered in all patients who appear septic and are admitted for presumed acute pyelonephritis.

4. **Complete blood count with differential.** Leukocytosis and a left shift are seen with acute pyelonephritis and sometimes with acute prostatitis. They are seldom seen in urethritis, cystitis, or chronic prostatitis.

5. **Urethral discharge.** In both men and women, the discharge should be gram-stained and cultured on Thayer-Martin medium. The presence of intracellular gram-negative diplococci on Gram's stain is sufficient presumptive evidence of gonorrhea in men and warrants therapy. In women with endocervical discharge, cultures for gonorrhea should be obtained. Alternatively, a specimen can be sent for a nucleic acid amplification test (NAAT) for gonorrhea. Discharge should also always be sent for NAAT for *C trachomatis* as well.

6. **Urine test for gonorrhea and chlamydia.** If the pelvic exam is unobtainable or unacceptable, an NAAT may be performed on the urine for gonorrhea and chlamydia.

7. **Vaginal discharge.** Wet mount to look for *T vaginalis,* which have flagella and, when viewed on a wet mount, move rapidly and erratically. *Clue cells,* or activated squamous cells coated with bacteria, indicate bacterial vaginosis. The presence of hyphae,

indicating infection with *C albicans,* should be assessed on a slide of vaginal discharge treated with 2–3 drops of 10% potassium hydroxide. Cervical swabs can also be sent for culture, DNA probe, or ligase chain reaction tests for chlamydia and gonorrhea.

C. Radiologic and other studies. Full urologic evaluation is indicated in men with pyelonephritis, recurrent infections, or other complicating factors. Women who have had more than two recurrences of pyelonephritis, as well as women in whom complicating factors such as anatomic abnormalities are suspected, should also undergo full urologic evaluation. An ultrasound, CT scan, or intravenous pyelography should be obtained in patients admitted for acute pyelonephritis if they are hypotensive on admission or remain febrile after 3 days of treatment with an appropriate antibiotic. An ultrasound or pelvic CT should also be obtained in patients with acute prostatitis who do not improve after 3 days of an appropriate antibiotic.

V. Plan

A. Acute pyelonephritis

1. **Suspected sepsis or intolerance to oral medications.** Administer a fluoroquinolone IV (Cipro 200–400 mg IV Q 12 hr). A third-generation cephalosporin such as ceftriaxone 1 g IV Q 24 hr is an alternative. If you suspect *Enterococcus* (more common with recurrence or in the presence of structural abnormalities), use ampicillin 1.5–2.0 g Q 4–6 hr and gentamicin 1.5–2.0 mg/kg IV loading dose; then give about 1.5 mg/kg IV Q 8–24 hr, depending on renal function (see aminoglycoside dosing, Section VII, Table 7–18, p 630). Once antibiotic susceptibility tests are known, the patient can be switched to oral medications after being afebrile for 24–48 hours. Duration of therapy should be 14 days.

2. **Hospitalization indications.** Include dehydration; inability to tolerate oral medications; concern about compliance; uncertainty about diagnosis; and severe illness with high fever, severe pain, and marked debility.

3. **Acute uncomplicated pyelonephritis.** A 7-day outpatient course of a fluoroquinolone antibiotic such as ciprofloxacin 500 mg PO bid. Other possibilities include amoxicillin/potassium clavulanate (Augmentin) and oral cephalosporins for 14 days. Trimethoprim (Bactrim) has fallen out of favor due to the high rate of resistance.

4. **Follow-up.** Urine cultures should be checked 2–3 weeks after therapy is completed.

B. Complicated UTI. These patients should be treated with a 7- to 14-day course of the same oral or IV agents as described above for uncomplicated pyelonephritis.

C. Lower UTI. In patients presenting with acute dysuria who are noted to have pyuria and bacteriuria on urinalysis, but do not have the clinical picture of acute pyelonephritis, an uncomplicated lower UTI (most likely cystitis) can be presumed and treated. A urine culture is not required in these patients. Studies indicate that trimethoprim-sulfamethoxazole (Bactrim) is the most efficacious treatment if local *E coli* resistance is < 20%. A 3-day regimen of Bactrim DS, 1 tablet PO bid, is sufficient for uncomplicated lower UTIs in women. A 7-day regimen should be considered for patients with diabetes mellitus, > 7 days of symptoms, a recent UTI, UTI with associated use of a diaphragm or spermicide, and UTIs in men. Alternative antibiotics for patients with a history of intolerance to sulfa are oral cephalosporins for 3 days or nitrofurantoin 100 mg qid for 7 days. If local *E coli* resistance to Bactrim > 20% ciprofloxacin and other fluoroquinolones are appropriate for a 3-day course. Otherwise, they are reserved as second-line agents for patients who have recurrences and treatment failures. A follow-up culture is also **not** necessary for acute uncomplicated lower UTIs unless they occur frequently.

D. Vaginitis. Therapy is directed to the specific cause of the vaginitis. For patients with bacterial vaginosis, metronidazole 500 mg PO bid for 7 days or metronidazole vaginal gel 1 application a day for 5 days is effective. For candida vaginitis, miconazole (Monistat) cream topically for 7 days is effective. An alternative is a single 150-mg oral dose of fluconazole (Diflucan). For trichomonal vaginitis, metronidazole 2 g PO in a single dose is recommended for the sex partner as well as the patient. Alternatively, treatment can be metronidazole 500 mg PO bid for 7 days. Topical Premarin cream is effective for atrophic vaginitis. The cream should be applied daily for 1 week and then 2–3 times a week thereafter.

E. Chlamydial urethritis. This should be suspected when dysuria and pyuria but no bacteriuria is present, and when the partner has symptoms. Doxycycline 100 mg bid for 7 days is effective. An alternative therapy is azithromycin 1 g PO in a single dose or ofloxacin 300 mg PO bid for 7 days. The partner should be evaluated and treated. Verify that women are not pregnant before prescribing doxycycline.

F. Gonococcal urethritis. With the emergence of penicillin resistance, ceftriaxone 125 mg IM or ofloxacin 400 mg PO is now recommended. Because of the frequent coexistence of chlamydial urethritis, azithromycin 1 g PO 1 dose or doxycycline 100 mg PO twice a day for 7 days should also be given. The patient's partner(s) should be evaluated and treated.

G. Acute prostatitis. Patients who are septic should be admitted and broad antibiotic coverage administered IV. If Gram's stain shows gram-positive cocci in chains, patients should be treated with intravenous ampicillin and gentamicin to cover *Enterococcus*. Patients with gram-negative rods in their urine should be treated with intravenous ceftriaxone and either a fluoroquinolone (PO or IV) or an aminoglycoside. Once the patient has been afebrile for 24–48 hours, the patient may be switched to oral antibiotics for a total of 2-4 weeks. Outpatient management usually involves either a fluoro-quinolone PO or trimethoprim-sulfamethoxazole DS PO for 2–4 weeks pending results of the urine culture for men over age 35. If under 35 years old, treatment covers gonorrhea/chlamydia with cef-triaxone 250 mg IM × 1 and doxycycline 100 mg PO bid × 10 days. Nonsteroidal anti-inflammatory drugs can be given to relieve pain, speed clearing of inflammation, and liquefy prostatic secretions.

H. Chronic prostatitis. Patients may respond to an oral agent such as a fluoroquinolone (Ciprofloxacin) or trimethoprim (Bactrim DS) for 4–12 weeks. Many patients have nonbacterial prostatitis and should be referred for urologic evaluation if symptoms do not resolve on a course of antibiotics.

I. Urethral syndrome. Identify foods or medications that cause symptoms. Alkalinization of urine may help some patients.

REFERENCES

Claudius HI: Dysuria in adolescents. West J Med 2000;172:201.

Gilbert DN, Moellering RC, Sande MA: *The Sanford Guide to Antimicrobial Therapy.* 33rd ed. Antimicrobial Therapy, Inc. (Hyde Park, VT);2003:15-23.

Hooton TM, Stamm WE: Diagnosis and treatment of uncomplicated urinary tract infection. Infect Dis Clin North Am 1997;11:551.

Johnson RE, Newhall WJ: Screening tests to detect *Chlamydia trachomatis* and *Neisseria gonorrhoeae* infections—2002. MMWR 2002;51:RR-15.

Lipsky BA: Urinary tract infections in men. Ann Intern Med 1989;110:138.

Orenstein R, Wong ES: Urinary tract infections in adults. Am Fam Physician 1999;59:1225.

Pappas PG: Laboratory in the diagnosis and management of urinary tract infections. Med Clin North Am 1991;75:313.

Stamm WE, Hooton TM: Management of urinary tract infection in adults. N Engl J Med 1993;329:1328.

21. FALLS

I. Problem. You are called to evaluate an 84-year-old woman with pneumonia who has fallen on her way to the bathroom.

II. Immediate Questions

A. What were the circumstances of the fall? Determine, if possible, exactly how the fall occurred: What activity was the patient doing, and how did she feel at the time of the fall? Causes of falls can be characterized as *intrinsic* (due to a condition of the patient, such as orthostatic hypotension) or *extrinsic* (due to an environmental cause, such as a slippery floor). In many cases, the causes are intermingled.

B. What symptoms (if any) does the patient have? Determine whether premonitory symptoms such as dizziness, palpitations, dyspnea, chest pain, weakness, confusion, incontinence, loss of consciousness, or tongue biting occurred. In addition, inquire about pain involving the head, neck, ribs, arms, back, or hips.

C. What are the vital signs? Hypotension and tachycardia may be associated with many conditions, such as acute infection, dehydration, or acute myocardial infarction (MI). Tachypnea may be noted with the above conditions or with a pulmonary embolus. Fever or hypothermia may be indicative of infection.

D. What medical conditions does the patient have? Many conditions predispose to dizziness. Diabetes mellitus may be associated with autonomic dysfunction leading to orthostatic hypotension; hyperglycemia can cause osmotic diuresis and lead to volume depletion. Parkinson's disease results in gait imbalance. Dementia is associated with an increased risk of falls. Chronic foot problems and arthritis affecting the lower extremities can also be factors.

E. What medications is the patient taking? Medication-related side effects such as dizziness, hypotension, or confusion may predispose to falls. Vasodilators and diuretics commonly cause hypotension and dizziness. Anxiolytics, antidepressants, sedatives, antipsychotics, and anticholinergics have also been associated with increased risk of falls.

III. Differential Diagnosis. With younger patients, the cause of the fall may be easily apparent. However, the differential diagnosis with an older patient may be extensive. The elderly frequently have many contributing causes of a fall.

A. Extrinsic causes. These result from the environment.
   1. **Slippery floors.** From water or urine.
   2. **Inadequate lighting.** Older patients may have cataracts or other ophthalmologic problems that impair vision.
   3. **Transfers.** A weakened patient attempting to make a transfer from the bed to a wheelchair may fall.
   4. **Bed side rails.** If side rails are placed up, a delirious patient attempting to climb over them can fall.
   5. **Walking aids not available.** A hospitalized patient may not have his or her cane or walker immediately available and may attempt to walk to the bathroom unaided.

B. Intrinsic causes
   1. **"Normal" aging.** Such as visual impairment (eg, presbyopia or cataracts). Patients with visual or hearing loss may be unable to move well in a new environment.
   2. **Neurologic**
      a. **Cerebrovascular accident with hemiparesis.** May result in decreased mobility.
      b. **Parkinson's disease.** May cause decreased mobility.
      c. **Dementia.** From any number of causes such as multi-infarct dementia, Alzheimer's disease, or hypothyroidism. The patient

with dementia may have poor judgment about his or her ability to move in a new environment.

d. **Seizures.** The patient usually functions normally after the seizure episode. Look for evidence of tongue biting or urinary incontinence.

e. **Carotid sinus hypersensitivity**

f. **Peripheral neuropathy.** Vitamin B_{12} deficiency is more common among the elderly. Also, consider peripheral neuropathy in a patient with a history of diabetes mellitus, thyroid disorders, or alcohol abuse.

g. **Vestibular dysfunction.** Inner ear problems may have associated attacks of vertigo, affecting balance.

3. **Cardiovascular.** See Section I, Chapter 59, Syncope, p 337.

   a. **Orthostatic hypotension.** Should be considered with dehydration, acute infections, gastrointestinal bleeding, or autonomic dysfunction (diabetes mellitus).

   b. **Arrhythmias.** Tachyarrhythmias or bradyarrhythmias should be considered, especially in the elderly or those with a history of heart disease. See Section I, Chapter 60, Tachycardia, p 345, and Section I, Chapter 8, Bradycardia, p 42.

   c. **Angina or MI.** Syncope or hypotension can be a sign of ischemic heart disease.

   d. **Vagal response disorders.** Valsalva (due to defecation, micturition, or other cause) may cause an increase in vagal tone, resulting in a decrease in heart rate and blood pressure, which then may result in a fall.

4. **Fluid/volume loss.** From any cause, including diuretic use, diarrhea, vomiting or nasogastric suction, GI hemorrhage, high fever, or decreased oral intake.

5. **Musculoskeletal disorders.** Degenerative joint disease or osteoarthritis is very common in the elderly. Deconditioning can be a problem, especially during hospitalization. In addition, a fall can cause a hip fracture, predisposing the patient to fall again. Proximal muscle weakness is common in the elderly.

6. **Metabolic disorders**

   a. **Hyperthyroidism.** Associated arrhythmias such as atrial fibrillation may affect function.

   b. **Hypoglycemia.** There may be associated diaphoresis, tachycardia, or syncope.

   c. **Electrolyte imbalance.** Hypokalemia or hypomagnesemia can lead to muscle weakness or arrhythmias. Hypercalcemia can cause confusion.

   d. **Diabetes mellitus.** Uncontrolled diabetes mellitus can cause an osmotic diuresis leading to volume depletion. Peripheral neuropathy and autonomic insufficiency causing orthostatic hypotension can result from longstanding diabetes mellitus.

      e. Metabolic encephalopathy. Uremia and hepatic failure can cause confusion.

7. **Psychological factors**

      a. Refusal of assistance or ancillary devices. Some patients may feel that they do not need a walker or assistance with transfer.

      b. Disorientation. From any number of causes, including dementia, acute bacterial infection, "sundowning," and intensive care unit psychosis. See Section I, Chapter 13, Coma, Acute Mental Status Changes, p 76.

      c. Depression. Depression may present as dementia. These patients may become increasingly immobile or less likely to notice obstacles or changes in their environment.

8. **Medications.** See II.E. above. Also, medications that may affect the vestibular system at either normal or toxic doses include aminoglycosides (gentamicin, tobramycin), aspirin, furosemide (Lasix), quinine, quinidine, and alcohol.

9. **Congestive heart failure.** Exercise tolerance may be limited, leading to a fall upon overexertion.

10. **Infection.** Any infection may be associated with a change in mental status, particularly in the elderly. Also, infections (eg, pneumonia) may cause weakness during hospitalization, and the patient may be unable to move about safely unassisted.

IV. Database

A. Physical examination key points

1. **Vital signs.** Look for hypotension, tachycardia or bradycardia, tachypnea, or an increase or decrease in the temperature from baseline. Check for orthostatic changes, a decrease in systolic blood pressure of 10 mm Hg, and/or an increase in heart rate of 20 bpm (16 bpm in the elderly) 1 minute after going from supine to a standing position.

2. **HEENT.** Look for evidence of trauma from the fall, such as soft tissue swelling and tenderness. Look for cataracts, which may impair vision.

3. **Extremities.** Look for evidence of fractures, such as an externally rotated and flexed hip, deformity of long bones, or swelling over these sites.

4. **Neurologic exam.** Examine for evidence of peripheral neuropathy or movement disorder (eg, Parkinson's disease). Perform a brief mental status exam and check for localizing findings to assess for possible subdural hematoma.

B. Laboratory data.
If there are obvious clues from the history and/or physical examination, an extensive laboratory evaluation may not be indicated.

1. **Complete blood count.** To evaluate for infection and anemia.
2. **Electrolytes.** Include blood urea nitrogen, creatinine, and glucose. Hypokalemia or hypomagnesemia can cause arrhythmias; hypercalcemia can cause confusion.
3. **Urinalysis.** Rule out infection, especially in older patients.
4. **Liver function tests.** Aspartate aminotransferase (AST), alanine aminotransferase (ALT), total bilirubin, and alkaline phosphatase or γ-glutamyltransferase (GGT) to rule out hepatic dysfunction.

C. **Radiologic and other studies**
   1. **Skeletal x-rays.** In elderly patients, the most common sites for significant fractures would be hip, humerus, distal radius, and ulna (Colles' fracture).
   2. **CT scan of head without contrast.** Because this test can be performed more quickly than an MRI, order if the patient has new neurologic deficits or confusion not explained by routine evaluation to rule out an acute bleed or to look for evidence of increased intracranial pressure.
   3. **Electrocardiography.** Look for evidence of ischemia, infarction, tachyarrhythmia, or bradyarrhythmia. Check the QT interval, especially if the patient is taking any medications that prolong the QT interval, such as amiodarone, sotalol, quinidine, or procainamide. A prolonged or a shortened QT interval can be secondary to hypocalcemia or hypercalcemia, respectively.

V. **Plan**
   A. **Prevention.** Preventive measures can greatly reduce the number of falls and are essential for good patient care. Environmental modifications include avoidance of restraints, if possible, and removal of obstacles that interfere with patient movement. Assistive devices used routinely, such as a walker, cane, or hearing aid, should be made available, if possible.
   B. **Medication modification.** Review all medications and reduce or eliminate those that may contribute to mental status changes or orthostatic hypotension or that may limit mobility.
   C. **Treat potential underlying causes.** Including but not limited to infection, cerebrovascular accident, myocardial ischemia or infarction, and gastrointestinal bleeding.
   D. **Observation.** The patient who has had a head injury should undergo a thorough neurologic examination by the physician and be monitored by neurologic checks by the nursing staff. Patients with abnormal vital signs should be monitored more frequently than the usual once per nursing shift. Patients should also be monitored for complaints of pain (eg, neck, back, arm, or hip) not present during the initial evaluation.
   E. **Physical therapy.** If the patient has gait imbalance or weakness, consult a physical therapist for a thorough gait and balance assessment and strengthening exercises.

REFERENCES

Fuller GF: Falls in the elderly. Am Fam Physician 2000;61:2159.
Kiel DP: The evaluation of falls in the emergency department. Clin Geriatr Med 1993;9:591.
King MB: Falls. In: Hazzard WR, Blass JP, Halter JB et al, eds. *Principles of Geriatric Medicine and Gerontology.* 5th ed. McGraw-Hill;2003:1517.
Mahoney JE: Immobility and falls. Clin Geriatr Med 1998;14:699.
Tinetti M, Speechley M: Prevention of falls among the elderly. N Engl J Med 1989;320:1055.

22. FEVER

I. **Problem.** You are called to see a 57-year-old man who has been hospitalized for 3 days and now has a fever of 39.5 °C (103.1 °F).

II. **Immediate Questions**

A. **Was the patient febrile on admission, implying community-acquired illness, or did the fever develop in the course of hospitalization (nosocomial)?** It is important to know whether this elevation in temperature signals the abrupt onset of fever or represents the gradual worsening of a prior fever. Fever above 40.0 °C (104.0 °F) requires immediate action.

B. **Does the patient have any other pertinent medical illnesses, or is he or she immunocompromised?** Such information is vital before you can properly assess the patient. Review should include all medical illnesses as well as previous surgeries. For example, a history of trauma that resulted in splenectomy places that patient at higher risk of infection with encapsulated organisms such as *Streptococcus pneumoniae*. Is there an underlying malignancy? Has the patient recently received chemotherapy? Is the patient taking or has he or she recently taken any other immunosuppressive medications such as prednisone or azathioprine? Also see Section I, Chapter 23, Fever in the HIV-Positive Patient, p 141.

C. **Are any indwelling catheters in place?** Indwelling Foley catheters, intravenous access sites, nasogastric tubes (which can predispose to sinusitis), and central venous catheter sites are frequent sources of nosocomial fever.

D. **Are there any associated symptoms?** The symptoms to ascertain include chills, rigors, night sweats, rash, myalgias, arthralgias, cough, sputum production, postnasal drainage, chest pain, headache, facial pain, dysuria, abdominal pain, nausea, vomiting, diarrhea, pain at an intravenous site, and change in mental status. Such questions may point toward a specific cause.

E. **What medications is the patient taking?** Ask whether the patient is taking any antipyretics or antibiotics. If the patient has been on antibiotics in the past 4 months, consider the possibility of *Clostridium dif-*

ficile colitis. Also consider a drug-induced fever and review all medications.

**F. Have any recent procedures such as bronchoscopy been car-
ried out, or has the patient recently received blood?** A fever up to
38.3 °C (101 °F) is common after bronchoscopy and transfusions.

**G. Are there any factors relating to the patient's psychosocial his-
tory that need to be assessed?** Inquire about recent travel, especially to countries with poor sanitation; HIV risk factors (intravenous
drug use; homosexual or bisexual male; promiscuous sexual activity;
or sexual intercourse with a prostitute, a person with AIDS, or HIV-
positive persons); exposure to dogs, cats, birds, ticks, and cattle; and
health of family members.

**H. Does the patient have significant valvular heart disease includ-
ing a prosthetic valve?** Significant valvular heart disease predisposes the patient to bacterial endocarditis. Be sure to inquire about
recent procedures, including dental work.

III. Differential Diagnosis. An exhaustive list is extraordinarily long; only
the major categories are presented here:

A. Infections
  1. **Bacterial**
  2. **Viral**
  3. **Mycobacterial**
  4. **Fungal**
  5. **Parasitic**
  6. **Protozoal**
  7. **Rickettsial**

B. Neoplasms. Solid tumors, especially with metastasis to the liver;
lymphoma; Hodgkin's disease; multiple myeloma; leukemia;
myelodysplastic syndromes. Fever with leukemia is often due to infection but may be caused by the primary disease, especially in
chronic myelogenous leukemia. Solid tumors causing fever include
renal cell and hepatocellular carcinoma, osteogenic sarcoma, and
atrial myxoma.

C. Connective tissue disease
  1. **Acute rheumatic fever**
  2. **Rheumatoid arthritis**
  3. **Adult Still's disease**
  4. **Systemic lupus erythematosus (SLE)**
  5. **Vasculitis.** Including hypersensitivity vasculitis, polymyalgia
     rheumatica, temporal arteritis, and polyarteritis nodosa.

D. Thermoregulatory disorders. Heat stroke, malignant hyperthermia,
thyroid storm, and malignant neuroleptic syndrome. Thyroid storm
may be a postoperative complication in a hyperthyroid patient. Features of malignant neuroleptic syndrome include hyperthermia, hy-

pertonicity of skeletal muscle, mental status changes, and autonomic nervous system instability in patients on neuroleptics.

E. Drug-induced fever. Potential culprits include antibiotics (especially beta-lactams, sulfonamides), sulfa-containing stool softeners, methyldopa, quinidine, hydralazine, procainamide, phenytoin, chlorpromazine, carbamazepine, anti-inflammatory agents such as ibuprofen, antineoplastic agents, and allopurinol. Other agents that may cause fever include steroids, antidopaminergic neuroleptic agents, sleep medications, sympathomimetics, cocaine, LSD, hallucinogens, ecstasy or MDMA (3,4-methylenedioxymethamphetamine), phencyclidine, and tricyclic antidepressants (increase thermoset point via action at the anterior hypothalamus). Withdrawal from ethanol, barbiturates, benzodiazepines, and sedative hypnotics also increases thermoset point via action at the anterior hypothalamus, as well as producing excessive muscular activity with consequent increased heat production. Dystonic reactions due to butyrophenones, phenothiazines, and metoclopramide can stimulate excess muscular activity as well. Salicylate toxicity can cause increased heat production. Parasympatholytic agents (anticholinergics, antihistamines, antiparkinsonism agents, phenothiazines, and tricyclic antidepressants) decrease sweating, resulting in decreased heat dissipation.

F. Miscellaneous disorders. Including pulmonary embolus with infarction, myocardial infarction, inflammatory bowel disease, and addisonian crisis (often results in hyothermia). Deep venous thrombosis, hematoma formation, alcoholic hepatitis, Jarisch-Herxheimer reaction, or central fever due to central nervous system (CNS) process.

G. Fever of unknown origin (FUO). Manifested by fever > 38.3 °C (101.0 °F) on several occasions for a duration of at least 3 weeks, with no definite etiology. When a cause is uncovered for an FUO, it usually falls into one of three categories: infection, malignancy, or autoimmune process.

H. Unknown source. 18% in one series of inpatients.

I. Factitious (self-induced) fever

IV. Database

A. Physical examination key points

1. **General appearance.** This factor can help determine whether the patient should receive empiric antibiotic therapy based on the most likely cause.

2. **Vital signs.** Take both oral and rectal temperatures. Neutropenia is a contraindication to taking rectal temperature. A rectal temperature should be taken to make sure the oral temperature is not falsely elevated secondary to recent consumption of a hot liquid or smoking. Check pulse and blood pressure to make sure

the patient is hemodynamically stable. Hypotension suggests sepsis or volume depletion, possibly secondary to the fever. (The heart rate should increase 9 bpm for each 1 °F increase in temperature.) If the heart rate does *not* increase (*pulse-temperature dissociation*), consider psittacosis (*Chlamydia psittaci*), brucellosis, typhoid fever (*Salmonella typhi*), atypical pneumonia (*Mycoplasma, Chlamydia pneumoniae, Legionella pneumophila*), malaria, drug fever, central fever, and lymphoma.

3. **Skin.** Check IV sites, if any. Examine skin for rashes; if a rash involves the palms and soles, consider Rocky Mountain spotted fever, secondary syphilis, and Stevens-Johnson syndrome (hypersensitivity drug reaction). Look for splinter hemorrhages under the fingernails, Osler nodes, and Janeway lesions, which suggest endocarditis.

4. **HEENT.** Look for evidence of conjunctivitis, sinusitis (can be caused by a nasogastric tube—the nasogastric tube may have been removed several days before onset of symptoms), otitis, and pharyngitis. Cotton-wool spots and flame hemorrhages on funduscopic examination could indicate systemic candidiasis, endocarditis, or cytomegalovirus. Conjunctival hemorrhages are seen with endocarditis as well as severe thrombocytopenia.

5. **Neck.** Check for meningeal signs, including Kernig's and Brudzinski's signs.

6. **Lymph nodes.** Including cervical, supraclavicular, epitrochlear, axillary, and inguinal nodes. Enlarged lymph nodes may suggest cause of fever such as lymphoma or focus the examination for a bacterial infection to a particular area.

7. **Lungs.** A unilateral increase in tactile fremitus, dullness to percussion, bronchial breath sounds, inspiratory crackles, egophony, and whispered pectoriloquy suggest pneumonia.

8. **Heart.** A murmur, especially a new regurgitant murmur, suggests endocarditis.

9. **Abdomen.** Listen for bowel sounds; palpate and percuss for signs of tenderness. Check for *Murphy's sign* (while palpating the right upper quadrant, tenderness is elicited and there is inspiratory arrest with deep inspiration), which is seen in cholecystitis. Examine for costovertebral angle tenderness suggesting pyelonephritis.

10. **Genitourinary system.** Exclude pelvic inflammatory disease or tubo-ovarian abscess in a female and epididymitis or orchitis in a male. Also check prostate for tenderness.

11. **Extremities.** Check intravenous sites for erythema and tenderness. Look for joint effusions or tenderness.

B. **Laboratory data**

1. **Complete blood count with differential.** An elevated WBC count and left shift and bandemia suggest an infectious etiology. Eosinophilia suggests drug reaction, neoplasm, rheumatologic

disease, or parasitic infection. A low WBC count may suggest overwhelming sepsis, a collagen vascular disease such as SLE, a viral infection, or a process that has replaced the normal bone marrow (lymphoma, carcinoma, or a granulomatous disease such as tuberculosis or histoplasmosis).

2. **Blood cultures.** Usually two sets; three sets if endocarditis is suspected. Fungal isolators are important if the patient is immunocompromised or has been on previous antibiotics with an indwelling catheter.

3. **Culture tips of central lines.** If a patient with a central venous catheter becomes febrile and diagnostic evaluation fails to reveal a source of infection, the venous catheter is assumed to be the culprit and must be removed. Be sure to culture the tip of the catheter. One may try to treat before removing the catheter in patients with indwelling intravenous catheters (eg, Hickman and Groshong catheters).

4. **Sputum Gram's stain and culture.** Request a Gram's stain and culture if there is a productive cough.

5. **Urinalysis and culture.** Rule out cystitis, prostatitis, or pyelonephritis. Sterile pyuria suggests tuberculosis, *Chlamydia, Ureaplasma,* SLE, or, if the WBCs are eosinophils (interstitial nephritis), a drug reaction.

6. **Miscellaneous tests.** In certain circumstances if clinically indicated, order liver function tests, erythrocyte sedimentation rate, C-reactive protein (CRP), hepatitis serologies, PPD and anergy screen, culture for acid-fast bacillus and fungus, examination of peripheral blood smear, *Legionella* titers, viral titers, fungal serologies, rapid plasma reagin (RPR), DFA stains for *Pneumocystis* and *Legionella, Legionella* urine antigen, *Histoplasma* urine antigen, stool stains for fecal leukocytes, enteric pathogens, *C difficile* toxin, antistreptolysin-O (ASO) titer, antinuclear antibody (ANA), lumbar puncture.

C. **Radiologic and other studies**

1. **Chest x-ray.** Should be obtained with a fever of unknown source.

2. **Sinus CT.** Should be obtained if sinus tenderness or discharge is present or if a nasogastric tube is or has recently been in place.

3. **Acute abdominal series.** Should be obtained if peritoneal signs are present or if bowel or viscus obstruction or perforation is suspected.

4. **Ultrasound.** To assess the gallbladder and biliary tree. Ultrasonography can also be used to detect abdominal, renal, and pelvic masses.

5. **HIDA scan.** If acute cholecystitis is suspected.

6. **Bone scan/MRI.** If osteomyelitis is suspected.

7. **CT scans.** To detect subphrenic, abdominal, pelvic, and intracranial lesions.

8. **Echocardiogram.** Especially if blood cultures are positive. Sensitivity is not high enough that a normal transthoracic echocardiogram rules out endocarditis; however, transesophageal echocardiography has a 90% sensitivity.

9. **Lumbar puncture.** In any patient with fever and unexplained mental status changes as well as any patient with suspected meningitis (see Section III, Chapter 10, Lumbar Puncture, p 440).

10. **Thoracentesis.** Should be performed with unexplained fever and a pleural effusion or with pneumonia and a pleural effusion (see Section III, Chapter 14, Thoracentesis, p 459).

V. Plan. The plan depends on the clinical setting. Many of the previously mentioned tests should be obtained only in certain circumstances and only if a previous workup has been unrevealing. The initial workup of a febrile patient late at night will not be as exhaustive as a more leisurely performed FUO evaluation.

A. Initial assessment

1. **Rule out hemodynamic instability.**

2. **Review medications.** Especially looking for any recent changes.

3. **Obtain appropriate cultures.** Blood cultures from at least two different sites if possible.

4. **Reduce patient's temperature.** Give antipyretics such as acetaminophen 650 mg PO or PR. If the patient has underlying cardiac disease, the temperature should be brought down quickly to avoid cardiac decompensation.

5. **Monitor for dehydration.** Insensible losses increase with a fever.

6. **Consider antibiotics.** If the patient is *hemodynamically stable* and there is no apparent source of infection, *it is often prudent to withhold antibiotics unless the patient is immunocompromised.* As noted in the differential, the causes of fever are many and often nonbacterial. Unneeded empiric antibiotics can confuse the issue in many cases.

B. Fever with hypotension. *Septic shock is a medical emergency.* Begin fluid resuscitation with normal saline through a large-bore IV or central line, place the patient in Trendelenburg position, begin appropriate broad-spectrum antibiotics, and transfer to an ICU. The antibiotics chosen should provide coverage for gram-positive and gram-negative aerobic and anaerobic bacteria unless the source of the sepsis is obvious. If the patient's blood pressure fails to respond to fluids, begin a dopamine infusion at 2–5 µg/kg/min. The use of high-dose IV steroids is warranted if you suspect addisonian crisis. Physiologic steroid replacement may be used with severe sepsis or septic shock. Decadron 10 mg IV Q 6 hr for 4 days should be given if meningitis is suspected.

C. IV catheter infection. Remove the offending peripheral IV, apply local heat, use anti-inflammatory agents if it is a peripheral site, and administer antibiotics. A first-generation cephalosporin (cephalothin or cephalexin) or nafcillin can be used. Vancomycin should be reserved for use in suspected or culture-proven methicillin-resistant *Staphylococcus aureus* (MRSA) infection or *Staphylococcus epidermidis*. If you feel a warm, tender, swollen vein or if the patient has a history of IV drug abuse, suspect septic thrombophlebitis. Obtain a surgery consultation immediately and begin antibiotics. If a central line is in place, change all line(s) to different site(s), culture the catheter tip(s), and begin antibiotics. Gram-positive organisms are likely causes.

D. **Pneumonia.** Initial treatment of pneumonia should be based on results of Gram's stain and the clinical picture. Recent guidelines suggest that community-acquired pneumonia in a normal host requiring hospitalization should be treated with a fluoroquinolone (such as levofloxacin or gatifloxacin) alone OR a third-generation cephalosporin (ceftriaxone or cefotaxime) PLUS a macrolide combination OR a beta-lactam/beta-lactamase inhibitor (such as Unasyn or Zosyn) PLUS a macrolide. With a severe community-acquired pneumonia (altered mental status, pulse > 125 bpm, respiratory rate > 30 per minute, systolic blood pressure < 90, temperature < 35 °C or > 40 °C), treatment should consist of a macrolide OR fluoroquinolone PLUS a third-generation cephalosporin OR beta-lactam/beta-lactamase inhibitor combination. If *Pseudomonas aeruginosa* infection is suspected (as in a patient with cystic fibrosis), then empiric therapy should provide double coverage consisting of an antipseudomonal agent (eg, piperacillin, piperacillin-tazobactam, imipenem, meropenem, or cefepime) plus ciprofloxacin OR an antipseudomonal agent plus an aminoglycoside PLUS a respiratory fluoroquinolone OR a macrolide. If the patient is allergic to penicillin, use aztreonam PLUS a fluoroquinolone (levofloxacin, gatifloxacin, or moxifloxacin) with or without an aminoglycoside. Hospital-acquired pneumonia or pneumonia in an immunocompromised host also requires broader coverage. Antipseudomonal coverage as outlined above must be considered. Caution is advised when administering aminoglycosides to patients with renal insufficiency. A Gram's stain can also be helpful in guiding therapy. If there are gram-positive cocci in clusters, the chosen antibiotic regimen should include vancomycin until the possibility of MRSA is excluded. Be sure to adjust the dose of vancomycin with renal insufficiency.

E. **Febrile, neutropenic patient.** If there is evidence of infection or fever with an absolute neutrophil count (ANC) below 500/μL, the patient should be pancultured immediately (body fluid cultures as indicated, eg, blood and urine) and broad-spectrum antibiotics initiated. The specific pathogens found are almost always pyogenic or enteric bacteria or certain fungi. These are usually endogenous to the patient and include *Staphylococcus* from skin and gram-negative organisms from the GI or urinary tract. In febrile neutropenic patients who were bacteremic, one study found that 46% of the isolated organisms were gram-positive (as high as 60–70% in one reference), 42% were gram-negative, and 12% were polymicrobial. Antibiotic coverage should therefore include both gram-positive and gram-negative bacteria. One may treat with one drug, such as ceftazidime, imipenem, cefepime, or meropenem; or two drugs, such as an aminoglycoside (amikacin, gentamicin, or tobramycin) plus an antipseudomonal beta-lactam (ceftazidime, piperacillin, ticarcillin, ticarcillin plus clavulanate). An aminoglycoside may be added, depending on how toxic the patient's condition appears. Vancomycin should be added if the patient is at high risk (catheter-related infection is suspected, significant mucosal damage from chemotherapy, use of prophylactic quinolone antibiotics, septic shock or cardiovascular compromise, colonization with penicillin- or cephalosporin-resistant *Streptococcus pneumoniae* or with MRSA, and positive blood cultures for gram-positive bacteria before determination of antibiotic susceptibility). An antifungal agent (amphotericin B) should be added on day 5–7 if the ANC remains < 500/mm^3 and the patient remains febrile despite antibiotics. When using vancomycin, aminoglycosides, and amphotericin B in patients on cisplatin or cyclosporine, monitor renal function closely. Neutropenia with infection is a medical emergency requiring immediate investigation and treatment.

F. Meningitis. *Meningitis is a medical emergency.* A lumbar puncture should be done as quickly as possible, especially if the patient has no history of a bleeding disorder and no focal neurologic deficits or papilledema and if you have no reason to suspect an intracranial abscess. Begin giving antibiotics as you are doing the lumbar puncture. Decadron 10 mg IV Q 6 hr × 4 days should be administered before or with the first dose of antibiotics. If for any reason there is a delay in performing the lumbar puncture (such as obtaining a CT scan of the head because of papilledema), the antibiotics should be administered immediately and not delayed until after the procedure. A third-generation cephalosporin such as cefotaxime (Claforan) or ceftriaxone (Rocephin) should be given for meningitis of unknown etiology. Empiric therapy for meningitis should also cover for *Listeria monocytogenes* (ampicillin) if the patient is immunocompromised or over 50 years old. Vancomycin should be included if there is a high rate of penicillin-resistant pneumococcus in the community. Vancomycin and ceftazidime would be recommended for patients with a CNS shunt, recent neurosurgery, or head trauma. Otherwise, antibiotic therapy should be adjusted based on the Gram's stain. Acyclovir should be added if herpes simplex virus meningoencephalitis is suspected.

G. Cholecystitis. Obtain an ultrasound and/or HIDA scan, begin antibiotics (ticarcillin/clavulanate or gentamicin plus ampicillin plus metronidazole, OR imipenem/cilastatin) and consult surgery.

H. Drug-induced fever. Discontinue all drugs that are possibly causing a drug fever, and substitute appropriate alternatives.

I. Thyroid storm. Treat with hydration, apply cooling blanket, and give saturated solution of potassium iodide (SSKI), beta-blockers (specifically propranolol), propylthiouracil, and glucocorticoids.

J. Addisonian crisis. Treat immediately with IV steroids such as dexamethasone 4 mg for 1 dose, perform Cortrosyn stimulation test, and then begin a glucocorticoid (hydrocortisone 100 mg IV push, then 100 mg IV Q 6–8 hr). Dexamethasone does not interfere with the Cortrosyn stimulation test.

K. Malignant neuroleptic syndrome. Treatment consists of discontinuation of the neuroleptic agents, general supportive measures, and consideration of dantrolene (Dantrium) 50 mg PO Q 12 hr.

L. Uncertain or unknown diagnosis. Remember to consider pulmonary infarction and myocardial infarction.

REFERENCES

Balk RA: Conundrums in the management of critically ill patients: Steroids for Septic Shock. Back from the dead? Chest 2003;124:1733.

Bohr D: Fever of unknown origin. In: Fletcher SW, Fletcher RH, Aronson MD, eds. UpToDate [CD-ROM]. Version 8.1. Wellesley, MA;2000. www.uptodate.com

de Gans J, van de Beek D. Dexamethasone in adults with bacterial meningitis. N Engl J Med 2002;347:1549.

Hughes WT, Armstrong D, Bodey GP et al: 1997 Guidelines for the use of antimicrobial agents in neutropenic patients and unexplained fever. Clin Infect Dis 1997;25:551.

Infectious Diseases Society of America: Update of practice guidelines for the management of community-acquired pneumonia in immunocompetent adults. Clin Infect Dis 2003;37:1405.

Mackowiak PA: Temperature regulation and the pathogenesis of fever. In: Mandell GL, Bennett JE, Dolin R, eds. *Principles and Practice of Infectious Diseases.* 5th ed. Churchill Livingstone;2000:604.

O'Grady NP, Barie PS, Bartlett JG et al: Practice guidelines for evaluating new fever in critically ill adult patients. Clin Infect Dis 1998;26:1042.

Quagliarello VJ, Scheld MW: Treatment of bacterial meningitis. N Engl J Med 1997;336:708.

23. FEVER IN THE HIV-POSITIVE PATIENT

I. Problem. A 35-year-old man presents to the emergency room with a fever to 102.5 °F for 2 days. The patient is known to be HIV-positive but has not yet had an AIDS-defining illness.

II. Immediate Questions

A. Have there been any constitutional symptoms, including headache, anorexia, weight loss, fatigue, or malaise? Any of these can occur periodically through the course of HIV and may occur more frequently in the late stages of the disease. Night sweats are sometimes reported and are most often secondary to an infectious process or lymphoma.

B. What is the fever history? When did it start? How high has the temperature risen? HIV-related fever is usually no higher than 102.0 °F. Symptoms such as chills and rigors are uncommon with HIV-related fever and are more often associated with bacterial infections. Elevation of temperature above 102 °F strongly suggests an opportunistic infection. Remember, however, that nonopportunistic pathogens (eg, *Streptococcus pneumoniae, Haemophilus influenzae*) are potential causes of pneumonia in an HIV-positive patient and should be considered as etiologic agents along with opportunistic pathogens.

C. Are there any specific symptoms? The physical examination and further laboratory testing will be directed by specific symptoms, such as a history of visual problems, dysphagia, cough and dyspnea, diarrhea, focal neurologic symptoms, mental status changes, or skin lesions. Headache may be a constitutional symptom or a symptom associated with specific central nervous system (CNS) diseases. About 50% of patients with *Toxoplasma gondii* infections of the CNS complain of headache.

D. Does the patient have AIDS? What was the last CD4 count? If the patient has AIDS, what was the indicator disease? This presentation could be a recurrence because many of the infectious agents associated with AIDS recur, such as *Pneumocystis carinii, Salmonella typhi, Cryptococcus neoformans,* and *T gondii.* Certain infections do not occur until the CD4 count is very low (< 50/mL), such as *Mycobacterium avium-intracellulare* (MAI).

III. Differential Diagnosis. There are multiple causes of fever in this setting. The HIV-positive patient is a special problem because you must consider not only opportunistic infections seen frequently in this population but also other causes of fever that occur in non–HIV-positive patients. (See Section I, Chapter 22, Fever, p 133.) Most opportunistic infections occur when the CD4 count is < 200/mL; they are especially common when the CD4 count is < 50/mL.

A. Drug fever. Antiretroviral agents rarely cause a fever, but zidovudine (AZT) and zalcitabine (ddC) may cause fever. Fever while on abacavir may represent a life-threatening hypersensitivity reaction. Antimicrobials, such as sulfonamides and beta-lactams, are common causes of fever. Relative bradycardia is the cardinal finding in drug fever (be sure to eliminate other causes of relative bradycardia [eg, use beta-blockers in the presence of another source of fever] in febrile patients before applying this in your differential).

B. Sinusitis. Bacterial sinusitis may occur at any time during the course of HIV infection but is more severe in the later stages. Presentation may include headache, fever, or congestion. Likely pathogens include *S pneumoniae, H influenzae,* and *Staphylococcus aureus.*

C. **Eye disease.** Retinitis can occur at low CD4 counts, especially < 50/mL. The most common cause of retinitis is cytomegalovirus (CMV). Presentation includes floaters, blurred vision, and visual field defects. Pain is not a symptom of CMV retinitis; fever is nonspecific and frequently absent. Patients with the above symptoms should immediately be seen by an ophthalmologist. CMV retinitis characteristically has a "spaghetti and cheese" appearance (whitish exudate with surrounding edema and hemorrhage). Other organisms that cause retinitis include varicella-zoster virus, *Toxoplasma,* and *P carinii.* Other eye diseases include optic neuritis, conjunctival Kaposi's sarcoma, and herpetic keratitis.

D. **Oral disease.** Oral disease rarely causes fever but may signify more widespread disease. For example, darkly pigmented nodular lesions on the hard palate suggest widespread Kaposi's sarcoma.

E. **Pulmonary disease.** Pulmonary disease with fever can be caused by a wide variety of bacteria, fungi, viruses, protozoa, and tumors.
 1. **Bacterial pneumonia.** Common organisms include *S pneumoniae*, *H influenzae, and S aureus.* In addition to fever, cough, pleuritic chest pain, sputum production, an increased white blood cell (WBC) count may be present. Focal infiltrates are usually seen on chest x-ray.
 2. **Acid-fast organisms.** Consider *Mycobacterium tuberculosis* (TB) if fever has been present for > 2 weeks. Remember that HIV patients may present more frequently with extrapulmonary signs and symptoms. (One study found mycobacteremia in 49% of TB patients with CD4 < 100.) TB occurs most frequently at CD4 counts < 500/mL, but it can occur at any time during the course of the disease regardless of the CD4 count. A negative PPD does not rule out TB, especially at low CD4 counts. Chest x-ray findings vary from the classic apical cavitary lesion to hilar adenopathy, nodules or infiltrates in any lung field, or a normal chest x-ray (21% in one series). MAI may also cause diarrhea as well as fever and pulmonary disease. Often MAI occurs very late in the course of the disease (CD4 counts < 50/mL).
 3. **Fungal infections.** *Pneumocystis carinii* pneumonia (PCP) tends to have a prodromal illness for 1–2 weeks. PCP is the most common indicator disease for AIDS. Progressive dyspnea, nonproductive cough, and fever are common symptoms. Diffuse bilateral interstitial pulmonary infiltrates are frequently seen on chest x-ray. An increased lactate dehydrogenase level may be present. With advanced HIV infection (CD4 < 50) other fungi also should be considered (eg, *Aspergillus*, *Coccidiodes*, *Cryptococcus*, *Histoplasma*).

F. **Cardiac disease.** Consider endocarditis, especially if a new murmur is present.

G. Gastrointestinal disease

1. **Esophagitis** generally presents with dysphagia. *Candida* esophagitis may or may not present with fever. Other common causes of esophagitis are CMV and herpes simplex virus.

2. **Diarrhea.** Often fever and abdominal pain accompany low-volume diarrhea and mucoid stools. Depending on the etiologic agent, blood may be present. *S typhi* often causes recurrent bacteremia and diarrhea. Other bacterial pathogens may include *Campylobacter jejuni, Shigella flexneri, Clostridium difficile,* and MAI, as well as enterotoxigenic *Escherichia coli.* CMV and a variety of parasites including *Cryptosporidium, Isospora belli,* and *Microsporidia* may cause diarrhea and fever. *Histoplasma capsulatum* can also cause diarrhea in HIV-positive patients.

H. Hepatobiliary/pancreatic disease

1. **Sclerosing cholangitis-like syndrome.** Fever, right upper quadrant pain, and progressive cholangitis have been described in patients with *Cryptosporidium,* CMV, *Microsporidia,* and *Cyclospora* infection involving the biliary tract.

2. **Hepatitis A, B, or C**

3. **Cholestatic hepatitis.** Secondary to MAI, TB, *H capsulatum, C neoformans.*

4. **Pancreatitis.** May occur as a result of an opportunistic infection, increased triglycerides, or drug toxicity (eg, pentamidine, didanosine, and stavudine, TMP-SMX).

I. Skin. Bacillary angiomatosis thought to be secondary to *Bartonella (Rochalimaea) henselae* causes firm purplish-to-reddish papules, subcutaneous nodules, or cellulitis-like plaques. Fever is unlikely unless there is a secondary infection. Herpes simplex virus type I or II may cause primary or recurrent erythematous/vesicular lesions with ulceration.

J. Neurologic disease. Many agents can cause a variety of neurologic complications, including meningitis, encephalitis, and mass lesions.

1. **Meningitis.** HIV can initially cause an aseptic meningitis. *C neoformans* is a common cause of meningitis. Presenting symptoms include fever, night sweats, and headaches. *M tuberculosis* as well as *S pneumoniae, H influenzae,* and *Neisseria meningitidis* need to be considered as etiologic agents.

2. **Encephalitis.** *T gondii* causes altered mental status, headache, fever, and focal neurologic findings.

3. **Mass lesions** can be caused by a variety of infectious agents (*T gondii, M tuberculosis, Nocardia asteroides, C neoformans, H capsulatum*) and noninfectious agents (primary CNS lymphoma, metastatic lymphoma, and Kaposi's sarcoma).

K. Malignant disease. Malignancies, including B-cell non-Hodgkin's lymphoma, Kaposi's sarcoma, and Hodgkin's lymphoma, may have associated fever.

L. Gynecologic complications. Gynecologic complications, including sexually transmitted disease (*Neisseria gonorrhoeae, Chlamydia trachomatis*), can cause fever as well as a vaginal discharge and pain.

IV. Database

A. Physical examination key points

1. **General appearance.** First, determine whether the patient appears ill or septic.
2. **Vital signs.** Should be evaluated for hypotension and tachycardia, either of which may be a sign of sepsis.
3. **HEENT.** Perform ophthalmologic exam to check for papilledema and signs of retinitis. Palpate sinuses for tenderness; inspect oral cavity for signs of candidiasis or hairy leukoplakia.
4. **Neck.** Check for neck stiffness as a sign of meningitis; however, meningeal signs are often absent in AIDS patients with meningitis. Palpate for lymphadenopathy. Check the jugular veins for distention to help assess fluid status.
5. **Lungs.** Percuss the lungs for dullness, which may occur with a focal infiltrate. Dullness at one base may indicate a pleural effusion. Auscultate for inspiratory crackles as a sign of consolidation.
6. **Heart.** Determine rate and note any murmurs.
7. **Abdominal exam.** Note any hepatomegaly or splenomegaly, and look for signs of peritoneal inflammation.
8. **Extremities/skin.** Note general appearance of the skin; look for any rashes, papules, or nodules.
9. **Genitourinary/rectal.** Inspect genitalia, noting presence and characteristics of any discharge. Examine the rectum for perineal abscess.
10. **Neurologic exam.** Should be *thorough,* including mental status examination.

B. Laboratory data.
Proceed with your workup based on findings from the history and physical examination. Many times specific aspects of the patient's history and physical will point you to a specific organ system. When only constitutional symptoms are present, diagnostic testing should include complete blood count and differential, CD4 count, HIV viral load, electrolytes, liver function tests, urinalysis, and blood for bacterial, acid-fast bacteria (AFB), and fungal cultures. Consider serum for cryptococcal antigen and urine for histoplasma antigen. A chest x-ray should also be obtained.

1. **Complete blood count with differential.** An elevated WBC count with an increase in banded neutrophils suggests a bacterial infection. The total WBC and lymphocyte count often decreases, especially late in HIV disease. In addition, many medications (eg, AZT, trimethoprim-sulfamethoxazole) can suppress the WBC count.

2. **Liver function tests** (aspartate aminotransferase, alanine amino-transferase, bilirubin, γ-glutamyltransferase, alkaline phosphatase). Look for abnormalities suggesting hepatitis, cholangitis, or liver involvement from a systemic disease.

3. **Arterial blood gases (ABG).** Essential in the evaluation of cough and dyspnea. Hypoxemia is almost universally present with PCP.

4. **Urinalysis.** Pyuria with bacteria suggests a urinary tract infection. Sterile pyuria could result from *M tuberculosis, Chlamydia, Ureaplasma,* or fungal involvement of the urinary tract.

5. **Electrolytes, blood urea nitrogen, and creatinine.** To help assess volume status.

C. **Other studies**

1. **Stool tests.** If diarrhea is present, obtain stool for WBCs, culture for enteric pathogens, *C difficile* toxin, fungal smear and culture, and AFB stain and culture. In addition, stool needs to be carefully examined for parasites such as *Cryptosporidium* and *Microsporidium.*

2. **Sputum studies.** Expectorated sputum should be sent for Gram's stain, culture and sensitivity, AFB stain and culture, and fungal stain and culture. *P carinii* can be diagnosed in about 10% of cases via a silver stain of expectorated sputum. Sputum for AFB smear and culture should be obtained in an HIV patient with a fever and cough even if the chest x-ray is normal.

3. **Blood cultures.** Essential in the evaluation of an HIV patient with a fever. Fungi and mycobacteria as well as bacteria are potential isolates.

4. **Serum cryptococcal antigen test.** Order this test if meningitis is suspected; 70–90% of patients with cryptococcal meningitis have a positive serum cryptococcal antigen test. It may also be helpful in a patient with a fever without neurologic symptoms or signs. Also, consider this test when CD4 count is < 50/mL.

5. **Lumbar puncture.** Should be performed with mental status change, meningeal signs, or focal neurologic findings. An imaging study should be done first to rule out a space-occupying lesion. Be sure to obtain cerebrospinal fluid (CSF) for cryptococcal antigen. The sensitivity of the AFB smear of CSF for diagnosing *M tuberculosis* increases with larger amounts of fluid (at least 10 mL) and with repeated lumbar punctures.

6. **Chest x-ray.** Essential in the initial evaluation of an HIV patient with a fever or cough and dyspnea. Look for infiltrates, pleural effusions, and cavitary lesions.

7. **CNS imaging.** Necessary with mental status changes and symptoms or signs of CNS disease such as papilledema. Look for a space-occupying lesion, which may be secondary to primary lymphoma, metastatic lymphoma, Kaposi's sarcoma, *T gondii,* or *M tuberculosis.* Magnetic resonance imaging is more sensitive than computerized tomography scans and is the preferred modality to image the CNS in this setting.

8. Bronchoscopy. With brushings and bronchoalveolar lavage. Essential in the evaluation of an HIV patient with an infiltrate on chest x-ray when sputum does not reveal the cause.

V. Plan. The treatment of various causes of fever in the HIV patient is beyond the scope of this book. Refer to references specific to this topic. Discussed below are the treatments for the more common causes of fever in the HIV patient and salient points.

A. General. See Section I, Chapter 22, Fever, V, p 138.

B. Specific infectious causes

1. *Pneumocystis carinii* pneumonia. First line of treatment is trimethoprim (TMP)-sulfamethoxazole (SMX) PO or IV (15–20 mg/kg/day TMP and 75–100 mg/kg/day SMX in 3–4 divided doses Q day). Pentamidine 4 mg/kg/day Q day, or dapsone 100 mg/day with TMP, can be used. Atovaquone 750 mg bid is reserved for patients who cannot tolerate TMP-SMX or pentamidine. Corticosteroids (prednisone 40 mg bid for 5 days followed by a taper) should be given if the initial pO_2 is < 70 mm Hg.

2. *Mycobacterium tuberculosis.* Four first-line drugs should be used initially, including isoniazid (INH) 300 mg once Q day; rifampin 600 mg once Q day; pyrazinamide (PZA) 20–35 mg/kg/day, once Q day; and ethambutol 25 mg/kg or streptomycin 0.5–1 g Q day to 1 g twice weekly. There is an increasing incidence of multidrug-resistant tuberculosis, especially in HIV-infected patients. Strict respiratory isolation must be observed. Consider use of corticosteroids (prednisone 60 mg PO Q day for 1–2 weeks followed by a taper) with tuberculous meningitis.

3. **Cytomegalovirus retinitis.** Give ganciclovir or foscarnet.

4. **Cryptococcal meningitis.** Amphotericin B 0.7–1 mg/kg/day with flucytosine 100 mg/kg/day in divided doses every 6 hr or fluconazole 400 mg/day with or without flucytosine.

5. *Toxoplasma gondii* infection. Pyrimethamine and sulfadiazine or clindamycin. Also needed is folinic acid to prevent myelosuppression from the pyrimethamine.

REFERENCES

Bartlett JG, Gallant JE: *Medical Management of HIV Infection*, 2003 ed. Johns Hopkins;2003.

Bissuel F, Leport C, Perronne C et al: Fever of unknown origin in HIV-infected patients: A critical analysis of a retrospective series of 57 cases. J Intern Med 1994;236:529.

Carrier J: MAC infections in HIV infected patients. In: Fletcher SW, Fletcher RH, Aronson MD, eds. UpToDate [CD-ROM]. Version 8.1. Wellesley, MA;2000. www.uptodate.com

Falloon J: Pulmonary manifestations of human immunodeficiency virus infection. In: Mandell GL, Bennett JE, Dolin R, eds. *Principles and Practice of Infectious Diseases.* 5th ed. Churchill Livingstone;2000:1415.

Holloway RG, Kieburtz KD: Neurologic manifestations of human immunodeficiency virus infection. In: Mandell GL, Bennett JE, Dolin R, eds. *Principles and Practice of Infectious Diseases.* 5th ed. Churchill Livingstone;2000:1432.

Jones BE, Young SM, Antoniskis D, Davidson PT, Kramer F, Barnes PF: Relationship of the manifestations of tuberculosis to CD4 cell counts in patients with human immunodeficiency virus infection. Am Rev Respir Dis 1993;148:1292.

Keiper MD, Beumont M, Elshami A, Langlotz CP, Miller WT: CD4 T lymphocyte count and the radiographic presentation of pulmonary tuberculosis. A study of the relationship between these factors in patients with human immunodeficiency virus infection. Chest 1995;107:74.

Sande M, Volberding P: *Medical Management of AIDS.* 6th ed. Saunders;1999.

Sepkowitz K, Talzak E, Carrow M et al: Fever among outpatients with advanced human immunodeficiency virus infection. Arch Intern Med 1993;153:1909.

Sulkowski MS, Chaisson RE: Gastrointestinal and hepatobiliary manifestations of human immunodeficiency virus infection. In: Mandell GL, Bennett JE, Dolin R, eds. *Principles and Practice of Infectious Diseases.* 5th ed. Churchill Livingstone;2000:1426.

Vander Els N: Clinical features and diagnosis of TB in HIV infected patients. In: Fletcher SW, Fletcher RH, Aronson MD, eds. UpToDate [CD-ROM]. Version 8.1. Wellesley, MA;2000. www.uptodate.com.

24. FOLEY CATHETER PROBLEMS

See also Section III, Chapter 4, Bladder Catheterization, p 422.

I. Problem. The Foley catheter is not draining in a patient admitted 2 days previously for congestive heart failure.

II. Immediate Questions

    A. What has the urine output been? If the urine output has slowly tapered off, then the problem may be oliguria rather than a nonfunctioning Foley catheter. A Foley catheter that has never put out urine may not be in the bladder.

    B. Is the urine grossly bloody; are there any clots in the tubing or collection bag? Clots or tissue fragments, such as those present after prostate or bladder resection, can obstruct the flow of urine in a Foley catheter.

    C. Is the patient complaining of pain? Bladder distention often causes severe lower abdominal pain; bladder spasms are painful and may cause urine to leak out around the catheter rather than through the catheter.

    D. Was any difficulty encountered in catheter insertion? Problematic urethral catheterization should raise the possibility that the catheter is not in the bladder. Patients with known pathologic conditions (eg, urethral stricture, benign prostatic hypertrophy, prostate cancer) may be at higher risk of faulty catheter placement.

III. Differential Diagnosis

    A. Low urine output. It may be a result of dehydration, hemorrhage, or acute renal failure, as well as a host of other causes (see Section I, Chapter 51, Oliguria/Anuria, p 283).

  B. Obstructed Foley catheter
    1. Kinking of catheter or tubing
    2. Clots, tissue fragments. Most common after transurethral resection of the prostate or bladder tumor. Grossly bloody urine suggests that a clot has formed. Tea-colored or rusty urine suggests that an organized clot may be present even though the urine is no longer grossly bloody. Bleeding often accompanies "accidental" catheter removal with the balloon still inflated and with a coagulopathy.
    3. Sediment/stones. Chronically indwelling catheters (usually > 1 month) can become encrusted and obstructed. Calculi can lodge in the catheter.

  C. Improperly positioned Foley catheter. Improper positioning is much more common in males. In traumatic urethral disruption associated with a pelvic fracture, the catheter can pass into the periurethral tissues. Strictures or prostatic hypertrophy may cause the end of the catheter to be positioned in the urethra and not the bladder. Improper catheter placement technique can cause a false passage.

  D. Bladder spasms. The patient may complain of severe suprapubic pain or pain radiating to the end of the penis. With a spasm, urine may leak around the sides of the catheter. Spasms are common after bladder or prostate surgery or surgery near the bladder. Spasms may be the only catheter complaint or may be so severe as to obstruct the flow of urine.

  E. Bladder disruption. Resulting from blunt abdominal trauma or operative complication or caused by severe distention secondary to a blocked catheter.

  F. Inability to deflate Foley balloon. Rare with modern catheters. All catheters should be test inflated and deflated before insertion.

IV. Database
  A. Physical examination key points
    1. Vital signs. Check for tachycardia or hypotension, which is characteristic of hypovolemia and may explain the low urine output.
    2. Abdominal exam. Determine whether the bladder is distended (suprapubic dullness to percussion with or without tenderness). This may be indicative of an obstructed Foley catheter. Percuss the bladder to help identify distention.
    3. Genital exam. Bleeding at the meatus suggests urethral trauma or partial removal of the catheter with the balloon inflated.
    4. Rectal exam. A "floating prostate" suggests urethral disruption.
    5. General. Look for signs of hypovolemia causing low urine output, such as poor skin turgor (which may be a normal variant in the elderly) and dry mucous membranes.

  B. Laboratory data. Most problems are usually mechanical in nature, so laboratory data are somewhat limited in this setting.

1. **Blood urea nitrogen (BUN), serum creatinine.** Elevations may be seen with cases of renal insufficiency. An elevated BUN-to-creatinine ratio (> 20:1) suggests volume depletion.
2. **Coagulation studies.** Especially if bleeding is present. See Section I, Chapter 12, Coagulopathy, p 70.

C. **Radiologic and other studies.** In the acute setting of a Foley catheter problem, radiologic studies are usually not needed. Ultrasound may demonstrate a distended bladder or hydronephrosis in cases of obstructive uropathy, or ultrasound may be used to guide puncture of the balloon as a last resort. Cystogram may diagnose bladder preforation.

V. **Plan**

A. **Be sure the catheter is functioning.** A rule of thumb is that a catheter that will not irrigate is in the urethra and not in the bladder. Start by gently irrigating the catheter with aseptic technique using a catheter-tipped 60-mL syringe and sterile normal saline. This may dislodge any clots obstructing the catheter. If sterile saline cannot be satisfactorily instilled and completely aspirated, the catheter should be replaced. Catheter irrigation or changing the catheter in any patient who has undergone bladder or prostate surgery should not be done without input from the surgical team that performed the procedure.

B. **If the catheter irrigates freely, evaluate the patient for anuria.** See Section I, Chapter 51, Oliguria/Anuria,V, p 290.

C. **Bladder spasms.** Can be treated with oxybutynin (Ditropan, Ditropan XL, Oxytrol), tolterodine (Detrol, Detrol LA), propantheline (Pro-Banthine), or belladonna and opium (B&O) suppositories. (See Section VII, Therapeutics, p 576, 584, 513 for dosing.) Be sure to discontinue these medications before removing the catheter to allow normal bladder function.

D. **Techniques to deflate a Foley balloon that does not empty**
1. Cut off the valve; if this does not work, thread a 16F central venous catheter or 0.38 guidewire into the inflation channel, which may bypass the obstruction or perforate and deflate the balloon.
2. Injection of 5–10 mL mineral oil into the inflation port will cause balloon rupture in latex catheters in 5–10 minutes but NOT in silicone catheters. Follow-up cystoscopy is needed to make sure there are no retained fragments. (***Note***: Hyperinflation of the balloon to rupture it should not be done.)
3. As a last resort, ultrasound-directed transvesical needle puncture of the balloon may be needed.

REFERENCE

Shahbandi M, Parulkar BG: Foley catheter problems. In: Gomella LG, ed. *5 Minute Urology Consult.* Lippincott Williams & Wilkins;2000:50.

25. HEADACHE

I. **Problem.** You are called to the emergency room to evaluate a 58-year-old man who complains of a severe headache that has lasted for several hours.

II. **Immediate Questions**

A. **Has the patient experienced similar headaches before?** If the headache is similar to previous tension or migraine headaches, then the situation is unlikely to be urgent; however, if the headache is new or deviates from a previous pattern, several potentially serious conditions should be considered, including acute glaucoma, sinusitis, subarachnoid hemorrhage, meningitis, neoplasm, temporal arteritis, and early hypertensive encephalopathy.

B. **What are the patient's vital signs?** Although essential hypertension by itself is an infrequent cause of headache, it may exacerbate a preexisting vascular or tension headache. Diastolic blood pressures > 140 mm Hg can cause severe headache. A fever should alert the clinician to the possibility of subarachnoid hemorrhage, meningitis, temporal arteritis, or acute sinusitis.

C. **Is the patient taking any anticoagulants?** Does the patient have a predisposition to bleeding? Aspirin or coumadin increases the risk for an intracranial hemorrhage, especially with minor head trauma. Spontaneous intracranial bleeding occurs with platelet counts of less than $20,000/\mu L$.

III. **Differential Diagnosis.** A detailed, well-focused history is the most important tool for evaluating headache. Most headaches are secondary to either tension-type or migraine headaches. A headache may also be the only symptom of a more serious condition, such as an intracranial mass, temporal arteritis, meningitis, and subarachnoid hemorrhage.

A. **Tension-type headache**

1. **Episodic tension-type headache.** This is frequently described as a squeezing, "bandlike" tightness that is usually felt bilaterally. It may occur in the occipital, frontal, or bitemporal regions. Occasionally, patients with tension-type headaches describe a "throbbing" pain. This form of headache may last 30 minutes to 7 days; it is generally described as having a mild to moderate intensity. There is usually no aggravation from walking stairs or similar routine activities and no associated nausea or vomiting. Photophobia and phonophobia are absent, or only one is present.

2. **Chronic tension-type headache.** Same as tension-type headache, except for the number of days with such headaches: at least 15 days per month for at least 6 months

B. **Migraine headache.** Although the precise pathophysiology has not been fully ascertained, migraine is thought to be secondary to cerebral vasoconstriction followed by vasodilation. The initial vasoconstriction may be associated with a variety of neurologic deficits including visual disturbances (scotoma, zig-zag lines, bright lights), dysarthria, hemiparesis, and hemianesthesia. Of these, the visual phenomena are most common. These neurologic features generally last 5–30 minutes and are then followed by headache. The headache is usually pounding or throbbing but may be dull and boring. It is usually unilateral but may also occur bilaterally in any location. Anorexia, nausea, and vomiting are frequently associated. The attack may last several hours to 2–3 days and occasionally longer. Migraines are much more common in women. Three characteristic migraine patterns are recognized:

1. **Migraine without aura (common migraine).** This vascular headache is not preceded by neurologic deficits or visual disturbances. It is the most common type, especially in women.
2. **Migraine with aura (classic migraine).** The headache is preceded by visual deficits such as scotomata and field deficits, but can affect somatic sensation, speech, and motor function.
3. **Complicated migraine.** The headache is accompanied by neurologic symptoms including hemiplegia and ophthalmoplegia.

C. **Cluster headaches.** Cluster headaches are excruciating, usually unilateral, and frequently associated with ipsilateral nasal congestion, lacrimation, and conjunctival injection. Nausea, vomiting, photophobia, and phonophobia are absent in cluster headaches. Each headache typically lasts < 2 hours; however, multiple attacks can occur within a 24-hour period.

Onset shortly after falling asleep is common. Unlike migraine, cluster headaches most often affect men between the ages of 20 and 40. Recent data demonstrate a strong genetic component, at least in some families.

D. **Temporal arteritis.** Temporal arteritis should be considered in any patient older than 50 years presenting with a recent history of headache. Other symptoms such as malaise, weight loss, fever, and myalgias are frequently present. Jaw claudication is a classic symptom. It is especially important to ask about any new visual problems such as double or blurred vision. Temporal arteritis can cause sudden blindness as a result of inflammation of the ophthalmic artery. Early diagnosis and treatment with steroids are necessary to prevent this complication.

E. **Trigeminal neuralgia.** This condition is more common in the elderly. The pain is described as brief, but severe and jabbing. The pain is usually unilateral and localized to one or more divisions of the trigeminal nerve. Precipitants include talking, chewing, or having physical pressure exerted on a specific trigger area. The cause of trigeminal neuralgia is unknown.

F. **Cerebrovascular disease.** Headache can be a presenting complaint in some patients experiencing an acute stroke. When the internal carotid is involved, the headache is usually located in the frontal region; involvement of the vertebrobasilar system generally yields an occipital headache. The headache of a cerebrovascular accident may precede or follow focal neurologic symptoms.

G. **Sinusitis.** Headache is usually dull, aching, and frontally located. Pain is frequently worse in the morning when the patient awakens but improves as the sinuses drain during the day. If the patient displays an altered mental status or complains of a stiff neck, a complicated sinus infection should be suspected (brain abscess, meningitis, septic cavernous sinus thrombosis).

H. **Eye disease.** Glaucoma, keratitis, and uveitis all may cause headaches. The pain is usually dull and located in the periorbital or retroorbital regions.

I. **Dental disease.** The teeth are innervated by the second and third divisions of the trigeminal nerve; thus, disease involving these structures may cause pain referred to the face or head. Secondary muscle spasm may result.

J. **Temporomandibular joint disease.** Headache is usually unilateral on the side of face and head. It is described as "aching" in quality and is worsened with jaw movement.

K. **Mass lesions.** Both neoplasm and brain abscess can produce headache as a result of either increased pressure or distention of local structures. Any new neurologic deficit such as visual or motor loss or change in mental status should alert the clinician to the possibility of a mass lesion. Onset of new headache in a patient > 50 years suggests a mass lesion. Nonspecific features of headache resulting from a mass lesion include progressive worsening despite administration of analgesics; early-morning headache; headache exacerbated by coughing or sneezing; anorexia; and vomiting without nausea. It is important to note that these features also occur frequently with other types of headache, including chronic tension headache, migraine headache, cluster headache, and sinus headache.

L. **Subarachnoid hemorrhage.** The rupture of a cerebral aneurysm is associated with acute onset of a violent headache. The typical patient with a subarachnoid hemorrhage has a sudden onset of severe headache (frequently described as the worst headache of his or her life) that develops during exertion. Transient loss of consciousness or buckling of the legs often accompanies the headache. Vomiting soon follows. Between 20% and 50% of patients with documented subarachnoid hemorrhage report a distinct, unusually severe headache in the days or weeks before the index episode of bleeding, referred to as a warning headache. These so-called *thunderclap headaches* develop in seconds, achieve maximal intensity in minutes, and last hours to days.

The differential diagnosis includes subarachnoid hemorrhage, acute expansion, dissection, or thrombosis of unruptured aneurysms; cerebral venous sinus thrombosis; brief headaches during exertion and sexual intercourse; and benign thunderclap headaches. The physical exam may show retinal hemorrhages, restlessness, a diminished level of consciousness, and focal neurologic signs. Blood in the subarachnoid space may induce fever and nuchal rigidity resembling acute meningitis. Sentinel leaks (warning leaks) from a cerebral aneurysm are more subtle and frequently precede subsequent rupture. These headaches may be difficult to distinguish from tension headaches and may cause nonspecific symptoms such as myalgias or a stiff neck, which may be erroneously attributed to an acute viral illness.

M. Carotid or vertebral artery dissection. Unilateral head, face or neck pain, and a partial *Horner's syndrome* (miosis and ptosis without anhidrosis) with subsequent retinal or cerebral ischemia is the classic presentation of carotid artery dissection. The headache may be similar to the headache associated with subarachnoid hemorrhage (thunderclap headache) but the onset is usually insidious. Unilateral facial or orbital pain is common. Transient ischemic attacks or transient monocular blindness occurs hours to days after the onset of the pain. An occipital headache or neck pain followed by unilateral arm pain or weakness suggests vertebral artery dissection.

N. Acute febrile illness. Fever may cause a vascular-type throbbing headache that remits as the illness resolves. Any febrile patient in whom headache is a major complaint should also be suspected of having meningitis, especially if nuchal rigidity or other signs of meningeal irritation are present.

IV. Database

A. Physical examination key points

1. **Vital signs.** See II.B.
2. **HEENT**
   a. **Scalp.** Patients with both migraine and chronic tension headaches frequently complain of scalp tenderness, which may also suggest temporal arteritis.
   b. **Temporal arteries.** A diminished pulse or tender temporal arteries suggests arteritis; however, temporal arteries may feel normal to palpation in 30–40% of patients with temporal arteritis.
   c. **Eyes.** Examine for injected conjunctivae and excessive lacrimation, which occur with cluster headaches. Miosis and ptosis suggest carotid artery dissection as the cause of the headache. Examine the fundi for any signs of papilledema or optic nerve atrophy resulting from an intracerebral mass. Retinal hemorrhage may be observed after subarachnoid hemorrhage. Subhyaloid hemorrhages may be seen trapped behind

the vitreous humor at the edge of the optic disc, suggesting a sudden rise in intracranial pressure.

- **d. Sinuses.** Palpate or percuss the maxillary and frontal sinuses for tenderness.
- **e. Ears.** Examine the ears for signs of otitis media.
- **f. Mouth.** Examine dentition for painful teeth and the temporomandibular joint for crepitus, pain, or limited jaw opening.

3. **Neck.** Examine for any resistance to passive flexion of the neck, which suggests meningeal irritation from either subarachnoid hemorrhage or meningitis.

4. **Neurologic exam.** A detailed exam is mandated in any patient with a complaint of headache to identify localizing signs that would suggest a central nervous system mass lesion, meningitis, intracerebral hemorrhage, or carotid or vertebral artery dissection.

B. Laboratory data

1. **Complete blood count.** An elevated leukocyte count may suggest infection such as sinusitis or meningitis.

2. **Erythrocyte sedimentation rate (ESR).** Almost always > 50 mm/hr with temporal arteritis. However, on occasion the ESR is normal. If clinical suspicion is high, a temporal artery biopsy should never be deferred simply because of a normal ESR.

3. **Prothrombin time, partial thromboplastin time, and platelets.** Order these tests if you suspect or if the patient has an intracranial hemorrhage.

C. Radiologic and other studies. Neuroimaging should be performed in any patient with an acute onset of a severe headache (the "worst headache of my life"), with a chronic headache pattern that has recently changed in frequency or severity, or with progressive worsening of a headache despite appropriate therapy. Moreover, neuroimaging should be performed in any patient > 50 years with a new onset of headache or whose neurologic exam reveals focal findings. In addition, a head CT scan should be obtained in any patient who has onset of headache that is exacerbated with exertion, cough, Valsalva's maneuver, or sexual activity, or that awakens the patient at night, or in any patient who has an orbital bruit. Finally, neuroimaging should be performed in any patient with new onset of headache and a history of cancer or HIV.

1. **Sinus films or CT with coronal images.** If sinusitis is suspected.

2. **Head CT scan.** Helical CT angiography is useful in diagnosing carotid artery dissection and intracranial aneurysms.

3. **MRI.** Preferable when posterior fossa lesions or craniospinal abnormalities (eg, Arnold-Chiari malformation) are suspected or in a patient with HIV. MR angiography is replacing conventional angiography as the test of choice in diagnosing carotid or vertebral artery dissection and can be used to diagnose intracranial aneurysms.

　　4. **Lumbar puncture.** If meningitis is suspected, lumbar puncture should be performed and not delayed for a CT scan when papilledema is absent and the neurologic examination is nonfocal. Lumbar puncture should be performed when subarachnoid hemorrhage is suspected and CT results are negative, equivocal, or technically inadequate.

V. Plan. The initial goal in the management of headache is to exclude rare but potentially serious causes, such as brain tumor, subarachnoid hemorrhage, brain abscess, and meningitis. When these conditions have been excluded, treatment can be directed according to the type of headache. Only the management of tension-type headache, migraine headache, and cluster headache is discussed here.

A. Episodic tension-type headache

1. **Nonsteroidal anti-inflammatory drugs (NSAIDs).** Relief of pain can usually be obtained with simple analgesics such as aspirin, acetaminophen, and NSAIDs.

2. **Avoid analgesic combinations.** Such as ergotamines, caffeine, butalbital, and codeine.

B. Chronic tension-type headache. This condition is notoriously difficult to manage. As with episodic tension-type headache, avoid the chronic use of narcotic analgesics, which may result in narcotic dependence. In patients with chronic tension-type headache, the treatment goals are to initiate effective prophylactic treatment and to manage any residual headaches in a manner that prevents the frequent use of analgesics and the risk for progression to chronic daily headache syndrome.

　　Patients with chronic tension-type headache should limit their use of analgesics to two times weekly to prevent the development of chronic daily headache. Analgesics can be augmented with a sedating antihistamine, such as promethazine (Phenergan) and diphenhydramine (Benadryl), or an antiemetic, such as metoclopramide (Reglan) and prochlorperazine (Compazine). If this regimen is inadequate, the patient can try acetaminophen or aspirin combined with caffeine and butalbital. This combination is usually effective but is also the most common cause of chronic daily headache.

1. **A tricyclic antidepressant.** Amitriptyline (Elavil) 75 mg HS is one of the most useful agents for treating chronic tension headache. This medication should be used regardless of whether depression is overtly present. Start with 10–25 mg every night and increase the dose by 25 mg every 5–7 days to 75 mg.

2. **NSAIDs.** Aspirin 325–650 mg PO Q 6 hr, naproxen 275–550 mg Q 12 hr, or ibuprofen 400–600 mg PO Q 6 hr may be beneficial.

3. **Selective serotonin reuptake inhibitors (SSRIs).** Several of these agents (paroxetine [Paxil], venlafaxine [Effexor], and fluoxetine [Prozac]) have shown their efficacy in the prophylaxis of chronic tension-type headache in small studies.

4. **Massage of the neck and local application of heat.** When occipital, suboccipital, or cervical muscle spasm is present.
5. **Psychotherapy, relaxation therapy, and biofeedback.** May be used if preceding measures fail.
6. **Smoking cessation.** This is an important issue to address in patients with chronic tension-type headache.

C. **Migraine headache.** Several different medications are now administered in the management of acute migraine.

1. **NSAIDs.** For an early mild attack, treatment with a NSAID such as aspirin, ibuprofen 400–600 mg Q 4–6 hr, naproxen (Naprosyn) 550 mg Q 12 hr, tolfenamic acid, or the combination of acetaminophen, caffeine, and aspirin may be effective. Metoclopramide (Reglan) 10 mg PO can be given at this time to increase drug absorption and reduce nausea and vomiting. In addition, ketorolac, a parenteral NSAID, has been shown to be effective at 60 mg IM.

2. **Ergot alkaloids**
   a. **Dihydroergotamine.** There is good evidence for the efficacy and safety of intranasal dihydroergotamine (DHE) as monotherapy for acute migraine attacks
   b. *Caution:* Avoid administration of ergotamines in patients with peripheral vascular disease, coronary artery disease, hypertension, renal failure, hepatic disease, hyperthyroidism, and in pregnant patients. Do not use in patients on CYP3A4 inhibitors such as protease inhibitors, some macrolide antibiotics, or azole antifungals. Because ergot alkaloids decrease cerebral blood flow, they should be avoided in patients with complicated migraine.

3. **Triptans–serotonin agonists**
   a. **Sumatriptan (Imitrex) 6 mg SC.** Other regimens and routes are available. Sumatriptan has been found to be effective in relieving headache and accompanying symptoms (nausea, vomiting, and photo- and phonophobia). It is effective even when taken late during an attack. A second dose is usually not effective. *Caution:* The triptans are contraindicated in patients with known or suspected ischemic heart disease, a history of angina, ischemic or vasospastic (Prinzmetal's) angina, uncontrolled hypertension, peripheral vascular disease, recent monoamine oxidase inhibitor therapy, severe liver disease, and hemiplegic or basilar artery migraine. The safety of the triptans during pregnancy is unclear. Use with ergotamines is contraindicated.
   b. **Zolmitriptan (Zomig) 2.5 mg.** Give 1 tablet PO at the onset of headache. Repeat at 2 hours if the headache returns, not to exceed 10 mg in 24 hours. One study has found zolmitriptan, 2.5 mg and 5 mg, to be at least as effective as sumatriptan, 25 mg or 50 mg, in the acute treatment of migraine. *Caution:* See above for triptans.

     c. **Rizatriptan (Maxalt) 5–10 mg.** Give 1 tablet PO. Repeat at 2 hours if no relief. Do not exceed 30 mg in 24 hours. In patients on propranolol, use the 5-mg dose, not to exceed 15 mg in 24 hours. *Caution:* See above for triptans.

  4. **Isometheptene 65 mg/dichloralphenazone 100 mg/acetaminophen 325 mg (Midrin).** Give 2 capsules at onset of headache followed by 1 capsule Q 1 hour to maximum of 5 capsules in 24 hours.

  5. **Prochlorperazine (Compazine) 25 mg IV.** This medication has been shown in some controlled trials to be superior to DHE in migraine relief.

  6. **Prophylactic therapy.** Several medications can be used for prophylaxis of migraine, including propranolol 80–240 mg/day, timolol 20–30 mg/day, amitriptyline 30–150 mg/day, divalproex sodium 500–1500 mg/day, and sodium valproate 800–1500 mg/day. These medications are less useful in the management of an acute migraine and do not receive further discussion here.

D. Cluster headaches

  1. **Oxygen.** Inhalation by face mask at 7 L/min for 10 minutes has been reported to be successful in aborting a cluster headache. Greatest benefit is obtained in patients < 50 years with episodic cluster headache.

  2. **Sumatriptan.** Found to be effective in aborting cluster headache in some patients and is administered as described above for migraine headaches.

  3. **Zolmitriptan.** 10 mg PO has been reported as being well tolerated and shown to be significantly superior to placebo in episodic cluster headache patients.

  4. **Prophylactic therapy.** Verapamil, lithium carbonate, methysergide and cortisone are the standard of care for preventive therapy of cluster headache. Some recent observations indicate that valproic acid, topiramate, gabapentine, naratriptan and the local application of civamide or anesthesia of the greater occipital nerve may be effective in cluster headache.

REFERENCES

Abramowicz M, ed: Drugs for migraine. Med Lett Drug Ther 1995;37:17.

Bartleson JD: Treatment of migraine headaches. Mayo Clin Proc 1999;74:702.

Dalessio DJ: Diagnosing the severe headache. Neurology 1994;44:S6.

Dresser GK, Spence JD, Bailey DG: Pharmacokinetic-pharmacodynamic consequences and clinical relevance of cytochrome P450 3A4 inhibition. Clin Pharmacokinet 2000;38:41.

Edlow JA, Caplan LR: Avoiding pitfalls in the diagnosis of subarachnoid hemorrhage. N Engl J Med 2000;342:29.

Evans RW: Diagnostic testing for headache. Med Clin North Am 2001;85:865.

Gallagher RM, Dennish G, Spierings ELH et al: A comparative trial of zolmitriptan and sumatriptan for the acute oral treatment of migraine. Headache 2000;40:119.

Maizels M, Scott B, Cohen W et al: Intranasal lidocaine for treatment of migraine: A randomized, double-blind, controlled trial. JAMA 1996;276;4.

Matthew N: Cluster headache. Semin Neurol 1997;17;4.

May A, Leone M: Update on cluster headache. Curr Opin Neurol 2003;16:333.

Millea PJ, Brodie JJ: Tension-type headache. Am Fam Physician 2002;66;797.

Prudy RA: Clinical evaluation of a patient presenting with headache. Med Clin North Am 2001;85;865.

Schievink WI: Intracranial aneurysms. N Engl J Med 1997;336:28.

Schievink WI: Spontaneous dissection of the carotid and vertebral arteries. N Engl J Med 2001;344:898.

Snow V, Weiss K, Wall EM, Mottur-Pilson C; American Academy of Family Physicians; American College of Physicians-American Society of Internal Medicine: Pharmacologic management of acute attacks of migraine and prevention of migraine headache. Ann Intern Med 2002;137;840.

Welch KMA: Drug therapy for migraine. N Engl J Med 1993;329:1476.

26. HEART MURMUR

I. **Problem.** You are asked to see a 50-year-old man complaining of acute shortness of breath. The nursing staff notes a loud murmur.

II. **Immediate Questions**

A. **Is the murmur itself responsible for the problem, or is it a sign of some underlying problem?** Acute aortic or mitral regurgitation from endocarditis or acute mitral regurgitation resulting from rupture of a papillary muscle after a myocardial infarction (MI) could explain the patient's condition. Underlying medical conditions such as severe anemia, thyrotoxicosis, and pregnancy can also have associated functional flow murmurs related to increased cardiac output.

B. **Does the patient have known valvular disease?** Progression of valvular dysfunction may be the cause of deterioration in such a patient.

C. **Does the patient have known congenital heart disease?** In a patient with a history of a murmur, bicuspid aortic valve, atrial septal defect (ASD), ventricular septal defect (VSD), patent ductus arteriosus (PDA), and pulmonic valve stenosis (PS) should always be considered. Often, patients with mild PS or a small ASD are asymptomatic.

D. **Has the deterioration been chronic or acute?** Acute decompensation suggests an acute process such as endocarditis or myocardial ischemia. Chronic deterioration suggests increasing ventricular dysfunction from preexisting valvular disease.

E. **Is there a history of IV drug abuse, recent dental work, invasive procedures such as a colonoscopy or cystoscopy, evidence of embolism such as stroke, or a history of fever or chills?** These factors suggest endocarditis.

F. **Does the patient have any chest pain?** If so, it is important to characterize the chest pain. Chest pain is often seen with angina, aortic dissection, and pericarditis. (See Section I, Chapter 11, Chest Pain, p 60.) Angina is one of the three presenting symptoms of hemodynamically significant aortic stenosis. Syncope and dyspnea secondary to congestive heart failure (CHF) are the others.

G. **Does the patient have coronary artery disease, and if so, is this the cause of the murmur?** A recent MI with papillary muscle dysfunction or rupture may result in acute mitral regurgitation. An acute VSD or free wall rupture after an MI can cause a new murmur. Hypertrophic obstructive cardiomyopathy (also called idiopathic hypertrophic subaortic stenosis [IHSS]) and aortic dissection can cause angina.

III. Differential Diagnosis

A. **Murmur aggravated by an underlying problem**

1. **Flow murmur.** A flow murmur may be caused by or aggravated by a significant anemia or thyrotoxicosis and resultant high-outflow CHF.

2. **CHF with "secondary" mitral regurgitation.** This can result from a variety of conditions, most notably severe dilated cardiomyopathy.

3. **Murmur of aortic insufficiency with possible aortic dissection.** Always consider an underlying connective tissue disorder such as Marfan syndrome as well as severe hypertension.

4. **Noncardiac murmur.** Thyroid or carotid bruits, subclavian artery stenosis, venous hums, and pericardial or pleural friction rubs all can be mistaken for a cardiac murmur.

5. **A new murmur in a patient with known bacteremia or sepsis.** This is an ominous finding and requires emergent evaluation if associated with hypotension, heart block, or symptoms of a stroke.

B. **Coronary artery disease**

1. **Acute ischemia/injury with papillary muscle dysfunction.** Can cause reversible mitral regurgitation.

2. **Recent MI**

   a. **Acute severe mitral regurgitation secondary to ruptured chordae tendineae or head of a papillary muscle**

   b. **Acute VSD**

   c. **Acute rupture of the ventricular wall**

3. **Acute ischemia.** Leading to immediate, severe left ventricular dysfunction with pulmonary edema and new or worsening mitral regurgitation.

C. **Valvular heart disease**

1. **Mitral valve prolapse with ruptured chordae/papillary muscle head and CHF.** Arrhythmias (ventricular or atrial) may lead to decompensation.

2. **Mitral stenosis.** New-onset atrial fibrillation can lead to decompensation.

3. **Aortic stenosis.** With progression, it may result in angina, left ventricular dysfunction, syncope, or arrhythmias (especially ventricular).

4. **Hypertrophic obstructive cardiomyopathy.** Arrhythmias, angina, and dyspnea are common. Sudden death can occur and is often related to exertion.

5. **Prosthetic valve dysfunction.** A new regurgitation murmur is an alarming finding in a patient with a prosthetic valve.

6. **Severe stenosis or regurgitation of any valve (especially mitral or aortic).** Can lead to left ventricular dysfunction and associated symptoms over time.

D. **Congenital heart disease**
   1. **ASD/VSD with right-to-left shunt, causing systemic hypoxemia.** Results from pulmonary hypertension or Eisenmenger's syndrome.
   2. **New dysrhythmias in a patient with previously stable congenital defects.** Can cause acute deterioration, especially atrial fibrillation.

E. **Atrial myxoma.** A rare cause of a murmur. The patient may present with CHF, chest pain, syncope, arrhythmias, constitutional symptoms (eg, fever, weight loss) or an embolic event mimicking endocarditis, collagen vascular disease, or occult malignancy.

IV. **Database**

A. **Physical examination key points**
   1. **General.** Inability to lie flat suggests pulmonary edema, pericarditis, or pericardial effusion.
   2. **Vital signs**
      a. **Temperature.** Elevated temperature may indicate infection (endocarditis), although myocardial infarction can cause fever for up to a week. Also, any fever can cause or intensify a flow murmur.
      b. **Heart rate and rhythm.** Tachycardia is often associated with CHF, pain, infection, pericarditis, and perhaps arrhythmias (see Section I, Chapter 60, Tachycardia, p 345). Irregular rhythm may suggest atrial fibrillation or frequent premature atrial or ventricular beats as well as second-degree atrioventricular block (see Section I, Chapter 45, Irregular Pulse, p 251).
      c. **Blood pressure.** Hypertension or hypotension is often associated with angina or MI. Hypotension could occur with sepsis or hemodynamic collapse. A widened pulse pressure may suggest aortic insufficiency. *Pulsus paradoxus* (a difference of 10 mm Hg in systolic blood pressure between tidal inspiration and expiration) indicates pericardial tamponade.
      d. **Tachypnea.** Suggests CHF, or decreased perfusion or hypoxia from any cause such as a VSD with a right-to-left shunt.

3. **Neck**
   a. **Elevated jugular venous distention.** Suggests right-sided ventricular failure or pericardial tamponade.
   b. **A decrease in the carotid upstroke.** Suggests significant aortic stenosis. Also, the murmur of aortic stenosis radiates to the carotids bilaterally and should not be confused with bilateral carotid bruits, a venous hum, or a thyroid bruit.
4. **Cardiovascular.** Careful cardiac examination is essential. Palpate the carotid pulsations for the presence of a palpable thrill, and palpate the chest for displacement of the apical impulse. First (S_1) and second (S_2) heart sounds and splitting of S_2 must be characterized. The presence of a fourth heart sound (S_4) may suggest a recent MI, hemodynamically significant aortic stenosis, or longstanding hypertension. A third (S_3) heart sound is consistent with ventricular dysfunction.
   a. **Flow murmur.** A midsystolic murmur with normal carotid upstroke is present.
   b. **Aortic insufficiency.** A diastolic blowing murmur heard best at the right second intercostal space down to the left lower sternal border with the patient leaning forward in full expiration. This may occur with acute aortic dissection or acute bacterial endocarditis, or it may be chronic. The aortic component of S_2 may be soft or absent. The murmur of acute aortic insufficiency is usually soft in intensity and short in duration, is heard best at the left lower sternal border, and can easily be missed. The carotid upstroke is sharp, followed by a rapid downstroke (*Corrigan's, or water-hammer, pulse*).
   c. **Aortic stenosis.** This systolic murmur is crescendo-decrescendo and harsh in character; it is heard best at the right second intercostal space. Critical aortic valve stenosis is characterized by the absence of the aortic component of S_2, a palpable S_4 gallop at the apex, late peaking of the maximal intensity of the murmur, a palpable carotid thrill (usually over the left carotid artery), and a diminished and delayed carotid upstroke (*pulsus parvus et tardus*).
   d. **Mitral regurgitation.** It is heard best as a blowing pansystolic murmur at the apex, radiating to the axilla and occasionally into the midback. An intermittent murmur of mitral regurgitation may suggest intermittent papillary muscle dysfunction secondary to ischemia or other causes. The murmur of acute, severe mitral regurgitation may be short in duration and soft in intensity. Other findings associated with severe mitral regurgitation include an S_3 gallop, tachycardia, pulmonary rales, and signs of poor peripheral perfusion.
   e. **Mitral valve prolapse.** A midsystolic click followed by a late systolic murmur suggests mitral valve prolapse. A click or mur-

mur may be present together or singly. Squatting delays the onset of the click and murmur.

f. **Mitral stenosis.** This mid-diastolic murmur is heard best in the left lateral decubitus position with the bell of the stethoscope positioned over the apical impulse. An opening snap may be heard between S_2 and the diastolic rumble. Mitral stenosis is often missed, particularly in a sick patient. It is always an important consideration in ill patients with a history of rheumatic fever. A confirmatory transthoracic echocardiogram is usually indicated. An otherwise stable patient with mitral stenosis decompensates quickly when atrial fibrillation develops. Control of the ventricular heart rate to permit adequate diastolic filling is beneficial in controlling shortness of breath and pulmonary edema.

g. **Hypertrophic cardiomyopathy.** Characteristically, it causes a systolic murmur that might be confused with aortic stenosis, but actually represents reversible left ventricular outflow tract obstruction secondary to hypertrophy of the interventricular septum. The murmur is a crescendo-decrescendo systolic murmur that increases in intensity with the Valsalva maneuver and standing, and decreases in intensity with squatting. The murmur is best heard at the apex and left lower sternal border. An S_4 gallop is usually present. A bisferiens contour to the carotid pulse is characteristic (double peaking of the pulse). Again, rapid decompensation occurs in the face of new onset atrial fibrillation.

h. **ASD/VSD.** An ASD murmur may be difficult to hear. Widely fixed splitting of S_2 is a clue to the presence of an ASD. VSDs are usually heard over the entire precordium; the murmur is holosystolic and a thrill is frequently present.

i. **Atrial myxoma.** An apical diastolic or systolic murmur is encountered more frequently than a third heart sound (*tumor plop*).

5. **Extremities.** Examine distal pulses for a pulse deficit that may suggest dissection or embolic phenomena. Clubbing is seen in cyanotic heart disease and bacterial endocarditis. *Quincke's sign* (a to-and-fro movement seen in the capillary bed of the fingers when light pressure is applied to the distal fingertip) is seen in chronic severe aortic insufficiency.

6. **Neurologic exam.** Focal neurologic deficits may occur with subacute bacterial endocarditis, myoxma, and thrombus formation with embolus. Funduscopic exam should be done to survey for stigmata of embolic disease (*Roth spots*).

7. **Skin.** Look for evidence of IV drug use or embolic phenomena, such as subcutaneous nodules at the fingertips (*Osler's nodes*), splinter hemorrhages under the fingernails, and petechiae (partic-

ularly of the conjunctivae and mucous membranes), which may suggest bacterial endocarditis.

B. Laboratory data. Clearly, these depend on the history and exam. The order in which laboratory data are acquired depends on the clinical picture.

  1. **Complete blood count with differential.** Anemia can cause high-output CHF. A significantly elevated white blood cell (WBC) count with an increase in the percentage of banded neutrophils indicates the presence of a bacterial infection. An elevated WBC count can accompany an acute MI.

  2. **Blood culture.** Should be obtained if there is any question of endocarditis. Three sets of two cultures should be obtained over several hours if the patient is stable. If the patient is unstable, at least one set of blood cultures should be obtained before antibiotic therapy is initiated.

  3. **Arterial blood gases.** Acidosis (see Section I, Chapter 2, Acidosis, p 10) and hypoxia suggest significant left ventricular compromise and pulmonary congestion in an ill patient with a new murmur.

  4. **Thyroid function tests, electrolytes including magnesium, renal function tests.** These may determine the cause as well as reflect the effects of a disease process.

  5. **Markers of cardiac disease,** Elevations in creatinine kinase (particularly the MB fraction) and troponin is supportive of myocardial ischemia or infarction. Brain natriuretic peptide increases in acute as well as chronic ventricular dysfunction.

C. Radiologic and other studies

  1. **Electrocardiogram.** The most useful test to screen for myocardial ischemia, MI, or dysrhythmia, particularly atrial fibrillation. Keep in mind that the abrupt onset of atrial fibrillation in a person with compensated CHF, stable hypertrophic cardiomyopathy, or stable valvular disease may cause rapid decompensation.

  2. **Chest x-ray.** The cardiac silhouette may give a clue to valvular disease, such as left atrial enlargement in mitral stenosis. Increased vascularization, pleural effusion, Kerley A and B lines, and confluent alveolar densities are radiographic evidence of pulmonary edema. Other signs to look for are cardiac chamber enlargement, mediastinal widening, and the presence of prosthetic valves.

  3. **Echocardiogram.** In evaluating an acutely ill patient with a murmur that is not easily identified, the echocardiogram may be the single best source of information. It can accurately determine the presence and degree of valvular stenosis or regurgitation. The cause of the valvular problem can also be suggested. Atrial and ventricular septal defects can be detected.

  4. **Swan-Ganz catheterization.** From a diagnostic standpoint, one can obtain right atrial and pulmonary artery blood samples to di-

agnose a step up in oxygen saturation, confirming the diagnosis of acute VSD. Acute or severe mitral regurgitation can be suggested by the presence of significant V waves in the pulmonary capillary wedge pressure tracing.

V. Plan. Treatment is generally aimed at the condition that is either causing the murmur (MI, papillary muscle dysfunction, VSD, aortic insufficiency in the face of aortic root dissection) or aggravating the condition for which the murmur is a secondary finding (thyrotoxicosis, new-onset atrial fibrillation, endocarditis, thrombus on a mechanical valve, or anemia). While one is initiating therapy, consultation should be considered. When a patient is symptomatic from a cardiac murmur, a cardiology consult is appropriate.

A. **Relieve angina.** In patients with recurrent pulmonary edema secondary to ischemia, this may result in prompt improvement. See Section I, Chapter 11, Chest Pain, V, p 66.

B. **Maintain hemodynamic support**
   1. **Dopamine.** Can be used if an arterial vasoconstricting agent is needed. See Section I, Chapter 42, Hypotension (Shock), V, p 241.
   2. **Dobutamine.** Should be used if a positive inotropic drug is required.

C. **ICU monitoring.** Certain pathologic conditions may require arterial pressure monitoring (see Section III, Chapter 1, Arterial Line Placement, p 416) or continuous monitoring of right heart pressures and pulmonary wedge pressure (see Section III, Chapter 12, Pulmonary Artery Catheterization, p 449).

D. **Treatment of acute MI**
   1. **Pain relief.** Relieve pain with nitroglycerin, IV beta-blockers, and morphine sulfate. (See Section I, Chapter 11, Chest Pain, Section V, p 66; or Section VII, Therapeutics, pp 572, 617, and 568, respectively, for doses.)
   2. **Thrombolysis.** If indicated and if the patient is an appropriate candidate.

E. **Treatment of suspected endocarditis after obtaining three sets of blood cultures.** Initiate empiric antibiotic therapy, being mindful of the presence of bioprostheses (eg, valves, hips), IV drug abuse, or infective focus.

F. **Arrange for invasive evaluation if warranted.** The evaluation of an unknown heart murmur in a critically ill patient can be extremely complex. The basic goal is to determine the possible causes as quickly as possible. Emergent evaluation with an echocardiogram, aortic root contrast injection, or surgical consultation may be indicated, depending on the patient's condition.

REFERENCES

Banning AP: Valvular disease: The GP's key role. Practitioner 1999;243:740.
Braunwald E, Perloff JK: Physical examination of the heart and circulation. In: Braunwald E, Zipes DP, Libby P, eds. *Heart Disease: A Textbook of Cardiovascular Medicine.* 6th ed. Saunders;2001:45.
DeGowin RL, Brown DD: *DeGowin's Diagnostic Examination.* 7th ed. McGraw-Hill;2000:247.
Maisel A: B-type natriuretic peptide levels: Diagnostic and prognostic in congestive heart failure. What's next? Circulation 2002;105:2328.

27. HEMATEMESIS, MELENA

I. **Problem.** A 56-year-old man is admitted to the hospital because of pneumonia; you are called because he "vomited blood."

II. **Immediate Questions**

A. **What are the patient's vital signs?** Is there supine hypotension (indicates 30% volume loss)? Is there resting tachycardia (indicates 20% volume loss)? Are there orthostatic changes in his pulse or blood pressure (indicates 10% volume loss)? If the patient has supine hypotension or resting tachycardia, fluid resuscitation must begin immediately.

B. **Does the patient have adequate IV access?** With no indication of hemodynamic instability, one 16- to 18-gauge IV is adequate. In the presence of hemodynamic compromise, two large-bore (14–16 gauge) IVs should be in place.

C. **Is there a history of gastrointestinal problems? Is there a history of peptic ulcer disease (PUD), liver disease, or esophageal varices?** A history of these disorders may indicate the cause of the hematemesis; however, in only 50% of patients with known esophageal varices can upper GI bleeding be attributed to variceal bleeding. Has the patient ever been evaluated or treated for *Helicobacter pylori?*

D. **Is the patient taking any medications?** Review medications. Note in particular the use of nonsteroidal anti-inflammatory drugs (NSAIDs), aspirin, steroids, and anticoagulants. Anticoagulants may unmask significant pathology or aggravate insignificant lesions.

E. **Does the patient smoke or have a family history of PUD?** Both are risk factors for PUD.

F. **Does the patient have a history of alcohol abuse?** This suggests gastritis or varices as the source of bleeding. Peptic ulcer is still the most common cause of upper GI hemorrhage in heavy users of ethanol. Alcohol use is also a risk factor for a Mallory-Weiss tear.

G. **Is there a previous hematocrit?** It is important to establish a baseline with which to monitor the patient.

H. Is there a history of abnormal liver function studies? These are suggestive of occult liver disease.

I. What is the volume of hematemesis? Ask the nurse to save the emesis. This is important to establish the volume of hematemesis as well as to validate the presence of blood. A large amount indicates more urgency. Indiscriminate use of Hemoccult to document blood is not recommended. The visual appearance is much more reliable.

J. Has there been any melena or bright red blood per rectum? Acute upper GI tract blood loss of about 1 unit results in melena; 2 units may cause hematochezia. With rapid bleeding from an upper source, 10% of patients exhibit hematochezia.

III. Differential Diagnosis

A. PUD Accounts for 50% of upper GI hemorrhages. The use of NSAIDs is the single most important risk factor for PUD and bleeding.

B. Esophageal varices. Accounts for 10% of upper GI bleeding. Esophageal varices are associated with the highest morbidity and mortality rates of all causes of upper GI bleeding. See Section I, Chapter 28, Hematochezia, p 171.

C. Mallory-Weiss tear. Causes ~ 5–15% of upper GI bleeding. Associated with recent heavy alcohol intake in 30–60% of cases. Vomiting often precedes the hematemesis.

D. Acute hemorrhagic gastritis. Accounts for 15% of community-acquired upper GI hemorrhage. It is often associated with alcohol, NSAID use, and stress (severely ill ICU patients).

E. Carcinoma. Very seldom the cause of acute bleeding. Carcinoma is almost always found in patients over 50 years old.

F. Aortoenteric fistula. A rare cause of upper GI hemorrhage, but it can be quite dramatic. Aortoenteric fistula should be suspected in patients who have had aortic bypass graft surgery. Of these fistulae, 75% communicate with the duodenum (third portion). Aortoenteric fistula is generally preceded by a self-limited episode of bleeding ("herald bleed").

G. Non-GI sources that may be confused with a GI bleed. Especially epistaxis or hemoptysis with swallowing of the blood

IV. Database

A. Physical examination key points

1. **Vital signs.** Including orthostatic blood pressure and heart rate. *Orthostatic changes* are a decrease in systolic blood pressure of 10 mm Hg and/or an increase in heart rate of 20 bpm 1 minute after changing from supine to standing position. Vital signs need to be checked frequently until the patient is stable.

2. **Skin.** Spider telangiectasia, palmar erythema, and jaundice indicate underlying cirrhosis and possible varices. Poor skin turgor and absent axillary sweat may indicate volume depletion. Acanthosis nigricans and Kaposi's sarcoma are associated with GI malignancy.
3. **Eyes.** Scleral icterus suggests liver disease.
4. **Chest.** Gynecomastia suggests cirrhosis.
5. **Abdomen.** An increase in bowel sounds suggests upper GI bleeding. Hepatomegaly or splenomegaly suggests cirrhosis or cancer. An abdominal mass points to cancer. Tenderness in the epigastrium or left upper quadrant suggests PUD. Ascites may be seen with cirrhosis and associated esophageal varices.
6. **Genitourinary system.** Rectal examination to look for melena or bright red blood per rectum. Testicular atrophy may be secondary to cirrhosis/chronic liver disease.

B. **Laboratory data**
1. **Stat complete blood count.** This can be done by phlebotomy before your arrival. Differential is not necessary.
2. **Type and cross-match.** At least 4 units of packed red blood cells (PRBCs).
3. **A nasogastric tube for gastric lavage.** This procedure is essential for accurate diagnosis. The possibility of varices is not a contraindication. Lavage until clear or at least only pink-tinged. Note that although a negative nasogastric aspirate suggests another source for bleeding, it can be negative in up to 25% of patients with an upper GI bleeding.
4. **Hematocrit.** Serial hematocrits are helpful; however, in acute hemorrhage the hematocrit may not reflect the amount of blood loss. The hematocrit may fall precipitously after aggressive fluid resuscitation.
5. **Blood urea nitrogen (BUN) and creatinine.** An increased BUN/creatinine ratio is seen in upper GI bleeding and volume depletion.
6. **Prothrombin time (PT), partial thromboplastin time (PTT), and platelet count.** An elevated PT, PTT, or thrombocytopenia can interfere with stabilization of the patient. An elevated PT may be seen in chronic liver disease. Platelets and clotting factors are lost with rapid bleeding. Correction of coagulopathy is indicated in acute bleeding.

C. **Radiologic and other studies.** The source of bleeding must be identified so that specific therapy can be instituted.
1. **Upper GI endoscopy (EGD).** Essential to diagnosing upper GI tract bleeding. EGD should be performed as soon as possible after hemodynamic stabilization and adequate lavage.
   a. The optimal timing of EGD is not well established. Most experts believe that it should be performed within 24 hours. With

the multitude of available therapeutic interventions, however, earlier endoscopy is considered preferable. The urgency of the procedure is based on the severity and/or the ongoing nature of bleeding.

b. It is important in patients with known alcoholic liver disease to distinguish varices from other sources of upper GI bleeding and to direct therapy.

c. Endoscopic appearance predicts outcome. Without endoscopic therapy, complications are as follows:

    i. Active bleeding—55% rebleeding and 11% mortality

    ii. Visible vessel—43% rebleeding and 11% mortality

    iii. Adherent clot—22% rebleeding and 7% mortality

    iv. Flat pigmented lesion—10% rebleeding and 3% mortality

    v. Clean base—< 5% rebleeding and 2% mortality

2. Colonoscopy Should be performed if no convincing source of bleeding is noted on EGD. Although melena is classically attributed to upper GI blood loss, colonic lesions, especially proximal ones, can produce melena.

3. Capsule endoscopy. New technology useful in evaluating obscure GI bleeding and small bowel disease. It is not indicated in cases of acute GI hemorrhage.

4. Technetium-labeled bleeding scan. This is the next examination to be ordered if upper and lower endoscopies are normal. It can detect very slow bleeding (0.5 mL/min). Localization is only fair and needs to be documented with endoscopy or angiography.

5. Angiography. Localization is very good, but patients must be bleeding fairly rapidly (1–2 mL/min) to detect the source. Angiography can also treat with selective intra-arterial infusion of vasopress or embolization.

V. Plan

A. Monitoring. The first step in management is to determine whether the patient should be monitored in an ICU. The following are guidelines for admission to the ICU.

1. Clearly documented frank hematemesis.

2. Coffee-ground emesis *and* either melena or hematochezia.

3. Hemodynamic instability, either hypotension, tachycardia, or orthostatic hypotension.

4. A drop in hematocrit of 5 points after fluid resuscitation.

5. A significant unexplained increase in the BUN when GI bleeding is suspected.

6. High-risk patient: advanced age, inpatient status at time of bleed, recurrent or evidence of persistent bleeding, major comorbidity (hepatic, renal, pulmonary, or cardiac disease).

B. Volume resuscitation. If massive bleeding is evident, place two large-bore (14- or 16-gauge) IV lines. Begin IV fluids containing normal saline at a rate to maintain hemodynamic stability. Transfuse PRBCs when available for massive bleeding to keep the hematocrit above 30%. With massive bleeding, consider transfusing typed non—cross-matched blood.

C. **Surgical consultation.** Essential in the management of upper GI tract hemorrhage. It should be obtained within the first few hours of the patient's arrival. If hemodynamic stability cannot be achieved, immediate surgical intervention may be necessary.

D. **Specific treatment.** The management of various sources of upper GI hemorrhage depends on the diagnosis.

1. **PUD.** Pharmacologic therapy with proton pump inhibitors has recently been shown to help prevent rebleeding. Pantoprazole is the only proton pump inhibitor with an IV form available in the United States. H_2-receptor antagonists (ranitidine [Zantac], cimetidine [Tagamet], and famotidine [Pepcid]) are not recommended for acute hemorrhage. Endoscopic therapies are effective for controlling bleeding and preventing rebleeding. They include thermal probe, injection therapy, electrocoagulation, and laser. If evidence of *Helicobacter pylori* infection is present (positive rapid urease test, histology, antibody or breath test), treatment with appropriate antibiotics is indicated.

2. **Acute hemorrhagic gastritis or esophagitis.** Acid reduction therapy. (See V.D.1.)

3. **Mallory-Weiss tear.** No specific therapy beyond supportive care. Thermal or electric probes have been used successfully.

4. **Esophageal varices.** Give octreotide bolus of 25–50 μg, followed by a continuous infusion of 25–50 μg/hour. If octreotide fails, then balloon tamponade should be considered. Endoscopic therapies include band ligation (preferred) and injection sclerotherapy.

5. **Aortoenteric fistula.** Surgical intervention is necessary.

REFERENCES

Besson I, Ingrand P, Person B et al: Sclerotherapy with and without octreotide for acute variceal bleeding. N Engl J Med 1995;333:555.

Cappell MS, ed: High risk gastrointestinal bleeding, Part I. Gastroenterol Clin North Am 2000;29:1.

Cappell MS, ed: High risk gastrointestinal bleeding, Part II. Gastroenterol Clin North Am 2000;29:275.

Consensus Conference: Therapeutic endoscopy and bleeding ulcers. JAMA 1989;262:1369.

Gisbert JP, Gonzalez L, Calvet X et al: Proton pump inhibitors versus H2-antagonists: A meta-analysis of their efficacy in treating bleeding peptic ulcer. Aliment Pharmacol Ther 2001;15:917.

Khuroo MS, Yattoo GN, Javid G et al: A comparison of omeprazole and placebo for bleeding peptic ulcer. N Engl J Med 1997;336:1054.

Laine L, Cook D: Endoscopic ligation compared with sclerotherapy for treatment of esophageal variceal bleeding: A meta-analysis. Ann Intern Med 1995;123:280.

Leighton JA et al. Obscure gastrointestinal bleeding. Gastrointest Endosc 2003;58:650.

Rockall TA, Logan RF, Devlin HB et al: Risk assessment after acute upper gastrointestinal hemorrhage. Gut 1996;38:316.

Rocky D: Gastrointestinal bleeding. In: Felman M, Friedman LS, Sleisenger MH, eds. *Gastrointestinal and Liver Disease: Pathophysiology/Diagnosis/Management.* 7th ed. Saunders;2002:211.

28. HEMATOCHEZIA

I. **Problem.** A 38-year-old man comes to the emergency room and states, "I have just passed a lot of blood from my bowels."

II. **Immediate Questions**

A. **What are the patient's vital signs?** Is there supine hypotension (indicates 30% volume loss)? Is there resting tachycardia (indicates 20% volume loss)? Are there orthostatic changes in his pulse or blood pressure (indicates 10% volume loss)? If the patient has supine hypotension or resting tachycardia, resuscitation must begin immediately.

B. **Does the patient have IV line access?** With no indication of hemodynamic instability, one 16- to 18-gauge IV line is adequate. In the presence of hemodynamic compromise, two large-bore IVs should be in place.

C. **Is there a history of previous gastrointestinal (GI) bleeding?** Ask about a history of diseases associated with lower GI bleeding, such as diverticular disease, colon polyps or carcinoma, inflammatory bowel disease, hemorrhoids, and other anal diseases. Inquire about prior upper GI bleeding and also peptic ulcer disease (PUD).

D. **What medications is the patient taking?** Ask specifically about steroids, nonsteroidal anti-inflammatory drugs (NSAIDs), and anticoagulants.

E. **Does the patient have a history of alcohol abuse?** This suggests the possibility of an upper GI source of bleeding such as varices or gastritis.

F. **What is the most recent hematocrit?** Obtain this information from previous visits. This will establish the baseline value with which to compare future hematocrits.

G. **What is the volume of bright red blood per rectum?** Ask the nurse to save the specimen or specimens for your inspection. This is important for establishing the presence and volume of blood loss. A large volume of blood suggests the need for immediate action.

H. **Has there been hematemesis?** Acute severe upper GI blood loss may result in hematochezia.

III. **Differential Diagnosis**

A. **Anorectal (hemorrhoids/fissures/rectal ulcers).** These account for 4% of all episodes of hematochezia and are usually not brought to the attention of a physician. They are rarely significant but may be of concern in the presence of portal hypertension.

B. Diverticular disease. Responsible for 33% of all lower GI bleeds and 30–50% of all significant bleeds. Prevalance is age dependent with < 5% noted at age 40, 30% at age 60, and 65% at age 85.

C. Angiodysplasia. This condition is much more common in the elderly, causing approximately 10% of significant lower GI bleeding. Considered by some to be the most common cause of lower GI bleeding in patients over 65. Also seen with renal failure.

D. Upper GI bleeding. Upper GI sources are responsible for 10% of hematochezia. Hematochezia from an upper GI bleed represents at least a 2-unit bleed and is almost always associated with hemodynamic instability *requiring ICU monitoring*. Upper GI bleeding must be ruled out before surgical exploration for hematochezia. See Section I, Chapter 27, Hematemesis, Melena, p 166.

E. Neoplasia including carcinoma and polyps. Causes 1–2% of significant lower GI tract bleeding.

F. Inflammatory bowel disease (IBD). Infrequent cause of significant lower GI tract bleeding. Bleeding is more likely with ulcerative colitis than with Crohn's disease. Bleeding from IBD is more common in younger patients.

G. Bowel ischemia. Ischemic colitis is frequently seen in the elderly and may be associated with risk factors for ischemia such as peripheral vascular disease (PVD). However, often there is no definite predisposing condition found, and the situation is usually reversible. This is in contrast to acute small bowel ischemia, which is frequently associated with predisposing factors such as atrial fibrillation, PVD, or a hypercoagulable state and is usually not spontaneously reversible.

IV. Database

A. Physical examination key points

1. **Vital signs.** Including orthostatic blood pressure and heart rate. A decrease in systolic blood pressure of 10 mm Hg, or an increase in the heart rate by 20 bpm 1 minute after movement from a supine position to standing, indicates volume depletion. Vital signs may need to be rechecked frequently. An irregularly irregular pulse suggests ischemic colitis caused by emboli secondary to atrial fibrillation.

2. **Skin.** Telangiectasias or melanotic lesions on palms or soles suggest Osler-Weber-Rendu disease and Peutz-Jeghers syndrome, respectively. Look for peripheral stigmata of chronic liver disease and lesions associated with GI cancer (acanthosis nigricans, Kaposi's sarcoma).

3. **HEENT.** Vascular malformations on lips or buccal mucosa suggest angiodysplasia or Osler-Weber-Rendu disease. Scleral icterus suggests chronic liver disease.

4. **Heart.** Aortic stenosis is associated with angiodysplasia.
5. **Abdomen.** Bruits suggest atherosclerosis and thus possible ischemic colitis. Hyperactive bowel sounds may indicate upper GI tract bleeding. Check for masses (cancer) or tenderness (midepigastric area: PUD). Hepatomegaly and splenomegaly suggest portal hypertension (varices) or cancer.
6. **Rectum.** Check for hemorrhoids for a mass and to document blood in the rectal vault (melena, bright red blood, or guaiac-positive stools).

B. **Laboratory data**
   1. **Nasogastric (NG) tube placement.** Obtain a quick aspirate for coffee-ground material. Testing for occult blood is not helpful because the placement of the NG tube is sufficient to cause occult blood positivity.
   2. **Stat complete blood count; type and cross-match.** Changes in the indices may also be helpful in differentiating acute from chronic bleeding.
   3. **Serial hematocrits.** Can be spun without phlebotomy. Serial hematocrit values are helpful, but the hematocrit does not always reflect the amount of blood loss because equilibration with extravascular fluid may take several hours.
   4. **Type and cross-match.** At least 4 units of packed red blood cells (PRBCs).
   5. **Blood urea nitrogen (BUN) and creatinine.** An increased BUN/creatinine ratio is seen in upper GI bleeding or volume depletion.
   6. **Prothrombin time (PT), partial thromboplastin time (PTT), and platelet count.** An elevated PT or PTT or thrombocytopenia can interfere with stabilization of the patient. An elevated PT may be seen in chronic liver disease. Platelets and clotting factors decrease with brisk bleeding and massive transfusions.

C. **Radiologic and other studies**
   1. **Anoscopy and flexible sigmoidoscopy.** Look for bleeding hemorrhoids or rectal mass.
   2. **Colonoscopy.** Preferred exam for diagnosis and treatment of suspected lower GI bleed. Colonoscopy should be performed after large-volume oral preparation.
   3. **NG tube.** For gastric lavage. NG tube should be placed if the NG aspirate is positive for blood.
      The NG tube may also be used for a rapid colon purge (over 1–2 hours) in the setting of acute lower GI bleeding. It is much easier to have the purge solution poured into the tube than to rely on the patient to drink it.
   4. **Upper GI endoscopy.** An upper GI source must be ruled out before surgery. In upper GI bleeds, 10% of upper GI endoscopies have a negative NG aspirate.
   5. **Technetium-labeled bleeding scan.** This is the next examination to be ordered if upper and lower endoscopies are normal. This scan

can detect very slow bleeding (0.5 mL/min). Localization is only fair and needs to be documented with endoscopy or angiography.

6. **Angiography.** Localization is very good, but patients must be bleeding fairly rapidly (1–2 mL/min) for the source to be detected by angiography. This procedure can also treat with selective intra-arterial infusion of vasopressin.

V. Plan

A. **Monitoring.** The primary question in managing bleeding patients is the necessity of ICU monitoring. The following are guidelines for admission to the ICU:

1. Clearly documented frank hematochezia (> 100 mL).
2. Coffee-ground emesis or positive NG aspirate and hematochezia.
3. Any indication of hemodynamic instability (tachycardia, hypotension, or orthostasis).
4. Drop in hematocrit > 5 percentage points after fluid resuscitation.
5. Significant increase in BUN when GI bleeding is suspected.
6. High-risk patient: advanced age, inpatient status at time of bleed, recurrent or evidence of persistent bleeding, major comorbidity (hepatic, renal, pulmonary, or cardiac disease).

B. **Volume resuscitation.** If massive bleeding is evident, place two large-bore (18-gauge or larger) peripheral or central lines. Begin IV fluids containing normal saline at a rate to maintain hemodynamic stability. With massive bleeding, transfuse PRBCs when available. Blood should be given to maintain a hematocrit above 30%.

C. **Surgical consultation.** Contact early in the management, especially if brisk bleeding is encountered.

D. **Establish source of bleeding.** The source of bleeding must be identified to institute specific therapy.

1. If bleeding is brisk, start with NG aspirate. If positive, evaluate for upper GI source. If negative, proceed with colonoscopy. If endoscopy is negative and bleeding remains brisk, proceed to angiography and then bleeding scan. Angiography may also be a therapeutic modality. If all tests fail to reveal the site, and the bleeding remains brisk, then the patient requires laparotomy. A negative NG aspirate for blood should not dissuade evaluation of the upper GI tract for the bleeding source (usually by upper GI endoscopy) before surgical exploration for hematochezia.
2. If the bleeding has stopped and the NG aspirate is negative, proceed first with colonoscopy after prep. Colonoscopy is rarely helpful during brisk bleeding. If the colonoscopy is negative, do an upper GI endoscopy and then angiography. *Note:* If at any point the patient becomes unstable and is difficult to stabilize with IV fluids and blood, surgery is indicated.
3. The tempo of the evaluation is dictated by the rate of the patient's bleeding and overall stability.

REFERENCES

Brandt LJ, Boley SJ: Intestinal ischemia. In: Feldman M, Friedman LS, Sleisenger MH, eds. *Gastrointestinal and Liver Diseases Pathophysiology/Diagnosis/Management.* 7th ed. Saunders;2004:2321.

Cappell MS, ed: High risk gastrointestinal bleeding, Part I. Gastroenterol Clin North Am 2000;29:1.

Cappell MS, ed: High risk gastrointestinal bleeding, Part II. Gastroenterol Clin North Am 2000;29:275.

Dusold R, Burke K, Carpentier W, Dyck WP: The accuracy of technetium-99m-labeled red cell scintigraphy in localizing gastrointestinal bleeding. Am J Gastroenterol 1994;89:345.

Jensen DM, Machicado GA: Diagnosis and treatment of severe hematochezia: The role of urgent colonoscopy after purge. Gastroenterology 1988;95:1569.

Jensen DM, Machicado GA, Jutabha R et al: Urgent colonoscopy for the diagnosis and treatment of severe diverticular hemorrhage. N Engl J Med 2000;340:78.

Rockey DC: Gastrointestinal bleeding. In: Feldman M, Friedman LS, Sleisenger MH, eds. *Gastrointestinal and Liver Diseases: Pathophysiology/Diagnosis/Management.* 7th ed. Saunders;2002:211.

Rogers BH. Endoscopic diagnosis and therapy of mucosal vascular abnormalities of the gastrointestinal tract occurring in elderly patients and associated with cardiac, vascular, and pulmonary disease. Gastrointest Endosc 1980;26:134.

Zuccaro G Jr: Management of the adult patient with acute lower gastrointestinal bleeding. Am J Gastroenterol 1998;93:1202.

Zuckerman DA, Bocchini TP, Birnbaum EH: Massive hemorrhage in the lower gastrointestinal tract in adults: Diagnostic imaging and intervention. AJR Am J Roentgenol 1993;161:703.

Zuckerman GR, Prakash C: Acute lower intestinal bleeding. Part II: Etiology, therapy, and outcomes. Gastrointest Endosc 1999;49:228.

29. HEMATURIA

I. Problem. A 51-year-old man has red blood cells noted on urinalysis 3 days after undergoing a total hip replacement.

II. Immediate Questions

A. Is there a history of gross hematuria? Microscopic hematuria may have been present for a long time without the patient's being aware of it, suggesting a chronic or acute process. Gross hematuria will not have gone unnoticed by the patient and likely represents an acute process or a process that has previously been evaluated.

B. Does the patient have a Foley catheter in place? Irritation of the bladder mucosa by a Foley catheter is a common cause of hematuria, as are trauma during placement and manipulation of the catheter by the patient. Other causes should be investigated if the hematuria does not completely clear after removal of the catheter.

C. Has the patient had recent abdominal surgery? This raises the question of an injury to the urinary tract and is usually apparent the night of surgery.

D. **Does the patient have abdominal pain or fever?** Abdominal pain may suggest an inflammatory or infectious cause. Colicky pain radiating from the flank to the groin suggests a renal stone. Infection is often accompanied by fever.

E. **Has there been a significant change in urine output?** A sudden decrease in urine output may indicate acute oliguric renal failure, obstruction, or renal vein thrombosis. See Section I, Chapter 51, Oliguria/Anuria, p 283.

F. **Does the patient have symptoms suggestive of urinary tract infection (UTI)?** Dysuria, frequency, and urgency are common symptoms associated with a UTI.

G. **Is the patient taking anticoagulant medication?** Anticoagulation therapy may cause hematuria by unmasking significant urinary tract pathology.

H. **Has the patient been treated with antineoplastic agents such as cyclophosphamide (Cytoxan)?** Complications of cyclophosphamide therapy are hemorrhagic cystitis or secondary genitourinary tract tumors.

I. **Is there a history of urologic conditions?** A history of nephrolithiasis, genitourinary surgery, bladder cancer, or benign prostatic hypertrophy should be determined.

III. Differential Diagnosis

A. **Blood**
   1. **Coagulopathy.** See Section I, Chapter 12, Coagulopathy, p 70. Inheritable defects such as hemophilia, severe liver dysfunction, and pharmacologic anticoagulation are potential causes.
   2. **Hemoglobinopathy.** Sickle cell disease with crisis is frequently associated with gross hematuria.

B. **Kidneys**
   1. **Glomerular disease**
      a. **Primary.** Red cell casts characterize poststreptococcal glomerulonephritis, IgA nephropathy, Goodpasture's syndrome, idiopathic rapidly progressive glomerulonephritis.
      b. **Secondary.** Vasculitis associated with systemic lupus erythematosus (SLE), scleroderma, Wegener's granulomatosis, polyarteritis, hypersensitivity vasculitis, subacute bacterial endocarditis.
      c. **Hereditary.** Alport's syndrome, associated with sensorineural hearing loss and ocular abnormalities.
   2. **Interstitial disease**
      a. **Consequence of systemic diseases.** Diabetic nephrosclerosis, accelerated hypertension, SLE.
      b. **Consequence of pharmacologic therapy.** Analgesic nephropathy, heavy metals, heroin nephropathy.

3. **Infections**
   a. **Pyelonephritis**
   b. **Tuberculosis.** Characterized by sterile pyuria.
4. **Malformations**
   a. **Cystic.** Familial polycystic kidney disease, ruptured solitary cysts, medullary sponge kidney.
   b. **Vascular.** Suggested by findings of hemangiomas or telangiectasias elsewhere.
5. **Neoplasms.** Particularly renal cell carcinoma and more rarely transitional cell carcinoma.
6. **Ischemia**
   a. **Embolism.** Aortic atherosclerosis, cardiac arrhythmias, manipulation of the aorta (aortography, coronary angiography).
   b. **Thrombosis.** Nephrotic syndrome, neoplastic disease, coagulation disorders (antithrombin III, protein-C or protein-S deficiencies, lupus anticoagulant, and factor V Lieden).
7. **Trauma**

C. **Postrenal**
   1. **Mechanical**
      a. **Kidney stones.** Nephrolithiasis and urolithiasis.
      b. **Obstruction.** Prostatic hypertrophy (common cause in men over 50 years), posterior urethral valves, retroperitoneal fibrosis, ureteropelvic junction abnormalities, strictures.
   2. **Inflammatory.** Infection or regional inflammation.
      a. **Periureteritis.** Diverticulitis, pelvic inflammatory disease.
      b. **Cystitis.** Infectious or inflammatory, such as cyclophosphamide-induced hematuria, which is a medical emergency.
      c. **Prostatitis**
      d. **Urethritis**
   3. **Neoplasm.** Transitional cell carcinoma, adenocarcinoma of the prostate, squamous cell carcinoma of the penis.
   4. **Exercise.** Especially in marathon runners.

D. **False hematuria**
   1. **Vaginal/rectal bleeding**
   2. **Factitious.** Most common in patients demonstrating drug-seeking behavior and requesting narcotics for nephrolithiasis.

IV. Database

A. Physical examination key points

1. **Abdomen.** Examine for palpable masses indicative of tumors, polycystic kidneys, or diverticular abscess. Tenderness accompanies infection, infarction, sickle cell crisis, inflammatory processes, and obstruction.
2. **Urethral meatus.** Look for gross blood, especially in trauma patients, and evidence of recent instrumentation or superficial lesions.

3. **Rectum.** Critical in the trauma patient when a "free-floating" prostate may be found, signifying urethral disruption. More commonly, prostatitis or prostatic carcinoma is uncovered. Attention should also be given to possible hemorrhoids.
4. **Pelvis.** Check for another source of bleeding such as vaginitis, cervicitis, and menorrhagia.
5. **Skin.** Ecchymoses, petechiae, and rash are suggestive of vasculitis or a coagulation disorder.

B. **Laboratory data**
1. **Urinalysis.** Red blood cell (RBC) casts are seen only with glomerulonephritis. White blood cells (WBCs) or bacteria suggest an infectious cause; WBC casts suggest pyelonephritis. Crystals may be seen in association with stones. Red discoloration without RBCs suggest myoglobinuria; urine should be checked for myoglobin and a serum creatine phosphokinase carried out.
2. **Coagulation studies.** Prothrombin time, partial thromboplastin time, platelets.
3. **Hemogram.** An elevated WBC count suggests an infectious or inflammatory process. Microcytic anemia may suggest chronic blood loss; however, hematuria is an unusual cause of microcytic anemia.
4. **Urine culture.** Rule out bacterial infection. Cultures for acid-fast bacilli should be done if pyuria is present and bacteria cultures are sterile (assuming the patient is not receiving antibiotics). An acid-fast stain may be helpful; however, some common saprophytes are acid-fast staining.
5. **Blood urea nitrogen and creatinine.** To be used for baseline evaluation of renal function or to assess any change in renal function.
6. **Sickle cell screen.** Useful if the patient's status is previously unknown and this condition is being entertained as a cause of the hematuria.
7. **Urinary cytology.** May diagnose transitional cell carcinoma.

C. **Radiologic and other studies**
1. **Abdominal plain x-ray (kidney/ureter/bladder [KUB]).** Eighty percent of urinary calculi are radiodense. Also, the KUB may show an inflammatory process (ileus or loss of psoas shadow).
2. **Excretory urography (IV pyelography) or other contrast imaging.** A part of the evaluation in all patients without an active infection who can receive IV contrast without undue risk. The evaluation of painful hematuria in many centers includes spiral computed tomography (CT) scanning, which is highly sensitive for demonstrating nephrolithiasis. In the evaluation of painless hematuria, a CT IV pyelogram is often used instead of an excretory urogram.
3. **Retrograde urethrogram/cystogram.** Second-line study to be used in cases in which tumor, vesicoureteral reflux, posterior urethral valves, or traumatic disruption is suspected.

4. **Further studies.** Should be directed by clinical suspicion and the results of initial studies. Further studies may include a CT scan of the abdomen, ultrasound, magnetic resonance imaging, angiography, magnetic resonance angiography (especially useful if contrast is to be avoided), cystoscopy, and renal biopsy. With normal renal imaging, patients with hematuria should have cystoscopy. With proteinuria, RBC casts, or suggestion of upper tract disease, if the renal imaging is normal, a renal biopsy may be indicated.

V. **Plan.** Treatment depends on the cause. Keep in mind that apart from gross hematuria with or without clots (trauma, severe coagulopathy, cyclophosphamide-induced hematuria), the causes of hematuria are rarely emergencies; a thoughtful and careful evaluation can therefore be pursued over several days.

A. **Urinary tract infection.** See Section I, Chapter 20, Dysuria, V, p 126. The infection must be eradicated and a repeat urinalysis performed to rule out continued hematuria. If hematuria persists, further evaluation is necessary.

B. **Urolithiasis.** If the stone is expected to pass spontaneously (usually < 1 cm) and there are no complicating factors (infection, obstruction), expectant therapy with analgesics and hydration is appropriate. The urine should be strained.

C. **Neoplasms.** A complete urologic evaluation is recommended for assessing gross hematuria.

D. **Tuberculosis.** Treat appropriately with antibiotics. Initial therapy is usually with isoniazid (INH) 300 mg PO Q day, rifampin 600 mg PO Q day, and pyrazinamide 15–30 mg/kg with a maximum dose of 2 g Q day and ethambutol 15–25 mg/kg/day. The American Thoracic Society and the Centers for Disease Control and Prevention recommend a four-drug regimen for treatment until the results of drug susceptibility studies are available; or unless there is < 4% primary resistance to INH within the community. If so, an initial three-drug regimen is recommended. Long-term follow-up with IV pyelograms is necessary, because strictures are late sequelae and can lead to obstruction.

E. **Collecting system abnormality.** Usually requires surgical referral and repair.

F. **Coagulopathy.** Correct clotting factor deficiencies or adjust anticoagulant dose. Frequently, the coagulopathy induces bleeding from a preexisting abnormality. A thorough evaluation is usually indicated in a patient who has hematuria and a coagulopathy.

G. **Glomerulonephritis.** Most cases require a biopsy for definitive diagnosis, with therapy as appropriate for the underlying illness.

H. **Hemorrhagic cystitis.** Treat with continuous saline irrigation and occasionally a 1% alum irrigation. Also, hyperbaric oxygen can be used. The primary treatment is prevention, which includes hydration (oral or intravenous) and mesna (Mesnex).

REFERENCES

Cohen RA, Brown RS: Clinical practice, microscopic hematuria. N Engl J Med 2003;48:2330.

Mazhari R, Kimmel PL: Hematuria: An algorithmic approach to finding the cause. Cleve Clin J Med 2002;69:870.

Miller OF, Rineer SK, Reichard SR et al: Prospective comparison of unenhanced spiral computed tomography and intravenous urogram in the evaluation of acute flank pain. Urology 1998;52:982.

30. HEMOPTYSIS

I. **Problem.** A 60-year-old male smoker comes to the emergency room complaining of "spitting up blood" for 1 week.

II. **Immediate Questions**

A. **Is the patient truly experiencing hemoptysis?** Blood from a nasal, oral, or upper GI (ie, gastroesophageal) source may be aspirated to the larynx and then expectorated. Usually, sputum is intermixed with blood in hemoptysis.

B. **What is the volume of the hemoptysis?** Massive hemoptysis (> 600 mL/24 hr) connotes a life-threatening problem that demands immediate ICU admission as well as a rapid diagnostic evaluation.

C. **Has this happened before? If so, how frequently?** Patients with recurrent acute bronchitis or with mitral stenosis may have had multiple episodes of minor hemoptysis.

D. **What is the smoking history?** The higher the pack-years, the more likely the patient has chronic bronchitis or bronchogenic carcinoma.

E. **Is there a history of productive cough preceding the hemoptysis?** If the answer is yes, then the problem may be an infection such as acute bronchitis or bronchiectasis.

F. **Has there been any accompanying chest pain?** Pleuritic chest pain may be a symptom of pneumonia or a pulmonary embolism with infarction. Hemoptysis may accompany pulmonary edema from any number of causes.

III. **Differential Diagnosis**

A. **Pulmonary sources**

1. **Infection**

a. **Acute or chronic bronchitis.** Most common cause of hemoptysis.

b. **Pneumonia.** A necrotizing gram-negative or staphylococcal pneumonia can cause hemoptysis. Symptoms are acute.

c. **Lung abscess.** Often produces foul-smelling sputum.

d. **Bronchiectasis.** Seen in patients with recurrent episodes of respiratory infections, voluminous sputum production, and intermittent hemoptysis.

e. **Tuberculosis.** Usually apical infiltrates on chest x-ray. Symptoms are often chronic or subacute.

f. **Mycetoma (fungus ball).** A ball of *Aspergillus* fungus may form in a previously formed cavity. Look for the "crescent sign" on the chest x-ray.

2. **Neoplasm**

a. **Bronchogenic carcinoma.** Usually, the chest x-ray is abnormal, but it may be normal in up to 13% of patients with early lung cancer and hemoptysis.

b. **Bronchial adenoma. Carcinoid tumors are notorious for brisk hemoptysis. Chest radiograph may be normal.**

c. **Metastatic disease.** A history of cancer should be uncovered during the history. The chest x-ray will be abnormal—usually with multiple lesions.

3. **Vascular**

a. **Pulmonary embolism (PE) with infarction.** Only 10% of patients with PE present with hemoptysis, but pulmonary emboli are very common and should not be missed.

b. **Mitral stenosis.** May arise either from rupture of the pulmonary veins or from frank pulmonary edema.

c. **Cardiogenic pulmonary edema.** Surprisingly common, especially now that most cardiac patients are on some form of anticoagulation therapy.

d. **Arteriovenous malformation**

B. **Trauma**

1. **Pulmonary contusion**

2. **Bronchial or vascular tear**

3. **Retained foreign body.** Teeth and fillings sometimes find their way down into the bronchi.

C. **Systemic diseases**

1. **Anticoagulation**

a. **Drugs.** Warfarin (Coumadin), heparin, aspirin, streptokinase (Streptase), urokinase (Abbokinase), tissue plasminogen activator, and APSAC (anisoylated plasminogen streptokinase activator complex) or antistreplase (Eminase).

b. **Uremia**

c. **Thrombocytopenia.** Drugs, idiopathic thrombocytopenic purpura, cancer.

d. **Disseminated intravascular coagulation**

e. **Liver disease.** Severe liver disease can result in thrombocytopenia and also in a decreased production of coagulation factors.

2. **Autoimmune diseases**
   a. **Wegener's granulomatosis.** Look for renal changes (red cell casts, hematuria, proteinuria) and sinus disease. The chest x-ray often is abnormal. Bilateral nodular densities and cavitation are common.
   b. **Goodpasture's syndrome.** This disease also involves the kidney. Proteinuria, hematuria, and red cell casts may be present. Diffuse alveolar infiltrates are often present.
   c. **Systemic lupus erythematosus (SLE).** Lupus more frequently involves the pleura, but patients may develop life-threatening hemoptysis from lupus pneumonitis.

IV. Database

A. Physical examination key points

1. **Vital signs.** Look particularly for fever and signs of impending respiratory failure: respiratory rate above 30 per minute, abdominal paradox with inspiration, and accessory muscle use.
2. **HEENT.** Look carefully for a nasal or oropharyngeal source of bleeding.
3. **Chest.** Inspect and palpate for signs of trauma such as rib or clavicle fractures. Listen for a pleural rub, localized rales, or signs of consolidation.
4. **Heart.** An irregularly irregular pulse signifies atrial fibrillation and suggests mitral stenosis as a possible cause. Pulmonary embolus can also cause atrial fibrillation. An S_3 and jugular venous distention suggest congestive heart failure as a possible cause. Always listen carefully for the low diastolic rumble of mitral stenosis at the apex with the bell.
5. **Abdomen.** Palpate the epigastrium, liver, and spleen. Peptic ulcer disease or alcoholic liver disease could certainly cause GI bleeding, which might mimic hemoptysis.
6. **Extremities.** Examine lower extremities for signs of deep venous thromboses or edema. Look for cyanosis and clubbing. Clubbed fingers associated with hemoptysis generally imply either bronchiectasis or a pulmonary neoplasm.
7. **Skin.** Inspect the skin for petechiae, ecchymoses, angiomata, and rashes.

B. Laboratory data

1. **Complete blood count.** May reveal an anemia that could be caused by hemoptysis or, more likely, is related to hemoptysis. A normocytic anemia with a normal or low reticulocyte count may be secondary to anemia of chronic disease (eg, cancer). An elevated reticulocyte count indicates hemolytic anemia possibly secondary to SLE. An iron deficiency may indicate Goodpasture's syndrome.
2. **Platelet count, prothrombin time, and partial thromboplastin time.** All are indicated to rule out coagulopathy as a cause. See

Section I, Chapter 12, Coagulopathy, p 70. If platelet dysfunction is suspected, bleeding time will be prolonged in the presence of a normal platelet count.

3. **Blood urea nitrogen, creatinine, and urinalysis.** For rapid evaluation of "pulmonary-renal" syndromes (Goodpasture's syndrome, Wegener's granulomatosis, SLE, and vasculitis).

4. **Antineutrophil cytoplasmic antibodies (ANCA) and anti-glomerular basement membrane (anti-GBM) antibody.** May indicate Wegener's (especially cytoplasmic-staining ANCA or C-ANCA) and anti-GBM Ab is positive in 85% of patients with Goodpasture's syndrome.

5. **Arterial blood gases.** Check for adequate ventilation and oxygenation. If the patient has underlying pulmonary disease, respiratory failure may be precipitated by hemoptysis.

6. **Sputum examination.** If the sputum is purulent, Gram's stain and culture are helpful. For patients with upper lobe infiltrates or HIV, check sputa for acid-fast bacilli smear and culture.

7. **PPD (tuberculin) skin test.** To help rule out tuberculosis.

C. **Radiologic and other studies**
1. **Chest x-ray.** First and most important test after the history and physical. The pattern and location of any infiltrate, combined with the history and physical examination, will dictate the remainder of your workup.

2. **Ventilation/perfusion ($\dot{V}/\dot{Q}$) lung scan.** If pulmonary embolism is highly suspected, a V/Q scan must be done. Alternatively, a fast-track computed tomography (CT) scan can be done. However, small peripheral pulmonary emboli may be missed with this imaging modality at present.

3. **Angiography.** If PE is suspected and ($\dot{V}/\dot{Q}$) scans are not clearly positive or negative, then pulmonary angiography is indicated. Angiography may also be indicated for the diagnosis of pulmonary arteriovenous malformations.

4. **Chest CT scan including CT angiography.** This provides a much better anatomic view of pulmonary pathology compared with chest radiographs and also reveals lesions not seen previously. However, the CT scan is only indicated acutely when looking for an aortic dissection and PE. CT angiography (helical or spiral and electron-beam) are about 90% sensitive and 90% specific for detecting proximal (main, lobar, and segmental) pulmonary artery emboli. CT angiography is poor at detecting subsegmental emboli.

5. **Electrocardiogram.** May show atrial fibrillation. A right axis shift and/or right bundle branch block may suggest a PE. Classically, a PE produces an S wave in lead I, and a Q wave and inverted T wave in lead III ($S_1Q_3T_3$).

6. **Bronchoscopy.** Patients with unclear sources of hemoptysis, massive hemoptysis, or the suspicion of a neoplasm require

fiberoptic bronchoscopy. The earlier it is done, the more likely the source of bleeding will be identified.

V. Plan

A. Intensive care unit
   1. **Massive hemoptysis**
   2. **Present or impending hypoxemic or hypercarbic respiratory failure**

B. Establish IV access. Death comes from asphyxia rather than hemorrhage, but IV medications are needed.

C. Always protect the airway. This may require early intubation.

D. Correct any coagulopathy. See Section I, Chapter 12, Coagulopathy, V, p 73.

E. Fiberoptic bronchoscopy. Arrange early if the diagnosis is in doubt or hemoptysis continues.

F. Consult. Obtain a thoracic surgery consultation if the patient has massive or continuous hemoptysis. Medical management of massive hemoptysis is associated with a high mortality rate.

G. Cough suppression. Retard the cough reflex with codeine-based drugs, and place the patient on quiet bed rest.

H. Treat the underlying disease state
   1. **Lung cancer.** Can be treated surgically if there are no metastases and the pulmonary reserve is adequate. Otherwise, radiation or laser therapy can rapidly control bleeding.
   2. **Infections.** Treat with antibiotics as dictated by Gram's stain and clinical picture. If a necrotizing pneumonia is present, consider methicillin-resistant *Staphylococcus aureus* or *Pseudomonas* infection and treat accordingly.
   3. **Pulmonary emboli.** Treat acutely with heparin. See Section I, Chapter 11, Chest Pain, V, p 66.
   4. **Diffuse alveolar hemorrhage or a pulmonary-renal syndrome.** 1000 mg methylprednisolone (Solu-Medrol) IV may control bleeding, pending definitive workup.
   5. **Nonsurgical patients with localized bleeding.** Bronchial arteriography followed by embolism may be lifesaving. However, collateral circulation to the spinal arteries or carotids must be excluded before embolization.

REFERENCES

Cahil BC, Ingbar DH: Massive hemoptysis-assessment and management in clinics. Clin Chest Med 1994;15:147.

Ryu JH, Swensen SJ, Olson EJ et al: Diagnosis of pulmonary embolism with use of computed tomographic angiography. Mayo Clin Proc 2001;76:59.

31. HYPERCALCEMIA

I. **Problem.** A 60-year-old man is admitted for severe diffuse bone pain and is found to have a calcium level of 5.5 mEq/L or 2.75 mmol/L (normal: 4.2–5.1 mEq/L or 2.10–2.55 mmol/L).

II. **Immediate Questions**

A. **What other symptoms are present?** The classic presentation of primary hyperparathyroidism is "stones, bones, moans, and groans" from renal calculi, osteitis fibrosa, constipation, and neuropsychiatric problems, respectively. Renal calculi and osteitis fibrosa are seldom associated with hypercalcemia of malignancy because both result from longstanding hypercalcemia. Hypercalcemia causes a variety of nonspecific symptoms including fatigue, weakness, polyuria, polydipsia, bone pain, constipation, nausea, vomiting, anorexia, and mental status changes ranging from confusion to coma.

B. **Does the patient have any condition that could be related to hypercalcemia?** Hypertension, peptic ulcer, and nephrolithiasis are associated with hyperparathyroidism.

C. **Is the patient on any medications that might cause hypercalcemia?** Thiazide diuretics, vitamin D, and exogenous sources of calcium are possible causes.

D. **Is there a family history of hypercalcemia?** One cause is familial hypocalciuric hypercalcemia. There are also three syndromes of multiple endocrine neoplasia (MEN) that are inherited in an autosomal dominant pattern. *MEN I* includes primary hyperparathyroidism, hypersecretion of pancreatic islet hormones, pituitary adenoma, and possibly other endocrine tumors. *MEN IIA* consists of primary hyperparathyroidism, medullary carcinoma of the thyroid, and pheochromocytoma. Hyperparathyroidism is rare in *MEN IIB*.

E. **Has the patient been noted to have elevated calcium in the past?** Longstanding hypercalcemia suggests primary hyperparathyroidism. Malignant disease is usually associated with recent-onset hypercalcemia.

III. **Differential Diagnosis**

A. **Primary hyperparathyroidism.** About 20% of patients with hypercalcemia have hyperparathyroidism, usually from a single hyperfunctioning adenoma. An elevated calcium, a low phosphate, and elevated or relatively elevated parathyroid hormone are characteristic findings. Most patients in whom hyperparathyroidism is diagnosed are asymptomatic.

B. **Malignant disease.** The most common cause of hypercalcemia in hospitalized patients is cancer, usually from bony metastasis or often from humoral factors produced by a tumor.

1. **Metastatic carcinoma to bone.** Breast, lung, and renal cell carcinoma.
2. **Hematologic malignancies.** Direct bone involvement with multiple myeloma and lymphoma.
3. **Humoral factors.** Prostaglandins, parathyroid hormone-related protein, and osteoclast-activating factor. These factors are most commonly seen with bronchogenic non–small cell carcinoma, renal cell carcinoma, breast cancer, T-cell or B-cell lymphoma, hepatoma, melanoma, and multiple myeloma.

C. **Medications**
1. **Thiazide diuretics.** These agents increase renal reabsorption of calcium.
2. **Vitamin D intoxication.** A fat-soluble vitamin that increases intestinal absorption, increases mobilization from bone, and increases renal reabsorption of calcium.
3. **Vitamin A intoxication.** Another fat-soluble vitamin that is a rare cause of hypercalcemia; causes increased bone reabsorption.
4. **Exogenous calcium.** For example, calcium carbonate, which is found in certain antacids.

D. **Granulomatous diseases—sarcoidosis.** These conditions are marked by increased sensitivity to vitamin D.

E. **Milk-alkali syndrome.** From increased intake of calcium and alkali. Milk-alkali syndrome results in hypercalcemia, hypocalciuria, hyperphosphatemia, renal failure, and metastatic calcifications.

F. **Immobilization.** Prolonged bed rest increases bone reabsorption, resulting in hypercalcemia and osteoporosis.

G. **Recovery from acute renal failure.** Thought to be from secondary hyperparathyroidism.

H. **Chronic renal failure**

I. **Endocrinopathies**
1. **Hyperthyroidism.** Bone reabsorption induced by thyroid hormone.
2. **Acromegaly**
3. **Adrenal insufficiency**

J. **Paget's disease.** The calcium level is usually normal but may increase with immobilization.

K. **Familial hypocalciuric hypercalcemia.** An autosomal dominant condition causing lifelong hypercalcemia with normal urinary calcium excretion.

IV. **Database**

A. **Physical examination key points**
1. **Vital signs.** There may be associated hypertension.
2. **Skin.** Excoriations may occur as a result of pruritus from metastatic calcifications in the skin.

3. **Lymph nodes.** Lymphadenopathy suggests carcinoma, hematologic malignancy, or sarcoidosis.
4. **HEENT.** An enlarged thyroid gland suggests hyperthyroidism.
5. **Chest.** Look for evidence of lung carcinoma.
6. **Abdomen.** An enlarged liver or spleen suggests metastatic carcinoma, a hematologic cancer, or sarcoidosis.
7. **Musculoskeletal exam.** Bone pain with palpation or percussion points to carcinoma or Paget's disease. Myopathy from hypercalcemia can cause proximal muscle weakness.
8. **Neurologic exam.** Impaired mentation, weakness, and hyporeflexia may result from hypercalcemia.

B. **Laboratory data**
1. **Repeat levels for calcium along with a serum albumin or obtain an ionized calcium level.** Always confirm an elevated calcium level and the severity of the hypercalcemia before initiating therapy. Keep in mind that a high-normal total calcium may signify hypercalcemia in the presence of marked hypoalbuminemia. A calcium value must be corrected in the presence of hypoalbuminemia. Normally, the total calcium decreases by 0.2 mmol/L, or 0.4 mEq/L, for every 1 g/dL decrease in the serum albumin from normal levels (4.0 g/dL) without changing the ionized calcium level. Symptoms of hypercalcemia usually develop at 6.5–7.0 mEq/L, or 3.25–3.5 mmol/L.
2. **Phosphorus.** The phosphorus level is low in primary hyperparathyroidism; it is elevated in vitamin D intoxication.
3. **Arterial blood gases.** A decrease in the pH will increase the ionized calcium mostly by displacing calcium bound to albumin. A metabolic acidosis may also be seen with adrenal insufficiency, a potential cause of hypercalcemia. An increase in the pH is seen in milk-alkali syndrome and possibly with thiazide diuretics if there is associated volume depletion.
4. **Alkaline phosphatase.** This value is increased in primary hyperparathyroidism, Paget's disease, and bony metastases.
5. **Blood urea nitrogen and creatinine.** Renal insufficiency exacerbates hypercalcemia or may be secondary to hypercalcemia.
6. **Total protein and albumin.** An increased total protein-to-albumin ratio suggests multiple myeloma. If the total protein-to-albumin ratio is elevated, then quantitative immunoglobulins and serum and urine protein electrophoresis should be ordered.
7. **Amylase and lipase.** Hypercalcemia can cause pancreatitis. If abdominal pain is present, pancreatitis should be ruled out.
8. **Urinalysis.** Hematuria may arise from renal cell carcinoma or secondary to nephrolithiasis.

C. **Radiologic and other studies**
1. **Chest x-ray.** Bilateral hilar adenopathy implies sarcoidosis. Also, carcinoma or lymphoma may be detected by chest x-ray. Os-

teopenia of the vertebral column may be evident on the lateral film.

2. **Abdominal x-rays.** May reveal renal calcifications as a result of hypercalcemia; other findings may suggest carcinoma.

3. **Bone films.** These are especially useful if there is localized bone pain; they may reveal osteolytic/osteoblastic lesions from carcinoma or the osteolytic lesions of multiple myeloma. If lesions are present, a bone scan would be helpful to reveal extent of the disease. A bone scan will be negative in a patient with multiple myeloma because of the absence of associated osteoblastic activity.

4. **Skull films and skeletal survey.** Obtain if multiple myeloma is suspected. These films classically reveal multiple punched-out lesions and may also be helpful in detecting subperiosteal resorption resulting from primary hyperparathyroidism, especially evident on hand films.

5. **Electrocardiogram.** Associated shortening of QT interval and lengthening of PR interval.

V. Plan. Lower the calcium level and then treat the underlying disorder. Treat more aggressively with severe hypercalcemia > 7.0 mEq/L, or 3.5 mmol/L, or when the patient is symptomatic. Treatment is directed at decreasing the release of calcium from bone or increasing deposition in bone, decreasing absorption from the gastrointestinal tract, and increasing excretion renally or through chelation.

A. Restrict calcium intake and encourage mobilization

B. Treat underlying causes

C. Institute saline diuresis. This is usually the initial step. Patients with moderate to severe symptomatic hypercalcemia are frequently volume-depleted. It is essential to restore the patient's volume and then to maintain a urine output of at least 2 L/day. Sodium increases calcium excretion by inhibiting proximal tubule reabsorption. Administration of large volumes of normal saline can be hazardous in the elderly or in patients with renal failure or with left ventricular dysfunction.

D. Administer medications

1. **Furosemide (Lasix).** Dosage is 20–80 mg IV Q 2–4 hr. You frequently administer the furosemide concomitantly with normal saline. Furosemide is a calciuric agent; however, calcium excretion is not promoted if volume depletion develops. Follow urinary output closely as well as monitor the volume of normal saline administered and daily weights. Older patients with tenuous cardiac conditions may need hemodynamic monitoring in an ICU if vigorous saline diuresis is attempted. Potassium chloride should be added to the saline solution after rehydration to maintain normokalemia. Also, monitor for hypomagnesemia and correct if necessary. **Caution:** Thiazide diuretics should *never* be used be-

cause they may actually worsen the hypercalcemia through enhanced distal tubular reabsorption of calcium.

2. **Bisphosphonates.** These agents inhibit osteoclastic activity. Pamidronate disodium (Aredia) is superior to etidronate (Didronel), the first drug in this class approved to treat hypercalcemia. Pamidronate 60–90 mg is given intravenously over 4–24 hours. Hypokalemia, hypomagnesemia, and hypophosphatemia can occur. Calcium levels decline in 2 days, with nadir at 7 days and duration of action of approximately 2 weeks. Use in combination with calcitonin if rapid reduction is desired.

3. **Plicamycin (Mithramycin).** Give 25 µg/kg in 1 L of normal saline over 3–6 hours. This agent inhibits bone reabsorption; effect may not manifest for 12–24 hours, with a peak action at 48–96 hours. The dose can be repeated at 24–48 hours for 3–4 total doses. Nausea and renal, hepatic, and bone marrow toxicity (thrombocytopenia) can occur.

4. **Calcitonin.** This agent is rapid-acting, but weak; it inhibits bone reabsorption and increases urinary excretion of calcium. Usually, calcitonin administration is only a temporary measure because resistance to the calcium-lowering effect often develops. An effective dose is 4 U/kg Q 12 hr IM or SC (salmon calcitonin). Side effects include nausea, vomiting, flushing, and allergic reactions.

5. **Corticosteroids.** Hydrocortisone 50–75 mg Q 6 hr decreases calcium absorption from the GI tract and inhibits bone reabsorption. It also may inhibit growth of lymphoid cancers. Corticosteroids are effective for treating hypercalcemia associated with sarcoidosis, vitamin D intoxication, and hematologic cancers (multiple myeloma, lymphoma, leukemia). *Note*: Onset of action is relatively slow.

6. **Intravenous phosphates.** These drugs work by increasing deposition of calcium in bone and soft tissues and decreasing bone reabsorption. Use of these drugs can result in metastatic calcification, renal failure, and death. They are contraindicated in patients with renal insufficiency and should be reserved for life-threatening hypercalcemia resistant to other measures.

E. Dialysis. This is a treatment of last resort.

REFERENCES

Case Records of the Massachusetts General Hospital (Case 38-2002). N Engl J Med 2002;347:1952.

Edelson GW, Kleerekoper M: Hypercalcemic crisis. Med Clin North Am 1995;79:79.

Marx SJ: Hyperparathyroid and hypoparathyroid disorders. N Engl J Med 2000;343:1863.

Mundy GR, Guise TA. Hypercalcemia of malignancy. Am J Med 1997;103:134.

Popovtzer MM: Disorders of calcium, phosphorus, vitamin D and parathyroid hormone activity. In: Schrier RW, ed. *Renal and Electrolyte Disorders*. 6th ed. Lippincott-Raven;2003:216.

32. HYPERGLYCEMIA

I. Problem. A 44-year-old man is admitted because of chest pain. His glucose is 428 mg/dL, or 23.79 mmol/L.

II. Immediate Questions

  A. What are the patient's vital signs? Fever may indicate sepsis, which can exacerbate hyperglycemia. Hypotension or tachycardia may indicate volume depletion common in diabetic ketoacidosis (DKA) and hyperosmolar syndromes. Tachypnea may be due to Kussmaul respirations in DKA.

  B. Is the patient known to be diabetic? A history of diabetes should make the clinician consider factors such as noncompliance with medication/diet, sepsis, acute stress, glucocorticoid use, and myocardial infarction (MI), which can result in poor control of hyperglycemia. The absence of a history of diabetes should make one consider all of the preceding factors as unmasking latent carbohydrate intolerance, as well as the possibility of laboratory error.

  C. If the patient is diabetic, what medications is he or she taking and when was the last meal in relation to the time of phlebotomy? Before one modifies the regimen, it is important to know whether the patient is receiving large or small amounts of insulin and whether he or she is receiving oral hypoglycemic agents. In addition, it is important to know whether the blood sugar was drawn randomly (and therefore could be postprandial) or whether it represents a fasting level.

III. Differential Diagnosis

  A. Diabetes mellitus

   1. **Type 1 (previously called juvenile diabetes or insulin-dependent diabetes).** Patients with type 1 diabetes require insulin even when not eating, although in lower doses. They are more likely to be thin or normal in weight, young, and "brittle" and are prone to DKA. *Diabetic ketoacidosis* may be defined as a blood sugar level > 300 mg/dL (16.68 mmol/L), urine ketones that are strongly positive, and a serum bicarbonate < 17 mmol or a pH < 7.30.

   2. **Type 2 (previously called adult-onset diabetes or non–insulin-dependent diabetes mellitus).** Patients with type 2 diabetes tend to be obese and older and are more prone to hyperosmolar hyperglycemic syndromes than to ketoacidosis. Weight loss may normalize carbohydrate metabolism initially. Some patients can be managed with diet and exercise alone, although data from the United Kingdom Prospective Diabetes Study indicate that type 2 diabetes usually progresses to require oral agents and eventually insulin.

   3. **Gestational diabetes.** Glucose intolerance associated with pregnancy. Close monitoring and tight control are important to improve outcome of mother and infant.

B. Acute stress. With mild carbohydrate intolerance, acute events such as sepsis, MI, trauma, and surgery may cause relatively marked hyperglycemia. Some patients do not require therapy after the acute event has resolved.

C. Exogenous glucose load. Hyperalimentation and peritoneal dialysis.

D. Medications. Exogenous or endogenous glucocorticoids (Cushing's syndrome), thiazide diuretics, and other agents may cause hyperglycemia or unmask latent carbohydrate intolerance.

E. Pancreatic disease. Severe acute pancreatitis or longstanding chronic pancreatitis with endocrine pancreatic insufficiency.

F. Spurious hyperglycemia. Drawing blood above an IV line that contains dextrose; mislabeling; or inadvertently switching blood from different patients results in inaccurate finger-stick glucoses. When in doubt, immediately repeat the test before treating.

IV. Database

A. Physical examination key points

1. **Vital signs.** Include orthostatic blood pressure and pulse to evaluate volume status. A decrease in systolic blood pressure of 10 mm Hg and/or an increase in heart rate of 20 bpm suggest volume depletion in younger patients. In patients over 75 years there may be up to 25 mm systolic orthostatic drop normally, and a pulse increase of 16 bpm signifies volume depletion. Fever implies sepsis. *Kussmaul respirations* (deep, regular respirations, whether slow or fast) suggest DKA.

2. **HEENT.** Fruity odor on breath suggests ketones and DKA. Funduscopic exam may show diabetic retinopathy, which suggests long-standing disease and increases the likelihood of other diabetic complications such as nephropathy and neuropathy.

3. **Lungs.** Evaluate for signs of pneumonia. Follow-up lung exams for rales are important in assessing volume.

4. **Heart.** Listen for associated findings of ischemia/MI, such as a third (S_3) or fourth (S_3) heart sound, or murmur of mitral insufficiency.

5. **Peripheral vascular system.** Listen for bruits.

6. **Abdomen.** Evaluate for cause of sepsis. Rebound tenderness suggests peritonitis. A positive Murphy's sign (see Section I, Chapter 1, Abdominal Pain, p 1) suggests acute cholecystitis, which is more common in diabetics.

7. **Extremities.** Check for foot ulcers and cellulitis.

8. **Neurologic exam.** A clouded sensorium suggests more severe disease (ketoacidosis or hyperosmolar syndrome).

B. Laboratory data

1. **Serum glucose.** Significantly elevated finger-stick glucose should be further evaluated with a serum glucose.

2. **Complete blood count.** Leukocytosis with a left shift suggests the presence of infection. An elevated WBC count may be seen in DKA without an associated infection or sepsis, but a left shift, toxic granulation, and vacuolization suggest a bacterial infection.

3. **Serum electrolytes, blood urea nitrogen and creatinine, phosphorus, calcium, magnesium, amylase.**
   a. Even though serum potassium may be normal or even high, total body potassium is often depleted and potassium repletion is indicated. Initially, normal or elevated potassium decreases with insulin administration and with correction of acidosis if present.
   b. Serum sodium is spuriously lowered by hyperglycemia. Several correction formulas have been proposed; a recently proposed formula follows:

   Corrected plasma sodium = measured plasma sodium + [change in plasma glucose ÷ 42]

   c. Serum bicarbonate is low and the anion gap is elevated in DKA.
   d. Creatinine may be falsely elevated in the presence of serum ketones. Both blood urea nitrogen and creatinine may be elevated as a result of profound volume depletion or diabetic nephropathy.
   e. Phosphate may fall with treatment and should be monitored, although routine prophylactic treatment with phosphate is not recommended. When needed, oral phosphate is preferred.
   f. Calcium may be low with acute pancreatitis.
   g. Magnesium may be low, especially in DKA. Magnesium deficiency may contribute to relative insulin resistance.
   h. An elevated amylase or lipase may indicate pancreatitis; ketone bodies may factitiously elevate the serum amylase.

4. **Arterial blood gases (ABG).** To evaluate the degree of acidemia. A careful look at the pH, pCO_2, and serum bicarbonate often reveals more than one acid–base disorder. (See Section I, Chapter 2, Acidosis, p 10.)

5. **Urine or serum for ketones.** This helps to distinguish between DKA and hyperosmolar coma. Acetoacetate is the ketone that is measured on standard tests; however, β-hydroxybutyrate is the predominant ketone in DKA. Initially, the level of ketones may not decrease or may actually increase as β-hydroxybutyrate is metabolized to acetoacetate.

6. **Cultures**. If sepsis is suspected, appropriate cultures should be ordered.

C. **Radiologic and other studies**
   1. **Chest x-ray.** To evaluate for pneumonia and congestive heart failure (CHF).

2. **Electrocardiogram (ECG).** To rule out MI as a cause of difficult-to-control diabetes.
3. **Miscellaneous studies.** Depending on clinical suspicion; for example, computed tomography scan of the abdomen is recommended if intra-abdominal abscess is suspected.

V. **Plan.** Management depends on the clinical setting and severity of hyperglycemia. This section is divided into four parts on the basis of severity.

A. **Type 2 diabetes with a serum glucose** < 450 mg/dL, or 25.0 mmol/L (no ketones, no metabolic acidosis, and patient is not critically ill or in the ICU or CCU).
   1. **Insulin.** Initially, may use sliding scale regular insulin Q 6 hr based on results of finger-stick glucoses. For a typical regimen, see Table 1–7. Patients already receiving insulin may be continued on their usual dose with supplemental sliding scale insulin or have their usual dose increased.
   2. **Oral hypoglycemic agents.** Some patients with type 2 diabetes mellitus may be managed with oral hypoglycemic agents, especially when the glucose is below 300 mg/dL (16.68 mmol/L).
      a. **Metformin.** An excellent drug, with a low risk of hypoglycemia. It is the only oral agent shown to reduce macrovascular complications. However, metformin should be avoided in patients whose serum creatinine is > 1.4 or in patients with CHF. Some diabetologists avoid using metformin in the inpatient setting or in unstable patients because of the risk of lactic acidosis. Caution is advised with ethanol abuse. Metformin should be held for 48 hours after intravenous contrast and after surgery.
      b. **Sulfonylureas.** These are often used for first-line treatment; generic sulfonylureas are less expensive. Meglitinides such as repaglinide (Prandin) act similarly to the sulfonylureas.
      c. **Thiazolidinediones.** Thiazolidinediones such as pioglitazone (Actos) and rosiglitazone (Avandia) potentiate the action of insulin by decreasing insulin resistance. The thiazolidinediones need to be monitored for potential hepatic toxicity. In fact, the

TABLE I–7. SLIDING SCALE OF INSULIN DOSAGE FOR HYPERGLYCEMIA.

Glucose Level	Insulin (Short-Acting/Regular)
<180 mg/dL (10.00 mmol/L)	0 U SC
180–240 mg/dL (10.00–13.34 mmol/L)	3–5 U SC
240–400 mg/dL (13.34–22.23 mmol/L)	8–10 U SC
>400 mg/dL (>22.23 mmol/L)	10–15 U SC[1]

[1]Follow with a stat serum glucose and notify the house officer of result.
SC, subcutaneous.

prototypic agent troglitazone was removed from the market for this reason. Obtain baseline serum transaminases, then again every 2 months for the first year and periodically thereafter.

   d. **Alpha-glucosidase inhibitors:** Acarbose (Precose) and Miglitol (Glyset) may be used for mild hyperglycemia or in combination with other agents. The main side effects are flatulence and diarrhea.

   e. **Other drugs.** Orlistat (Xenical) is a hepatic and pancreatic lipase inhibitor that results in significant weight loss, which may in turn result in improved glycemic control. Combination therapy with different classes of oral agents and/or bedtime insulin is becoming more common.

3. **Diet.** In the short term, an 1800-calorie American Diabetes Association diet is useful, although other modified diets may be appropriate in certain settings. The importance of diet is controversial. A nutritious diet low in simple sugars and fat usually suffices. If there is a complicating condition such as a foot ulcer that requires positive nitrogen balance for resolution, be sure the patient receives adequate calories and protein.

B. **Hyperosmolar, hyperglycemic nonketotic syndrome, glucose > 600 mg/dL, or 33.35 mmol/L (no ketones, no metabolic acidosis)**

   1. **Aggressive management.** The ICU is often required. Depressed mental status is a marker of a more serious situation.

   2. **Saline**

      a. **Rate of administration.** Hypotension due to volume depletion (hypovolemic shock) should be treated with IV normal saline and given as rapidly as possible until hypotension resolves. Less profound volume depletion may be treated with 500–1000 mL of NS in the first hour, after which the rate is decreased to 250–500 mL/hr until signs of volume depletion resolve. Obviously, caution is indicated, particularly in smaller or older patients and those with limited cardiac and renal reserve. These patients need frequent (every 1–2 hours) assessment of volume status with orthostatic blood pressure and pulse, and auscultation for a S_3 and rales.

      b. **Concentration.** Some clinicians prefer switching from NS to half-normal saline after the first liter, or alternating half-normal saline with NS. When the blood sugar reaches 250–300 mg/dL (13.90–16.68 mmol/L), IV fluids are switched to D5 half-normal saline or half normal saline at a rate based on volume assessment.

   3. **Potassium.** If serum potassium is < 5.5 mmol/L, add 20–30 mEq/L at a rate not to exceed 10–15 mEq/hr. Follow levels Q 4 hr. Keep serum potassium at 4.0–5.0 mmol/L.

   4. **Insulin.** There are many ways of giving insulin. Continuous IV infusion drip of short-acting (regular) insulin is preferred. An initial

dose of 0.15 U/kg of short-acting (regular) insulin is given as a bolus and is followed immediately by a continuous-infusion drip at 0.1 U/kg/hr. This should be adjusted to ensure that blood glucose is falling at least 10% per hour. If IV access is not readily available, then administer regular insulin intramuscularly; or, if shock is not present, rapid-acting insulin aspart, insulin lispro, or regular insulin may be used subcutaneously.

5. **Lab work.** Serum glucose measurements are needed Q 1–2 hr. Magnesium should be checked initially and repeated if there are signs of magnesium deficiency. Potassium should be checked Q 2-4 hr, and phosphorus Q 6–12 hr.

6. **Dextrose in IV fluids.** When glucose falls to the range 250–300 mg/dL (13.89–16.68 mmol/L), some authors recommend decreasing the insulin drip and changing IV fluids to D5 half-normal saline, with the goal of maintaining the glucose at 100–200 mg/dL (5.56–11.12 mmol/L). Other authors recommend discontinuing the continuous insulin drip, resuming the patient's usual insulin regimen, and using half-normal saline with potassium to continue fluid-electrolyte repletion.

C. **Diabetic ketoacidosis.** Hyperglycemia with ketonuria and low serum bicarbonate. This is a medical emergency, often requiring management in the ICU setting. In the setting of profound ketoacidosis, patients are less responsive to insulin and larger doses are required. Volume repletion is essential.

1. **IV fluids.** In the setting of shock, normal saline is administered as rapidly as possible until blood pressure rises. In patients who are not hypotensive, administer 500 to 1000 mL of NS in the first hour followed by 200 mL to 500 mL per hour until volume status improves. The same volume assessment parameters should be followed as in hyperosmolar coma, described earlier (see V.B.2.a.). Some authors prefer switching or alternating half-normal saline with NS. When serum glucose levels reach 250–300 mg/dL (13.89–16.68 mmol/L), change to D5 half-normal saline; or half normal saline (add 40 mEq of potassium per liter) at a rate based on volume assessment.

2. **Insulin.** Recent guidelines of the American Diabetes Association recommend a bolus of 0.15 U/kg of regular insulin followed by a continuous infusion of 0.1 U/kg/hr with a desired decrease in glucose by 50–75 mg/dL/hr. If the glucose does not decrease by at least 50 mg/dL/hr, the rate of the continuous infusion is doubled every hour until the glucose decreases by the desired rate. When the glucose is 250–300 mg/dL, the continuous infusion of insulin is decreased to 0.05–0.1 U/kg/hr and the intravenous fluids are changed to include 5% dextrose. A continuous infusion of insulin is maintained until the metabolic acidosis in DKA resolves (ketones are cleared) or until mental status changes and hyperosmolarity resolves.

3. **Potassium.** Potassium depletion is almost always present in DKA, even if the measured serum potassium is elevated. If serum potassium is < 5.5 mEq/L, potassium 20–30 mEq /L is given in IV fluids at a rate not to exceed 15 mEq/hr unless the patient's heart rhythm is being continuously monitored. If hypokalemia is present initially, this implies profound potassium depletion and IV potassium chloride is started immediately. Potassium 10–15 mEq/hr is given to maintain serum potassium at 3.0–5.0 mmol/L. Doses of potassium > 15 mEq/hr should not be administered without continuous cardiac monitoring. Potassium is osmotically active, so that adding 40 mEq per liter of normal saline will give an osmolality approximately equal to ¾ NS.

4. **Bicarbonate.** Its use is controversial and most clinicians are more conservative than in the past. One approach is to use bicarbonate to correct the pH to 7.00. For pH 6.90–7.00, give 44 mmol over 1–2 hr; for pH < 6.90, give 88 mmol of sodium bicarbonate over 1–2 hr. Administration of sodium bicarbonate should be considered if life-threatening hyperkalemia (with ECG changes) is present, or if there is significant acidosis without an elevated anion gap.

5. **Lab work.** Glucose should be repeated Q 1–2 hr, and electrolytes Q 4–6 hr. Magnesium should be checked initially, and phosphate initially and after 6–12 hr. An ABG measurement should be obtained Q 2–4 hr if acidosis is severe, or if the patient requires sodium bicarbonate. Serum/urine ketones may be of some use, although increasing ketones may be spurious (see IV.B.5, p 192).

6. **Associated conditions.** Treat any associated condition such as sepsis, MI, or stress appropriately. Recent evidence suggests the importance of glucose control in critically ill patients in the ICU, even those without diabetes mellitus. Target glucose values in this setting are 90–145 mg/dL (5.0–8.0 mmol/L).

D. **Guidelines for management of hyperglycemia in diabetes.** Evidence suggests that close management ("tight" control) of diabetes will lower the incidence of complications. Current recommendations for patients with diabetes are to maintain the glucose of 80–120 mg/dL before meals and a hemoglobin A_3 level < 6.5%. Such tight control necessitates self-monitoring of finger-stick glucoses, multiple insulin administrations per day, or use of a continuous-infusion insulin pump.

E. **Hyperglycemia in the setting of critical illness.** Maintaining near normal glucose levels with insulin reduces morbidity in patients with severe acute illness during the perioperative period and in the setting of acute MI. Consider IV insulin in these settings. One protocol is as follows:

1. Initial units of insulin per hour in infusion = (plasma glucose-60) × 0.03.

2. Measure glucose hourly; recalculate and adjust insulin infusion rate hourly as below:

   a. If plasma glucose > 140 mg/dL, increase formula multiplier by 0.01.

   b. If plasma glucose < 100 mg/dL, decrease multiplier 0.01.

   c. Treat hypoglycemia if plasma glucose < 80–100 mg/dL. Give D50 using formula: 100-plasma glucose × 0.3 = #cc D50 to be given IV push. Re-measure plasma glucose in 30 minutes and repeat D50 treatment if needed.

REFERENCES

American Diabetes Association: Clinical practice recommendations. Diabetes Care 2001;24(entire suppl 1).

American Diabetes Association: Standards of medical care for patients with diabetes mellitus. Diabetes Care 2000;23(suppl 1):S32.

Brown G. Dodek P: Intravenous insulin nomogram improves blood glucose control in the critically ill. Crit Care Med 2001;29:1714.

DeFronzo RA: Pharmacologic therapy for type 2 diabetes mellitus. Ann Intern Med 1999;131:281.

Finney SJ, Zekveld C, Elia A, Evans TW: Glucose control and mortality in critically ill patients. JAMA 2003;15;290:2041.

Lebovitz HE: Oral therapies for diabetic hyperglycemia. Endocrinol Metab Clin North Am 2001;30:909.

Nathan DM: Clinical practice. Initial management of glycemia in type 2 diabetes mellitus. N Engl J Med 2002;347:1342.

The Diabetes Control and Complications Trial Research Group: The effect of intensive treatment of diabetes on the development and progression of long-term complications in insulin-dependent diabetes mellitus. N Engl J Med 1993;329:977.

33. HYPERKALEMIA

I. Problem. A 64-year-old man with diabetes admitted for a myocardial infarction is found to have a potassium (K^+) level of 7.1 mmol/L.

II. Immediate Questions

A. What are the patient's vital signs? Hyperkalemia can result in life-threatening ventricular arrhythmias. Obtain an electrocardiogram (ECG) immediately.

B. What is the urine output? Acute oliguric renal failure is the most common cause of potentially fatal hyperkalemia. Evaluate urine output and renal function tests.

C. Is the patient receiving potassium in an intravenous (IV) solution? Supplemental potassium administration is the most common cause of severe hyperkalemia in hospitalized patients, and the risk is greater with IV potassium. Standard IV solutions often contain 20 mEq/L potassium; hyperalimentation solutions may contain more. Stop all exogenous potassium until the problem is resolved.

D. Is the patient on any medications that could elevate the potassium? Potential causes include potassium-sparing diuretics such as spironolactone (Aldactone), triamterene (Dyrenium), and amiloride (Midamor); nonsteroidal anti-inflammatory drugs (NSAIDs); angiotensin-converting enzyme (ACE) inhibitors, and trimethoprim-sulfamethoxazole can also cause hyperkalemia.

E. Is the lab result correct? If hyperkalemia is unexpected or inconsistent after the preceding questions are answered, consider pseudohyperkalemia, especially if the ECG shows no changes of hyperkalemia. There are several causes of factitious hyperkalemia, the most common being from the tourniquet used to draw blood. A tight tourniquet around an exercising extremity can elevate the potassium as much as 2.0 mmol/L. Hemolysis of a blood sample before the chemical determination is another common source of error. Extreme leukocytosis (> 70,000) or thrombocytosis (> 1,000,000) can also elevate the serum potassium. If this is a possibility, obtain a plasma potassium.

III. Differential Diagnosis. In general, true hyperkalemia results from one of three mechanisms: a shift of potassium from intracellular to extracellular space, impaired renal excretion of potassium, or increased exogenous potassium intake.

A. Increased exogenous intake. High-potassium foods, potassium salts (salt "substitutes," ie, sodium-free salt), or large doses of potassium penicillin are examples of exogenous sources of potassium. Hyperkalemia in this setting usually occurs in patients on potassium-sparing diuretics, ACE inhibitors, or NSAIDs.

B. Increased potassium release from cells. Shifts from intracellular to extracellular space.

  1. Insulin deficiency. Occurs with diabetic ketoacidosis.

  2. β_2-adrenergic blockade. In patients with renal disease, propranolol and labetolol, but not atenolol, which is selective for B_1, can raise potassium levels by about 1 mEq/L. At higher doses, atenolol becomes less B_1 selective and can cause hyperkalemia.

  3. Acute metabolic acidosis. Metabolic acidosis can cause hyperkalemia by shifting intracellular potassium into plasma. This occurs with diarrhea when bicarbonate is lost or by infusion of acids such as arginine hydrochloride, which may be used to assess growth hormone reserves or to treat metabolic alkalosis.

  4. Tissue breakdown. Any condition associated with rapid destruction of cells results in the release of potassium into the extracellular fluid. Examples include rhabdomyolysis, burns, massive hemolysis, and tumor lysis.

  5. Digitalis intoxication. A massive overdose of digitalis is a rare cause of hyperkalemia. This results from inhibition of the sodium/potassium–dependent ATPase pump, and intracellular potassium is lost.

6. **Succinylcholine.** Mild increases in serum potassium occur with this commonly used muscle relaxant. In patients with tissue destruction or neuromuscular disease, life-threatening hyperkalemia may occur. Succinylcholine causes cell membrane depolarization, resulting in intracellular-to-extracellular shifts in potassium.

7. **Hyperosmolality.** Administration of hypertonic mannitol or saline results in major increases in serum osmolality and thus may cause hyperkalemia.

8. **Hyperkalemic periodic paralysis.** This rare, inherited disorder is characterized by spontaneous episodes of hyperkalemia and muscle weakness.

C. **Impaired renal excretion of potassium**

1. **Chronic renal failure.** Most patients with chronic renal failure maintain normal potassium balance until renal function is severely impaired. However, when this condition is challenged with a potassium load or potassium-sparing diuretics (spironolactone, triamterene, amiloride), ACE inhibitors (enalapril, lisinopril), or NSAIDs (indomethacin, ibuprofen), the patient's adaptive mechanisms are inadequate to prevent hyperkalemia.

2. **Acute renal failure.** Hyperkalemia complicates oliguric renal failure because of the flow-dependent distal tubular potassium secretion. Acute renal failure often occurs in the setting of increased potassium load (trauma, blood transfusions, or postoperative hypercatabolic state).

3. **Adrenal insufficiency.** Adrenal insufficiency, in particular hypoaldosteronism, results in reduced renal ability to excrete potassium.

4. **Hyporeninemic hypoaldosteronism.** Hyperchloremic metabolic acidosis (type IV renal tubular acidosis) as well as hyperkalemia is present. Mild renal insufficiency secondary to diabetic nephropathy or interstitial nephropathy is also seen. This condition may be aggravated by administration of NSAIDs or potassium-sparing diuretics.

5. **Heparin.** Long-term anticoagulation with heparin may lead to hyperkalemia, probably through the inhibition of aldosterone synthesis.

6. **Potassium-sparing diuretics.** Hyperkalemia secondary to triamterene or spironolactone is usually seen with underlying renal insufficiency. But there have been cases, especially in diabetics, in which patients with normal renal function developed hyperkalemia.

7. **NSAIDs.** See III.C.1.

8. **ACE inhibitors.** See III.C.1.

9. **Systemic lupus erythematosus (SLE), renal transplantation, sickle cell disease.** Patients with these disorders may demonstrate an isolated defect in renal potassium excretion thought to be secondary to aldosterone resistance.

10. **Trimethoprim-sulfamethoxazole (TMP-SMX).** High-dose TMP-SMX therapy used for the treatment of *Pneumocystis carinii* pneumonia in HIV-infected patients may result in life-threatening hyperkalemia. Standard-dose TMP-SMX has subsequently been shown to increase serum potassium when used to treat various infections, especially with concomitant renal insufficiency. Trimethoprim acts like amiloride to block sodium channels in the distal nephron, decreasing renal potassium excretion.

IV. Database

A. Physical examination key points

1. **Cardiovascular exam.** The conduction system of the heart is most vulnerable to hyperkalemia, which may result in bradycardia, ventricular fibrillation, or asystole.
2. **Neuromuscular exam.** Skeletal muscle paralysis may occasionally dominate and result in weakness, tingling, and hyperactive deep tendon reflexes.

B. Laboratory data

1. **Electrolytes.** Low bicarbonate may indicate a metabolic acidosis. Low sodium may result from aldosterone deficiency.
2. **Plasma potassium.** Obtain if the serum level is in doubt.
3. **Blood urea nitrogen (BUN) and creatinine.** Assess renal function.
4. **Arterial blood gases (ABG).** Along with a serum bicarbonate, an ABG is essential in establishing the acid–base status.
5. **Platelets and white blood cell count.** Marked elevations may cause factitious hyperkalemia.
6. **Serum creatine phosphokinase.** To detect rhabdomyolysis.
7. **Digoxin level.** If indicated.
8. **Serum aldosterone level.** Indicated after initial workup. Lack of stimulation with volume depletion is consistent with mineralocorticoid deficiency.

C. Other studies. *An ECG is a must!* The cardiac abnormalities that occur with hyperkalemia are initially tall, peaked T waves in the precordial leads, followed by decreased amplitude of the R wave, widened QRS complex, prolongation of the PR interval, and then decreased amplitude and disappearance of the P wave. Finally, the QRS blends into the T wave, forming the classic sine wave. Ventricular fibrillation and asystole may follow.

V. Plan. Hyperkalemia should be treated as an emergency if the serum potassium has reached 7 mmol/L, although cardiac or neuromuscular symptoms may mandate urgent treatment at lower potassium levels.

A. Acute treatment

1. Calcium is the initial treatment in the emergency setting. Calcium antagonizes the membrane effects of hyperkalemia and restores

normal excitability within 1–2 minutes. Calcium chloride 10% at 5–10 mL or 10% calcium gluconate at 10–20 mL should be given IV over 3–5 minutes.

2. Potassium can be quickly shifted into cells by the administration of alkali or glucose plus insulin.

   a. Sodium bicarbonate (1 ampule [44 mmol] of bicarbonate) may be administered IV over several minutes.

   b. A 50-g ampule of dextrose and 15 U of IV regular insulin may be given (3 g glucose for every 1 U of regular insulin).

B. **Further treatment.** Note that calcium, alkali, glucose, and insulin do not lower the total body potassium. Once the patient is stabilized, the total body potassium needs to be reduced.

   1. Potassium-binding resins may be used when the immediate life-threatening cardiac manifestations are under control. Kayexalate may be given orally, 40 g in 25–50 mL of 70% sorbitol every 2–4 hours; or rectally, 50–100 g in 200 mL water as a retention enema for 30 minutes every 2–4 hours.

   2. Hemodialysis and peritoneal dialysis are definitive measures for controlling hyperkalemia in renal failure.

REFERENCES

Acker CG, Johnson JP, Palevsky PM et al: Hyperkalemia in hospitalized patients. Arch Intern Med 1998;158:917.

Black RM : Disorders of acid base and potassium balance. In: Dale DC, ed. *ACP Medicine 2001*. Section 10, Nephrology.

Greenberg S, Reiser IW, Chou S-Y et al: Trimethoprim-sulfamethoxazole induces reversible hyperkalemia. Ann Intern Med 1993;119:291.

Perazella MA: Drug-induced hyperkalemia: Old culprits and new offenders. Am J Med 2000;109:307.

Perazella MA, Mahnensmith RL: Hyperkalemia in the elderly. J Gen Intern Med 1997;12:646.

Velazquez H, Perazella MA, Wright FS et al: Renal mechanism of trimethoprim induced hyperkalemia. Ann Intern Med 1993;119:296.

34. HYPERNATREMIA

I. **Problem.** The clinical chemistry lab calls to tell you that the 65-year-old female patient admitted with pneumonia has a serum sodium of 155 mmol/L (normal: 136–145 mmol/L).

II. **Immediate Questions**

A. **Is the patient awake, alert, and oriented? Or, is the patient lethargic and confused?** The major signs and symptoms of hypernatremia are lethargy, which may lead to coma or convulsions; and neuromuscular irritability, including tremors, rigidity, and hyperreflexia. Mortality and symptoms are related to the level and acuity of the hypernatremia. Mortality in adults is increased with the sodium levels above 160 mmol/L.

B. **What medications is the patient taking?** Mannitol can cause an osmotic diuresis, resulting in hypernatremia with low total body sodium. Exogenous steroids and salt tablets can cause an increase in the total body sodium.

C. **What are the patient's intake/output values for the past few days?** A loss of total body water by fluid deprivation (inadequate thirst mechanism or inadequate administration of fluids) or from sweating can cause hypernatremia.

D. **Are there any underlying medical conditions?** Certain diseases, such as diabetes insipidus (DI) (central or nephrogenic), hyperaldosteronism, and Cushing's syndrome, are associated with hypernatremia. Recent cerebral trauma or neurosurgery can be a cause of central DI.

E. **Does the patient have a condition that prevents access to water?** Dehydration can result from inadequate access to water secondary to being bedridden or inadequate thirst mechanism from central nervous system (CNS) dysfunction.

F. **Is the lab value accurate?** As with any lab result that is unexpected, the abnormal laboratory value could be an error. It may be prudent to repeat the test.

G. **What is the composition of fluids administered?** Check sodium content of fluids; hypertonic solutions (eg, hypertonic dialysate) can cause hypernatremia. If the patient is on tube feedings, be sure there is adequate free water (300 mL/day).

H. **Is there a history of polyuria and polydipsia?** Diabetes mellitus and DI can cause hypernatremia.

III. **Differential Diagnosis.** The differential diagnosis is best considered in light of the possible causes of hypernatremia: a loss of water and sodium, a loss of total body water, and, rarely, an increase in total body sodium.

A. **Water and sodium loss.** Significant sodium loss with even greater loss of water.
   1. **Renal losses** (urine [Na^+] > 20 mmol/L)
      a. **Osmotic diuresis**
         i. **Mannitol**
         ii. **Hyperglycemia**
         iii. **Urea**
      b. **Diuretics.** For example, thiazide diuretics and furosemide.
      c. **Postobstructive diuresis.** Caused by relief of longstanding bilateral ureteral (nephrolithiasis, cervical carcinoma) and bladder outlet obstruction (prostatic hypertrophy).
      d. **Acute tubular necrosis.** Polyuric phase.
      e. **Intrinsic renal disease**

    2. Extrarenal losses (urine [Na⁺] < 20 mmol/L)

      a. Cutaneous losses

        i. Fever. Losses of 500 mL/24 hr for each degree centigrade increase above 38.3 °C (101 °F).

        ii. Burns

        iii. Profuse sweating

      b. Gastrointestinal losses

        i. Vomiting

        ii. Nasogastric suction

        iii. Diarrhea. Hypotonic diarrhea in children. Also, with the use of lactulose when the number of stools per day exceeds the recommended 2–3.

        iv. Fistulae

B. Water losses without loss of sodium (urine [Na⁺] is variable)

    1. Renal losses

      a. Central diabetes insipidus. Results from failure to produce adequate amounts of antidiuretic hormone (ADH). If the thirst mechanism is intact and the patient has free access to water, hypernatremia may be minimal. Central diabetes insipidus may be idiopathic or caused by CNS surgery, trauma, infection, or tumor (metastatic or primary).

      b. Nephrogenic. ADH is not effective in nephrogenic hypernatremia, which may be congenital or caused by sickle cell disease, hypokalemia, hypercalcemia, polycystic kidney disease; or by drugs (lithium, alcohol, phenytoin, and glyburide).

    2. Extrarenal losses

      a. Pulmonary losses. Insensible losses, especially in intubated patients who are not receiving adequate humidification or in patients with increased respiratory rates.

      b. Cutaneous losses. Fever or sweating.

C. Increase in total body sodium without a change in total body water (urine [Na⁺] > 20 mmol/L).

    1. Increase in mineralocorticoids or glucocorticoids

      a. Exogenous steroids (eg, prednisone)

      b. Primary aldosteronism

      c. Cushing's syndrome. Cushing's disease, bilateral adrenal hyperplasia, or ectopic adrenocorticotropin production.

      d. Exogenous steroids

    2. Administration of hypertonic sodium

      a. Sodium chloride tablets

      b. Hypertonic dialysate

      c. Hypertonic sodium bicarbonate. Given during resuscitation after cardiopulmonary arrest.

      d. Hypertonic sodium chloride fluids ("hot salt," 3% NaCl)

      e. Improper mixed formulas or tube feedings

      f. Ingestion of sea water

      g. **Hypertonic saline enemas**
      h. **Sodium chloride–rich emetics**
      i. **Intrauterine injection of hypertonic saline**

IV. Database

A. Physical examination key points

1. **Vital signs.** Check for orthostatic changes in blood pressure and heart rate. A decrease in systolic blood pressure of 10 mm Hg and/or an increase in heart rate of 20 bpm 1 minute changing from a supine to a standing position points to volume depletion. Also, a decrease in weight suggests volume depletion.
2. **Skin.** Check turgor; poor turgor suggests volume depletion. Remember that poor skin turgor can be a normal variant in the elderly.
3. **Mouth.** Dry mucous membranes suggest volume depletion.
4. **Neurologic exam.** Look for signs of irritability, muscle twitching, hyperreflexia, or seizures. A thorough neurologic examination needs to be done, since CNS trauma, infection, or tumor can cause DI.

B. Laboratory data

1. **Serum sodium.** Normal 136–145 mmol/L. Follow closely, especially if sodium is > 160 mmol/L.
2. **Urine osmolality.** > 700 mOsm/L suggests insufficient water intake with or without extrarenal water losses or an osmoreceptor defect. A urine osmolality between 700 mOsm/L and the serum osmolality suggests partial central DI, osmotic diuresis, diuretic therapy, acquired (partial) nephrogenic DI, or renal failure. A urine osmolality < serum osmolality suggests complete central DI or nephrogenic DI.
3. **Spot urine sodium.** In hypernatremia with water and sodium loss, a level < 20 mmol/L suggests extrarenal loss. In hypernatremia with water loss without loss of sodium, the spot sodium in extrarenal losses is variable.
4. **Water deprivation/vasopressin.** If you suspect DI. The patient is fluid-deprived until the plasma osmolality is 295 mOsm/kg or greater; or if, on three consecutive hourly urines, the osmolality does not increase; or, if the patient loses 3% to 5% of his or her body weight. Five units of aqueous vasopressin is then given, either IM or SC.
   a. **Normal subjects.** Urine concentrates with fluid deprivation and no change occurs with vasopressin.
   b. **Complete central DI.** Urine does not concentrate with fluid deprivation. There is a significant increase in urine osmolality after vasopressin.
   c. **Nephrogenic DI.** Urine does not concentrate with deprivation, and there is no change in urine osmolality with vasopressin.

C. Radiologic and other studies.
A computed tomography scan of the head to rule out a CNS lesion may be helpful if central DI is suspected.

V. Plan. The overall plan is to slowly decrease the serum sodium toward normal. Only hyperacute hypernatremia (hypernatremia < 12 hours) may be treated rapidly. Too rapid a correction of the sodium in hypernatremia may result in cerebral edema, seizures, and herniation, leading to death. The rate of correction of the sodium should not exceed 0.7 mmol/L/hr or about 10% of the serum sodium concentration per day. Specific treatment depends on whether there is a loss of sodium and water, a loss of water, or an increase in total body sodium.

   A. Water and sodium loss. Represents significant volume depletion. With shock, replenish volume with normal saline. If the patient is hemodynamically stable, replace volume with hypotonic saline (half-normal saline).

   B. Water loss without loss of sodium. Calculate the free water deficit:

      Weight (kg) × 0.60 = total body water
      Water deficit = total body water × 1 −[desired (Na^1)/Measured (Na$^+$)]

      Give half of the calculated free water deficit in the first 12 hours and the remainder in the next 24 hours. Include maintenance fluids.

   C. Increase in total body sodium. Remove excess sodium, either by giving free water and diuretics or by dialysis with hypotonic dialysate.

   D. Treatment of underlying cause
      1. Central DI. After correction of free water deficit, begin vasopressin.
      2. Diabetes mellitus. Treat with insulin and IV fluids (see Section I, Chapter 32, Hyperglycemia, V, p 193).
      3. Nephrogenic DI. After correction of free water deficit, begin thiazide diuretic and low-salt diet. Remove offending agent, if appropriate.

REFERENCES

Adrogue HJ, Madias NE: Hypernatremia. N Engl J Med 2000;342:1493.
Berl T, Schrier RW: Disorders of water metabolism. In: Schrier RW, ed. *Renal and Electrolyte Disorders.* 6th ed. Lippincott-Raven;2003:1.
Palvevsky PM, Bhagrath R, Greenberg A: Hypernatremia in hospitalized patients. Ann Intern Med 1996;124:197.

35. HYPERTENSION

   I. Problem. A 37-year-old woman complains of having a severe occipital headache for the past 6 hours. Her blood pressure is 220/140.

  II. Immediate Questions

   A. Is there a history of hypertension? You need to know if the patient is being treated for hypertension and regularly sees a physician. Previously, what were the highest blood pressure levels?

   B. What is the patient's medical regimen? Determine what medications the patient is taking and whether she is compliant. For example, she may have stopped taking clonidine (Catapres) or a short-acting beta-blocker such as propranolol (Inderal), which can cause severe rebound hypertension. Hypertensive crisis can occur in people taking a monoamine oxidase inhibitor who ingest certain cheeses or wine containing tyramine. Ingestion of street drugs such as cocaine or amphetamines can also cause hypertensive crisis.

C. Is the patient experiencing any other symptoms besides headache? A patient with severe hypertension who has a headache with mental status changes may have hypertensive encephalopathy, which is a medical emergency. Hypertensive encephalopathy is more common in patients whose blood pressure suddenly rises, as with toxemia of pregnancy. Other manifestations of end-organ damage from malignant hypertension include myocardial infarction, angina pectoris, dyspnea (left ventricular dysfunction), dissecting aortic aneurysm, visual loss, nausea, vomiting, seizures, focal neurologic deficits, and a decrease in urinary output.

III. Differential Diagnosis. Hypertension can be classified as essential or secondary (describes the cause); and as accelerated or malignant (describes urgency). Patients with malignant hypertension often have a secondary cause of hypertension. In patients with malignant hypertension, the first concern is to lower the blood pressure.

A. Essential. Comprises 90–95% of all hypertension. There is no underlying cause.

B. Secondary

1. **Renovascular.** From fibromuscular dysplasia (usually women 20–30 years old) and atherosclerosis (usually men older than 50).
2. **Primary aldosteronism.** Hypertension with unexplained hypokalemia.
3. **Cushing's disease.** Characteristic findings include moon facies, truncal obesity, purple striae, a buffalo hump, hirsutism, and easy bruising. Hypernatremia and hypokalemic metabolic alkalosis are common.
4. **Pheochromocytoma.** Usually episodic hypertension. The hypertension often has associated diaphoresis, palpitations, pallor, and headache.
5. **Coarctation of the aorta.** This should be suspected in any young person presenting with hypertension. Blood pressures are often higher in the right arm, and femoral pulses are often absent or diminished
6. **Primary renal disease**
7. **Hyperthyroidism.** Systolic hypertension primarily.
8. **Hypothyroidism.** Diastolic hypertension.
9. **Heavy ethanol use or withdrawal.** May cause or aggravate underlying hypertension. Hypertension associated with withdrawal is secondary to hyperadrenergic state.

10. Drugs
  a. **Estrogens**
  b. **Other prescription medications.** Cyclosporine, nonsteroidal anti-inflammatory drugs, corticosteroids, and erythropoietin occasionally cause hypertension.
  c. **Over-the-counter medications containing sympathomimetics.** For example, decongestants (pseudoephedrine) and weight loss medications (ephedrine and ephedra) may elevate the blood pressure.
  d. **Illicit drugs.** Phencyclidine (PCP), amphetamines, and cocaine.
11. Postoperative conditions. Multifactorial, including hypoxia, pain, anxiety, volume overload, hypothermia, and medications.
12. Gestational
13. Hyperparathyroidism
C. Miscellaneous diseases. Other diseases can cause a marked elevation in blood pressure; or they may be the consequence of long-standing, poorly controlled hypertension.
  1. **Cerebrovascular accident.** If the patient has had a stroke resulting in marked elevation of blood pressure, the physician is not quite as aggressive in lowering the blood pressure. A sudden marked drop in blood pressure can extend a stroke, so blood pressure should be lowered cautiously in the acute phase of stroke.
  2. **Subarachnoid hemorrhage.** Patients classically complain of the worst headache of their life.
  3. **Aortic dissection.** "Tearing" chest pain, often radiating to the back, and most severe at onset. There is usually a history of hypertension.
  4. **Congestive heart failure/pulmonary edema**
  5. **Angina pectoris/myocardial infarction.** See Section I, Chapter 11, Chest Pain, p 60.
D. Accelerated hypertension. Markedly elevated blood pressure with no current life-threatening problem secondary to the hypertension.
E. Malignant hypertension. Usually a markedly elevated blood pressure with an associated serious complication, such as hypertensive encephalopathy, angina pectoris, myocardial infarction, aortic dissection, or cerebrovascular accident; proteinuria, hematuria, and red blood cell casts may be present.

IV. Database
A. Physical examination key points
  1. **Vital signs.** Take blood pressure in both arms, feel both radial pulses, and check for a radial-femoral pulse lag. Such maneuvers may point to aortic dissection or coarctation.
  2. **Eyes.** Look for evidence of papilledema, hemorrhages, exudates, severe arteriolar narrowing, and arteriovenous nicking. Pa-

pilledema is usually present with malignant hypertension, but it can occur in other conditions with increased intracranial pressure.
3. **Lungs.** Rales may indicate congestive heart failure.
4. **Heart.** Palpate the apical impulse for displacement. Listen for a third heart sound (S_3) indicative of left ventricular dysfunction; a fourth heart sound (S_4) often seen with longstanding hypertension or a recent myocardial infarction; and a murmur of aortic insufficiency, which can occur in aortic dissection.
5. **Neurologic exam.** Assess the patient's mental status and look for any focal deficits that may indicate a cerebrovascular accident. Confusion and somnolence progressing to coma are hallmarks of hypertensive encephalopathy. Be sure to check reflexes; unilateral hyperreflexia may indicate an intracranial event.

B. **Laboratory data**
  1. **Electrolytes, blood urea nitrogen (BUN), glucose, and creatinine.** To rule out evidence of renal insufficiency, hypokalemia, or hyperglycemia. Hypokalemia occurs in Cushing's disease, primary hyperaldosteronism, and renovascular hypertension. Hyperglycemia can be a manifestation of a pheochromocytoma, Cushing's disease, or stress. Mild renal insufficiency occurs with hypertensive nephropathy, whereas marked renal insufficiency potentially suggests a secondary cause of hypertension.
  2. **Urinalysis.** To look for proteinuria, hematuria, and red cell casts for evidence of a secondary cause or hypertensive nephropathy.
  3. **Complete blood count and examination of peripheral blood smear.** Red blood cell fragments, or *schistocytes,* occur in microangiopathic hemolytic anemia resulting from malignant hypertension.

C. **Radiologic and other studies**
  1. **Chest x-ray.** To look for cardiomegaly, congestive heart failure, and mediastinal widening, suggesting proximal aortic dissection. Rib notching and obliteration of the aortic knob suggest coarctation of the aorta.
  2. **Electrocardiogram.** To look for ischemic changes and left ventricular hypertrophy.
  3. **CT scan.** If the patient has mental status changes or focal neurologic findings, a CT scan must be performed to exclude a thromboembolic stroke or subarachnoid hemorrhage.

V. **Plan**

A. **Hypertensive emergency.** Treatment must be initiated within minutes if possible. Hospitalization and parenteral drug therapy is necessary.
  1. **Admission to an ICU.** Intravenous (IV) and arterial lines should be placed.
  2. **Appropriate therapy.** Initiated once therapeutic goals are established. The goal of immediate therapy is to reduce mean arterial

blood pressure by no more than 25% within minutes to 2 hours. Overly aggressive reduction of blood pressure beyond these levels can lead to cerebral hypoperfusion and worsening neurologic deficits. This is particularly important in patients who have a stroke or a transient ischemic attack, who are more susceptible to abrupt falls in blood pressure.

   a. Nitroprusside is commonly used in hypertensive crises. It reduces preload and afterload when given in a dose of 0.25–10 µg/kg/min as a continuous IV infusion. It has the advantage of immediate onset and is easily titrated. Disadvantages include the need for constant monitoring; also, prolonged use is associated with thiocyanate toxicity. ***Caution:*** Avoid use in the presence of azotemia.

   b. IV labetalol, an alpha- and beta-blocker, is infused at 20 mg IV over 2 minutes followed by 40–80 mg at 10-minute intervals, to a total dose of 300 mg; **OR** 2 mg/min IV as a constant infusion. Potential disadvantages include beta-blocking side effects. ***Caution:*** Avoid labetalol use in the presence of acute heart failure.

   c. For suspected pheochromocytoma, IV labetalol, phentolamine, or phenoxybenzamine can be used.

   e. Hypertension associated with aortic dissection should be controlled with IV labetalol, esmolol, or verapamil (see Section I, Chapter 11, Chest Pain, V, p 66).

3. Treatment of accelerated hypertension. Can be treated with oral medications. Clonidine 0.1 mg PO can be used; repeat the dose every 1–2 hours. You may just want to increase the patient's current medications and follow him or her closely. ***Caution:*** Calcium channel–blocking agents other than sustained-release formulations have fallen into disfavor because of the increased mortality associated with their long-term use. Other oral agents such as beta-blockers and angiotensin-converting enzyme inhibitors can also be used. You must closely monitor the blood pressure to avoid wide fluctuations in blood pressure and to avoid hypotension.

4. Treatment of hypertension. A thorough discussion of hypertension is beyond the scope of this book. Please refer to any number of references including those listed here.

REFERENCES

Coates ML, Rembold CM, Farr BM: Does pseudoephedrine increase blood pressure in patients with controlled hypertension? J Fam Pract 1995;40:22.

Kaplan NM: *Clinical Hypertension.* 6th ed. Williams & Wilkins;1994.

The Seventh Report of the Joint National Committee on Detection, Evaluation, and Treatment of High Blood Pressure. JAMA 2003;289,2560.

36. HYPOCALCEMIA

I. **Problem.** A 54-year-old man admitted for an acute myocardial infarction (MI) has a calcium of 3.5 mEq/L, or 1.75 mmol/L (normal: 4.2–5.1 mEq/L, or 2.10–2.55 mmol/L).

II. **Immediate Questions**

A. **Are there any symptoms relevant to the low calcium?** Asymptomatic hypocalcemia usually does not require emergent treatment. Signs and symptoms of hypocalcemia may include peripheral and perioral paresthesias, Trousseau's and/or Chvostek's signs (see IV.4.a. and b.), confusion, muscle twitching, laryngospasm, tetany, and seizures.

B. **Does the low calcium level represent the true ionized calcium?** Most laboratories report the total serum calcium, but it is the ionized calcium level that is important physiologically. The total serum calcium level decreases by 0.2 mmol/L, or 0.4 mEq/L, for every 1 g/dL decrease in the serum albumin level without changing the ionized calcium level. Calculate the adjusted total calcium level or order an ionized calcium level.

C. **Does the patient have a history of neck surgery?** Surgical removal or infarction of the parathyroid glands is one of the more common causes of hypocalcemia. Look for a scar on the neck.

III. **Differential Diagnosis.** The causes of low ionized serum calcium can be categorized as parathyroid hormone deficits, vitamin D deficits, and loss or displacement of calcium.

A. **Parathyroid hormone (PTH) deficits**
   1. **Decreased PTH level**
      a. **Surgical excision or injury.** Including thyroid surgery.
      b. **Infiltrative diseases of the parathyroid gland.** For example, hemochromatosis, amyloid or metastatic cancer.
      c. **Idiopathic**
      d. **Irradiation.** To the neck to treat lymphoma.
   2. **Decreased PTH activity**
      a. **Congenital.** Pseudohypoparathyroidism: resistance to PTH at the tissue level.
      b. **Acquired.** Hypomagnesemia.

B. **Vitamin D deficiency**
   1. **Malnutrition**
   2. **Malabsorption**
      a. **Pancreatitis**
      b. **Postgastrectomy**
      c. **Short-gut syndrome**
      d. **Laxative abuse**
      e. **Sprue**
      f. **Hepatobiliary disease with bile salt deficiency**

3. **Defective metabolism**
   a. **Liver disease.** Failure to synthesize 25-hydroxyvitamin D.
   b. **Renal disease.** Failure to synthesize 1,25-dihydroxyvitamin D.
   c. **Anticonvulsant treatment with phenobarbital or phenytoin (Dilantin).** Possibly from an increase in the metabolism of vitamin D in the liver leading to a vitamin D deficiency.

C. **Calcium loss or displacement**
   1. **Hyperphosphatemia.** Increases bone deposition of calcium.
      a. **Acute phosphate ingestion**
      b. **Acute phosphate release by rhabdomyolysis or tumor lysis**
      c. **Renal failure**
   2. **Acute pancreatitis**
   3. **Osteoblastic metastases.** Especially breast and prostate cancer.
   4. **Medullary carcinoma of the thyroid.** Increased calcitonin.
   5. **Decreased bone resorption.** Overuse of actinomycin, calcitonin, or mithramycin.
   6. **Miscellaneous disorders.** Sepsis, massive transfusion, hungry bone syndrome, toxic shock syndrome, and fat embolism.

IV. **Database**

A. **Physical examination key points**
   1. **Skin.** Dermatitis with chronic hypocalcemia.
   2. **HEENT.** Cataracts with chronic hypocalcemia. Laryngospasm is rare but life-threatening. Look for surgical scars on the neck.
   3. **Neuromuscular exam.** Confusion, spasm, twitching, facial grimacing, and hyperactive deep tendon reflexes all indicate symptomatic hypocalcemia.
   4. **Specific tests for tetany of hypocalcemia**
      a. **Chvostek's sign.** Present in 5–10% of normocalcemic patients. Tapping on the facial nerve near the zygoma will elicit a twitch in hypocalcemic patients.
      b. **Trousseau's sign.** Inflate a blood pressure cuff above the systolic pressure for 3 minutes and watch for carpal spasm.

B. **Laboratory data**
   1. **Serum electrolytes.** Particularly calcium, phosphate, potassium, and magnesium. Calcium must be interpreted in terms of the serum albumin (see II.B, p 210). Hypomagnesemia and hyperkalemia may potentiate the effects of hypocalcemia.
   2. **Serum albumin.** See II.B.
   3. **Blood urea nitrogen and creatinine.** To rule out renal failure.
   4. **Parathyroid hormone level.** A low normal level is inappropriately low in the presence of true hypocalcemia.
   5. **Vitamin D levels.** 25-hydroxyvitamin D and 1,25-dihydroxyvitamin D.

      6. Urinary cyclic adenosine monophosphate. May indicate evidence of PTH resistance.

      7. Fecal fat. To evaluate for steatorrhea.

  C. Radiologic and other tests

    1. Electrocardiogram. A prolonged QT interval and T-wave inversion can occur with marked hypocalcemia, as can various arrhythmias.

    2. Bone films. May show bony changes of renal failure or osteoblastic metastases.

V. Plan. Assess for tetany, which can potentially progress to laryngeal spasm or seizures, and requires immediate treatment. Otherwise, establish the diagnosis by testing blood for calcium, albumin, magnesium, phosphate, and PTH levels, and begin appropriate oral therapy.

  A. Emergency treatment. Emergency treatment is usually needed for a calcium level below 1.5 mmol/L (3 mEq/L) to prevent fatal laryngospasm. Give 100–200 mg of elemental calcium IV over 10 minutes in 50–100 mL of D5W; follow with a 1–2 mg/kg/hr infusion for 6–12 hours. Use caution in patients on digoxin because calcium may potentiate the effect of digoxin, resulting in heart block.

    1. 10% calcium gluconate. One 10-mL ampule contains 23.25 mmol (93 mg) of calcium. Give 10–20 mL initially; follow with the infusion.

    2. 10% calcium chloride. One 10-mL ampule contains 68 mmol (272 mg) of calcium. Give 5–10 mL IV, being careful to avoid extravasation, which can cause skin to slough; then start an infusion.

    3. 10% calcium gluceptate. One 5-mL ampule contains 90 mg of elemental calcium. One can deliver 900 mg of calcium in 500 mL of fluid by adding 10 ampules to 450 mL of D5W.

  B. Chronic therapy. With primary PTH deficiency the goal is to give 2–4 g of oral calcium daily in four divided doses, adding vitamin D as necessary. With vitamin D disorders, vitamin D must always be supplemented.

    1. Calcium carbonate. There is 240 mg of calcium per 600-mg tablet.

    2. Calcium citrate and lactate tablets and calcium glubionate syrup are available.

    3. Vitamin D. Ergocalciferol (vitamin D_2) 50,000 U/d or dihydrotachysterol (vitamin D_2 analogue) 100–400 μg/day or calcitriol (1,25-dihydroxy-vitamin D_3) 0.25–1.0 μg/day.

    4. Magnesium. Patients on parenteral nutrition need at least 4–7 mg/kg/day of magnesium.

  C. Magnesium deficiency. See Section I, Chapter 39, Hypomagnesemia, V, p 224.

    1. In an emergency, one can give 10–15 mL of $MgSO_4$ 20% solution IV over 1 minute, followed by 500 mL of $MgSO_4$ 2% solution in D5W over 4–6 hours.

2. More typically, 6 g (49 mEq, or 24.5 mmol) of $MgSO_4$ in 1000 mL of D5W is given IV over 4 hours, followed by 6 g every 8 hours × 2, followed by 6 g every day.

REFERENCES

Bushinsky DA, Monk RD: Calcium. Lancet 1998;352:306.

Carlstedt F, Lind L: Hypocalcemic syndromes. Crit Care Clin 2001;17:139.

Marx SJ: Hyperparathyroid and hypoparathyroid disorders. N Engl J Med 2000;343:1863. (See correction of Figure 2: N Engl J Med 2001;344:240.)

37. HYPOGLYCEMIA

I. **Problem.** A 33-year-old woman was admitted for diabetic ketoacidosis (DKA) 24 hours ago. The patient's finger-stick glucose is now 50 mg/dL, or 2.78 mmol/L.

II. **Immediate Questions**

A. **What are the patient's vital signs? Is the patient symptomatic?** Assessment of current status and vital signs allows the resident to evaluate the urgency of the situation; that is, is there time for a repeat finger-stick or blood glucose, or should therapy be instituted immediately? Patients with hypoglycemia can have multiple symptoms. Early symptoms include headache, hunger, palpitations, tremor, and diaphoresis. As hypoglycemia progresses, abnormal behavior (such as combativeness) and slurred speech mimicking ethanol intoxication is followed by loss of consciousness, seizures, and even death. Beta-blockers can mask the early adrenergic symptoms of hypoglycemia (but diaphoresis, a cholinergic response, is usually still present). Patients with longstanding diabetes mellitus may also lose the ability to perceive hypoglycemia.

B. **What medications is the patient taking?**

1. The dose, route, and type of insulin are important in determining the timing and severity of the hypoglycemia. Patients on intermediate-acting insulin (NPH or Lente) generally have a peak effect between 6 and 16 hours, whereas those on rapid-acting insulin (regular) given subcutaneously peak at 2–6 hours. Ultra-short-acting insulin (Humalog, Humulin) has an onset of action of 15 minutes and peaks at 1 hour. Insulin glargine (Lantus) is a long-acting insulin analogue that has a delayed onset of action and a constant, peakless, 24-hour (or longer) duration of effect. Inhaled insulin, insulin lispro, and insulin aspart, peak at 45–75 minutes. Only regular insulin is used intravenously. IV bolus insulin produces its maximum effect in 30 minutes. Patients on continuous IV infusion insulin drips and continuous SC insulin (by insulin pump) can show very rapid decreases in their serum glucose, although the total dose received may be relatively small.

2. Some patients have different responses to rapid-acting and intermediate-acting insulin such that the peak effect is extended to
18–24 hours for intermediate-acting insulin and to 6–12 hours or
longer for regular insulin.

3. Knowing the amount, type, and route of administration of insulin
helps to determine the likelihood of worsening or recurring hypoglycemia after treatment, as well as the necessary changes in the
insulin regimen. If a patient is on an oral hypoglycemic agent, it is
important to know which one. Longer-acting agents increase the
risk of recurrent hypoglycemia for hours or even a day, especially
in older patients or those who are fasting.

C. **Is there IV access?** It is necessary to determine that IV access is
available to administer D50 if needed and to ascertain whether the
patient is receiving intravenous fluids containing dextrose.

D. **When was the patient's last meal or snack?** If the patient has
eaten a meal within an hour from the time that the finger-stick was
obtained, the situation will be less urgent because the meal may be
treating the hypoglycemia.

III. Differential Diagnosis

A. Medications

1. **Insulin.** Check for accidental overdose, as when insulin is given
to the wrong patient; or administration of the wrong type of insulin
or administration by the wrong route; or intentional overdose (eg,
Munchausen syndrome).

2. **Oral hypoglycemic agents.** Especially chlorpropamide (Diabinese), and glyburide (DiaBeta) in older adults.

3. **Other medications.** Acetaminophen (Tylenol), pentamidine (Pentam), haloperidol (Haldol), quinine, and salicylates can cause hypoglycemia.

4. **Ethanol.** Ethanol intoxication may cause hypoglycemia; in addition, many alcoholics may be glycogen-depleted prior to alcohol
consumption because of inadequate food intake and they may become hypoglycemic with fasting.

4. **Drug interactions.** The activity of oral hypoglycemic agents is increased when taken with nonsteroidal anti-inflammatory drugs,
sulfonamides, or monoamine oxidase inhibitors. Angiotensin converting enzyme inhibitors may increase insulin sensitivity leading
to hypoglycemia.

B. Reactive hypoglycemia. This form of hypoglycemia occurs after
eating. It is found in 5–10% of patients who have undergone partial
to complete gastrectomies, as well as de novo in the general population.

C. Severe liver disease. With massive liver destruction, glycogen
stores are easily depleted.

D. Insulinoma. Pancreatic islet cell tumor. Insulinoma may be malignant. Serum insulin or C-peptide levels are helpful in establishing the diagnosis.

E. Endocrinopathies. These include Addison's disease, pituitary insufficiency, and myxedema.

F. Renal disease. This usually occurs in the setting of combined uremia and malnutrition. Insulin clearance decreases with renal failure.

G. Sepsis. Hypoglycemia is more likely in the setting of septic shock.

H. Malnutrition/prolonged fasting. Hypoglycemia is common in protein calorie malnutrition (kwashiorkor).

I. Abrupt discontinuation of total parenteral nutrition (TPN). This diagnosis is more likely if the TPN solution contains insulin.

J. Factitious hypoglycemia. This may occur as a result of either a marked elevation in the white blood cell count (*leukocyte metabolism*) or prolongation of contact of serum with red blood cells. Be suspicious of self-induced hypoglycemia if the patient has access to insulin or oral hypoglycemic agents.

K. Neoplasms. Retroperitoneal sarcoma, hepatocellular carcinoma, and small cell carcinoma of the lung can cause hypoglycemia by production of insulin-like hormone, impaired glycogenolysis, or glucose consumption.

L. Other causes. These include glycogen storage disease, hereditary fructose intolerance, carnitine deficiency, anorexia nervosa, and akee fruit poisoning.

IV. Database

A. Physical examination key points

1. **Vital signs.** Hypertension and tachycardia may be caused by increased catecholamines as a response to hypoglycemia. This adrenergic response may be be blunted or eliminated in the presence of beta-blockers.

2. **Skin.** Diaphoresis is a common cholinergic response to hypoglycemia that is not generally eliminated by beta-blockers.

3. **Neurologic exam.** The patient's sensorium and orientation are often altered. (See Section I, Chapter 13, Coma, Acute Mental Status Changes, p 76.) Tremor at rest and with intention may be present. Unconsciousness and seizures indicate need for urgent treatment. Hypoglycemia occasionally presents with focal neurologic findings.

B. Laboratory data

1. **Serum glucose.** This is the most critical test; in general, a glucose level below 50 mg/dL and the presence of symptoms are diagnostic of hypoglycemia. Finger-stick values should always be confirmed by serum glucose measurements because finger-stick

glucoses are prone to error secondary to strips that have been exposed to air, inappropriate preparation of the finger with povidone-iodine (Betadine), presence of alcohol on the finger, incorrect timing, or an uncalibrated machine. In the presence of symptoms, blood should be obtained immediately, but treatment should not be withheld pending results or because of a delay in obtaining blood.

2. **Electrolytes, blood urea nitrogen and creatinine, liver function studies, complete blood count, urinalysis.** In the setting of hypoglycemia with no history available, obtain these test results to evaluate for common causes listed in the differential diagnosis.

3. **Drug screens.** Look specifically for oral hypoglycemics as well as for ethanol, salicylates, acetaminophen, and antipsychotics (eg, haloperidol).

4. **Serum insulin.** Results may indicate either exogenous insulin administration or insulinoma.

5. **C-peptide.** Helps to differentiate between insulinoma and exogenous insulin administration. The C-peptide level is elevated with an insulinoma and low with the administration of exogenous insulin.

C. **Radiologic and other studies.** These may be indicated in specific circumstances to rule out infection, insulinoma, malignancy, or pituitary lesion.

V. Plan

A. **Administer glucose.** Do not wait for the results of the serum glucose if you strongly suspect the diagnosis. It is best to draw blood before administering glucose; however, you should proceed with treatment if there will be a significant delay before blood can be obtained and the patient is markedly symptomatic. If the patient is awake and able and willing to take fluids, glucose should be given orally. Otherwise, administer IV glucose.

1. Orange juice with added sugar is usually readily available. Specific glucose-containing liquids are stocked on most hospital floors and may be substituted for orange juice. For mild hypoglycemia, 8 ounces of 2% milk or a package of saltines with juice may be adequate and may not result in "overshoot" hyperglycemia. If glucose tablets are used, 15–30 g are administered orally.

2. Give 25–50 g (½ to 1 ampule) of 50% dextrose (D50) IV push; repeat in 5 minutes if no response. If there is no response after the second ampule, the diagnosis should be seriously questioned and other causes for the symptoms should be considered, such as hypoxia, transient ischemic attack, and ethanol or drug intoxication or overdose.

3. If the patient is unable to take glucose PO, and IV access is not immediately available, give glucagon 0.5–1 mg IM or SC (may induce vomiting; be prepared to protect the patient's airway).

4. Start maintenance IV fluids with D5W at 75–100 mL/hr, especially if the hypoglycemia may recur, such as that resulting from glyburide use or sepsis.

5. Follow serial glucoses frequently. Depending on the severity of the hypoglycemia, repeat glucose after treatment and again in 1–2 hours according to the results.

B. Adjust medications. Review schedule and dosing of insulin and/or oral hypoglycemics. Consider use of metformin (Glucophage) for patients with type 2 diabetics (less likely to cause hypoglycemia). See Section VII, Therapeutics, pp 556, 613, and 564.

C. Miscellaneous. If the patient is not taking hypoglycemic agents, then consider other causes listed in the differential diagnosis and evaluate accordingly.

REFERENCES

Cryer PE, Davis SN, Shamoon H: Hypoglycemia in diabetes. Diabetes Care 2003;26:1902.
Cryer PE, Fisher JN, Shamoon H: Hypoglycemia. Diabetes Care 1994;17:734.
Service FJ: Hypoglycemia. Endocrinol Metab Clin North Am 1997;26:937.

38. HYPOKALEMIA

I. **Problem.** A 72-year-old woman with hypertension develops profound muscle weakness after 3 days of vomiting and diarrhea. Her serum potassium is 2.5 mmol/L (2.5 mEq/L).

II. **Immediate Questions**

A. **What are the patient's vital signs?** Although cardiac arrhythmias rarely occur with hypokalemia without underlying heart disease, even mild to moderate hypokalemia can induce cardiac arrhythmias in the presence of cardiac ischemia, congestive heart failure, or left ventricular hypertrophy. Premature atrial contractions (PACs), premature ventricular contractions (PVCs), or ventricular arrhythmias may be suggested by examination of the pulse.

B. **What medications is the patient taking?** The most common cause of hypokalemia is medications. Medications, especially diuretics, can cause renal potassium wasting. Also, remember that digitalis toxicity is potentiated by hypokalemia.

C. **Has the patient had vomiting, diarrhea, nasogastric suction, or excessive sweating?** Gastrointestinal sources are possible causes of potassium loss. A prolonged, elevated temperature or delirium tremens can result in hypokalemia from sweating.

III. **Differential Diagnosis.** In general, hypokalemia is caused by cellular shifts or by renal or gastrointestinal losses.

A. **Hypokalemia resulting from inadequate potassium intake**. Low potassium dietary content is unusual in the United States and other developed countries because potassium is found in most foods.

B. **Hypokalemia resulting from cellular shifts**
   1. **Alkalosis.** Both respiratory alkalosis and metabolic alkalosis are associated with hypokalemia. Hyperventilation during surgical anesthesia can cause acute respiratory alkalosis and produce significant hypokalemia.
   2. **Familial periodic paralysis.** This rare, inherited disease is characterized by intermittent attacks of varying severity, ranging from muscle weakness to flaccid paralysis.
   3. **Barium poisoning.** Ingestion of soluble barium salts may cause profound hypokalemia, muscle paralysis, and cardiac arrhythmias, probably as a result of intracellular shifts, although associated vomiting and diarrhea may contribute.
   4. **Treatment of megaloblastic anemia.** Treatment of severe pernicious anemia (hematocrit < 20%) with vitamin B_{12} causes an acute reduction in serum potassium as a result of the rapid uptake of potassium because of the marked increase in bone marrow activity.
   5. **Leukemia.** Hypokalemia may be produced by sequestration of potassium ions by rapidly proliferating blast cells.
   6. **Transfusions.** Administration of previously frozen washed red blood cells may cause hypokalemia due to the uptake of potassium by these cells.
   7. **Drugs.** Drugs with ß$_2$-sympathomimetic activity, including decongestants (pseudoephedrine), bronchodilators (albuterol), and inhibitors of uterine contractions (terbutaline), can cause hypokalemia. The standard dose of albuterol reduces the serum potassium by 0.2–0.4 mmol/L, and a second dose within 1 hour reduces it by almost 1 mmol/L. Theophylline, caffeine, verapamil intoxication, chloroquine intoxication, and insulin overdose may produce clinically significant hypokalemia.
   8. **Hyperthyroidism.** Severe hypokalemia can occur rarely in association with hyperthyroidism. It results in sudden onset of severe muscle weakness and paralysis and is most commonly seen in patients of Asian descent.

C. **Hypokalemia resulting from abnormal losses**
   1. **Gastrointestinal potassium losses**
      a. **Diarrhea.** Diarrhea from virtually any cause may result in hypokalemia. But severe hypokalemia secondary to diarrhea is suggestive of colonic villous adenoma or non–insulin-secreting pancreatic islet cell tumors.
      b. **Vomiting.** Potassium concentration in gastric contents is low. The loss of large volumes of gastric secretions would be required to cause hypokalemia. Hypokalemia seen with vomiting is due to renal, not gastric, losses (see below).

  c. **Clay ingestion.** Reported to be relatively common in the southeastern United States. Clay binds potassium, resulting in potassium being excreted in the stool.
2. **Potassium losses from skin**
   a. **Excessive sweat.** Patients engaging in intense physical exercise in hot, humid environments can lose over 10 liters of sweat per day. Potassium losses can be substantial despite potassium content of sweat being only 5 mEq/L.
   b. **Burns.** In a severely burned patient, local tissue breakdown leads to the release of intracellular potassium. The potassium content of fluid lost through the skin after extensive burns may greatly exceed that of plasma.
3. **Hypokalemia resulting from renal losses**
   a. **Diuretics.** The most common cause of hypokalemia is diuretic therapy. Loop diuretics, thiazides, and acetazolamide (Diamox) all may cause hypokalemia.
   b. **Vomiting.** Although gastric contents contain some potassium ions, the major loss through vomiting occurs in the urine. The loss of gastric hydrogen ions generates metabolic alkalosis, which stimulates potassium ion secretion. The sodium and water losses from vomiting cause volume depletion and stimulate aldosterone secretion.
      In cases of surreptitious vomiting (*bulimia*), hypokalemia, metabolic alkalosis, volume depletion, and a low urine chloride suggest the diagnosis.
4. **Renal losses caused by excess mineralocorticoid**
   a. **Primary aldosteronism.** Should be suspected in hypertensive patients who are hypokalemic before institution of diuretic therapy, or in those who become profoundly hypokalemic (< 2.5 mmol/L) with diuretics.
   b. **Cushing's syndrome.** Fifty percent of patients with Cushing's syndrome have hypokalemia. Hypertension and metabolic alkalosis are also seen.
   c. **Ectopic adrenocorticotropic hormone production.** Most commonly seen with small cell carcinoma of the lung.
   d. **Adrenogenital syndrome.** *11-Hydroxylase deficiency* is manifested by virilization in the female, precocious puberty in the male, hypokalemia, metabolic alkalosis, and hypertension. 17-Hydroxylase deficiency is a rare form of congenital hyperplasia of the adrenal glands associated with hypokalemia and hypertension.
   e. **Licorice ingestion.** Natural licorice contains glycyrrhizic acid, which has potent mineralocorticoid activity. Affected patients clinically resemble those with primary aldosteronism.
   f. **Hyperreninemic states.** Hypokalemia is accompanied by hypertension and metabolic alkalosis in renal vascular hypertension, malignant hypertension, and renin-producing tumors. It is

distinguished from primary aldosteronism by an elevated plasma renin.

g. **Bartter's syndrome.** A rare disorder characterized by hypokalemia, metabolic alkalosis, elevated renin and aldosterone levels, and normal blood pressure.

h. **Liddle's syndrome.** A rare disorder characterized by hypokalemia, hypertension, metabolic alkalosis, low plasma renin, and low urinary aldosterone.

i. **Type I (distal) renal tubular acidosis.** Characterized by hyperchloremic metabolic acidosis and hypokalemia. It results from an inability to maintain a hydrogen ion gradient.

j. **Type II (proximal) renal tubular acidosis.** Impaired proximal bicarbonate reabsorption results in distal delivery of bicarbonate and urinary loss of potassium ions as well as bicarbonate.

k. **Antibiotics.** Carbenicillin and ticarcillin, administered as sodium salts, enhance potassium ion excretion. Amphotericin B alters distal tubule permeability, resulting in hypokalemia.

l. **Magnesium depletion.** This may increase mineralocorticoid activity, but the pathophysiology is unknown.

m. **Ureterosigmoidostomy.** Hypokalemic hyperchloremic metabolic acidosis occurs because of an exchange mechanism in the colon. Ureteral implantation into a loop of ileum is now performed.

IV. Database

A. Physical examination key points

1. **Cardiovascular.** Irregular pulse may represent an arrhythmia (PACs or PVCs), or digitalis toxicity.

2. **Abdomen.** Look for distention and the presence of bowel sounds. Ileus secondary to hypokalemia may be present. Abdominal examination may reveal a cause of vomiting.

3. **Neurologic exam.** Weakness, blunting of reflexes, paresthesias, and paralysis may be seen.

B. Laboratory data

1. **Serum electrolytes.** Hypomagnesemia may coexist or may cause the hypokalemia.

2. **Arterial blood gases.** Look for alkalosis.

3. **Urine potassium, chloride, and sodium.** If the patient is not taking diuretics, a low urine sodium or chloride indicates volume depletion. A relatively high urine potassium in the face of hypokalemia indicates renal losses.

4. **Digoxin level.** A must if the patient is on digoxin. Hypokalemia may potentiate digoxin toxicity.

C. Radiologic and other studies.
An electrocardiogram may show digitalis effect or manifestations of hypokalemia ranging from PACs and PVCs to life-threatening ventricular arrhythmias. A U wave is a common finding.

V. Plan. The degree of hypokalemia cannot be used as a rigid determinant of the total potassium ion deficit. It has been estimated that in a normal adult, a decrease in serum potassium from 4 to 3 mmol/L corresponds to a 100- to 200-mmol decrement in total body potassium. Each additional fall of 1 mmol/L in serum potassium represents an additional deficit of 200–400 mmol.

A. Parenteral replacement

1. **Indications.** Should be considered in the following situations: digoxin toxicity or significant arrhythmias, severe hypokalemia (< 3.0 mmol/L), and inability to take oral replacements (NPO, ileus, nausea, and vomiting). Ideally, parenteral solutions should be administered through a central venous catheter. In most other cases, hypokalemia can be safely corrected in a slow, controlled fashion with oral supplementation. Unfortunately, supplemental potassium administration is also the most common cause of severe hyperkalemia in hospitalized patients, and the risk is greatest with intravenous potassium.

2. **Implementation.** The maximum concentration of potassium chloride used in peripheral veins should generally not exceed 40 mmol/L because of the sclerosing effect of potassium (especially high concentrations) on the veins, although in an emergent situation 60 mmol/L can be attempted. Potassium chloride 20 mmol diluted in 50–100 mL D5W or normal saline can be infused over 1 hour through a central line safely, with doses repeated as needed when severe depletion or life-threatening hypokalemia is present. Special care must be taken to ensure slow infusion of high doses. For lesser degrees of hypokalemia that require parenteral replacement, 10–15 mmol/hr can be infused peripherally.

3. **Monitoring.** With large total replacement doses, check serum potassium every 2–4 hours to avoid hyperkalemia. Cardiac monitoring in an ICU is required if arrhythmias are present, or for rapid infusions of potassium chloride. *Caution:* Cardiac monitoring is required for rates that exceed 10–15 mmol/hr.

B. Oral replacement. Generally indicated for asymptomatic, mild potassium depletion (potassium usually > 3.0 mmol/L). Oral replacements include liquids and powder. Slow-release pills typically contain 8–10 mmol per tablet and thus are not usually appropriate for repletion therapy. The replacement rate should be 40–120 mmol/day in divided doses, depending on the patient's weight and level of hypokalemia. Maintenance therapy, if needed, should be given in doses of 20–80 mmol/day, using the preparation best tolerated by the patient. With normal renal function, it is difficult to induce hyperkalemia through the oral administration of potassium. An important exception is the use of potassium supplements with potassium-sparing diuretics or with angiotensin-converting enzyme inhibitors.

C. **Replacement of ongoing losses.** Large amounts of nasogastric aspirate should be replaced milliliter for milliliter with D5 half-normal saline with 20 mmol/L potassium chloride every 4–6 hours.

D. **Refractory cases.** Rarely, hypokalemia is not correctable because of concomitant hypomagnesemia (see Section I, Chapter 39, Hypomagnesemia, V, p 224).

REFERENCES

Black RM: Disorders of acid base and potassium balance. In: Dale DC, ed. ACP Medicine 2001;Section 10: *Nephrology*.

Cohn JN, Kowey PR, Whelton PK, Prisant M: New guidelines for potassium replacement in clinical practice. Arch Intern Med 2000;160:2429.

Gennari FJ: Hypokalemia. N Engl J Med 1998;339:451.

39. HYPOMAGNESEMIA

I. **Problem.** A 40-year-old man complaining of chest pain is admitted to rule out myocardial infarction. A magnesium level returns at 0.8 mEq/L (normal: 1.5–2.1 mEq/L).

II. **Immediate Questions**

A. **What are the patient's vital signs?** Magnesium deficiency is associated with cardiac arrhythmias, including atrial fibrillation, other supraventricular tachycardias, ventricular tachycardia, and ventricular fibrillation. Determining that the patient is not in any immediate distress and does not have hypotension or a tachyarrhythmia is essential.

B. **Is the patient tremulous or currently having a seizure?** Tremor, tetany, muscle fasciculations, and seizures all are associated with magnesium deficiency. Determining the presence or absence of these neurologic symptoms help to guide the urgency of treatment.

III. **Differential Diagnosis.** The diagnosis of magnesium deficiency, in general, rests on a high degree of suspicion, clinical assessment, and measurement of serum magnesium. It is important to recognize that serum magnesium levels do not always correlate well with intracellular magnesium levels. Thus, it is possible to have total body or intracellular magnesium depletion with normal (or even high) serum magnesium levels. For this reason, some experts have suggested that an initial 24-hour urine collection for magnesium, or a 24-hour urine magnesium retention test after parenteral administration of magnesium, be done to determine whether magnesium depletion is truly present. Although such tests may be useful in specific settings, an acutely ill patient is generally treated based on the serum level and sound clinical judgment.

A. **Hypocalcemia.** The signs and symptoms of hypocalcemia are similar to those of hypomagnesemia, and both problems often coexist.

Hypocalcemia that does not correct with IV supplementation suggests the presence of magnesium deficiency.

B. **Hypokalemia.** Potassium depletion often coexists with hypomagnesemia and can cause arrhythmias and muscle weakness, similar to those found in hypomagnesemia. Hypokalemia that does not correct with potassium repletion suggests magnesium depletion.

C. **Lab error.** More likely if a colorimetric assay is used. When in doubt, ask the lab to repeat the test and controls.

D. **Causes of hypomagnesemia**
   1. **Increased excretion**
      a. **Medications.** Especially diuretics, antibiotics (ticarcillin, amphotericin B), pentamidine, aminoglycosides, foscarnet, *cis*-platinum, and cyclosporin may cause hypomagnesemia.
      b. **Alcoholism.** Very common cause. Hypomagnesemia results from decreased intake and renal magnesium wasting.
      c. **Diabetes mellitus.** Commonly seen in diabetic ketoacidosis.
      d. **Renal tubular disorders.** With magnesium wasting.
      e. **Hypercalcemia/hypercalciuria**
      f. **Hyperaldosteronism, Bartter's syndrome, Gitelman's syndrome**
      g. **Excessive lactation**
      h. **Marked diaphoresis**
   2. **Reduced intake/malabsorption**
      a. **Starvation.** A common cause.
      b. **Bowel bypass or resection**
      c. **Total parenteral nutrition without adequate magnesium supplementation**
      d. **Chronic malabsorption syndrome.** Such as pancreatic insufficiency.
      e. **Chronic diarrhea**
   3. **Miscellaneous**
      a. **Acute pancreatitis**
      b. **Hypoalbuminemia**
      c. **Vitamin D therapy.** Resulting in hypercalciuria.
      d. **Postparathyroidectomy** as part of the hungry bone syndrome

IV. **Database**

A. **Physical examination key points**
   1. **Vital signs.** Blood pressure and pulse to evaluate for hypotension and tachyarrhythmias. While taking blood pressure, leave cuff inflated above the systolic blood pressure for 3 minutes to check for carpal spasm (*Trousseau's sign*).
   2. **HEENT.** Check for *Chvostek's sign* (tapping over the facial nerve produces twitching of the mouth and eye). Nystagmus may be present.

3. **Heart.** Check for rate and regularity of rhythm.
4. **Abdomen.** Evaluate for evidence of pancreatitis, such as absent bowel sounds and tenderness. Stigmata of chronic liver disease such as hepatosplenomegaly, caput medusae, ascites, spider angiomas, and palmar erythema suggest chronic alcohol abuse.
5. **Neurologic exam.** Hyperactive reflexes, muscle fasciculations, muscle weakness seizures, and tetany can occur. Hyperactive reflexes may also be seen with alcohol withdrawal and hypocalcemia.
6. **Mental status.** Psychosis, depression, and agitation may be present.

B. **Laboratory data**
1. **Serum electrolytes, glucose, calcium, and phosphorus.** Hypomagnesemia frequently accompanies other electrolyte abnormalities, especially hypocalcemia, hypokalemia, and alkalosis. If the patient is an alcoholic, then hypophosphatemia is also likely. Patients with diabetes are prone to develop hypomagnesemia (especially with diabetic ketoacidosis).
2. **24-hour urine for magnesium.** May be helpful if the diagnosis is in question or if there is a suspicion of renal magnesium wasting.
3. **Magnesium retention test.** Using either parenteral or oral magnesium. This test may be helpful in certain subsets of patients in whom either the diagnosis is in question or malabsorption is suspected.
4. **Miscellaneous.** As indicated. Liver function studies in alcoholics and serum amylase if pancreatitis is suspected.

C. **Radiologic and other studies.** Electrocardiographic findings may include prolongation of the PR, QT, and QRS intervals as well as ST depression and T-wave changes. Rhythm disturbances include supraventricular arrhythmias (especially atrial fibrillation) as well as ventricular tachycardia and ventricular fibrillation. Arrhythmias may be particularly common if the patient is taking digoxin, has coexisting myocardial ischemia, or recently underwent cardiopulmonary bypass.

V. **Plan.** The urgency of treatment depends on the clinical setting. The patient who is having neurologic or cardiac manifestations should be treated urgently with parenteral IV therapy. Asymptomatic individuals may be treated with oral magnesium, although many clinicians treat magnesium levels < 1.0 mEq/L with parenteral magnesium even though there is not always a good correlation between serum levels and intracellular levels.

A. **IV magnesium sulfate.** Magnesium sulfate 1 g (2 mL of a 50% solution of $MgSO_4$) equals 98 mg of elemental magnesium, which is equal to 8 mEq $MgSO_4$ or 4 mmol Mg^{++}. With tetany, status epilepticus, or significant cardiac arrhythmias, then 2 g of magnesium sulfate (16 mEq) can be given IV over 10–20 min. For slightly less urgent situations, 1–2 g/hr (not to exceed 12 g in the first 12 hours) may be given with close hemodynamic and electrocardiographic monitoring including checking of deep tendon reflexes Q 3–4 hr. Deep tendon reflexes (DTRs) typically decrease with magnesium replacement; toxicity is suggested by diminished or absent DTRs. Magnesium should be administered only in life-threatening situations with renal insufficiency; monitoring of DTRs is required every hour. For less urgent replacement, the infusion can be slowed so that the patient receives approximately 4–6 g of magnesium sulfate in the first 24 hours as long as signs and symptoms of hypomagnesemia are improving. Selected patients may require more or less magnesium. Subsequently, 5–6 g of magnesium sulfate may be given Q 24 hr to replenish body reserves over 3–4 days.

In the setting of acute myocardial infarction, some clinicians feel that therapeutic (rather than replacement) administration of magnesium may prevent arrhythmias, limit damage from reperfusion injury, and have a favorable impact on hemodynamics. Other authors and the recent MAGIC study dispute these claims. Protocols for administration vary, but one popular protocol is to give 2 g magnesium sulfate IV over 5 minutes followed by 13–16 g over 24 hours as a constant infusion. Patients often experience a flushing sensation with rapid infusions. An overdose of magnesium may occur in the setting of renal failure or renal insufficiency and also accidentally (several formulations are available in different concentrations—particular attention must be made to correct dosing). Magnesium overdose complicated by respiratory arrest, shock, or asystole should be initially treated with 1–2 g IV calcium gluconate (100–200 mg elemental calcium) over 3 minutes followed by 15 mg/kg over 4 hours. Physostigmine 1 mg given over 1 minute has also been used. Initial treatment can be followed by dialysis, or saline and furosemide diuresis.

B. **IM magnesium sulfate.** Give 1–2 g IM Q 4 hr for 5 doses during the first 24 hours (following the patient's clinical status and serum levels as described earlier). This can then be followed by 1 g IM Q 6 hr for 2–3 days. Many patients complain about pain with the injections.

C. **Oral magnesium: SlowMag (magnesium chloride) and MagTab (magnesium lactate) are sustained-release formulations providing 5–7 mEq per tablet; 2–4 tablets per day for mild depletion, 6–8 tablets per day for more severe depletion. Magnesium oxide (20 mEq of magnesium per 400-mg tablet).** Give 1–2 tablets per day for chronic maintenance therapy (may cause diarrhea, especially at higher doses).

D. **Miscellaneous.** Treat other electrolyte disorders, especially hypocalcemia (see Section I, Chapter 36, Hypocalcemia, V, p 212), hypokalemia (see Section I, Chapter 38, Hypokalemia, V, p 221) and hypophosphatemia (see Section I, Chapter 41, Hypophosphatemia, V, p 236), as well as other underlying illnesses.

REFERENCES

Agus ZS: Hypomagnesemia. J Am Soc Nephrol 1999;10:1616.

Antman EM: Early administration of intravenous magnesium to high-risk patients with acute myocardial infarction in the Magnesium in Coronaries (MAGIC) Trial: a randomised controlled trial. Lancet 2002;360:1189.

40. HYPONATREMIA

I. **Problem.** A 50-year-old man is admitted for evaluation of a right pulmonary hilar mass. The serum sodium is 118 mmol/L (normal: 136–145 mmol/L).

II. **Immediate Questions**

A. **Is the patient symptomatic from the hyponatremia?** Patients with hyponatremia may be asymptomatic, or they may have central nervous system (CNS) symptoms or signs ranging from lethargy, anorexia, nausea, vomiting, agitation, and headache to marked disorientation, seizures, and death. Muscle cramps, weakness, and fatigue are also common.

B. **Are there any recent sodium levels to document the chronicity of the hyponatremia?** The rate of development and magnitude of hyponatremia correlates directly with the severity of the symptoms. Acute changes in sodium levels are more likely to produce more severe symptoms.

C. **Is there any evidence of volume depletion?** Orthostatic changes in blood pressure and heart rate suggest volume depletion.

D. **Does the patient have a history of vomiting or diarrhea?** Vomiting and diarrhea can cause wasting of sodium and extracellular fluid, resulting in hyponatremia.

E. **Is there any history of renal disease, congestive heart failure (CHF), cirrhosis, or nephrotic syndrome?** Any of these edematous states suggests an excess of sodium accompanied by an even greater excess of total body water.

F. **Is there any history of hypothyroidism or adrenal insufficiency?** Hypothyroidism and hypoadrenalism cause renal wasting of sodium, even in the face of hyponatremia.

G. **Is the patient taking any medications that could cause the hyponatremia?** Diuretics can cause hyponatremia by inducing sodium deficits in excess of water deficits. Chlorpropamide, clofibrate, nicotine, narcotics, cyclophosphamide, vincristine, nonsteroidal anti-inflammatory drugs (NSAIDs), antipsychotic medications (eg, haloperidol and thioridazine), tricyclic antidepressants, selective serotonin reuptake inhibitors (SSRIs), angiotensin-converting enzyme (ACE) inhibitors and anticonvulsants such as carbamazepine (Tegretol) may cause hyponatremia. Mannitol used to treat elevated intracranial pressure or glaucoma can cause a low serum sodium by shifting water from the intracellular space to the hypertonic extracellular space.

H. Is there any pulmonary disease? Pneumonia, tuberculosis, lung carcinoma, and other pulmonary pathology may cause the syndrome of inappropriate antidiuretic hormone secretion (SIADH).

I. Is there any CNS disease? Meningitis, encephalitis, brain abscess, tumors, trauma, and a variety of other diseases can cause SIADH.

J. Is there a history of weight loss, cough, and hemoptysis? SIADH has been associated with bronchogenic carcinoma as well as several other cancers.

K. Is there any history of hyperlipidemia or hyperproteinemia? Either can cause a low serum sodium without extracellular fluid hypertonicity. This condition is also called *pseudohyponatremia*.

L. Is there a history of diabetes? A markedly elevated glucose can lower the serum sodium. The serum sodium is diluted by water moving from the intracellular space to the hypertonic extracellular space. Correction of the hyperglycemia corrects the hyponatremia.

M. Has the patient recently undergone a colonoscopy? In a recent study of 40 patients undergoing colonoscopy, 10 had elevated levels of serum arginine vasopressin and 3 patients developed hyponatremia of 130 mmol/L or lower.

N. Is the lab value correct? If the sodium level is unexpected, repeat the test.

III. Differential Diagnosis. (See Figure I–4.) The initial differentiation is between true hyponatremia with hypotonicity and laboratory artifact (pseudohyponatremia), as well as dilutional effects that result in isotonic or hypertonic hyponatremia. True hyponatremia may be classified according to the volume status of the patient: hypovolemic, euvolemic, or hypervolemic (see IV.A).

A. Laboratory error. If the serum sodium concentration is unexpected, laboratory error should always be considered as a potential cause.

B. Pseudohyponatremia due to space-occupying compounds. Lipids are the most common cause. For every increase in triglycerides of 1 g/dL, sodium falsely decreases by 1.7 mmol/L. The lab can ultracentrifuge the specimen to determine the correct plasma sodium level. Proteins are also a common cause of pseudohyponatremia (Waldenström's macroglobulinemia and multiple myeloma). A 1 g/dL increase in protein falsely lowers the sodium by 1 mmol/L, plus some true reduction occurs via the accumulation of cationic proteins in multiple myeloma.

C. Dilutional. This is not a true pseudohyponatremia but rather a hypertonic hyponatremia resulting from the intracellular-to-extracellular

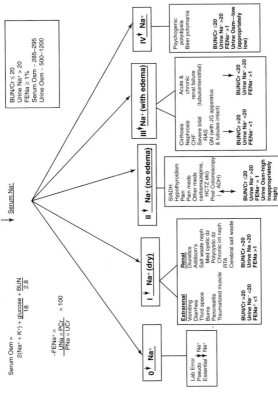

Figure I-4. Differential diagnosis of hyponatremia. ADH, antidiuretic hormone; BUN, blood urea nitrogen; CHF, congestive heart failure; Chron int neph, chronic interstitial nephritis; Cr, creatinine; GN, glomerulonephritis; HCTZ, hydrochlorothiazide; JG, juxtaglomerular; Med cystic dz, medullary cystic disease; Pseudo, pseudohyponatremia; RAS, renal artery stenosis; RTA, renal tubular acidosis; SIADH, syndrome of inappropriate antidiuretic hormone.

movement of water. Diabetes mellitus is the most common cause. The expected decrease in serum sodium is 2.4 mmol/L for each 100 mg/dL of glucose > 100 mg/dL. Other nonglucose solutes can cause the same effects (eg, mannitol or glycerol). If the calculated serum osmolality differs from the measured serum osmolality by > 10 mOsm/kg, then it can be inferred that another solute is present.

D. Essential hyponatremia. This is an uncommon congenital disorder in which the osmostat is set for a serum sodium that is lower than the normal range. However, it is normal for the patient. It is a benign condition that does not require treatment. Previous serum sodium values and the exclusion of other conditions causing the hyponatremia are required to make this diagnosis.

E. Acute water intoxication (hypotonic hyponatremia). Occurs when the water intake exceeds maximal urinary free water excretion. Urine osmolality should be < 120 mOsm/kg (specific gravity < 1.003) if maximal urinary dilution is present. This can occur by inappropriate administration of IV fluids or tube feedings, extensive use of tap water enemas, excessive swallowing of water during swimming or bathing, or abnormal water consumption (eg, in psychiatric patients). Treated by restricting water intake.

F. Hypovolemic hyponatremia
1. **Extrarenal losses** (spot urinary sodium < 10 mmol/L)
   a. **GI fluid losses.** Result from vomiting, diarrhea, drainage tubes, and fistulae. In surreptitious or bulimic vomiting, the urinary chloride is usually < 10 mmol/L.
   b. **Third-space fluid loss.** May occur in pancreatitis, peritonitis, muscle trauma, effusions, or burns.
   c. **Skin.** Fluid may be lost through burns, cystic fibrosis, or heat stroke. Sweating secondary to vigorous exercise can cause marked losses of water and sodium. Resulting increases in antidiuretic hormone leads to retention of ingested water.
2. **Renal losses** (spot urinary sodium > 20 mmol/L)
   a. **Diuretic usage.** Caused by thiazides and loop diuretics; often associated with hypokalemia and metabolic alkalosis. With surreptitious diuretic use, urine chloride is > 20 mmol/L.
   b. **Renal disorders.** Renal tubular acidosis, medullary cystic disease, polycystic disease, and chronic interstitial nephritis can cause hyponatremia.
   c. **Addison's disease.** Characterized by mineralocorticoid deficiency. Hyperkalemia, low urinary potassium, and metabolic acidosis are present.
   d. **Osmotic diuresis.** Most commonly caused by hyperglycemia or mannitol.
   e. **Cerebral salt wasting.** Inappropriate renal sodium wasting associated with a CNS disorder, most commonly subarachnoid hemorrhage, also seen in bacterial and tuberculous

meningitis. Mediated through atrial natriuretic hormone or cerebral natriuretic peptide.

G. Euvolemic hyponatremia

1. **SIADH.** The diagnosis is based on the findings of low serum osmolality, elevated urine sodium (> 20 mmol/L), and concentrated urine (osmolality near normal) after ruling out hypothyroidism and hypoadrenalism and confirming euvolemia.

   a. **Carcinoma.** Small cell lung carcinoma is the most common, but many others can also cause SIADH.

   b. **Pulmonary disease.** Pneumonia, tuberculosis, tumor, atelectasis, and pneumothorax.

   c. **CNS disorders.** Include trauma, tumors, infections (eg, meningitis and encephalitis), cerebrovascular accidents, and psychoses.

   d. **Stress.** Including perioperative stress.

   e. **Drugs.** See II.G. There are reports of SSRIs causing SIADH, especially in the elderly, as well as ACE inhibitors.

   f. **Postoperative conditions.** Anesthesia, stress from surgery, and postoperative pain as well as narcotics cause an increase in antidiuretic hormone.

   g. **After colonoscopy.** May cause transient hyponatremia.

2. **Hypothyroidism**

3. **Glucocorticoid deficiency**

4. **Hypopituitarism**

5. **Psychogenic polydipsia and beer potomania.** Differentiated from G.1.–G.4 (above) in that psychogenic polydipsia and beer potomania have a low urine osmolality, whereas the other conditions are marked by inappropriately high urine osmolality.

   Note: In addition to the above, there is a new postulated cause of hyponatremia seen after intracranial surgery. The proposed mechanism involves an extracellular-to-intracellular shift of sodium in exchange for potassium.

H. Hypervolemic hyponatremia

1. **CHF.** Urine sodium is < 10 mmol/L.

2. **Cirrhosis.** Urine sodium is < 10 mmol/L.

3. **Renal disease**

   a. **Chronic renal failure.** Urine sodium > 20 mmol/L.

   b. **Nephrotic syndrome.** Urine sodium < 10 mmol/L.

IV. Database

A. Physical examination key points.

Assessment of volume status is essential.

1. **Vital signs.** Evaluate for orthostatic blood pressure and heart rate changes. A decrease in systolic blood pressure of 10 mm Hg, and/or an increase in heart rate of 20 bpm 1 minute after changing from a supine to a standing position points to volume deple-

tion. Tachypnea may suggest volume overload and pulmonary edema.

2. **Skin.** Tissue turgor is diminished and mucous membranes may appear dry with volume depletion. Poor skin turgor can be a normal variant in the elderly. Edema suggests volume overload. Jaundice, spider angiomas, and caput medusae suggest cirrhosis.

3. **HEENT.** Assess internal jugular venous pressure. When the patient's bed is elevated at 30 degrees, the veins will be flat with volume depletion and markedly engorged with volume overload.

4. **Lungs.** Crackles may be heard with CHF. Noncardiogenic pulmonary edema is seen in marathon runners with hyponatremia and is thought to be secondary to the resulting cerebral edema.

5. **Heart.** An S_3 gallop suggests CHF.

6. **Abdomen.** Hepatosplenomegaly and ascites suggest cirrhosis. A hepatojugular reflux may be present in CHF.

7. **Neurologic exam.** Decreased deep tendon reflexes (DTRs), altered mental status, confusion, coma, or seizures may be present after a rapid fall in serum sodium or from a chronically low serum sodium. If hyponatremia is chronic, the neurologic and mental status exams may be normal, even with levels < 120 mmol/L. A delay in the relaxation phase of DTRs is seen in hypothyroidism.

8. **Extremities.** Clubbing may be present with lung cancer.

B. **Laboratory data**

1. **Electrolytes.** Other abnormalities may coexist. Hypokalemia can potentiate hyponatremia as sodium shifts into cells in exchange for potassium. Hypokalemia and an increase in serum bicarbonate are seen with diuretic use. Hyperkalemia and a decrease in serum bicarbonate are seen in Addison's disease.

2. **Spot urine electrolytes and creatinine.** Obtain before any diuretic treatment.

3. **Urine and serum osmolality.** Serum osmolality is normal in cases of laboratory artifact but decreased in true hyponatremia. Serum osmolality is increased in hypertonic hyponatremia secondary to mannitol or glucose. Serum osmolality is low with SIADH.

4. **Liver function tests.** To detect liver disease.

5. **Thyroid function.** Hypothyroidism must be ruled out before diagnosing SIADH.

6. **Cortisol levels, ACTH stimulation test.** Glucocorticoid deficiency must be ruled out before diagnosing SIADH, as well.

7. **Cultures.** Cultures and stains as indicated.

C. **Radiologic and other studies**

1. **Chest x-ray.** Look for CHF, lung cancer, pneumonia, and tuberculosis. Noncardiogenic pulmonary edema is seen in marathon runners with hyponatremia.

2. **Head computer tomography scan.** If indicated.

V. Plan. The cause and the presence and severity of symptoms guide therapy. Aggressive treatment of severe symptoms (eg, coma) is discussed below, as are specific therapies for certain diagnoses.

   A. Emergency treatment. Usually for severe CNS symptoms (eg, seizures or coma).

   1. **Normal saline (NS) and furosemide 1 mg/kg.** Use a combination of NS and diuretics to achieve a net negative free water deficit in hyponatremia associated with euvolemic or hypervolemic conditions. Use NS by itself if the hyponatremia is associated with volume depletion. Carefully document fluid intake and output. Supplement fluids with potassium as needed. Too-rapid correction of sodium can be deleterious, resulting in central pontine myelinolysis. Correct sodium level *rapidly* (> 1.0 mmol/L/hr) to 120–125 mmol/L; then *slowly* correct sodium level (< 0.5 mmol/L/hr) over the next 24–48 hours to normal.

   For hypovolemic states, calculate the total amount of sodium required to increase the sodium to a desired level, use the following formula:

   $$\text{Sodium required (mmol)} = (\text{desired sodium [Na]} - \text{actual serum [Na]}) \times \text{TBW}$$

   $$\text{TBW} = \text{weight (kg)} \times 0.60$$
   $$\text{TBW} = \text{total body water}$$

   To estimate the increase in serum sodium concentration for a given amount of saline administered, the following equation can be used:

   $$\text{Increase in serum [Na}^+] = \frac{(\text{IV fluid [Na}^+] - \text{serum [Na}^+]) \times \text{IV fluid volume}}{\text{TBW}}$$
   $$\text{TBW} = \text{weight (kg)} \times 0.60$$
   $$\text{TBW} = \text{total body water}$$

   2. **Hypertonic saline (3%: contains 513 mEq of Na per liter).** This preparation is rarely needed. Hypertonic saline can replace NS in the above treatment regimens. Extreme care must be taken in using hypertonic saline because of the potential for serious complications (eg, pulmonary edema and central pontine myelinolysis) secondary to overly rapid correction of hyponatremia.

   B. Hypovolemic hyponatremia

   1. **Treat by replacing volume and sodium.** Give NS IV.

   2. **Potassium.** In cases of diuretic abuse, repletion of lost body potassium is also necessary.

   C. Euvolemic hyponatremia. (Patient is not edematous.) In cases of SIADH, restrict patient's water intake to 800–1000 mL daily. Give demeclocycline (300–600 mg bid PO) for chronic SIADH, such as that resulting from neoplasms. Onset of medication action may take up to 1 week.

D. Hypervolemic hyponatremia. (Patient is edematous.) Restrict IV and oral fluids.

1. **CHF.** Treat with digoxin, diuretics (eg, furosemide), ACE inhibitors, and sodium restriction.

2. **Nephrotic syndrome.** Give steroids (if the cause is steroid-responsive), restrict sodium and water intake, and increase patient's protein intake. Furosemide is commonly used.

3. **Cirrhosis.** Treat with restriction of sodium and water, and diuretics. Initially, give spironolactone 100 mg PO Q day, increasing dose 100 mg Q 2–3 days up to 400 mg Q day. Furosemide is often used with spironolactone, especially when is present (40 mg furosemide is given with 100 mg of spironolactone, increasing by 40 mg with increasing doses of spironolactone; 40 mg Q AM, 80 mg Q AM, 80 mg Q AM and 40 mg Q PM and 80 mg bid). A portosystemic shunt is needed in only 5–10% of patients to control ascites.

4. **Renal failure.** Treat with sodium and water restriction, loop diuretics, and dialysis, if indicated.

REFERENCES

Adrogue HJ, Madias NE: Hypernatremia. N Engl J Med 2000;342:1493.

Ayus CJ, Varon J, Arieff AI: Hyponatremia, cerebral edema, and noncardiogenic pulmonary edema in marathon runners. Ann Intern Med 2000;132:711.

Berl T, Schrier RW: Disorders of water metabolism. In: Schrier RW, ed. *Renal and Electrolyte Disorders.* 6th ed. Lippincott-Raven;2003:1.

Cohen CD, Keuneke C, Schiemann U et al: Hyponatremia as a complication of colonoscopy. Lancet 2001;357:282.

Fabian TJ, Amico JA, Kroboth PD et al: Paroxetine-induced hyponatremia in older adults. Arch Intern Med 2004;164:327.

Van Amelsvoort T, Bakshi R, Devaux CV et al: Hyponatremia associated with carbamazepine and oxcarbazepine therapy: A review. Epilepsia 1994;35:181.

Weisberg LS: Pseudohyponatremia: A reappraisal. Am J Med 1989;86:315.

41. HYPOPHOSPHATEMIA

I. Problem. A 26-year-old male with type 1 diabetes was admitted 6 hours ago for treatment of diabetic ketoacidosis (DKA) and now has a serum phosphate level of 1.0 mg/dL.

II. Immediate Questions

A. Are there any symptoms related to the low phosphate? Serum phosphate levels below 1.0 mg/dL require prompt treatment regardless of symptoms. Above that level, check for symptoms related to low phosphate, such as numbness or tingling, muscle weakness, anorexia, confusion, irritability, seizures, and skeletal pain. Muscle weakness, mental status changes, and hematologic abnormalities are common findings.

B. What treatment is the patient receiving? Hypophosphatemia usually results from phosphate shifts within the body. This is most often a consequence of medical treatment, such as hyperalimentation, correction of DKA, or refeeding of malnourished or alcoholic patients. Antacids also can cause hypophosphatemia by binding phosphate in the gut.

C. Does the patient consume alcohol? Chronic alcoholism is a common cause of hypophosphatemia secondary to poor intake and possible increased renal excretion, especially if hypomagnesemia is also present.

III. Differential Diagnosis. A low serum phosphate level usually results from a combination of increased renal loss, increased intestinal loss, or intracellular shift of phosphate—the latter being the most common.

A. Intracellular shift of phosphate. Alkalosis from any cause. See Section I, Chapter 3, Alkalosis, p 19.

B. Increased intestinal phosphate loss
   1. **Phosphate-binding antacids**
   2. **Malabsorption, vomiting, diarrhea, malnutrition**

C. Increased renal phosphate loss
   1. **Acidosis.** Including untreated DKA.
   2. **Hyperparathyroidism, renal tubular disease, hypokalemia, hypomagnesemia, diuretics**

D. Multifactorial
   1. **Alcoholism and liver disease.** All three mechanisms.
   2. **Vitamin D deficiency or resistance.** Renal and intestinal loss.
   3. **Treatment of DKA and severe burns.** Renal and intracellular shift.

IV. Database
   A. Physical examination key points
      1. **Vital signs**
         a. **Temperature.** Heat stroke can cause hypophosphatemia from intracellular shifts. Sepsis occurs more frequently with hypophosphatemia because of leukocyte dysfunction.
         b. **Respiratory rate.** Hyperventilation with resulting alkalosis is a cause of extracellular-to-intracellular shifts of phosphate.
      2. **HEENT.** Check for thyromegaly. Thyrotoxicosis can also cause extracellular-to-intracellular shifts of phosphate.
      3. **Heart.** A reversible congestive cardiomyopathy may result from hypophosphatemia. Look for a laterally displaced apical pulse and third heart sound (S_3).
      4. **Lungs.** Listen for rales as evidence of cardiomyopathy. Acute hypophosphatemia can also result in acute respiratory failure.

    5. **Neurologic exam.** Confusion and coma may be present. Sensory examination may be abnormal secondary to related paresthesias.

    6. **Musculoskeletal exam.** Check for diffuse muscle weakness. Tenderness suggests rhabdomyolysis; however, the phosphate may increase to extremely high levels secondary to rhabdomyolysis.

B. Laboratory data

    1. **Serum electrolytes.** Especially bicarbonate and potassium. An elevated bicarbonate may suggest a metabolic alkalosis; a low bicarbonate may represent compensation for a chronic respiratory alkalosis. Alkalosis results in extracellular-to-intracellular shifts of phosphate. Hypokalemia can cause hypophosphatemia.

    2. **Arterial blood gases and pH.** Alkalosis (either metabolic or respiratory) results in intracellular shifts of phosphate. A metabolic acidosis with an increased anion gap and an elevated glucose suggests DKA, which can have associated hypophosphatemia. An elevated pCO_2 also suggests respiratory failure, which can occur as a result of hypophosphatemia.

    3. **Calcium, magnesium, and glucose levels.** A low calcium level may suggest vitamin D deficiency or osteomalacia. High calcium suggests hyperparathyroidism or thiazide diuretic use, which can cause hypophosphatemia. Hypomagnesemia results in increased phosphate excretion.

    4. **Glucose.** There is increased urinary excretion of phosphate in DKA.

    5. **Uric acid.** Hypophosphatemia can be seen with acute gout; however, the uric acid level may be high, normal, or low in acute gout.

    6. **Liver enzymes, albumin, bilirubin, and creatine phosphokinase (CK).** Hypophosphatemia may cause liver dysfunction. CK should be checked to rule out rhabdomyolysis from severe hypophosphatemia, especially if muscle tenderness is present or develops.

    7. **Complete blood count with differential.** An elevated white blood cell (WBC) count with a left shift suggests a bacterial infection. As a result of WBC dysfunction, patients with hypophosphatemia are more susceptible to bacterial infections.

    8. **Peripheral smear.** Severe hypophosphatemia can cause hemolysis.

    9. **Platelet count.** Thrombocytopenia and platelet dysfunction can result.

C. Radiologic and other studies

    1. **Bone films.** May show pseudofractures.

    2. **Chest x-ray.** Possible complications of hypophosphatemia such as congestive cardiomyopathy and respiratory failure are indications for a chest x-ray.

    3. **Electroencephalogram (EEG).** An EEG may be needed to evaluate seizures or encephalopathy, which are possible complications.

V. Plan. If the phosphate level is < 1.0 mg/dL, start IV replacement therapy immediately. If the level is 1.0–1.5 mg/dL and the patient is symptomatic, start IV replacement therapy. Otherwise, oral treatment is usually sufficient.

A. Intravenous treatment

1. If the hypophosphatemia is recent and uncomplicated, give 0.08 mmol/kg (2.5 mg/kg) IV over 6 hours. Sodium phosphate and potassium phosphate IV solutions both contain 3 mmol of phosphate per milliliter.

2. If the hypophosphatemia is longstanding or complicated, give 0.16 mmol/kg (5.0 mg/kg) IV over 6 hours.

3. In either case, consider using 25–50% higher doses if the patient is symptomatic, but do not exceed 0.24 mmol/kg (7.5 mg/kg) or 16.9 mmol (525 mg) for a 70-kg patient.

4. Recheck the phosphate level promptly after the 6-hour infusion, and reassess the patient's need for further replacement.

B. Oral replacement

1. Neutra-Phos tablets contain 250 mg phosphorus (8 mmol) per tablet; Neutra-Phos powder contains 0.1 mmol phosphate per milliliter.

2. Milk contains modest amounts of phosphate. Skim milk has slightly more phosphate and may be better tolerated for those who are lactose intolerant (Table I–8).

3. Fleet enema solution and Fleet Phospho-Soda contain buffered sodium phosphate and can be administered orally. Fleet enema solution contains 1.4 mmol/mL. Administer 15–30 mL, tid–qid (50–150 mmol/24 hr). Fleet Phospho-Soda contains 4.15 mmol/mL phosphate. An estimated two-thirds of orally administered phosphate is absorbed.

C. Precautions

1. It may be necessary to give calcium supplements to hypocalcemic patients who are being given phosphate.

2. Do not give calcium and phosphate through the same IV line.

3. Beware of causing hyperphosphatemia, hypotension, hyperkalemia, osmotic diuresis, or hypernatremia.

TABLE I–8. AMOUNT OF PHOSPHATE IN AN 8-OZ SERVING OF MILK.

Milk	Phosphorus[1] (mg/8-oz. serving)
Skim	247
Whole	227

[1] 250 mg of elemental phosphorus = 8 mmol phosphate.

REFERENCES

Shiber JR, Mattu A: Serum phosphate abnormalities in the emergency department. J Emerg Med 2002;23:395.

Subramanian RMB, Khardori R: Severe hypophosphatemia: Pathophysiologic implications, clinical presentations, and treatment. Medicine 2000;79:1.

42. HYPOTENSION (SHOCK)

I. **Problem.** A 75-year-old woman presents with confusion, nausea, abdominal pain, and weakness. Her blood pressure is 70/50 mm Hg.

II. **Immediate Questions**

A. **What are all of the patient's vital signs?** Confirm the blood pressure in both arms manually. An arterial line may be useful. Either severe bradycardia or tachycardia can be the primary problem, or tachycardia can be associated with the cause of the hypotension. Fever suggests sepsis, but hypothermia can also be seen in sepsis, myxedema, and addisonian crisis. Tachypnea may be seen in cardiogenic shock, pulmonary embolus (PE), and sepsis. Hypopnea is often associated with sedative or narcotics overdosage, to which the elderly may be most sensitive.

B. **What is the patient's mental status?** Confusion or altered mental staus may be an indicator of inadequate perfusion of vital organs. These symptoms could also result from the administration of narcotics or sedatives, particularly in the elderly in whom symptoms can occur with "usual" doses.

C. **What are the patient's usual medications and when were they last taken? Have any medications been started recently?** All antihypertensive medications (angiotensin-converting enzyme inhibitors, direct vasodilators, calcium channel blockers, beta-blockers and central-acting antihypertensive agents) significantly lower blood pressure, especially in the setting of volume depletion or with concomitant use of diuretics. Review all intravenous (IV) medications that may have been or are being administered, including nitroprusside, nitroglycerin, nicardipine, esmolol, fenoldopam, and phenytoin. Anaphylaxis to a new drug should be considered, especially if there is respiratory distress. Diuretics alone rarely cause significant volume depletion sufficient to cause hypotension, but they can augment the effects of other drugs, especially in the elderly.

D. **Are there any accompanying symptoms?** A history of bleeding, vomiting, diarrhea, polyuria, polydipsia, dysuria, cough, chest pain, or abdominal pain may suggest the underlying cause of hypotension. Chest discomfort and dyspnea suggest PE or myocardial ischemia/infarction. Dyspnea may be the only symptom of cardiac ischemia/infarction, especially in the elderly.

III. Differential Diagnosis. *Hypotension* is a relative term and must be individualized to the patient. An elderly hypertensive patient may not tolerate a systolic blood pressure (SBP) of 100 mm Hg, but in others, SBP of 90 mm Hg may be normal. *Shock* is a condition in which the blood pressure is inadequate to provide required tissue perfusion. The following are subcategories of shock.

A. Hypovolemic
   1. Hemorrhagic
      a. Traumatic. Trauma patients may lose a large volume of blood internally (chest, abdomen, and pelvis), which may not be readily apparent. A thorough exam and high index of suspicion are necessary to guide diagnostic testing.
      b. Postoperative or postprocedural. Hemorrhage may occur after percutaneous biopsy (liver, kidney, or lung) or after central venous line placement, angiography, or cardiac catheterization/percutaneous transluminal angioplasty.
      c. Miscellaneous. Gastrointestinal (GI) bleeding, ruptured aneurysm, ruptured ovarian cyst, or ectopic pregnancy.
   2. Fluid losses. Severe vomiting, diarrhea, perspiration, extensive burns, diuresis, and "third-space losses" (peritonitis or pancreatitis) may result in significant hypovolemia.

B. Vasogenic. Inappropriate loss of vascular tone may develop as a result of sepsis, anaphylaxis, adrenal insufficiency, acidosis, central nervous system injury, or medications, or it may occur postprandially (especially in the elderly).

C. Cardiogenic. Acute cardiac failure most commonly occurs as a result of acute myocardial infarction (MI) or profound ischemia, and it may occur with decompensated congestive heart failure (CHF). Cardiac arrhythmia (supraventricular, ventricular, or various degrees of heart block), tension pneumothorax, pericardial tamponade, and PE can cause hypotension.

D. Neurogenic. An increase in vagal stimulation from a variety of causes, including spinal cord injury and pain can result in inapproriate bradycardia and vasodilation.

IV. Database

A. Physical examination key points
   1. Vital signs. Temperature, blood pressure, pulse, respiratory rate, and orthostatic changes (if feasible; do not try to stand a patient with SBP < 90 mm Hg). A decrease in SBP of 10 mm Hg or an increase in heart rate of 20 bpm from supine to standing position (or both) after 1 minute are indicative of volume depletion.
   2. Skin. Poor skin turgor suggests volume depletion, but it may be a normal variant in the elderly. Cool, clammy skin indicates car-

diogenic or hypovolemic shock, whereas warm, moist skin signifies vasodilation (sepsis). Burns and trauma should be apparent with close inspection.

3. **Neck.** Jugular venous distention (JVD) and pulsations may be helpful in determining volume status and cardiac rhythm, as well as in diagnosing cardiac tamponade or tension pneumothorax. JVD with the latter two conditions does not decrease with inspiration. Coexisting cardiac or pulmonary disease makes this exam difficult to interpret.

4. **Chest.** Tracheal deviation suggests tension pneumothorax. Wheezing or stridor may indicate anaphylaxis (see Section I, Chapter 4, Anaphylactic Reaction, p 25) or acute exacerbation of chronic obstructive pulmonary disease. Rales and wheezes can occur with cardiac failure or pneumonia. Chest percussion may help diagnose pneumothorax, pleural effusion, hemothorax, and pneumonia.

5. **Heart.** Auscultate for a murmur and palpate for a thrill or a change in the apical impulse. A new thrill or systolic murmur may indicate a ventricular septal defect (VSD) or papillary muscle dysfunction complicating an acute MI. Loss of a palpable apical pulse suggests a pericardial effusion. A third heart sound (S_3) is heard with left ventricular failure; a new fourth heart sound (S_4) suggests acute myocardial ischemia.

6. **Abdomen.** Rebound tenderness or positive Murphy's sign and absence of bowel sounds suggest sepsis from an abdominal source. (See Section I, Chapter 1, Abdominal Pain, p 1.) Absent bowel sounds and tenderness may be present with a large GI bleed. A pulsatile mass suggests a leaking aortic aneurysm. Ecchymoses may be seen with retroperitoneal bleeding from a variety of causes such as hemorrhagic pancreatitis or retroperitoneal hemorrhage, but are rare.

7. **Rectum.** Hematochezia or occult blood indicates GI blood loss.

8. **Female genitalia.** A gynecologic exam in women of childbearing age is mandatory to rule out a ruptured ectopic pregnancy or pelvic infection.

9. **Extremities.** Instability of pelvis or femurs suggests a fracture, which can result in significant bleeding into either the pelvis or the thigh. Edema may indicate volume overload or venous/lymphatic obstruction. Inspect for inflammation of vascular access sites suggesting iatrogenic infection/sepsis.

10. **Neurologic exam.** Altered mental status may indicate inadequate cerebral hypoperfusion as well as suggest possible causes (cerebrovascular accident).

B. **Laboratory data**
  1. **Complete blood count.** The initial hematocit may appear normal or stable with acute blood loss, but serial hematocrits may indi-

cate blood loss as intravascular volume is replaced. An elevated white blood cell count and differential with a "left shift" may indicate sepsis. A low platelet count may point to disseminated intravascular coagulation (DIC), suggesting sepsis.

2. **Serum electrolytes.** A low serum bicarbonate could be caused by a lactic acidosis secondary to decreased perfusion. Severe acidosis, hyperkalemia, and hypokalemia may cause an arrhythmia. Refractory lactic acidosis most often suggests an abdominal catastrophe such as bowel infarction.

3. **Prothrombin time, partial thromboplastin time.** A coagulopathy may indicate DIC, hepatic dysfunction, or excessive anticoagulation.

4. **Arterial blood gases.** Early sepsis may produce a respiratory alkalosis, and a metabolic acidosis will develop with progression of the infection. Metabolic acidosis also develops in shock as a result of poor tissue perfusion. Severe acidosis (pH < 7.20) may inhibit the effectiveness of vasopressors and cause arrhythmias. Hypoxemia may also require ventilatory support.

5. **Creatine phosphokinase with isoenzymes and troponin-I and troponin-T.** Obtain if MI or myocarditis is suspected, as well as to rule out myocardial injury secondary to the hypotension.

6. **Type and cross-match.** Blood should be made ready for transfusion if hemorrhage is suspected.

7. **Pregnancy test.** To rule out ectopic pregnancy in women of childbearing age.

8. **Blood, sputum, urine, and other cultures as indicated.** If sepsis is suspected.

9. **Nasogastric (NG) aspirate.** To assess for upper GI bleeding. A negative NG aspirate does not rule out upper GI bleeding because a small percentage of duodenal bleeding does not reflux into the stomach.

C. **Radiologic and other studies**

1. **Chest x-ray.** May indicate the source of sepsis or identify CHF. It may be diagnostic for pneumothorax or hemothorax.

2. **Electrocardiogram.** Myocardial infarction/ischemia or arrhythmias can be detected.

3. **Pulmonary artery catheter (Swan-Ganz).** Very helpful in evaluating and treating shock. Hemodynamic measurements may be used to aid the diagnosis and management of the hypotensive patient (see Table III-3, p 451). Swan-Ganz catheter is also useful when ruling out cardiac tamponade when there is equalization of intracardiac pressures. The right atrial pressure equals the elevated right ventricular diastolic pressure.

4. **Angiography/digital subtraction angiography/high-resolution CT scan.** All these modalities can detect a PE, and CT scans detect pericardial effusion. Abdominal angiograms may be helpful in detecting the source of GI bleeding, particularly in lower GI bleed-

ing. CT scanning detects abdominal aortic anuerysm and determines whether rupture or leaking has occurred.

5. **Nuclear scans.** A ventilation/perfusion ($\dot{V}/\dot{Q}$) lung scan may aid in diagnosing PE, but is less sensitive/specific than CT scanning. Radiolabeled red blood cell scans may help identify sources of GI bleeding.

6. **Echocardiogram.** A noninvasive test to evaluate global ventricular function and valvular function and to rule out mechanical defects such as VSD or ruptured papillary muscle. Pericardial effusion resulting in tamponade can also be identified.

7. **Paracentesis, thoracentesis, culdocentesis, pericardiocentesis.** As indicated.

V. **Plan.** Establish adequate tissue perfusion as soon as possible. Generally, an SBP > 90 mm Hg is adequate. Signs of adequate perfusion include an improved mental status and a urine output of 0.5–1.0 mL/min.

A. **Emergency management**
1. Control external hemorrhage with direct pressure.
2. Establish venous access, preferably two large-bore (14- to 16-gauge) peripheral IV lines or a central venous line (jugular, subclavian or femoral).
3. Trendelenburg position (supine with feet elevated) or pneumatic antishock garment (PASG or MAST) may be useful in hypovolemic shock.
4. Insert Foley catheter to monitor urinary output.
5. Administer supplemental oxygen and ventilatory support as needed.
6. Severe metabolic acidosis (pH < 7.10) should be corrected. See Section I, Chapter 1, Acidosis, III. C.

   Remember that an ampule of sodium bicarbonate is hyperosmolar. After several ampules, it is prudent to start an isotonic bicarbonate drip for persistent acidosis. A bicarbonate drip is made by adding 2.5 ampules of sodium bicarbonate (50 mEq/50 mL) to 1 L of D5W. Respiratory acidosis can be corrected by improving minute ventilation (V_e) to reduce pCO_2.
7. Swan-Ganz catheterization with hemodynamic monitoring aids in the differential diagnosis of shock as well as with fluid management. See Section III, Chapter 12, Pulmonary Artery Catheterization, p 449.

B. **Hypovolemic shock**
1. Administer fluids (IV normal saline or lactated Ringer's solution) and administer packed red blood cells if HCT < 30%, using blood pressure, urine output, and central filling pressures (pulmonary capillary wedge pressure [PCWP]) as a guide for further therapy. Give IV fluid bolus of 250–500 mL followed by either a second fluid bolus or maintenance IV fluids at 200–250 mL/hr.
2. Use vasopressor agents such as norepinephrine and dopamine if hypotension persists despite a fluid challenge sufficient to achieve

adequate filling pressures (PCWP 16–18 mmHg). If SBP is 70–90 mm Hg, begin dopamine at a dose of 2.5–5.0 μg/kg/min and increase up to 20 μg/kg/min or begin norepinephrine, 1–20 μg/min.

C. Neurogenic shock

1. Institute moderate IV fluid administration See V.B. Avoid volume overload.
2. Low-dose vasopressors may be necessary. Use an alpha agent such as phenylephrine (Neo-Synephrine) 100–180 μg/min initially; the usual maintenance dosage is 40–60 μg/min. Or, use norepinephrine (see V.B.).

D. Vasogenic shock

1. **Septic shock.** Identify and treat the source of the infection.
   a. Administer IV fluids and vasopressors as indicated.
   b. Broad-spectrum antibiotics are generally used if a specific source cannot be readily identified. Gram's stain of infected fluid will guide antibiotic choice. See Section I, Chapter 22, Fever, V, p 138.
2. **Anaphylactic shock.** See Section I, Chapter 4, Anaphylactic Reaction, p 25.
   a. Remove precipitating agent as soon as possible.
   b. Immediately administer epinephrine 0.3 mL of 1:1000 SC or IM. Depending on the BP, the onset of action may be delayed by the subcutaneous route. For IV resuscitation, 10 mL of 1:10,000 (10 mg) is administered. If epinephrine is given by a peripheral IV, the IV line should be subsequently flushed with 20 mL of fluid. If IV access is not available, epinephrine can be delivered via an endotracheal tube. The dose for this route should be twice the IV dose.
   c. Maintain an adequate airway.
   d. An antihistamine such as diphenhydramine (Benadryl) 25 mg IM or IV, and corticosteroids such as hydrocortisone 100–250 mg IV, can also be given.
3. **Addisonian crisis.** Give hydrocortisone 100 mg IV bolus, then 100 mg IV every 6 hours, if this diagnosis is suspected. Obtain a cortisol level before instituting therapy.

E. Cardiogenic shock

1. Cardiogenic shock is usually complicated and more difficult to manage than hypovolemic or septic shock; therefore, hemodynamic monitoring with a Swan-Ganz catheter is mandatory. See Section III, Chapter 12, Pulmonary Artery Catheterization, p 449.
2. Initial priority should be given to establishing an adequate perfusion pressure (SBP > 90 mm Hg) while hemodynamic monitoring catheters are placed.
3. Once cardiac hemodynamics have been evaluated, appropriate use of diuretics (IV furosemide, bumetanide), cardiac inotropes (dopamine, dobutamine, milrinone), vasopressors (dopamine,

norepinephrine; see V.B.2.), antiarrhythmics, and intra-aortic balloon counterpulsation (IABP) can be instituted. IABP may be most effective at reversing cardiogenic shock.

4. Pericardiocentesis is indicated if there is hemodynamic compromise secondary to pericardial tamponade.

5. If a tension pneumothorax is present, a 14- to 16-gauge needle should be placed in the second or third intercostal space just superior to the rib in the midclavicular line until a chest tube can be placed.

6. Treat any tachyarrhythmia or bradyarrhythmia (see Section I, Chapter 60, Tachycardia, V, p 351; Section I, Chapter 8, Bradycardia, V, p 45; and Section I, Chapter 45, Irregular Pulse, V, p 254).

REFERENCES

Hollenberg SM, Kavinsky CJ, Parrillo JE: Cardiogenic shock. Ann Intern Med 1999;131:47.

Jansen RWMM, Lipsitz LA: Postprandial hypotension: Epidemiology, pathophysiology, and clinical management. Ann Intern Med 1995;122:286.

43. HYPOTHERMIA

I. **Problem.** You are called to the emergency room to see a patient with a temperature of 32.0 °C (89.6 °F).

II. **Immediate Questions**

A. **Does the patient have any possible source of infection?** Septic patients may be hypothermic. Look for evidence of pneumonia, urinary tract infection, or any other cause of bacteremia. One study found that 41% of patients admitted for hypothermia had a serious infection.

B. **Is there a history of other medical problems?** Hypothyroidism, hypoglycemia, hypopituitarism, and hypoadrenalism all may present with hypothermia. Alcohol also predisposes humans to environment-induced hypothermia.

C. **What is the clinical setting? Does the patient have a history of exposure to cold weather or inadequate heating or clothing?** The very young and very old are susceptible to hypothermia as a result of environmental exposure.

D. **Is the patient taking any medications?** Barbiturates and phenothiazines impair hypothalamic thermoregulation. Alcohol is a vasodilator and central nervous system (CNS) depressant, thus increasing the risk for hypothermia from environmental exposure. The use of insulin, thyroid medication, or steroids may also suggest a cause. Beta-blockers and clonidine can impair the body's ability to compensate for hypothermia.

III. Differential Diagnosis

    A. Sepsis. Bacteremia must be ruled out.

    B. Environmental exposure. Was the patient found outdoors or in an unheated building? Such patients frequently have concomitant alcoholism, drug addictions, and mental illnesses.

    C. Metabolic abnormalities

        1. Myxedema. Thermoderegulation resulting in hypothermia associated with hypothyroidism may have concomitant mental status changes including coma. There is often a precipitating event.

        2. Hypoglycemia. This condition has many potential causes (see Section I, Chapter 37, Hypoglycemia, p 213). It may also be associated with overwhelming sepsis or depleted glycogen stores due to chronic alcohol consumption, profound liver disease, or adrenal insufficiency.

        3. Adrenal insufficiency. May be acute or chronic. The patient often has a history of steroid ingestion. Adrenal insufficiency may be secondary to metastatic carcinoma or may be idiopathic.

        4. Uremia. Easily ruled out by checking blood urea nitrogen (BUN) and creatinine.

        5. Hypopituitarism. Can result in hypoadrenalism and hypothyroidism and can also cause hypoglycemia.

    D. CNS dysfunction

        1. Cerebrovascular accident. Look for focal neurologic findings such as motor weakness or sensory deficit, unilateral hyperreflexia, or plantar extension with Babinski reflex.

        2. Head trauma. A history and careful examination of head, eyes, ears, nose, and neck should reveal any recent injury.

        3. Spinal cord transection. Paraplegia or quadriplegia on examination. These patients have impaired thermoregulation and are predisposed to hypothermia. They are essentially poikilothermic.

        4. Wernicke's encephalopathy. This condition is characterized by a triad of ophthalmoplegia, mental status changes, and ataxia. It is secondary to thiamine deficiency from decreased intake associated most often in the United States with chronic alcohol ingestion.

        5. Drug ingestion. See II.D.

        6. Miscellaneous. Other diagnoses to consider are generalized erythroderma, protein–calorie malnutrition, and anorexia nervosa.

IV. Database

    A. Physical examination key points

        1. Vital signs. Record the core temperature accurately with a rectal or bladder thermometer; make sure that it is a low-recording thermometer. Standard thermometers may not record temperatures lower than 34.4 °C (93.8 °F). Keep in mind that hypotension and bradycardia frequently occur in hypothermia.

2. **Skin.** Look for evidence of frostbite, diffuse erythroderma, burns, or insulin injection sites. Hyperpigmentation (especially in the creases of the palms) suggests primary adrenal insufficiency.
3. **Heart.** Heart sounds may be distant, slow, or absent.
4. **Lungs.** Respirations may be slow and shallow. Look for signs of pneumonia.
5. **Abdomen.** Ileus may occur with hypothermia.
6. **Neurologic exam.** Look for signs of head trauma. Check pupil reactivity; pupils are often sluggish and react slowly to light. Occasionally in this setting, pupils are nonreactive to light. Mental status may vary from mental slowing to confusion and coma. Check deep tendon reflexes, which may be absent with severe hypothermia. A slow relaxation phase points to hypothyroidism.

B. **Laboratory data**
   1. **Complete blood count.** Hypothermia can cause hemoconcentration and leukocytosis. Leukocytosis or leukopenia with an increase in banded neutrophils suggests sepsis.
   2. **Platelet count.** A low platelet count can occur with either secondary sequestration or disseminated intravascular coagulation (DIC) caused by either hypothermia or associated with sepsis. (See Section I, Chapter 61, Thrombocytopenia, p 355.)
   3. **Prothrombin time (PT), partial thromboplastin time (PTT).** Elevation of the PT and PTT is consistent with DIC, which can be a complication of hypothermia or associated with sepsis. (See Section I, Chapter 12, Coagulopathy, p 70.)
   4. **BUN and creatinine.** To rule out uremia. The BUN:creatinine ratio may be increased secondary to hemoconcentration.
   5. **Glucose.** Hypoglycemia may be the cause of hypothermia or associated with the underlying cause.
   6. **Thyroxine (T_4) and thyroid-stimulating hormone (TSH).** You need to rule out hypothyroidism. T_4 can be low in the euthyroid sick state, but TSH is usually normal.
   7. **Cortrosyn stimulation test.** See Section II, ACTH Stimulation Test, p 369. This test is used to rule out adrenal insufficiency, since a single cortisol level can be misleading. Also, be sure to check adrenal reserve in all patients with severe hypothyroidism.
   8. **Arterial blood gases (ABG).** Most experts no longer recommend correction of ABG for hypothermia.
   9. **Blood cultures.** Rule out sepsis.
   10. **Serum and urine drug screen.** Rule out barbiturates or phenothiazines as possible causes.

C. **Radiologic and other studies**
   1. **Chest x-ray.** Obtain to rule out pneumonia as a source of infection. Pneumonia is also the most common sequela of hypothermia during the recovery period.

2. **Electrocardiogram (ECG).** Hypothermia can promote myocardial irritability and cause conduction abnormalities. The ECG may show T-wave inversion and PR, QRS, and QT prolongation as well as the unique *Osborn wave*, which closely follows the QRS complex. Continuous ECG monitoring is important with a temperature below 32 °C (89.6 °F) because of the risk of cardiac arrhythmias. Atrial fibrillation is common.

Junctional bradycardia can also occur. Ventricular tachycardia and fibrillation occur frequently at temperatures below 30 °C (86.0 °F).

V. Plan

A. General support

1. **For moderate/severe hypothermia (< 32 °C), admit to an intensive care unit.** Make sure the patient is hemodynamically stable. If ventricular fibrillation occurs, cardiopulmonary resuscitation should be instituted and continued until the core temperature rises (see Section I, Chapter 9, Cardiopulmonary Arrest, V, p 49). In this clinical setting, the statement "A patient is not dead until they are warm and dead" applies.

2. If you suspect hypothermia secondary to environmental exposure, place an IV line to replace fluids because chronic hypothermia leads to volume depletion. The IV fluids can be warmed to 43 °C (109.4 °F).

3. Other therapeutic measures depend on the clinical setting. If sepsis is a possibility, begin antibiotics immediately.

4. Give IV steroids if you suspect Addison's disease or IV thyroxine if you suspect possible myxedema coma.

5. Some clinicians advocate administration of 100 mg thiamine IV, an ampule (50 mL) of 50% dextrose solution (D50), and 2 mg of naloxone (Narcan) to all comatose hypothermic patients. Narcotic overdose should be suspected with bradypnea and pin-point pupils. Empiric dextrose administration is controversial because the administration of D50 has been associated with poorer outcomes in patients with anoxic or ischemic coma. Some experts recommend IV dextrose only if an immediate finger-stick glucose is low.

B. Rewarming techniques

1. In cases of environmental exposure, remove the patient from the cold environment and use some insulating material such as blankets. Patients with mild hypothermia (body temperature, 32.2 ° to 35 °C) and no circulatory compromise can be treated with passive rewarming.

2. Patients with moderate (body temperature, 28 ° to < 32.2 °C) or severe hypothermia (temperature, < 28 °C) should be treated with active rewarming. Some aggressive rewarming techniques are

controversial. Active *external* rewarming with an electric blanket may produce hypovolemic shock through peripheral vasodilation or cause "afterdrop" in core temperature through movement of the cold blood to the body core. External rewarming may also worsen a metabolic acidosis.

3. Such concerns have led to the use of active *core* rewarming for patients with core temperatures below 32 °C (89.6 °F), especially in the setting of chronic hypothermia secondary to environmental exposure. Active core rewarming techniques currently recommended include inhalation of warmed oxygen, use of warm IV fluids, and use of cardiopulmonary-bypass circuit.

REFERENCES

Browning RG, Olson DW, Stueven HA et al: 50% dextrose: Antidote or toxin? Ann Emerg Med 1990;19:683.

Danzl DF, Pozos RS: Accidental hypothermia. N Engl J Med 1994;331:1756.

Lazar HL: The treatment of hypothermia. N Engl J Med 1997;337:1545.

Lewin S, Brettman LR, Holzman RS: Infections in hypothermic patients. Arch Intern Med 1981;141:920.

Reuler JB: Hypothermia: Pathophysiology, clinical settings and management. Ann Intern Med 1978;89:519.

Scott MG, Heusel JW, LeGrys VA et al: Electrolyte and blood gases. In: Burtis CA, Ashwood ER, eds. *Tietz Textbook of Clinical Chemistry*. 3rd ed. Saunders;1999:1056.

Walpoth BH, Walpoth-Aslan BN, Mattle HP et al: Outcome of survivors of accidental deep hypothermia and circulatory arrest treated with extracorporeal blood warming. N Engl J Med 1997;337:1500.

Weinberg AD: Hypothermia. Ann Emerg Med 1993;22:370.

44. INSOMNIA

I. **Problem.** A patient hospitalized for lower-extremity cellulitis complains of lying awake for hours at night.

II. **Immediate Questions**

A. **What is the patient's mental status?** Delirium and dementia both can present with sleep disturbance. Delirium frequently results in a reversal of the normal sleep–wake cycle. It is important to avoid treatment with sedatives or hypnotics because they may actually worsen the symptomatology. Because some causes of delirium are potentially life-threatening, aggressive evaluation of delirious patients is warranted. (See Section I, Chapter 13, Coma, Acute Mental Status Changes, p 76.)

B. **Is the patient kept awake by pain?** Painful stimuli result in a state of increased arousal that interferes with sleep and escalates the cycle of sleep disturbance and pain. Common examples include rheumatoid arthritis, in which a worsening of morning stiffness is associated with sleep disturbance, and fibrositis, in which symptoms can be reproduced by disturbing delta sleep in normal subjects.

C. What is the patient's daytime sleep pattern? Certainly, a patient who sleeps for extended periods during the day will not be able to fall asleep readily at night. Sleep hygiene interventions may be helpful.

D. Does the patient take hypnotic medications regularly? What are his or her current medications? Virtually all hypnotic agents show a tolerance effect with chronic use and a disruption of the sleep patterns that can interfere with normal sleep. Abrupt withdrawal of these agents almost invariably results in sleep disturbance, often termed *rebound insomnia*. It is also important to remember that withdrawal from barbiturates can be associated with convulsions and death. Remember to ask specifically about over-the-counter preparations. In addition to self-administered preparations, many medications prescribed in the hospital can interfere with normal sleep; a thorough review of the patient's medication record is warranted.

E. What are the patient's food and beverage habits? Ingestion of stimulant-containing beverages (coffee, tea, some soft drinks) and foods (some cheeses) can interfere with sleep. Cigarette smoking and alcohol consumption both have deleterious effects on normal sleep patterns. Alcohol use and withdrawal are also associated with sleep disturbance and are frequently not reported.

F. Does the patient have difficulty lying flat? Most often this is related to a cardiopulmonary condition and is often associated with dyspnea.

G. What is the patient's customary sleep pattern? Many clues to the cause of sleep disturbance can be derived from a careful history of the sleep–wake cycle, including duration of periods of arousal and associated symptoms. Prolonged sleep latency is frequently associated with chronic or situational anxiety. Early-morning awakening is often seen with major depression, but may also be related to alcohol use. Frequent awakening with urinary urgency may be secondary to prostatic hypertrophy with bladder outlet obstruction, hyperglycemia with polyuria, or mobilization of fluid in a patient with congestive failure or chronic venous stasis and insufficiency. Awakening after a period of sleep with shortness of breath requiring a prolonged upright posture before resumption of sleep suggests left ventricular failure.

III. Differential Diagnosis

A. Medical causes

1. **Delirium.** Evaluate the patient for systemic illnesses, sepsis, and liver dysfunction; also consider drug toxicities.
2. **Pain.** Control of this symptom frequently relieves the sleep disturbance.

3. **Cardiac disorders.** Ventricular dysfunction, arrhythmias, and is-chemia can cause sleep disturbances. Ask about orthopnea, paroxysmal nocturnal dyspnea, dyspnea on exertion, palpitations, pre-syncope, syncope, and angina.

4. **Respiratory disorders.** Sleep disturbance can be seen in pa-tients with asthma, chronic obstructive airway disease, cystic fi-brosis, sarcoidosis, pneumonia, and sleep apnea. Sleep apnea is most frequently seen in patients who are morbidly obese. Central apnea syndrome is not necessarily related to body habitus. These patients are frequently unaware of their frequent arousals and in-stead complain of excessive daytime drowsiness.

5. **Periodic limb movements or restless legs syndrome.** These disorders should be considered in patients with evidence of kick-ing during sleep or an uncomfortable sensation in their legs inter-fering with sleep continuity.

6. **Hyperthyroidism.** Associated symptoms and signs include weight loss, hyperdefecation, heat intolerance, anxiety, tachycar-dia, and tremor.

B. **Drugs/toxins**
1. **Tolerance to sleep medications from chronic usage**
2. **Abrupt withdrawal of sedative or hypnotics or antidepressant medications**
3. **Alcohol abuse.** Secondary disruption of appropriate sleep pat-terns may occur as a result of chronic consumption or sudden withdrawal.
4. **Tobacco use**
5. **Caffeine ingestion.** When inquiring about the patient's beverage consumption, keep in mind that many soft drinks contain caffeine.
6. **Stimulant use or abuse**

C. **Psychiatric causes**
1. **Depressive illness.** Either bipolar or unipolar. Hallmarks are de-creased sleep with no perception of sleep deficiency and early-morning awakening, respectively.
2. **Anxiety disorders.** Generally manifested by a prolonged sleep latency.

D. **Situational causes.** Frequently related to hospitalization.
1. **Noise.** The ICU environment and talkative or emotionally dis-tressed roommates are cited as common offenders.
2. **Frequent disruptions.** Nursing duties such as administration of medications, recording of vital signs, and hygienic activities often interrupt patients' sleep.
3. **Anger.** The patient may be troubled by unexpressed anger over illness or anger toward staff or family.
4. **Anxiety.** This is a short-term response, usually related to the pa-tient's medical condition or disorienting environment.

IV. **Database.** The most important components of the database in evaluating insomnia are the patient's history and an evaluation of his or her mental status.

   A. Physical examination key points

      1. Cardiopulmonary exam. Rales, elevated jugular venous pressure, displaced point of maximal impulse, S_3 gallop, and peripheral edema all suggest congestive heart failure.

      2. Respiratory exam. Wheezing suggests obstructive airway disease but can be seen with pulmonary edema.

      3. Neurologic exam. Conduct a mental status examination for evidence of anxiety, depression, delirium, and dementia.

   B. Laboratory data. The cause of insomnia is very often determined without the use of laboratory tests.

      1. Screening chemistries. Include hepatic and renal function tests to evaluate for possible delirium.

      2. Thyroid hormone levels. If indicated by clinical presentation. (See III.A.6.)

      3. Urine drug screen. To be obtained in patients in whom drug use is strongly suspected but denied.

   C. Radiologic and other studies. Chest x-ray is indicated if congestive heart failure or pneumonia is suspected. Rarely a sleep study (polysomnography) is needed.

V. **Plan.** It is most important to determine the medical, psychological, or situational causes of the patient's sleeplessness. Most cases are secondary to a situational cause and do not represent a pathologic situation. In cases in which there is no contraindication to their use, it is reasonable to include a sleeping medication to be taken as needed with admission orders. When a specific cause is determined, it should be remedied if possible rather than treating the sleeplessness symptomatically.

   A. Nonmedical treatments. These measures are often as effective as medical treatment and lack side effects. They include minimizing disturbances, trying to maintain the patient's normal waking and sleeping times, eliminating roommate problems when possible, eliminating caffeine and tobacco use, and minimizing noise from monitors or other hospital equipment.

   B. Symptomatic treatment

      1. Oral sleeping medication. Choices include the benzodiazepines, benzodiazepine receptor agonists, chloral hydrate, and antihistamines. Barbiturates are not recommended.

         a. Benzodiazepines. These agents are most frequently used for short-term treatment of insomnia. Newer hypnotics such as estazolam (ProSom) 0.5–2.0 mg, zolpidem (Ambien) 5–10 mg, and zaleplon (Sonata) 5–10 mg PO nightly are effective; reports suggest less disturbance of rapid-eye-movement

(REM) sleep and lower abuse potential than with older benzo-diazepines. Other older, rapidly absorbed, short half-life agents such as triazolam (Halcion) 0.125–0.25 mg PO every night; or temazepam (Restoril) 15–30 mg PO and flurazepam (Dalmane) 15–30 mg PO every night can be used.

b. Chloral hydrate. Available in both oral and rectal forms; the dose is 500–1000 mg by either route. Do not use in patients with hepatic or renal failure.

c. Antihistamines. Be conscious of anticholinergic side effects, particularly in the elderly.

    i. **Diphenhydramine (Benadryl)** 25–50 mg PO or IM.

    ii. **Hydroxyzine (Vistaril)** 25–50 mg PO or IM.

d. Antidepressants. Many have significant anticholinergic side effects and should be used with caution in the elderly. Also, be aware of cardiac side effects.

    i. **Amitriptyline (Elavil).** Give 25–50 mg PO Q HS. Has significant anticholinergic side effects; most useful when chronic pain syndromes accompany sleep disturbance.

    ii. **Imipramine (Tofranil).** Give 75 mg PO Q HS. Requires the same precautions as with amitriptyline but is less useful in chronic pain.

    iii. **Desipramine (Norpramin).** Give 50 mg PO every night. It may have fewer anticholinergic side effects.

    iv. **Trazodone (Desyrel).** Give 25–50 mg PO Q HS.

2. Alternative therapies. Valerian, kava, and others are not to be recommended because of inadequate research regarding their effectiveness and because of concerns over the quality and consistency of concentration of the preparations of the various manufacturers. Melatonin, which has been extensively studied, has vasoconstrictive properties, and cardiovascular disease is a contraindication.

REFERENCES

Hardman JG, Limbird LE, eds: *Goodman & Gilman's The Pharmacological Basis of Therapeutics.* 10th ed. McGraw-Hill;1996.

McCrae CS, Lichstein KL: Secondary insomnia: diagnostic challenges and intervention opportunities. Sleep Med Rev 2001;5:47.

Meyer TJ: Evaluation and management of insomnia. Hosp Pract 1998;33:75.

Morin CM, Daley M, Ouellet MC: Insomnia in adults. Curr Treat Options Neurol 2001;3:9.

45. IRREGULAR PULSE

See also Section I, Chapter 60, Tachycardia, p 345, and Section I, Chapter 8, Bradycardia, p 42.

I. Problem. A 77-year-old man with mental status changes is reported to have an irregular pulse.

II. Immediate Questions

A. What is the patient's heart rate? The heart rate, as well as the degree of irregularity, can assist the physician in developing a differential diagnosis of the irregular heart rhythm. For example, an irregularly irregular rhythm with an apical pulse of greater than 100 beats per minute suggests atrial fibrillation.

B. What are the patient's other vital signs? Low systolic blood pressure (less than 90 mm Hg) would signal an urgent situation. (See Section I, Chapter 42, Hypotension, p 237.)

C. Has the patient been noted to have an irregular pulse before? A previous history of "skipped heartbeats" suggests a chronic problem. The sporadic occurrence of isolated premature atrial contractions (PACs) or premature ventricular contractions (PVCs) may be chronic. This is a common benign condition associated with several medical problems or with the use of a variety of medications. It can be seen occasionally in otherwise healthy persons.

D. Is there any history of previous cardiac disease? A history of mitral stenosis hints to atrial fibrillation related to left atrial enlargement, whereas a history of previous myocardial infarction (MI) or longstanding hypertension with left ventricular hypertrophy or dilated cardiomyopathy suggests ventricular arrhythmias.

E. What medication is the patient taking? Ask specifically about medications (eg, digoxin, antiarrhythmic agents, diuretics, bronchodilators [especially theophylline], and tricyclic antidepressants). Digoxin can cause atrioventricular (AV) heart block with variable conduction. Diuretic-induced hypokalemia and hypomagnesemia as well as the use of antiarrhythmic drugs can cause both PACs and PVCs, which may be responsible for an irregular rhythm. Many asthma drugs and other stimulants to the heart can cause an irregular heartbeat.

III. Differential Diagnosis

A. Premature contractions

   1. PACs. These contractions can result from acute illnesses. Think of PACs in patients with a significant history of tobacco, alcohol, or caffeine use. PACs may occasionally lead to sustained supraventricular tachycardia, but usually they do not require acute therapy in the absence of sustained supraventricular tachyarrhythmia.

   2. PVCs. The prevalence of benign isolated PVCs increases with age. PVCs are also seen with serious infections and illnesses; during acute myocardial ischemia; with stress; with use of many types of anesthetic drugs; and with excessive use of tobacco, alcohol, caffeine, or other cardiac stimulants. PVCs may also be seen with hypoxemia, metabolic or respiratory acidosis or alkalosis, hypokalemia, and hypomagnesemia. Patients with hypertrophic cardiomyopathy and mitral valve prolapse may have frequent multifocal nonsustained runs of ventricular ectopy that are considered risk factors for sudden cardiac death. The presence of isolated PVCs does not increase mortality in the absence of underlying organic heart disease and therefore usually does not require any specific therapy.

B. **Sinus arrhythmia.** Sinus arrhythmia occurs in almost every age group and is usually a normal variant. Treatment is rarely indicated or required. Sustained tachyarrhythmias rarely occur in otherwise healthy patients with sinus arrhythmia. The P-wave and QRS morphologies appear normal. Think about medications and other external cardiac stimulants.

C. **Sinoatrial exit block.** This is defined by the absence of a normally timed P wave, resulting in a pause that is a multiple of the P-to-P interval. This rhythm can be seen with vagal nerve stimulation, during acute myocarditis or acute MI, or with fibrosis of the conduction system. It can be related to the use of several cardiac drugs such as quinidine, procainamide, and digitalis. Syncope is a rare outcome.

D. **Atrial fibrillation.** Defined as chaotic atrial depolarizations and a grossly irregular ventricular response, atrial fibrillation can be seen in patients with apparently normal hearts. Or, it can be seen in patients with rheumatic heart disease, acute myocardial ischemia or infarction, myocarditis, pericarditis, hypertrophic and dilated cardiomyopathies, hypertensive heart disease, acute alcohol intoxication, pulmonary embolism, and thyrotoxicosis. The resting ventricular response is usually between 100 and 160 bpm. It may, however, be < 100 bpm in the presence of AV node disease or certain medications.

E. **Atrial flutter.** The pulse may be irregular if the AV node conduction varies; however, the pulse during atrial flutter is frequently rapid and usually regular. Atrial flutter is associated with the same diseases as atrial fibrillation.

F. **Second-degree AV block.** Both Mobitz type I (Wenckebach) and Mobitz type II second-degree heart block can bring about an irregular pulse if the atrial-to-ventricular conduction is variable. Second-degree heart block can be seen with acute MI, degenerative disease of the cardiac conduction system, viral myocarditis, acute rheumatic fever, and Lyme disease. Mobitz type I second-degree AV block can be seen during times of increased parasympathetic tone, such as with painful stimuli. In this circumstance, it does not indicate disease of the intracardiac conduction system.

IV. **Database**

A. **Physical examination key points**

1. **Vital signs.** Palpate the brachial or carotid pulses to determine the heart rate and assess the degree of cardiac irregularity. The brachial,

carotid, and femoral artery pulses are preferred for palpation over more peripheral pulses. Be careful to avoid mistaking a heartbeat with a variable pulsation amplitude from an irregular cardiac rhythm. Variations in pulsation amplitude can be seen during severe pulmonary bronchospasm, during an extensive MI, with decompensated congestive heart failure, with acute aortic insufficiency, or with pericardial tamponade. Prompt action must be taken if hypotension is present. A fever may suggest an infection, which can have associated PVCs or PACs. Several specific infections (eg, acute rheumatic fever and acute Lyme disease) can cause AV node block.

2. **Heart.** AV node block with an associated murmur might suggest acute rheumatic fever. An S_4 gallop suggests acute MI. Several cardiac arrhythmias may be present with an acute MI, including PVCs and PACs, variable degrees of AV block, atrial fibrillation, and atrial flutter. If atrial fibrillation is present, listen for the diastolic rumble of mitral stenosis at the cardiac apex. It is best heard using the bell of the stethoscope, with the patient in the left lateral decubitus position.

B. **Laboratory data**
   1. **Electrolytes.** Rule out hypokalemia. A low serum bicarbonate suggests metabolic acidosis.
   2. **Arterial blood gases.** If PVCs are present, exclude hypoxemia and severe acidemia or alkalemia.
   3. **Medications.** A recent serum digoxin level is imperative if the patient is taking this medication. Digitalis intoxication can cause PVCs, sinoatrial exit block, or second-degree heart block. Consider measuring serum levels of other medications, such as quinidine, procainamide, and theophylline. An elevated digoxin level can occur if the level is obtained while the drug is in the distribution phase (6–8 hours).

C. **Electrocardiogram (ECG) and rhythm strip**
   1. Be sure to include a long rhythm strip to catch the pattern of the responsible arrhythmia.
   2. Identify all the P waves that are present and note their timing and their relation to the QRS complexes. P waves are best seen in leads I, II, aVR, aVF, and V1. You may need to examine several rhythm strips from different leads to correctly identify the cardiac rhythm.
   3. Be certain to examine the ECG for evidence of myocardial ischemia; drug effects such as prolongation of the QT interval; and for the electrocardiographic changes of pulmonary embolism (S_1, Q_3, T_3, acute right bundle branch block, acute right-axis deviation), and for pericarditis (diffuse ST-elevation with upward concavity, T-wave inversion, and PR-segment depression).

V. **Plan.** Many of the cardiac arrhythmias that result in a detectably irregular pulse do not need emergent therapy; however, they should be identified and predisposing conditions treated appropriately. Possible exceptions to this statement include the following:

A. **Frequent or multifocal PVCs after an MI or with impaired left ventricular function.** Be sure to exclude predisposing conditions, such as hypokalemia, hypoxemia, hypomagnesemia, acidosis, alkalosis, and myocardial ischemia. Beta-blockers are the agents of choice because they are the only class of drugs proven to decrease the incidence of sudden cardiac death in postinfarction patients. Beta-blockers may cause or worsen congestive heart failure, particularly in patients with impaired left ventricular function. If treatment with an antiarrhythmic drug is considered, that consultation with a cardiac electrophysiologist is recommended before starting the patient on any long-term antiarrhythmic drug therapy. This recommendation is based on the results of the Cardiac Arrhythmia Suppression Trial (CAST) study, which showed that the pro-arrhythmic side effects of some of these medications (eg, encainide, flecainide, moricizine) might increase rather than decrease the risk of sudden cardiac death.

B. **Mobitz type II second-degree AV block.** This condition frequently progresses to third-degree heart block; therefore, exclusion of reversible causes and placement of a temporary transvenous pacemaker should be considered.

C. **Atrial fibrillation and flutter.** See Section I, Chapter 60, Tachycardia, V, p 351.

REFERENCES

Cardiac Arrhythmia Suppression Trial (CAST) Investigators: Preliminary report: Effect of encainide and flecainide on mortality in a randomized trial of arrhythmia suppression after myocardial infarction. N Engl J Med 1989;321:406.

Falk RH: Atrial fibrillation. N Engl J Med 2001;344:1067.

Miller JM, Zipes DP: Management of the patient with cardiac arrhythmias. In: Braunwald E, Zipes DP, Libby P, eds. *Heart Disease: A Textbook of Cardiovascular Medicine.* 6th ed. Saunders;2001:700.

Wagner GS, ed: *Marriott's Practical Electrocardiography.* 9th ed. Williams & Wilkins;1994.

46. JAUNDICE

I. **Problem.** A 66-year-old woman is admitted because of icteric sclerae and abdominal pain.

II. **Immediate Questions**

A. **What are the patient's vital signs?** Fever and tachycardia with or without hypotension can indicate sepsis associated with ascending cholangitis. This is a medical emergency and requires immediate aggressive intervention.

B. **Does the patient have diabetes?** Diabetes is a significant risk factor for ascending cholangitis.

C. **Is there a history of alcoholism or chronic alcohol use?** Cirrhosis may be a source of jaundice.

D. **Is there a history of intravenous (IV) drug abuse, high-risk sexual activities such as men having sex with men, or exposure to hepatitis?** Viral hepatitis could be the source of the jaundice. A viral prodrome is often elicited.

E. **Is there associated abdominal pain?** A history of postprandial right upper quadrant or epigastric pain, especially with radiation to the back, may represent biliary colic. Abdominal pain can also be associated with cancer.

F. **Is there a history of previous biliary surgery?** Jaundice may occur as a result of a retained common duct stone or biliary stricture.

G. **What medications is the patient taking?** Inquire about nonprescription as well as prescription drugs. Consider intentional as well as unintentional overingestion of acetaminophen.

H. **Is the patient taking any herbal preparations?** Ask the patient about herbs specifically because he or she may not consider them as drugs. Also ask the patient to bring in the container; the patient may only recall the primary ingredient but many preparations contain multiple active substances. Chaparral, comfrey, germander, willow bark, and others have caused liver disease.

I. **Has the patient been exposed to toxins?** The patient's occupation and hobbies are important. Examples of toxins include *Amanita phalloides,* carbon tetrachloride, and Ecstasy.

III. **Differential Diagnosis.** The differential diagnosis of jaundice can be classified as either surgical or medical.

A. **Surgical: extrahepatic biliary obstruction.** This category includes carcinoma and common bile duct stones. Biliary obstruction may lead to cholangitis and potentially life-threatening sepsis.

B. **Medical**

1. **Alcoholic liver disease.** Alcoholic cirrhosis is usually seen after at least 10 years of heavy ethanol ingestion. Check for stigmata of chronic liver disease (palmar erythema, spider telangiectasias, gynecomastia, and testicular atrophy). Frequently, a reversible, inflammatory element of alcohol injury called *alcoholic hepatitis* is present. This inflammatory entity can coexist with cirrhosis or may exist alone. Many of the features associated with severe alcoholic hepatitis such as ascites and jaundice remit after several months of abstinence.

2. **Viral hepatitis.** Consider viral hepatitis with a history of IV drug abuse, exposure to persons with jaundice, sexual promiscuity,

male homosexual activity, travel to endemic areas, or recent history of transfusion.

3. **Other medical causes of hepatitis.** Autoimmune disorders or drugs such as isoniazid and halothane.

4. **Hemolysis.** Rarely raises the bilirubin over 5 mg/dL. Look for an increased reticulocyte count and an increased indirect bilirubin.

5. **Primary biliary cirrhosis.** Usually found in middle-aged women, who present with jaundice, fatigue, and pruritus.

6. **Drugs.** May cause hepatitis, cholestasis, or hemolysis. Phenothiazines and estrogens are common causes of cholestasis.

7. **Total parenteral nutrition (TPN).** Associated with high carbohydrate loads, usually from long-term TPN.

8. **Pregnancy.** Acute fatty liver of pregnancy is a rare disorder that usually occurs in the third trimester. Symptoms include a prodrome of headache, fatigue, nausea, vomiting, and abdominal pain. Jaundice may follow the prodrome.

9. **Postoperative cholestasis.** Diagnosis of exclusion.

10. **Sepsis.** Diagnosis of exclusion.

IV. **Database.** An experienced clinician can make an accurate diagnosis with history, physical examination, and simple laboratory tests 85% of the time.

A. **Physical examination key points**

1. **Vital signs.** A fever with rigors may suggest ascending cholangitis.

2. **Skin.** Palmar erythema and telangiectasia point toward chronic liver disease. Look for needle marks or "tracks" suggestive of IV drug abuse.

3. **Breasts (in males).** Gynecomastia is consistent with chronic liver disease.

4. **Abdomen.** The physical exam should be centered on the abdomen. Look for hepatomegaly or palpable gallbladder (*Courvoisier's sign*), which may indicate malignant obstruction. The presence or absence of abdominal tenderness, particularly right upper quadrant tenderness, and *Murphy's sign* (tenderness in the right upper quadrant during inspiration with palpation) should be documented. Ascites may be present with cirrhosis.

5. **Rectum/genitourinary system.** A rectal exam should be done; look for occult blood. Testicular atrophy may be present in patients with chronic liver disease.

B. **Laboratory data**

1. **Liver function studies.** Including transaminases (AST and ALT), bilirubin total and fractionated, alkaline phosphatase, and γ-glutamyl transpeptidase (GGT). There are two basic patterns in liver function tests: hepatocellular and hepatocanalicular. The hepatocellular pattern is characterized by AST and ALT 10 times the

upper limits of normal with much smaller increases in alkaline phosphatase or GGT and bilirubin. Conversely, the hepato-canalicular pattern is suggested when the alkaline phosphatase or GGT is 5–10 times normal with relatively normal transaminases. Bilirubin is also more commonly elevated. Transaminases > 300 almost never occur in alcoholic liver disease without the combined effect of some other toxin such as acetaminophen (Tylenol). Bilirubin levels > 20 are very suggestive of extrahepatic cholestasis. An elevated indirect bilirubin suggests hemolysis; an elevated total bilirubin secondary to hemolysis alone seldom exceeds 5 mg/dL.

2. **Amylase.** Significant elevations in amylase (> 10 times the upper limits of normal) are suggestive of biliary disease.

3. **Prothrombin time (PT).** Increased PT that corrects with the administration of vitamin K suggests fat-soluble vitamin malabsorption, which can be seen in any condition in which bile quantities are reduced in the bowel lumen, such as intra- or extra-hepatic biliary obstruction. Response to vtiamin K is associated with preserved synthetic function of the liver.

4. **Hepatitis serology.** Hepatitis B surface antigen, hepatitis B IgM core antibody, hepatitis A IgM antibody, and hepatitis C antibody. (See Section II, Laboratory Diagnosis, Hepatitis Tests, pp 389–391.)

5. **Other tests.** Antinuclear (ANA), antimitochondrial, and anti–smooth muscle antibody tests may be helpful. The triad of antimitochondrial antibody, elevated alkaline phosphatase, and an elevated class M immunoglobulin is consistent with primary biliary cirrhosis. A high ANA, a high anti–smooth muscle antibody, or both are seen in autoimmune hepatitis. In a patient younger than 40, Wilson's disease should be considered. Iron overload should be considered; elevated ferritin and transferrin saturation are characteristic. α_1-Antitrypsin deficiency can also cause chronic liver disease in adults; phenotype testing and biopsy are useful.

C. **Radiologic and other studies**

1. **Ultrasound or computed tomography (CT).** Should be the first studies in patients with intermediate or low risk for extrahepatic biliary obstruction. Ultrasound and CT are good primarily for detecting dilated ducts, pancreatic masses, and stones in the gallbladder. Detection of stones in the common bile duct is uniformly poor with both of these tests.

2. **Endoscopic retrograde cholangiopancreatography (ERCP) and percutaneous transhepatic cholangiogram (PTC).** Tests of first choice for patients believed to have a high risk for extrahepatic obstruction. Selection of ERCP or PTC is based on local expertise and the clinical situation. ERCP is recommended in patients with ascites, coagulation abnormalities, a history of failed

percutaneous transhepatic cholangiography, a suspicion of sclerosing cholangitis, and a planned sphincterotomy. It is also the test of choice when carcinoma of the pancreas is suspected, because a biopsy can be done. Indications for PTC include patients with dilated ducts, previous gastric surgery with Billroth II anastomosis, a previous failed ERCP, or a mass involving the proximal bile duct.

3. **Liver biopsy.** Liver biopsy is often performed in the evaluation of viral hepatitis. It may occasionally reveal an unsuspected diagnosis such as metastatic tumor. Liver biopsy may also be used for prognostic purposes.

4. **Nuclear scan (HIDA).** This scan is generally not very useful in the diagnosis of jaundice, but it is very helpful if acute cholecystitis is suspected.

5. **Magnetic resonance cholangiopancreatography (MRCP).** MRCP offers a noninvasive alternative to ERCP for diagnostic purposes. A normal MRCP may eliminate the need to subject the patient to an invasive procedure. However, ERCP offers the benefit of being both diagnostic and theraputic in regard to biliary obstruction.

V. **Plan.** The tempo of diagnostic evaluation is dictated by the severity of the patient's illness. If acute cholangitis is suspected, the evaluation must proceed emergently. Patients with signs of liver failure, including significant coagulopathy-hepatic encephalopathy, acidosis, and renal failure, require management in an ICU. Early indentification of these patients and referral to a liver transplantation program emergently are key parts of appropriate care.

A. **Medical: hepatocellular cholestasis**
   1. **Viral hepatitis.** Patients who are dehydrated or vomiting or have significant coagulopathy need admission for treatment with IV fluids, vitamin K, and fresh-frozen plasma.
   2. **Alcoholic liver disease.** Requires aggressive supportive care, entailing dietary restriction of protein, full evaluation of any coagulopathy (see Section I, Chapter 12, Coagulopathy, V, p 73), and treatment of associated electrolyte deficiencies that are often encountered in alcoholics (eg, hypokalemia, hypomagnesemia, and hypophosphatemia). Thiamine, folate, and multivitamins may be needed. In a patient with ascites, a paracentesis should be performed (see Section III, Chapter 11, Paracentesis). With ascites, prophylactic antibiotics are recommended to prevent peritonitis if the total protein in the ascitic fluid is < 1 g/dL or if the patient had a previous episode of spontaneous bacterial peritonitis. Norfloxacin 400 mg per day; ciprofloxacin 750 mg per week; or trimethoprim-sulfamethoxazole DS, 1 pill per day, 5 days per week should be given indefinitely.

B. Surgical: extrahepatic cholestasis. Extrahepatic biliary obstruction can be conceptualized in two forms: chronic and acute.

1. Chronic extrahepatic cholestasis. Usually accompanied by biliary ductal dilation, which can be demonstrated by various techniques.

2. Acute biliary obstruction. Jaundice due to acute biliary obstruction, usually by a gallstone, can be more difficult to evaluate. Noninvasive imaging studies such as ultrasound or CT fail to reveal evidence of obstruction in 25–75% of such cases. The diagnosis of extrahepatic obstruction is frequently suggested by accompanying clinical features such as right upper quadrant pain, fever, sepsis, and the presence of cholelithiasis.

Although noninvasive tests are usually the first line of imaging, if clinical suspicion of acute extrahepatic biliary obstruction is high, proceeding with ERCP first may be appropriate. ERCP is both a diagnostic and therapeutic modality in this setting. If ERCP fails, percutaneous drainage of the biliary tract can be attempted.

C. Hemolysis. Treat underlying cause.

REFERENCES

Frank BB: Clinical evaluation of jaundice. JAMA 1989;262:3031.

Friedman LS, Emmett BK, eds. *Handbook of Liver Disease*. Churchill Livingstone;1998.

Kamath PS: Clinical approach to the patient with abnormal liver function tests. Mayo Clin Proc 1996;71:1089.

Lidofsky S: Jaundice. In: Feldman M, Friedman LS, Sleisenger MH, eds. *Gastrointestinal and Liver Diseases: Pathophysiology/Diagnosis/Management*. 7th ed. Saunders;2002:249.

Moseley RH: Evaluation of abnormal liver function tests. Med Clin North Am 1996;80:887.

Rösch T et al: A prospective comparison of the diagnostic accuracy of ERCP, MRCP, CT and EUS in biliary strictures. Gastrointest Endosc 2002;55:870.

47. JOINT SWELLING

I. Problem. A 35-year-old woman is admitted with right knee swelling and pain.

II. Immediate Questions

A. Is there a previous history of joint swelling? A history of multiple joint involvement suggests a cause resulting in polyarthritis rather than monarthritis. Remember that many diseases causing a polyarthritis can present initially as a monarthritis. The pattern of joint involvement may suggest the cause; for example, the first metatarsophalangeal (MTP) joint in gout or the distal interphalangeal (DIP) joint and proximal interphalangeal (PIP) in osteoanthritis. Joint involvement that is similar on both sides of the body (symmetric) is more common in rheumatoid arthritis and in systemic lupus erythematosus (SLE), whereas an asymmetric arthritis is more common in psoriatic arthritis and seronegative spondyloarthritis. In rheumatoid arthritis, the metacarpophalangeal (MCP) and PIP joints are commonly involved. The history of onset, such as acute, chronic, or migratory, may be helpful in diagnosis.

B. Is there a history of trauma? Trauma to the joint would lead the clinician to consider fracture, ligamentous tear, loose body, or dislocation. A sport and occupational history is essential.

C. Does the patient have any constitutional symptoms? Fever suggests septic arthritis, although infection must be considered in any case of monarticular arthritis even without fever. Patients with rheumatoid arthritis, SLE, adult Still's disease, and polyarticular gout can also present with fever. Malaise, fatigue, and weight loss suggest a systemic arthritis. Morning stiffness of significant duration (> 1 hour) suggests inflammatory arthritis.

D. Are there any other systemic symptoms? It is important to obtain a full rheumatic disease systems review. A photosensitive rash suggests SLE, whereas diarrhea may occur with inflammatory bowel disease (IBD) or enteropathic spondyloarthritis (reactive arthritis). A partial list of systemic symptoms would include rash, alopecia, Raynaud's phenomenon, oral or genital ulcers, urethritis or cervicitis, diarrhea, eye inflammation, sicca symptoms, weakness, and central nervous system (CNS) disturbances.

E. What is the patient's medical and family history? Inquire about recent febrile illnesses, tick bites, and other events, because the patient may not associate these symptoms with the onset of arthritis. A medication history may provide a clue to diagnosis (eg, hemarthrosis associated with warfarin therapy); or a positive family history may suggest arthritis associated with psoriasis, hemoglobinopathy, or coagulopathy. Travel to an endemic region may suggest Lyme disease.

III. Differential Diagnosis. Arthritis is classified as being either monarticular or polyarticular. Subclassification is often based on the joint fluid analysis (see Section IV). Remember that an arthritis that is generally polyarticular can present as a monarticular arthritis.

A. Monarticular arthritis

1. **Infection.** May be bacterial, viral, fungal, or tuberculous.
2. **Trauma.** Causes include loose foreign bodies, fracture, plant thorn synovitis, and internal derangement.
3. **Hemarthrosis.** Causes include hemoglobinopathy, coagulopathy, anticoagulation therapy, and pigmented villonodular synovitis.
4. **Tumors.** Consider osteogenic sarcoma, metastatic tumor, synovial osteochondromatosis, and paraneoplastic syndromes.
5. **Crystals.** Types of crystals associated with arthritis include those found in gout (first MTP involvement characteristic), pseudogout,

calcium oxalate, and hydroxyapatite crystals. Pseudogout may be hereditary or associated with hyperparathyroidism, hemochromatosis, hypothyroidism, hypomagnesemia, or hypophosphatasia.

6. **Noninflammatory diseases.** These include avascular necrosis, which is often associated with a history of trauma, steroid use, alcohol use, or sickle cell anemia; osteoarthritis; endocrine disorders; amyloid; osteochondritis dissecans; and neuropathy.

7. **Inflammatory–connective tissue diseases.** Rheumatoid arthritis or Reiter's syndrome. Any inflammatory arthritis can begin as a monarthritis.

B. **Polyarticular arthritis**

1. **Infection or associated with systemic infection**

   a. **Gonococcal infection.** Frequently associated with a migratory arthritis, tenosynovitis, and a pustular rash.

   b. **Lyme disease.** Associated with both an acute arthritis and a late chronic destructive arthritis.

   c. **Rheumatic fever.** Primarily lower-extremity large joints. In the adult, arthritis is rarely migratory.

   d. **AIDS.** Septic arthritis, Reiter's syndrome, and a lupus-like presentation with nondestructive polyarthritis, rash, pleuritis, and CNS symptoms all have been described.

   e. **Subacute bacterial endocarditis**

   f. **Chronic active hepatitis.** Chronic hepatitis B and C infections are associated with arthritis alone or with polyarteritis nodosa or mixed essential cryoglobulinemia.

2. **Crystals.** Examples are crystals found in gout and pseudogout, as well as hydroxyapatite crystals.

3. **Metabolic disorders.** Causes include hypothyroidism, acromegaly, hemochromatosis, ochronosis (alkaptonuria, associated degenerative arthritis sparing the small joints, pigmentation of the skin and sclera, and urine turning black with time or alkalinization), hemophilia, and hyperparathyroidism. Hyperparathyroidism and hemochromatosis are associated with pseudogout.

4. **Noninflammatory diseases**

   a. **Osteoarthritis.** Consider when DIP and carpal-metacarpal joints of hands are involved.

   b. **Intestinal bypass surgery.** Rare now with present surgical techniques.

5. **Inflammatory arthritis**

   a. **Seronegative spondyloarthropathies.** These can be defined as arthropathies characterized by sacroiliitis and/or spondylitis, asymmetric peripheral arthritis and enthesopathies (inflammation of sites of tendon insertions). This group includes ankylosing spondylitis, reactive arthritis (triggered by an enteric or urogenital infection), psoriatic arthritis, arthritis associated with inflammatory bowel disease and undifferentiated spondyloarthropathies.

b. **Psoriatic arthritis.** Can involve joints in both arms or legs, but the joints tend to be different on each side in contrast to rheumatoid arthritis, which involves the same joints on both sides of the body. Psoriatic arthritis, unlike rheumatoid arthritis, can affect the DIP joints.

c. **Juvenile rheumatoid arthritis (JRA).** Also called adult Still's disease. The features are high spiking fever once or twice a day, usually evening, arthralgias or arthritis, myalgias, and a salmon pink macular or maculopapular evanescent rash often occurring with fever.

d. **Rheumatoid arthritis.** A symmetric arthritis characteristically involves the MCP and PIP joints of the hands.

e. **SLE.** Resembles rheumatoid arthritis but is rarely an erosive arthritis.

f. **Scleroderma.** Significant joint swelling is uncommon.

g. **Polychondritis**

h. **Mixed connective tissue disease.** Defined by the finding of a positive antiribonuclear protein (anti-RNP) antibody. This disorder includes features of rheumatoid arthritis, scleroderma, polymyositis, and SLE.

i. **Sarcoidosis.** An acute migratory arthritis frequently associated with tenosynovitis and erythema nodosum, and a chronic pauciarticular form involving the knees and ankles.

j. **Vasculitis.** Leukocytoclastic vasculitis and larger vessel vasculitides such as Churg-Strauss syndrome, Wegener's granulomatosis, polyarteritis nodosa, and Behçet's syndrome can rarely present with arthritis.

k. **Parvovirus (B19).** Symmetric involvement of MCPs, PIPs, knees, wrists, and ankles with arthralgias or frank arthritis. Anti-B19 IgM may be elevated only 2 months after infection. Ten percent of adults may have prolonged symptoms.

l. **Paraneoplastic.** Usually presents as a monarthritis if due to metastatic disease to the joint. Polyarthritis has been associated with occult malignancy of breast and lung. Dermatomyositis can be associated with solid tumors and can be associated with arthritis.

m. **Polymyalgia rheumatica.** Presents with pain in muscles of shoulders, neck, and pelvic girdle. Peripheral arthritis or diffuse edema of the hands can occur.

IV. Database

A. **Physical examination key points.** Physical exam must be complete. Systemic disease must be ruled out as the cause of the arthritis; there can be no shortcuts.

1. **Skin.** A rash may indicate the cause of the joint swelling. For evidence of psoriasis, frequently overlooked areas include under the

hairline or rectum. Telangiectasia, nailfold infarcts, palmar erythema, and livedo reticularis suggest connective tissue disease or vasculitis. Nodules are seen in rheumatoid arthritis and gout, and painful nodules are seen with bacterial endocarditis. Bluish-black pigmentation suggests ochronosis.

2. **Eyes.** Retinal abnormalities (hemorrhages) may suggest an infectious cause such as subacute bacterial endocarditis. Scleral pigmentation may be seen with ochronosis.

3. **Mouth.** Oral and nasal ulcers point to SLE or Behçet's syndrome.

4. **Musculoskeletal system.** All major joints should be examined for range of motion, tenderness, deformity, and swelling. True swelling (arthritis) must be present rather than bone pain, muscle pain, or pain from bursitis, tendinitis, or torn ligaments or menisci.

B. **Laboratory data**

1. **Complete blood count with differential.** To rule out infection and to identify anemia or thrombocytopenia if a systemic arthritis is considered.

2. **Joint fluid analysis**

   a. Any initial presentation of arthritis should be evaluated with joint aspiration if possible. (See Section III, Chapter 3, Arthrocentesis [Diagnostic & Therapeutic], p 418.) Fluid should be sent for Gram's stain, as well as bacterial, acid-fast bacillus, and fungal cultures if indicated. Also obtain a crystal exam and cell count with differential. A white blood cell (WBC) count of 0–300 is normal, 300–2000 is noninflammatory, 2000–75,000 indicates an inflammatory process, and > 100,000 indicates septic arthritis; however, cell counts from a bacterial source may be as low as 5000 WBC/mL. A differential count with a predominance of neutrophils suggests septic arthritis, whereas lymphocytosis suggests leukemia or tuberculosis. These values are only guidelines, since there is considerable overlap in all these diseases.

   b. Gram's stain smears are positive in only 66% of subsequent culture-proven cases of septic arthritis. Therefore, a negative result does not exclude the possibility of infection. The monosodium urate crystals of gout are rod-shaped, negatively birefringent crystals (3–10 μm) seen within WBCs during active disease and often extend beyond the cell wall. The crystal is yellow when parallel with the slow ray of the compensator. Calcium pyrophosphate dihydrate (CPPD) crystals are rhomboid-shaped, positively birefringent crystals that are blue when parallel with the slow ray of the compensator. The crystal is usually contained within the WBC. Calcium hydroxyapatite crystals are small (< 1 μm), minimally birefringent, irregularly shaped cytoplasmic inclusions that appear under light microscopy as "shiny coins" when extracellular. Calcium hydroxyapatite crystals are more commonly associated with acute episodes of bursitis, tendinitis, or periarthritis seen in chronic renal failure patients or in older women with the progressive destructive arthritis of Milwaukee shoulder syndrome.

3. **Other cultures.** Cultures of urine and blood should be obtained if septic arthritis is considered. If gonorrhea is considered, obtain cervical/urethral, rectal, and pharyngeal specimens.

4. **Creatinine.** Often obtained because many drugs, especially non-steroidal anti-inflammatory drugs (NSAIDs), used in treatment are contraindicated if creatinine is elevated.

5. **Urinalysis.** Proteinuria, red blood cells, and casts may indicate a systemic cause such as SLE.

6. **Rheumatic disease workup.** If a collagen vascular disease is suspected, obtain a Westergren erythrocyte sedimentation rate (ESR), C-reactive protein (CRP), antinuclear antibodies (ANA), and rheumatoid factor (RF). Tests for anti–double-stranded DNA (anti-DSDNA), extractable nuclear antigens (anti-RNP, anti-Smith, anti-SSA(Ro), anti-SSB(La), complement (CH50, C3, C4), and cryoglobulin are usually not obtained initially. Measurement of hepatitis B and C serologies or antineutrophil cytoplasmic antibody (ANCA) may be considered if the history is suggestive. A positive C-ANCA is highly suggestive of Wegener's granulomatosis. HLA-B27 is rarely helpful.

C. **Radiologic and other studies.** Plain films of the involved joints are often helpful, especially if the arthritis is chronic. If normal, the films can serve as a baseline as the arthritis progresses. Films of the hands and feet are particularly helpful when rheumatoid arthritis is considered.

V. **Plan.** Treatment depends on the type of arthritis diagnosed. An individual discussion of each type is beyond the scope of this book.

A. **Drug therapy.** Ensure from the patient's history and laboratory tests that there are no contraindications to the medication chosen. The patient must be informed of side effects. The most commonly prescribed medications (NSAIDs) are contraindicated in patients with elevated creatinine, a history of hypersensitivity reaction to aspirin or NSAIDs, platelet abnormalities, and possibly peptic ulcer disease. In the elderly, one must be aware of the CNS side effects. The selective COX-2 inhibitors (rofecoxib [Vioxx] and celecoxib [Celebrex]) are less likely to cause gastrointestinal toxicity. The COX-2 inhibitors, however, have the same renal toxicity as other NSAIDs. Avoid using celecoxib in patients with an allergy to sulfa drugs.

B. **Supportive measures.** Depending on the diagnosis, heat or ice therapy, specific exercises, splinting, and physical therapy may be indicated.

C. **Septic arthritis**

1. Daily drainage of joint fluid is absolutely necessary. If the joint is not easily drained, open drainage may be necessary. Gram's stain helps to direct the initial choice of antibiotic pending cultures.
2. If gonococcal arthritis is suspected, ceftriaxone should be given. (See Section VII, p 490.)
3. In nongonococcal bacterial arthritis, gram-positive cocci on Gram's stain should be treated with a penicillinase-resistant penicillin or vancomycin if methicillin-resistant *Staphylococcus aureus* is prevalent or if *Staphylococcus epidermidis* is suspected. An aminoglycoside and an antipseudomonal penicillin or third-generation cephalosporin would be used for gram-negative bacilli. If the Gram's strain is negative in a compromised host, use broad-spectrum coverage for both gram-positive and gram-negative organisms.

REFERENCES

Baker DG, Schumacher HR: Acute monarthritis. N Engl J Med 1993;329:1013.
Klippel JH, ed: *Primer on the Rheumatic Diseases.* 12th ed. Arthritis Foundation;2001.

48. LEUKOCYTOSIS

I. **Problem.** A 63-year-old woman is admitted for hypoxemia, bilateral pulmonary infiltrates, and fever. Broad-spectrum intravenous (IV) antibiotics are begun after appropriate cultures are obtained. Her white blood cell (WBC) count remains about 25,000–30,000/µL.

II. **Immediate Questions**

A. **What is the patient's current clinical status?** Elevated WBC counts are often associated with infection; look for associated fever, rigors, hypotension, and tachycardia.

B. **Have any intervening clinically relevant episodes of physical stress occurred since admission?** Hypotension and other signs of shock can be associated with leukocytosis. The use of mechanical ventilation or resuscitative measures can stimulate leukocytosis.

C. **Is there a history suggestive of prior underlying systemic illness?** Weight loss, prior sustained fevers, night sweats, chronic cough or dyspnea, hemoptysis, myalgias, and bone pain all are suggestive of chronic illnesses such as mycobacterial or fungal infections, connective tissue diseases, or possibly a neoplastic disorder. A history of new symptoms argues against a chronic or subacute illness.

D. **Are there any prior complete blood counts with which to compare this leukocyte count?** Again, the presence or absence of prior leukocytosis aids in the evaluation. Sustained leukocytosis over weeks or months strongly implies a chronic or subacute process, whether it is an infection such as an abscess or tuberculosis (TB), or a neoplasm.

E. Is there evidence of infection that has not been addressed, such as intra-abdominal (abscess), genitourinary, or central nervous system infection? Pulmonary infiltrates may represent adult respiratory distress syndrome occurring as a reaction to underlying sepsis, such as from an abdominal infection. Acute infectious causes of leukocytosis must be excluded, since they are so readily treatable.

F. Is the patient on any medication such as granulocyte colony-stimulating factor (G-CSF), granulocyte-macrophage colony-stimulating factor (GM-CSF), or any other growth factors used to stimulate WBC production that are now commonly used in a variety of oncologic or hematologic conditions? Has the patient received one of these growth factors recently? In addition, other medications such as vasopressors and glucocorticoids can cause demargination and subsequent leukocytosis. Lithium also causes a benign reversible leukocytosis.

G. Does the patient have a history of an underlying hematologic disorder? Symptoms such as paresthesias, pruritus, cyanosis in response to changes in ambient temperature, and easy bruising or bleeding all are suggestive of a primary bone marrow pathology.

H. Does the patient have a history of abdominal trauma or surgery or, specifically, splenectomy? The postsplenectomy state is often associated with a baseline WBC count that is above normal. In addition, after splenectomy the patient has a greater risk for developing sepsis, especially from encapsulated organisms such as *Streptococcus pneumoniae* and *Haemophilus influenzae*.

III. Differential Diagnosis. There are numerous causes of leukocytosis. It is a normal response to many noxious emotional and physical stimuli. *Leukocytosis* is defined as a WBC count > 10,000/μL. A broad division of causes separates leukocytosis into acute and chronic.

A. Acute

1. **Bacterial infection.** Either localized or generalized (sepsis).
2. **Other infections.** Mycobacteria, fungi, certain viruses, rickettsiae, and even spirochetes.
3. **Trauma**
4. **Myocardial infarction (MI), pulmonary embolism/infarction, mesenteric ischemia/infarction, or peripheral vascular disease with ischemia**
5. **Vasculitis, antigen–antibody complexes, and complement activation**
6. **Physical stimuli.** Extremes of temperature, seizure activity, and intense pain are associated with increased WBC counts.
7. **Emotional stimuli.** Occasionally can trigger acute leukocytosis.
8. **Drugs.** Can often cause or contribute to leukocytosis, especially vasopressor agents, corticosteroids, lithium, G-CSF, and GM-CSF.

B. Chronic
   1. **Persistent infections.** Often the same infection that caused the acute leukocytosis.
   2. **Partially treated or occult infections.** Osteomyelitis, subacute bacterial endocarditis, and intra-abdominal abscess often present as chronic leukocytosis.
   3. **Mycobacterial or fungal infections.** These are notorious for promoting a sustained leukocytosis, often with little other clinical pathology at initial evaluation.
   4. **Chronic inflammatory states.** Rheumatic fever, connective tissue disease such as systemic lupus erythematosus (SLE), thyroiditis, myositis, drug reactions, and pancreatitis all can chronically elevate the WBC count.
   5. **Neoplastic processes.** Solid tumors and lymphoproliferative disorders can have an associated chronic leukocytosis.
   6. **Primary hematologic disorders.** These include myeloproliferative disorders (eg, polycythemia vera), myelodysplasia, leukemias, chronic hemolysis, and asplenic states.
   7. **Congenital disorders (including Down's syndrome).** May be associated in rare cases with chronic leukocytosis.
   8. **Drugs.** These are less common causes. Potential offending agents include glucocorticoids and lithium.
   9. **Overproduction of adrenocorticotropic hormone or thyroxine.** May cause chronic elevation of the baseline WBC count.

IV. Database
   A. Physical examination key points
   1. **Vital signs.** Be especially careful to check for fever or hypothermia, which suggests infection or sepsis. Fever can also indicate a neoplastic process, infarction of various tissues, or a connective tissue disorder. (See Section I, Chapter 22, Fever, p 133.) Hypotension may occur with sepsis.
   2. **General.** Look for evidence of acute distress or a chronic disease state (cachexia, digital clubbing, bitemporal wasting).
   3. **Lymph nodes.** Check for palpable lymph nodes and note their character. Soft and tender nodes are most consistent with an infectious cause. Rubbery and generalized nodes are most often seen with lymphoproliferative disorders such as lymphoma. Hard, fixed, and localized nodes suggest carcinoma.
   4. **Skin/mucosa.** Petechiae or ecchymoses suggest sepsis with disseminated intravascular coagulation, primary bone marrow pathology with altered platelet number or function, or a clotting disorder or vasculitis.
   5. **Lungs.** Inspiratory rales imply pneumonitis or pneumonia. Diminished breath sounds and dullness to percussion suggest a pleural effusion or empyema. A pleural rub may accompany infectious or

malignant processes or other conditions such as thromboembolism and SLE.

6. **Heart.** Tachycardia is consistent with acute stress. The presence of a new murmur, particularly with fever, is suggestive of bacterial endocarditis. Look for evidence of volume overload, sometimes triggered by an infection or occasionally associated with leukemias or myeloproliferative disorders.

7. **Abdomen.** Tenderness or rebound suggests an acute abdominal process such as perforation or infarction of a viscus.

8. **Genitourinary/gynecologic exam.** Flank, pelvic, or prostate tenderness is suggestive of acute infection.

9. **Neurologic exam.** Altered mental status, confusion, seizures, and focally abnormal deep tendon reflexes all can be seen in a variety of situations associated with leukocytosis, including meningitis (infectious or neoplastic), sepsis, leukemias, lymphomas, and solid malignancies.

B. **Laboratory data**

1. **Blood.** *Personally reviewing the peripheral blood smear is absolutely critical.* Look for a coexisting anemia, polycythemia, and abnormal platelet count. Leukocytosis with a "left shift," Döhle bodies, and toxic granulation suggests an acute infection, whereas a normal differential pattern implies a nonbacterial cause. A lymphocytosis points to a viral illness, lymphoma, or leukemia. An increase in monocytes is often seen with carcinoma or TB. Eosinophilia suggests connective tissue disease, possible drug reaction, or possible parasitic infection. Promyelocytes, myelocytes, or an increase in basophils is consistent with myeloproliferative disorders (leukemias most commonly), although severe infections, toxic insults, and inflammation can result in the release of early myeloid forms. (However, > 5% blasts are usually not seen except in leukemias.)

2. **Liver function tests.** Can be elevated in patients with acute hepatitis, sepsis, leukemia, lymphoma, or metastatic carcinoma.

3. **Electrolytes.** Acute infection (especially pneumonia) and chronic infection involving the lung (TB, *Legionella*) or central nervous system (tuberculous or fungal meningitis) can cause the syndrome of inappropriate antidiuretic hormone release, resulting in hyponatremia.

4. **Arterial blood gases.** A metabolic gap acidosis can accompany sepsis, leukemia, or solid tumors.

5. **Cultures.** Blood, urine, cerebrospinal fluid, sputum, and other cultures are vital to rule in or exclude an infectious cause.

C. **Radiologic and other studies**

1. **Chest x-ray.** Check chest x-ray for evidence of acute pneumonic process, mass lesion, or a mediastinal abnormality.

2. **CT scan.** Can be used to localize an abscess, to define the extent of any suspicious masses or adenopathy, and to determine the presence or extent of organomegaly.
3. **Tumor markers.** Tests like terminal deoxynucleotidal transferase, leukocyte alkaline phosphatase (LAP), and vitamin B_{12} level, as well as tests for monoclonal antibodies to carcinomas, can be quite useful. Frequently with a sustained leukocytosis, the LAP score can be one of the most useful initial lab tests to distinguish between an infectious/inflammatory cause and a myeloproliferative disorder. The LAP score is usually elevated in infectious processes, whereas it is classically low in chronic myelogenous leukemia and variable in the other myeloproliferative disorders. The LAP score is also elevated in polycythemia vera.
4. **Bone marrow aspiration and biopsy.** May be required to exclude a primary marrow disorder, metastatic tumor, or chronic infections. Cytogenic studies can be performed to look specifically for myelodysplasia and for myeloproliferative disorders such as leukemias or lymphomas. At times, this is the only way to differentiate between a reactive bone marrow and chronic myelogenous leukemia.

V. Plan. The cause of the increased WBC count, of course, guides therapy. When obvious acute stress (infection, trauma, and inflammation) is not present, chronic infections, inflammation, carcinoma, or primary marrow pathology must be considered. As mentioned, strict attention to history, clinical presentation, and physical examination together with personal review of the peripheral blood smear is absolutely vital for the initial evaluation of leukocytosis. The overlooked or inappropriately treated infection can be catastrophic. For specific treatment of the various causes of leukocytosis, refer to any general reference.

REFERENCES

Arnold SM, Patchell R, Lowy AM et al: Paraneoplastic syndrome. In: Devita VT, Hellman S, Rosenberg SA, eds. *Cancer: Principles and Practice of Oncology.* 6th ed. Lippincott Williams & Wilkins;2001:2511.
Curnutte JT, Coates TD: Leukocytosis and leukopenia. In: Hoffman R, Benz EJ, Shattil SJ et al, eds. *Hematology: Basic Principles and Practice.* 3rd ed. Churchill Livingstone;2000:720.
Dale DC: Neutropenia and neutrophilia. In: Beutler E, Lichtman MA, Coller BS et al, eds. *William's Hematology.* 6th ed. McGraw-Hill;2001:823.

49. LEUKOPENIA

I. Problem. A 39-year-old man with a history of schizophrenia is placed on clozapine. Two months later, he returns with complaints of fever and chills. He appears toxic, and his white blood cell (WBC) count is 1000/μL.

II. Immediate Questions

A. What is the absolute neutrophil count (ANC)? *Neutropenia* is defined as an absolute neutrophil count < 1500/L (ANC = % segmented and banded neutrophils × total WBC count divided by 100). At ANCs < 1000/L, the risk of infection begins to increase. Neutropenia can be mild (ANC 1000–1500), moderate (ANC 500–1000), or severe (ANC < 500). This definition of neutropenia holds true for people of most ages and ethnic groups with a few exceptions (see II.J).

B. Has the patient reported any fever, gastrointestinal complaints, or viral symptoms or any other signs of infection? Several viral (infectious hepatitis, mononucleosis, HIV) and bacterial (salmonella, bacillary dysentery) illnesses, and rickettsial infections have been associated with neutropenia. Neutropenic patients also are susceptible to infections that can be life-threatening if left untreated; therefore, neutropenia should be investigated by a thorough review of symptoms and physical examination.

C. What is the patient's occupation? Has the patient been exposed to any chemicals? Farmers and gardeners may be exposed to insecticides (DDT, lindane, chlordane) that can cause leukopenia. A painter, dry cleaner, or chemist may be exposed to benzene.

D. Has the patient received any antineoplastic drugs or radiation therapy? Myelosuppression is often an expected result of chemotherapy. Radiation is a direct myelosuppressant.

E. What are the patient's medications? Several commonly used drugs have been documented to cause neutropenia, including semisynthetic penicillins, phenothiazines, sulfonamides, phenytoin, cimetidine, clozapine, captopril, and ranitidine.

F. Has the patient noted any tea-colored urine? Paroxysmal nocturnal hemoglobinuria (PNH) and hepatitis may be associated with pancytopenias including aplastic anemia.

G. Does the patient have a history of alcohol abuse or any history of cirrhosis? Ethanol is a direct myelosuppressant and can cause leukopenia. Folate deficiency, which can occur in alcoholics, may also cause leukopenia. Hypersplenism and sequestration of WBCs as well as platelets is seen with cirrhosis.

H. Is there any psychiatric history or history of anorexia nervosa? Several medications (eg, phenothiazines) used in the treatment of psychiatric disorders can cause leukopenia. Anorexia nervosa and starvation can cause leukopenia; however, the mechanism is unknown.

I. Does the patient have rheumatoid arthritis? *Felty's syndrome* is the constellation of splenomegaly, neutropenia, and rheumatoid arthritis.

J. What is the patient's ethnic background? African Americans and Yemenite Jews may have a normal racial variant of leukopenia.

K. What is the patient's sexual and drug history? Patients with high-risk sexual behavior and intravenous (IV) drug users are at increased risk for HIV infection, which can cause leukopenia.

L. Has the patient experienced recurrent, cyclic fevers? Cyclic neutropenia is a rare form of neutropenia involving fluctuations of the neutrophil count at fairly regular 3-week intervals. The only clue may be unexplained recurrent fevers every 3 weeks.

III. Differential Diagnosis. The causes of neutropenia can be grouped into three broad categories: (1) *bone marrow failure* (defective neutrophil production or maturation); (2) accelerated neutrophil removal; and (3) neutrophil redistribution. This classification can be useful in directing the choice of laboratory studies and management. Most acquired causes of neutropenia are due to infection, drugs, or immune disorders.

A. Inadequate bone marrow production

1. **Acute leukemia.** About 25% of acute cases of leukemia present with pancytopenia.

2. **Myelodysplastic syndromes.** The bone marrow is normally hypercellular or normocellular, but the WBCs fail to reach the circulation.

3. **Megaloblastic syndromes.** Both vitamin B_{12} and folate deficiencies can result in neutropenia. There is increased intramedullary destruction of blood cells.

4. **Marrow infiltration**
   a. **Metastatic cancer**
   b. **Granulomatous diseases**

5. **Drugs.** Benzene, alkylating agents (melphalan), doxorubicin (Adriamycin), and antimetabolites (methotrexate).

6. **Radiation.** A direct marrow toxin.

7. **Aplastic anemia**

8. **Cyclic neutropenia**

9. **Racial or familial neutropenia**

10. **Infections.** In cases of infectious mononucleosis, 20–30% of patients have moderate neutropenia. Other viral infections (HIV, hepatitis A or B) and particularly overwhelming bacterial infections may have a direct myelosuppressive effect.

11. **Starvation/anorexia nervosa**

12. **PNH**

B. Accelerated removal/consumption

1. **Drug induced**
   a. **Immune.** Such as hydralazine (Apresoline), quinidine, quinine, cefoxitin (Mefoxin), and nafcillin.
   b. **Nonimmune.** Such as phenacetin, indomethacin (Indocin), phenytoin, chloramphenicol, cimetidine, ranitidine, and phenothiazines.

2. **Hemodialysis and cardiovascular bypass.** Exposure of blood to a dialysis coil of cellophane or nylon fiber appears to activate the complement pathway. This increases neutrophil adhesion, causing neutrophils to sequester in pulmonary capillaries.

3. **Felty's syndrome.** Neutropenia associated with seropositive rheumatoid arthritis and splenomegaly suggests this diagnosis.

4. **Infection.** At times, the peripheral requirements for neutrophils during overwhelming sepsis can exhaust the marrow reserves. This is particularly true in the debilitated patient, such as a patient with chronic alcohol abuse.

C. **Redistribution of neutrophils**

1. **Enhanced neutrophil margination.** Endotoxemia in gram-negative sepsis can give rise to rapid margination of neutrophils to the tissue.

2. **Hypersplenism.** Refers to the clinical situation in which, in the presence of splenomegaly and a relatively normal bone marrow, there is a decrease of one or more cell lines in the peripheral blood because of sequestration in the spleen.

IV. **Database**

A. **Physical examination key points**

1. **Vital signs.** Fever suggests infection. Hypotension may be a sign of sepsis.

2. **Skin.** Petechiae are consistent with Rocky Mountain spotted fever or disseminated intravascular coagulation. Rash may be seen in connective tissue diseases or with certain bacterial infections such as *Neisseria gonorrhoeae* and *N meningitidis*.

3. **HEENT.** Temporal wasting and oral thrush may occur in acquired immunodeficiency syndrome (AIDS). Nuchal rigidity suggests meningitis.

4. **Lymph nodes.** Lymphadenopathy can be seen in both malignant and infectious processes, including HIV infection.

5. **Lungs.** Pneumonia with overwhelming sepsis may cause or be secondary to neutropenia. Inspiratory crackles, increased tactile and vocal fremitus, and egophony suggest pneumonia.

6. **Abdomen.** Hepatosplenomegaly can be a sign of malignancy (leukemia or lymphoma), infection, or hypersplenism.

7. **Joints.** Look for classic findings of rheumatoid arthritis, such as symmetric swelling of the proximal interphalangeal and metacarpophalangeal joints. Rheumatoid nodules on the extensor surface of the arms near the elbows are also a classic sign.

B. **Laboratory data**

1. **Complete blood count with differential.** The presence of anemia and thrombocytopenia along with leukopenia may suggest B_{12} or folate deficiency, aplastic anemia, PNH, ethanol abuse, or leukemia. The mean corpuscular volume is increased with B_{12} or folate deficiency.

2. **Blood and urine cultures.** Obtain if an infectious process is suspected.

3. **Liver function test and hepatitis serologies.** Obtain if hepatitis is suspected. Also, an elevated lactate dehydrogenase level may suggest B_{12} deficiency or lymphoma.

4. **Peripheral blood smear.** Dysplastic, degranulated neutrophils with pseudo–Pelger-Huët anomaly (a bilobed neutrophil) may suggest a myelodysplastic syndrome. Toxic granulation and Döhle bodies suggest infection. Neutrophils with five and six lobes point toward vitamin B_{12} or folate deficiency. Blasts are suggestive of leukemia.

5. **Leukocyte alkaline phosphatase (LAP) score.** Increased in certain infectious and inflammatory diseases and polycythemia vera. In contrast, the LAP score is decreased in chronic myelogenous leukemia.

6. **Rheumatoid factor and antinuclear antibodies (ANA).** Obtain ANA values if collagen vascular disease is suspected.

7. **Carotene (serum).** Elevated in anorexia nervosa and decreased in starvation.

8. **Vitamin B_{12} and folate levels.** To rule out megaloblastic anemia.

9. **Ham test/flow cytometry.** Although historically the Ham test has been the "gold standard" for the diagnosis of PNH, flow cytometry of erythrocytes using anti-CD59 or granulocytes using anti-CD55 and/or anti-CD59 antibodies has replaced this older technique once used for diagnosis. The underlying defect in PNH is a mutation in the *PIG-A* gene, an X-linked gene that has a role in the formation of the phosphatidylinositol anchor that attaches many different proteins to the surface of blood cells. In PNH, CD55, and CD59 are examples of surface proteins that are typically absent owing to the absence of the phosphatidylinositol anchor on the surface of the blood cells.

C. **Radiologic and other studies**

1. **Chest x-ray.** To rule out pneumonia if suspected.

2. **Sinus films, dental Panorex.** As indicated when looking for source of fever in a neutropenic patient.

3. **Lumbar puncture.** Indicated when meningitis (acute or chronic) is suspected.

4. **Bone marrow biopsy and aspiration.** This procedure can provide critical information about granulocyte aplasia, hypoplasia or dysplasia, infiltration of marrow, cellularity, and cellular maturation. A bone marrow biopsy and aspiration can be essential in diagnosing the cause of neutropenia. See Section III, Chapter 5, Bone Marrow Aspiration & Biopsy, p 423.

V. **Plan.** The major consequence of neutropenia is vulnerability to infection. The usual clinical manifestations of infection are often absent because of the lack of granulocytes (neutrophils). Thus, pneumonia may be present without a significant infiltrate on chest x-ray; meningitis may occur without pleocytosis or meningeal signs; and pyelonephritis may be present without pyuria. A heightened awareness for infection is extremely important in the neutropenic patient, because an untreated infection can be fatal. The specific clinical management of a neutropenic patient depends on the cause, duration, and degree of neutropenia as well as other comorbid medical conditions. An elderly myelodysplastic patient with bone marrow failure who has an ANC < 500 and high fever and also has diabetes is more seriously ill and has a higher risk of developing infectious complications than a young otherwise healthy woman who is postchemotherapy for breast cancer with nadir counts ANC of 1000 and low-grade temperature.

A. Emergent management

1. **Evidence of infection or fever with an ANC < 500/μL.** The patient should immediately be pancultured (body fluid cultures as indicated, such as blood and urine, etc), and broad-spectrum antibiotics should be initiated. The specific pathogens found are almost always pyogenic or enteric bacteria or certain fungi. These are usually endogenous to the patient and include staphylococci from skin and gram-negative organisms from the gastrointestinal tract or urinary tract. In febrile neutropenic patients who were bacteremic, one study found that 46% of the isolated organisms were gram-positive (as high as 60–70% in one reference); 42% were gram-negative; and 12% were polymicrobial. Antibiotics should therefore provide broad-spectrum coverage and include such choices as (a broad-spectrum semisynthetic penicillin or cephalosporin, such as cefepime, ceftazidime, imipenem, cefepime, or meropenem); or two drugs—an aminoglycoside (amikacin, gentamicin, or tobramycin) plus an antipseudomonal beta-lactam (cefepime, ceftazidime, piperacillin, ticarcillin, or ticarcillin plus clavulanate). An aminoglycoside may be added to a one-drug regimen, depending on how toxic the patient appears. Vancomycin should be added if the patient is at high risk (high risk is defined by the Infectious Disease Society of America as having catheter-related infection, significant mucosal damage from chemotherapy, use of previous prophylactic quinolone antibiotics, septic shock or cardiovascular compromise, colonization with penicillin- or cephalosporin-resistant *Streptococcus pneumoniae* or with methicillin-resistant *Staphylococcus aureus,* and positive blood cultures for gram-positive bacteria before determination of antibiotic susceptibility). The patient's response to antibiotics should be reevaluated every 48–72 hours. An antifungal agent should be considered on days 5–7 if the ANC remains < 500/mm^3 and the patient remains febrile despite antibiotics. Neutropenia with infection is a medical emergency requiring immediate investigation and treatment.

2. **Patients with ANC > 1000 may be considered for management with outpatient antibiotics.** This decision depends also on

the cause and duration of the neutropenia and any other ongoing medical problems.

3. **Identify any potential drugs or chemicals that may have induced the neutropenia; discontinue them.**

4. **Always wash your hands before touching the patient.** The patient should avoid exposure to fresh fruits or vegetables, flowers, live plants, and persons with active infections. Avoid rectal manipulation such as with digital examination or rectal temperature.

B. **Definitive care.** After the patient has had a complete history and physical exam, the cause of the neutropenia can usually be placed in one of the three broad categories discussed earlier (see III). Subsequent tests can be obtained to confirm a specific diagnosis. In general, regardless of the cause, supportive care is indicated for most of these patients (ie, antibiotics for infections and blood products for associated severe anemia or thrombocytopenia).

1. **Bone marrow failure.** For drug-induced neutropenia, remove the offending agent and give supportive care until the counts increase to normal or at least above the neutropenic range (generally within 1–2 weeks). Colony-stimulating factors (CSFs) are now available that can be used for drug-induced (ie, by chemotherapy) neutropenia to speed recovery. Specific guidelines have been established by the American Society of Clinical Oncology for the use of CSFs in cancer patients receiving chemotherapy for primary and secondary prophylaxis. In general, the CSFs are used as primary prevention with chemotherapeutic regimens that are significantly myelosuppressive to help decrease the incidence of febrile neutropenia. The CSFs are started approximately 24–72 hours after completion of the chemotherapy and are given until the ANC is > 10,000 following the neutrophil nadir. For use in the febrile patient with neutropenia, the CSFs may be used if the patient has clinical features of deterioration, profound neutropenia (ANC < 100), pneumonia, sepsis, hypotension, or a fungal infection. They are usually continued until ANC is > 10,000. The usual dosage is 5 µg/kg/day for G-CSF (filgrastim) and 250 µg/m^2/day for GM-CSF (sargramostim). The treatment for viral etiology or myelodysplastic syndromes is generally supportive care. The use of CSFs can be considered in myelodysplastic patients if patients are experiencing neutropenic infections.

2. **Consumption.** Treat bacterial infections as indicated. Immune-mediated consumption may require steroids. The patient with Felty's syndrome generally requires no specific treatment for the neutropenia unless he or she has recurrent infections. Then, splenectomy may be required.

3. **Redistribution.** Patients with hypersplenism are generally able to immobilize the sequestered neutrophils and thus fight off infection; subsequently, they do not require any specific therapy.

REFERENCES

American Society of Clinical Oncology: 2000 Update of recommendations for the use of hematopoietic colony-stimulating factors: Evidence-based, clinical practice guidelines. J Clin Oncol 2000;18;3558.

Baehner R. Overview of neutropenia. In: UpToDate, Rose, BD, ed. UpToDate. Wellesley, MA;2004.

Bodey GP, Buckley M, Sathe YS et al: Quantitative relationships between circulating leukocytes and infection in patients with acute leukemia. Ann Intern Med 1966;64:328.

Elting LS, Rubenstein EB, Rolston KV et al: Outcomes of bacteremia in patients with cancer and neutropenia: Observations from two decades of epidemiological and clinical trials. Clin Infect Dis 1997;25:247.

Hughes WT, Armstrong D, Bodey GP et al: 1997 Guidelines for the use of antimicrobial agents in neutropenic patients and unexplained fever. Clin Infect Dis 1997;25:551.

Shoenfeld Y, Alkan ML, Asaly A et al. Benign familial leukopenia and neutropenia in different ethnic groups. Eur J Haematol 1988;41:273.

50. NAUSEA & VOMITING

I. **Problem.** A 39-year-old man is admitted with diffuse abdominal pain and fever. Later that evening he has severe nausea and vomiting.

II. **Immediate Questions.** When you are evaluating nausea and vomiting, a careful history and a complete physical exam are important to rule out serious causes requiring prompt intervention, such as peritonitis and intracranial lesions.

A. **What are the patient's vital signs?** Fever suggests an inflammatory process such as gastroenteritis, peritonitis, or cholecystitis. Hypotension may be secondary to volume depletion or associated sepsis. Hypertension and bradycardia may reflect increased intracranial pressure.

B. **When do the nausea and vomiting occur? Are they related to meals?** Vomiting during or soon after a meal suggests psychogenic causes or may be seen with pyloric channel ulcer, pancreatitis, or biliary tract disease. If abdominal pain is relieved with vomiting, an ulcer is more likely. Vomiting an hour or more after a meal is more characteristic of pancreatitis or motility disorders, such as diabetic gastroparesis and postvagotomy. Nausea and vomiting early in the morning on arising are often associated with alcoholism, pregnancy, uremia, and increased intracranial pressure.

C. **What are the appearance and volume of the vomitus?** Large amounts of vomitus or secretions usually indicate partial or complete bowel obstruction, gastric atony, or, in rare cases, Zollinger-Ellison syndrome.

Technically, vomiting refers to forcible ejection of food from the stomach and, although it is commonly referred to as "vomiting," regurgitation of unacidified food implies esophageal abnormalties such as achalasia or diverticula.

The presence of bile indicates a patent pyloric channel. A fecal smell suggests lower intestinal obstruction. Occasionally, this can be seen with bacterial overgrowth in the proximal small intestine or a fistula. Blood or coffee-ground–appearing material points to an upper gastrointestinal (GI) bleed. Vomiting can also induce hematemesis secondary to a Mallory-Weiss tear. (See Section I, Chapter 27, Hematemesis, Melena, p 166.)

D. Does the patient consume alcohol? Does the patient take any non-steroidal anti-inflammatory drugs (NSAIDs)? Pancreatitis or acute gastritis can be caused by ethanol and result in nausea and vomiting. An NSAID such as ibuprofen (Motrin) may induce gastritis or ulcers.

E. Is there associated abdominal pain? This can be seen with most abdominal causes of nausea and vomiting. Knowing the location of the abdominal pain helps in determining the cause of the nausea and vomiting. (See Section I, Chapter 1, Abdominal Pain, p 1.)

III. Differential Diagnosis. Disorders that are associated with nausea and vomiting can be grouped as follows:

A. Intra-abdominal or thoracic etiology

1. **Gastric outlet obstruction.** Occurs in patients with a history of peptic ulcer disease (PUD), prior abdominal surgery, or neoplasms.

2. **Small or large bowel obstruction.** May be caused by fibrous bands and adhesions (usually after surgery), primary or secondary metastatic neoplasms, impacted feces, active inflammatory bowel disease (IBD)–related stricture, postoperative strictures, intestinal parasites, gallstones, incarcerated hernia, intussusception, or a volvulus.

3. **Pseudo-obstruction or functional (paralytic) ileus.** Results from failure of normal intestinal peristalsis. Causes include abdominal surgery; retroperitoneal or intra-abdominal hematomas; severe infections; renal disease; metabolic disturbances such as hypokalemia; or drugs, particularly anticholinergics. Chronic cases of pseudo-obstruction can result from abnormalities in either the enteric nervous system or the gut smooth muscle.

4. **PUD.** Local irritation or edema surrounding a pyloric channel ulcer can cause a mechanical obstruction.

5. **Pancreatitis.** Usually associated with abdominal pain that frequently (in > 50% of cases) radiates to the back. A computed tomography (CT) scan is helpful in demonstrating inflammation and pseudocyst formation. Retroperitoneal abscess formation can complicate pancreatitis.

6. **Biliary colic.** From distention of smooth muscle in bile ducts secondary to stones, inflammation, or neoplasms.

7. **Intestinal ischemia.** From local vascular compromise or from reduced cardiac output. Guaiac-positive stools are common findings.

8. **Pyelonephritis or nephrolithiasis**
9. **Hepatitis.** May be either viral or drug-induced.
10. **Appendicitis.** Often associated with right lower quadrant pain, fever, and leukocytosis with a left shift.
11. **Diverticulitis.** Lower abdominal pain and fever are common.
12. **Perforated viscus.** Usually presents as an acute abdomen.
13. **Pelvic inflammatory disease (PID)**
14. **Acute myocardial infarction (MI).** MI, especially involving the inferior wall, can present with nausea and vomiting; chest pain may be absent.

B. **Intracranial etiology**
1. **Tumor or mass lesions leading to increased intracranial pressure.** Consider an acute cerebral vascular accident, neoplasm, or subdural hematoma.
2. **Bacterial and viral meningitis**
3. **Migraine headache.** Usually a unilateral headache, with photophobia and history of similar headache. The affected patient may have a prodrome (eg, aura).
4. **Labyrinthitis**

C. **Metabolic etiology**
1. **Uremia.** Often associated with weight loss, lethargy, and intense pruritus.
2. **Hepatic failure.** From a variety of causes including cirrhosis, hypoxic injury, and drug-induced states such as acetaminophen overdose.
3. **Adrenal insufficiency.** Can occur in patients on chronic corticosteroid therapy that is suddenly discontinued or in such patients when stressed (surgery, serious infection) and the steroid dose is not increased. Associated symptoms include weakness, fatigue, hypotension, and abdominal pain.
4. **Metabolic acidosis.** See Section I, Chapter 2, Acidosis, p 10.
5. **Electrolyte abnormalities.** Hypercalcemia, hyperkalemia, and hypokalemia can cause nausea.
6. **Hypothyroidism with decreased intestinal motility or thyroid storm.** Weight gain, constipation, mental status changes, and dry skin suggest hypothyroidism. Weight loss, hyperdefecation, moist skin, hyperthermia, and mental status changes as well as a precipitating event are consistent with thyroid storm.

D. **Miscellaneous etiology**
1. **Drug-induced.** Major offenders are dopamine agonists such as L-dopa and bromocriptine (Parlodel), opiate analgesics such as morphine, digoxin (Lanoxin), and certain chemotherapy agents such as cisplatin (Platinol). Also consider alcohol, NSAIDs, and aspirin.
2. **Acute gastroenteritis.** Common in the outpatient setting with "food poisoning" from bacterial endotoxins. Diarrhea is often present. (See Section I, Chapter 17, Diarrhea, p 101.)

3. **Pregnancy.** Especially during the first trimester.
4. **Toxins**
5. **Psychogenic**
6. **Post–general anesthesia**
7. **Rumination.** Although distinct from vomiting, it is useful to consider rumination in the differential diagnosis. The term refers to involuntary, effortless, painless regurgitation of food into the mouth with subsequent re-chewing and re-swallowing. This may be pleasurable for the patient. The cause is unknown.

IV. Database

A. Physical examination key points

1. **Vital signs.** Hypotension may result from volume depletion or sepsis. Orthostatic blood pressure changes suggest volume depletion. An orthostatic decrease in blood pressure without an increase in heart rate suggests autonomic neuropathy, which may accompany diabetes with gastroparesis. Fever points to an inflammatory component, possibly infection. Tachycardia can result from associated pain.
2. **HEENT.** Look for signs of head trauma that would indicate an intracranial process. Scleral icterus suggests hepatic failure/hepatitis. Papilledema is consistent with an intracranial process or a hypertensive emergency. An enlarged thyroid gland occurs with hypothyroidism or hyperthyroidism.
3. **Skin.** Check the patient's skin turgor and mucous membranes to estimate volume status. Check for jaundice. Hyperpigmentation may be caused by adrenal insufficiency (*Addison's disease*).
4. **Chest.** Inspiratory crackles secondary to atelectasis can be associated with any intra-abdominal process limiting deep inspiration because of pain. Crackles may also suggest left ventricular dysfunction associated with MI.
5. **Abdomen.** See Section I, Chapter 1, Abdominal Pain, p 1.
6. **Rectum.** Check for fecal impaction, rectal masses, and occult blood. Tenderness on the right side is consistent with appendicitis. Blood can be secondary to diverticulitis, IBD, PUD, and gastritis; or it may result from vomiting (Mallory-Weiss tear).
7. **Female genitalia.** Examine for pain with cervical motion and cervical discharge that may suggest PID.
8. **Neurologic exam**
   a. Mental status changes may signify central nervous system (CNS) lesions, encephalopathy, sepsis or severe infection, or significant electrolyte disturbances.
   b. Focal neurologic findings such as weakness, unilateral hyperreflexia, or a positive Babinski's sign on one side suggest an intracranial process.
   c. Pain with flexion of the neck is consistent with meningeal inflammation secondary to either a subarachnoid bleed or

meningitis. A positive *Kernig's sign* also indicates meningeal irritation; it is obtained by flexing the patient's hip and knee to a 90-degree angle. Attempts to extend the leg at the knee will result in posterior thigh pain and resistance to movement.

B. Laboratory data

1. **Electrolytes.** Severe vomiting may lead to various electrolyte disturbances, such as hypokalemia, hypochloremia, and metabolic alkalosis.

2. **Complete blood count with differential.** A leukocytosis with an increase in banded neutrophils suggests an infection. An elevated hematocrit can be associated with volume depletion. Anemia suggests chronic GI blood loss or massive acute bleeding.

3. **Blood urea nitrogen and creatinine.** To determine whether uremia is present and to provide prognostic information in acute pancreatitis.

4. **Urinalysis.** Look for white blood cells and casts suggesting pyelonephritis. Red blood cells, especially with flank pain, may indicate nephrolithiasis.

5. **Liver function tests, transaminases (AST and ALT), total bilirubin, and alkaline phosphatase.** To rule out acute hepatitis and biliary tract obstruction.

6. **Amylase and lipase.** If pancreatitis is suspected.

7. **Arterial blood gases.** Needed to evaluate the presence of an acid–base disturbance as a cause or consequence of vomiting. Vomiting associated with an acid–base disturbance is almost always related to a serious underlying problem.

8. **Serum intact human chorionic gonadotropin (HCG) serum.** Pregnancy must always be ruled out in a woman of reproductive age. Strongly consider even in patients unlikely to be pregnant (eg, in perimenopausal patient or after tubal ligation) if no obvious source of nausea and vomiting is noted on noninvasive workup.

C. Radiologic and other studies

1. **Acute abdominal series (KUB).** Air–fluid levels are seen in obstruction; free air under the diaphragm indicates perforation. If the patient may be pregnant, defer KUB until the result of the HCG test is known.

2. **Electrocardiogram.** Helpful in evaluating for acute MI. ST-segment depression or elevation, T-wave inversion, or Q waves suggest myocardial ischemia or infarction. An electrocardiogram should be done early in evaluating an acute abdomen with vomiting.

3. **Barium studies:** Provide better structural information than plain radiography. They also provide information on GI motility and therefore are a useful adjunct to endoscopy.

4. **Endoscopy.** Important in the diagnosis of PUD or esophageal diverticula.

5. **Gastric emptying scan.** Useful in suspected gastroparesis, especially in patients with longstanding diabetes who have nausea and vomiting.
6. **CT abdomen and pelvis:** Especially useful in the evaluation of the solid organs including pancreas, liver, and kidneys.
7. **Abdominal ultrasound or HIDA scan.** These may aid in the diagnosis of cholecystitis, biliary duct obstruction, and abscesses. Biliary colic cannot be ruled out with a normal ultrasound.

V. Plan. Treatment of the underlying cause is essential in the management of nausea and vomiting. A nasogastric tube should be used for decompression if obstruction is present. Separate treatment of each cause is beyond the scope of this section. Commonly used medications are listed here.

A. Phenothiazines. Most commonly used antiemetics. Their principal mode of action is via depression of CNS dopamine receptors. Prochlorperazine (Compazine) 10 mg PO Q 4–6 hr or 25 mg PR; chlorpromazine (Thorazine) 25 mg PO Q 8 hr, and promethazine (Phenergan) 12.5–25 mg PO, PR, or IM Q 6–12 hr prn are effective agents. Extrapyramidal side effects can be treated with benztropine (Cogentin) 2 mg IV or diphenhydramine (Benadryl) 25 mg IV or IM Q 4–6 hr.

B. Butyrophenones. These agents also block CNS dopamine receptors. Give haloperidol (Haldol) 2 mg PO or IM Q 4–6 hr; or droperidol (Inapsine) 2–5 mg IV or IM Q 4–6 hr. Because droperidol has been associated with QT prolongation, care should be exercised with the use of this medication.

C. Miscellaneous drugs
1. **Ondansetron (Zofran).** A selective 5-HT_3-receptor antagonist, it is very effective prophylaxis for chemotherapy-induced and postoperative nausea and vomiting. The recommended adult oral dose is 8 mg (10 mL of oral solution) bid. 5-HT_3 receptor antagonists are not effective in treating nausea and vomiting once such symptoms occur.
2. **Metoclopramide (Reglan), high-dose.** At a dose of 1–2 mg/kg Q 4–6 hr, this constitutes a useful and very effective adjunct with cancer chemotherapy to prevent nausea and vomiting. It is effective for both prevention and treatment.
3. **Benztropine 2 mg PO or IV or diphenhydramine 25–50 mg PO or IM.** Should be given prophylactically to prevent extrapyramidal reactions with high doses of metoclopramide.

REFERENCE

Makau L: Nausea and vomiting. In: Feldman M, Friedman LS, Sleisenger MH, eds. *Gastrointestinal and Liver Diseases: Pathophysiology/Diagnosis/Management.* 7th ed. Saunders;2002:119.

51. OLIGURIA/ANURIA

I. **Problem.** You are called because a 68-year-old man admitted with pyelonephritis and diabetes mellitus type 2 has had only 100 mL of urine output over the last 8 hours.

II. **Immediate Questions.** A medical history and review of the patient's chart and hospital course are essential in evaluating and treating oliguria.

A. **Are there any serious or life-threatening conditions?** Oliguria may be associated with shock, hypotension, pulmonary edema, uremia, hyperkalemia, uncompensated metabolic acidosis, other electrolyte disorders, or the accullation of toxic levels of medications and/or metabolites.

B. **Is the patient in distress? Does he appear ill? Is he hemodynamically stable?** Oliguria may be an early manifestation of impending shock.

C. **What are the patient's serum chemistries and blood urea nitrogen (BUN) and creatinine levels?** Review the patient's lab results in the chart. What is the patient's baseline serum creatinine? Has the creatinine changed during hospitalization? An elevated creatinine suggests different causes compared with a normal or only slightly elevated creatinine, especially with an elevated BUN:creatinine ratio. Because of the reciprocal nature of serum creatinine in the estimate of glomerular filtration rate (GFR), small changes in low values of serum creatinine reflect a large loss of renal function. For example, if a patient with a baseline creatinine of 0.6 mg/dL develops a creatinine level of 1.2 mg, he or she has lost half of the renal function.

Other factors besides a decreased GFR may contribute to an elevated creatinine. Accelerated muscle breakdown as is seen in rhabdomyolysis increases creatinine production. At lower levels of GFR, the proportion of creatinine cleared by tubular secretion increases. Certain medications that compete for creatinine for tubular secretion such as cimetidine and trimethoprim raise serum creatinine without affecting GFR. An elevated BUN:creatinine ratio is seen in patients in the prerenal state and in those with increased catabolism, increased protein intake such as total parenteral nutrition, and gastrointestinal (GI) bleeding, and with the administration of glucocorticoids.

D. **What is the cause of the oliguria?** Prompt identification of the underlying cause or causes is essential to prevent or attenuate renal injury.

E. **What is the urine output?** *Oliguria* is defined as a 24-hour urine output of 100–400 mL. As a general rule, the minimal acceptable urine output is 0.5–1.0 mL/kg/hr. *Anuria,* less than 100 mL/day of urine, may indicate complete urinary obstruction, a catastrophic renal vascular event, bilateral cortical necrosis, severe rapidly progressive glomerulonephritis, or severe allergic interstitial nephritis (AIN; or acute interstitial nephritis), as may be seen with patients taking rifampin. A urine pattern of fluctuating decreased and increased urine output may indicate intermittent obstruction.

F. Are there any underlying diseases that could result in oliguria or renal failure? Congestive heart failure (CHF), cirrhosis, nephrotic syndrome, and "third spacing" of fluid (eg, pancreatitis) may decrease renal perfusion. Autoimmune disorders may affect the kidneys. Infections may cause renal failure through direct extension as well as through immune mechanisms. Diabetics, the elderly, and patients with preexisting renal insufficiency are at increased risk for acute renal failure (ARF).

G. Does the patient have any symptoms or predisposing conditions that suggest hypovolemia? Hypovolemia is a common cause of oliguria. Early diagnosis and prompt treatment are essential. Prolonged prerenal causes of oliguria may result in ischemic acute tubular necrosis (ATN). Diarrhea, vomiting, GI bleeding, high fever, and low oral intake are examples. Positional dizziness suggests hypovolemia.

H. Does the patient have a history of symptoms that suggest bladder outlet obstruction from prostatic hypertrophy? Has the patient recently had a Foley catheter? A history of hesitancy, difficulty initiating urination, and dribbling suggests prostatic hypertrophy.

I. Has the patient been exposed to any potentially nephrotoxic agents? Aminoglycosides, amphotericin B, radiocontrast agents, and certain chemotherapeutic agents may cause ATN. Cyclosporine, tacrolimus, angiotensin-converting enzyme inhibitors, and nonsteroidal anti-inflammatory drugs (NSAIDs) may cause renal vasoconstriction. Intratubular obstruction from deposition of crystals from acyclovir, sulfonamides, and methotrexate may occur. Several medications have been associated with AIN.

J. Is there a history of hematuria? Rapidly progressive glomerulonephritis may be associated with hematuria. Hematuria is a common sign of nephrolithiasis and bladder or renal cell carcinoma.

K. Is there any history of prolonged hypotension? This may lead to ischemic ATN.

L. Is there any history of abdominal, suprapubic, or flank pain? Suggests nephrolithiasis, urinary tract obstruction, infection, or a renal vascular event.

M. During the initial assessment, do the medications, IV fluids, and dietary orders need to be adjusted? Renally cleared medications may need to have the dose or dosing interval adjusted. Potassium may need to be removed from IV fluids.

N. Are any diagnostic procedures planned that involve radiocontrast agents? Radiocontrast dye will likely add further injury to the kidneys.

III. **Differential Diagnosis.** The differential diagnosis for acute oliguria and acute renal failure is identical and may be divided into prerenal, renal, and postrenal causes. Keep in mind that multiple causes may frequently contribute to the development of ARF.

   A. **Prerenal causes.** Relating to renal hypoperfusion. Prompt recognition and correction of prerenal azotemia are important in that renal hypoperfusion may lead to ischemic ATN. Prerenal ARF and ischemic ATN together account for about 75% of cases of ARF in hospitalized patients.
      1. **Shock/hypovolemia**
         a. **Hemorrhage.** From GI bleeding or trauma, or as a postoperative complication.
         b. **Inadequate fluid administration.** Fever, diarrhea, vomiting, poor oral intake without adequate fluid administration.
         c. **Sepsis.** Causes decreased renal perfusion from a decreased systemic vascular resistance.
      2. **Apparent intravascular hypovolemia.** A relative decrease in the effective circulating volume.
         a. **Third-space losses.** Pancreatitis, major burns, and after major operations.
         b. **CHF**
         c. **Cirrhosis.** Hepatorenal syndrome may be associated.
         d. **Nephrotic syndrome**
      3. **Vascular**
         a. **Renal artery occlusion (acute or chronic)**
         b. **Aortic dissection**
         c. **Emboli (such as cholesterol)**
   B. **Renal causes**
      1. **Acute tubular necrosis**
         a. **Ischemia.** Secondary to shock from any cause, including sepsis.
         b. **Toxins.** These may include medications (aminoglycosides, amphotericin B), contrast media, and heavy metals.
         c. **Transfusion reaction.** Causes intravascular hemolysis.
         d. **Myoglobinuria.** Secondary to rhabdomyolysis; often seen in alcoholics. Muscle tenderness, elevated creatine phosphokinase, and pigmented casts point to myoglobinuria.
      2. **AIN**
         a. **Drugs.** Beta-lactamase–resistant penicillins (eg, methicillin); also sulfonamides, fluoroquinolones, NSAIDs, and many others.
         b. **Hypercalcemia**
         c. **Uric acid.** Tumor lysis syndrome (chemotherapy for leukemia or lymphoma).

    d. Infections. Staphylococcal or streptococcal infections, legionnaires' disease, toxoplasmosis, tuberculosis, and others.
3. **Acute glomerular disease**
    a. **Malignant hypertension**
    b. **Emboli, thrombosis, disseminated intravascular coagulation**
    c. **Rapidly progressive glomerulonephritis**
    d. **Systemic diseases.** Wegener's granulomatosis, Goodpasture's syndrome, thrombotic thrombocytopenic purpura, systemic lupus erythematosus, scleroderma.

C. Postrenal causes
1. **Urethral obstruction.** Prostatic hypertrophy, catheter obstruction. Prostatic carcinoma is an unusual cause of postrenal obstruction.
2. **Bilateral ureteral obstruction.** Most often as a result of carcinoma or retroperitoneal fibrosis. Common cause of death in cervical carcinoma.
3. **Intratubular obstruction.** Precipitation of crystals from medications such as acyclovir, sulfonamides, and methotrexate or tumor lysis syndrome.

IV. Database

A. Physical examination key points. The physical examination may help determine the cause and/or identify possible complications of oliguria. Also, review oral and IV fluid input and urine output (and drains and number of stools) and daily weights to assess volume status.
1. **Vital signs**
    a. **Temperature.** Fever points to infection (possibly sepsis) or acute AIN.
    b. **Heart rate.** An irregularly irregular pulse is consistent with atrial fibrillation, a common cause of emboli.
    c. **Blood pressure**
        i. **Hypertension.** Malignant hypertension may cause acute renal failure. Volume overload from oliguria may cause hypertension. Also longstanding hypertension can be a cause of chronic renal insufficiency.
        ii. **Orthostatic changes.** It is most important to assess the patient for orthostatic blood pressure and pulse changes (a decrease in systolic blood pressure of 10 mm Hg or an increase in heart rate by 20 bpm 1 minute after movement from supine to standing position). Orthostatic hypotension without a change in heart rate can be found in the elderly secondary to autonomic insufficiency or in patients on beta-blockers who are volume-depleted. An imbalance in intake and output can cause volume depletion resulting in orthostatic changes in heart rate and blood pressure. Weight loss can be seen with volume depletion

       iii. **Pulsus paradoxus.** If uremic pericarditis is suspected, pulsus paradoxus may indicate impending tamponade.

2. **Skin.** Decreased tissue turgor, dry mucous membranes, and loss of axillary sweating may occur with volume depletion. The presence of purpura may indicate thrombotic thrombocytopenic purpura. A maculopapular rash may indicate an allergic drug eruption, which may be seen with AIN. Livedo reticularis may be seen with cholesterol emboli.

3. **HEENT.** On funduscopic examination look for exudates, hemorrhages, papilledema, Roth spots, and Hollenhorst plaques (cholesterol emboli).

4. **Neck.** Flat neck veins with the patient supine suggest volume depletion. There may be an increase in jugular venous pressure secondary to volume overload from oliguria/anuria. Failure of neck vein distention with inspiration (*Kussmaul's sign*) may be seen in pericardial tamponade.

5. **Pulmonary.** Rales suggest CHF, possibly from volume overload.

6. **Cardiac.** S_3 suggests CHF; a new-onset murmur may be seen in endocarditis.

7. **Abdomen.** Look for ascites or a distended bladder. A palpable enlarged bladder suggests bladder outlet obstruction. Bruits may indicate renal artery stenosis.

8. **Genitourinary system.** Examine males for an enlarged prostate. Remember that bladder outlet obstruction can occur even when the gland feels normal in size. In females, rule out a pelvic mass.

9. **Extremities.** Assess perfusion by skin color and temperature.

B. **Laboratory data.** See Section II, Table 11–7, p 412, for urinary indices used in evaluating renal failure.

1. **Urinalysis**
   a. High specific gravity suggests volume depletion or recent dye administration.
   b. Protein (large amount) or red blood cell casts suggest glomerular disease.
   c. Significant hematuria points toward renal embolization or ureteral calculi. White blood cell casts suggest pyelonephritis or severe inflammation (AIN). Eosinophils are seen with AIN; frequent granular casts are consistent with ATN. Uric acid crystals may be seen in acute uric acid nephropathy.

2. **Serum chemistries.** Compare the BUN and creatinine. If the BUN:creatinine ratio is > 20:1, a prerenal cause is likely, although obstruction may also cause a high ratio, as can GI bleeding and catabolic states. If the ratio is < 15:1 and the BUN and creatinine are elevated, a renal cause is likely. Note the presence of hyponatremia or hypernatremia, hyperkalemia, and a low bicarbonate—any of which may complicate acute renal insufficiency.

3. **Urine electrolytes and creatinine.** In the face of oliguria, a urinary sodium < 20 mmol/L suggests a prerenal cause; a urinary

sodium > 20 mmol/L suggests renal causes. The fractional excretion of sodium (FE_{Na}) is calculated as [urinary sodium × serum creatinine/urine creatinine × serum sodium] × 100. A FE_{Na} < 1 suggests volume depletion; a FE_{Na} > 1 suggests renal causes. Acute urinary tract obstruction and dye nephrotoxicity may also reduce the FE_{Na} to < 1.

C. Radiologic and other studies

1. **Kidneys, ureters, bladder.** Helpful in assessing for obstructing renal calculi or for emphysematous pyelonephritis with diabetes.

2. **Ultrasound.** Renal ultrasound is useful in determining renal size, the presence of stones, and the presence of hydronephrosis. Hydronephrosis may be absent in early obstruction. Bedside bladder ultrasound may be useful in detecting bladder outlet obstruction.

3. **Radionucleotide renal scans.** Technetium-labeled diethylene-triaminepentaacetic acid (DTPA) or mercaptoacetyltriglycine nuclear medicine studies can assess renal perfusion (thrombosis, infarction, or emboli) or renal function via renogram; through the excretory phase, they can assess for obstruction. Gallium scans may be positive in AIN.

4. **Central venous pressure line or pulmonary artery catheter.** For a more accurate assessment of volume status.

5. **Retrograde pyelogram (RPG).** If obstruction is suspected, an RPG can reveal the cause and specific location of the obstruction. In addition, ureteral stent placement at the time of the procedure can relieve the obstruction.

6. **Renal biopsy.** Useful in renal failure of unknown cause or of prolonged duration. Renal biopsy may diagnose rapidly progressive glomerulonephritis or vasculitis, or suspected interstitial disease of unknown etiology.

7. **Renal duplex Doppler.** May be useful in detecting renal artery disease, but is operator dependent.

8. **CT scan, intravenous pyelogram, arteriography.** Radiocontrast studies are best avoided in acute oliguria unless specifically indicated. For example, arteriography in suspected polyarteritis nodosa.

9. **MRI.** Useful in the diagnosis of renal vein thrombosis and avoids radiocontrast media.

10. **Chest x-ray.** May be useful to assess for pulmonary edema and heart size.

11. **Electrocardiogram.** Should be obtained in patients with hyperkalemia.

12. **Echocardiogram.** Useful to assess for suspected pericardial effusion and left ventricular function.

D. Other diagnostic and therapeutic maneuvers

1. **Urinary catheter.** Initially, if a urinary catheter is in place, make sure the catheter is working by irrigating with 50 mL sterile normal

saline (NS), using a catheter-tip syringe. The fluid should pass easily, and the entire amount should be aspirated. (See Section I, Chapter 24, Foley Catheter Problems, p 148). If no urinary catheter is in place and obstruction is suspected, an in-and-out bladder catheterization should be performed. If a large postvoid residual is obtained, the catheter should be left in place. If a patient has very little urinary output, an indwelling catheter should be avoided because of the risk of infection.

2. **Volume challenge.** It is appropriate in most cases of oliguria to administer a volume challenge of 500 mL of NS without potassium given over 30 minutes. With a fragile cardiorespiratory status or in the elderly, smaller boluses should be given and central venous catheters used to monitor volume status. Then adjust the IV rate accordingly.

3. **Diuretics.** The use of diuretics in an attempt to convert an oliguric ARF to a nonoliguric ARF has been advocated. However, no benefits in outcomes from this maneuver have been noted in clinical trials. It should be emphasized that a decrease in urine output should not automatically trigger a trial of diuretics. The patient's volume status needs to be carefully assessed, and diuretics need to be avoided if the patient is volume-depleted. Indiscriminate use of diuretics may lead to further volume depletion and exacerbation of renal failure. If the patient is volume-overloaded, one may try diuresis with loop diuretics ± thiazides pending initiation of dialysis (see Use of diuretics in renal insufficiency below). Dialytic therapy, if indicated, should not be delayed because of a trial of diuretics.

E. **Use of diuretics in renal insufficiency**

1. **Loop diuretics.** High doses of loop diuretics may be required to initiate a diuretic response with an intrinsic renal disease. One must be cautious of the adverse extrarenal effects of loop diuretics, such as ototoxicity. Large doses of bumetanide may be associated with severe myalgias. To help avoid such adverse effects, large doses of diuretic should be infused over approximately 30–60 minutes. Initial doses of furosemide (40–80 mg), bumetanide (1–2 mg), or torsemide (20–50 mg) can be tried. If urine output does not increase within 1 hour, the doses can be progressively doubled until maximal doses are achieved (furosemide 360–400 mg, bumetanide 8–10 mg, or torsemide 200 mg). If a diuresis is established, loop diuretics may be administered as needed. Volume status should be monitored carefully to prevent volume depletion. An alternative strategy is to administer a bolus of loop diuretic followed by a continuous infusion that may be titrated according to need. (For example, a bolus of 80–160 mg of furosemide can be followed by 20 mg/hr titrating up by 10 mg/hr every hour as needed to a maximum of 80 mg/hr; or a

bolus of 1–2 mg of bumetanide can be followed by an infusion of 0.5 mg/hr titrating up by 0.5 mg/hr to a maximal dose of 2 mg/hr.)

2. **Thiazide diuretics.** May be used synergistically with loop diuretics. Metolazone 5–10 mg PO may be tried. An alternative is IV chlorothiazide 500 mg infused over 30 minutes.

F. **Mannitol.** May be used to help establish a diuresis in cases of rhabdomyolysis, hemolytic transfusion reactions, acute uric acid nephropathy, contrast-induced oliguria, and other toxic nephropathies. A dose of 12.5–25 g (50–100 mL of a 25% solution) IV may induce an osmotic diuresis. Mannitol may cause hyponatremia or hypernatremia, hypokalemia, or volume overload. Volume status must be carefully monitored and appropriate replacement fluids administered.

G. **Dopamine.** Renal-dose dopamine is not recommended in the treatment of ARF.

V. **Plan**

A. **Management of specific causes of oliguria/ARF**

1. **Prerenal**

a. **Monitor volume replacement.** Give crystalloid to increase central venous pressure above 10 mm Hg or pulmonary capillary wedge pressure above 12–14 mm Hg. A hematocrit > 25–30% is adequate.

b. **Follow hourly urine output.** Give specific criteria, such as having the house officer called if urine output is < 0.5 mL/kg/hr. Remove potassium and magnesium from IV solutions. If hypokalemia or hypomagnesemia is present, replace judiciously, preferably by the oral route.

2. **Postrenal**

a. **Bladder outlet obstruction.** Manage acutely with a Foley catheter. There are several concerns with this therapy, including acute bladder decompression, postobstructive diuresis, and increased risk of infection. Rapid bladder decompression has been a concern in the past because of possibly triggering a vasovagal episode or bladder hemorrhage. However, studies have demonstrated that large changes in bladder pressure occur with the first 100–250 mL of urine output. Thus, intermittent clamping of the catheter is probably unnecessary.

b. **Postobstructive diuresis.** Occasionally, relief of obstruction is followed by a brisk diuresis. This is thought to be the result of volume overload and is physiologic. Volume depletion and electrolyte disturbances may occur. The usual therapy is IV maintenance fluids such as ½ normal saline or 0.45% NaCl at 75 mL/hr. Replacement of urine output with IV fluids milliliter per milliliter should be avoided.

c. **Risk of infection.** Intermittent, rather than continuous, bladder catheterization should be considered to reduce infection risk.

   d. Ureteral obstruction. Ureteral obstruction requires urologic consultation. The consultation is emergent if an infection is suspected in the obstructed kidney (*pyonephrosis*).
   3. **Renal causes.** Therapy for renal causes of oliguria/ARF should be directed at the specific cause. The most common cause of intrinsic renal failure in hospitalized patients is ATN.

A. **Management of ATN.** The therapy of ATN is supportive care (see V.B.1–4).

   In addition to supportive care, dialysis may be indicated in 85% of patients with oliguric (< 400 mL/24 hr) and in 30–40% of patients with nonoliguric (> 400 mL/24 hr) ATN. Consult with a nephrologist early when serum creatinine is ≥ 2.0 mg/dL. Important issues to discuss with nephrology are the timing of initiation, the mode of dialytic therapy, and the use of biocompatible membranes.

B. **Management of oliguria/ARF.** General measures include the following:
   1. **Fluid management.** Fluid management needs to be individualized. Excessive fluid resuscitation should be avoided. This may lead to "pseudoacute respiratory distress syndrome" in patients with sepsis who may have leaky pulmonary vasculature. In general, IV fluids should not contain potassium. Accurate records of fluid intake and output are essential. Serum electrolytes need to be followed carefully. If the patient has a metabolic acidosis with pH < 7.10, sodium bicarbonate should be added. Excessive hypotonic fluids may lead to hyponatremia.
   2. **Nutrition.** Patients with ARF need a diet restricted in potassium, sodium, protein, and total fluids. Use enteral rather than parenteral nutrition.
   3. **Medications.** Review the patient's medications and stop all nephrotoxic drugs. Doses of renally excreted drugs should be adjusted.
   4. **Hemodialysis or peritoneal dialysis.** Should be considered in the following circumstances: severe hypervolemia unresponsive to diuretics, intractable metabolic acidosis, severe hyperkalemia, pericarditis thought secondary to uremia, and severe uremic symptoms or encephalopathy.

VI. **Prevention of ARF**
   A. **Identify and monitor patients at risk for ARF.** The elderly and those with chronic renal disease, diabetes mellitus, CHF, cirrhosis, severe vascular disease, jaundice, and other conditions.
   B. **Avoid dehydration and hypotension.**
   C. **Judicious use of potentially nephrotoxic drugs.** NSAIDs, amphotericin B, aminoglycosides, and cyclosporine.
   D. **Use of low-osmolality contrast media**

E. **Limiting radiocontrast nephropathy**
   1. Use alternative diagnostic procedures that do not require radio-contrast such as ultrasound or MRI when appropriate.
   2. Limit the amount of contrast.
   3. Hydrate patients with 0.45% saline at 1 ml/kg 6–12 hours before and after contrast.
   4. Treat at-risk patients with oral acetylcysteine, 600 mg twice one day before and the day of the radiographic study.

REFERENCES

Cadnapaphornchai P, Alavalapti RK, McDonald FD: Differential diagnosis of acute renal failure. In: Jacobson HR, Striker GE, Klahr S, eds. *The Principles and Practice of Nephrology.* 2nd ed. Mosby;1995:555.

Esson ML, Schrier RW: Diagnosis and treatment of acute tubular necrosis. Ann Intern Med 2002;137:744.

Holley JL: Clinical approach to the diagnosis of acute renal Failure. In: Greenberg A, ed. *Primer on Kidney Diseases.* 3rd ed. Academic Press;2001:245.

Klahr S, Miller SB: Current concepts: Acute oliguria. N Engl J Med 1998;338:671.

Post TW, Rose BD: Approach to the patient with renal disease including acute renal failure. In: Fletcher SW, Fletcher RH, Aronson MD, eds. UpToDate [CD-ROM]. Version 8.2. Wellesley, MA;2000. www.uptodate.com

Rose BD: Optimal dosage of loop diuretics. In: Fletcher SW, Fletcher RH, Aronson MD, eds. UpToDate [CD-ROM]. Version 8.2. Wellesley, MA;2000. www._uptodate.com.

Rose BD: Rate of decompression of an enlarged bladder. In: Fletcher SW, Fletcher RH, Aronson MD, eds. UpToDate [CD-ROM]. Version 8.2. Wellesley, MA;2000. www.uptodate.com.

Rose BD: Urine output in urinary tract obstruction and postobstructive diuresis. In: Fletcher SW, Fletcher RH, Aronson MD, eds. UpToDate [CD-ROM]. Version 8.2. Wellesley, MA;2000. www.uptodate.com

Singri N, Ahya SN, Levin ML: Acute renal failure. JAMA 2003;289:747.

Thadhani R, Pascual M, Bonventre JV: Acute renal failure. N Engl J Med 1996;334:1448.

52. OVERDOSES

I. **Problem.** You are called to the emergency room to evaluate a 38-year-old woman who was found unconscious by her husband, with an empty pill bottle lying on the floor near her.

II. **Immediate Questions**

A. **Is the patient conscious? What are the vital signs?** Assessing the patient's hemodynamic and respiratory status is the first priority in managing overdoses. Many overdose patients require ventilatory and/or blood pressure support. Unconscious patients need to have rapid assessment of blood glucose and immediate treatment with thiamine. Naloxone should be considered with respiratory depression even before opiate toxicity is confirmed. Only in instances in which the health care team is at risk of exposure—as in certain cases of inhalation overdose or in cases of topical organophosphate exposure—should other interventions come first.

B. What is the agent responsible for the overdose? Although supportive measures are the primary concern in overdose management, discovering the causative agent can help predict possible toxicity and direct further care. A detailed history and physical exam should provide the clues necessary to answer this question. For a patient who is unreliable or has an altered mental status, an exhaustive investigation is necessary. Question the patient's family and friends, thoroughly search the patient's belongings and the site of the overdose, and contact the patient's physician or pharmacy to determine possible medications ingested. All packaging of medication or chemical ingested should be obtained and pill counts made. Remember that with intentional overdoses the likelihood is high that more than one substance was taken.

III. **Differential Diagnosis.** The possible causes of acute overdoses are numerous. One method of simplifying the classification of overdoses is to group toxins by their effects. Six toxic syndromes encompass most of the common agents causing overdoses. A small group of additional agents do not fit any of the categories and are considered separately. Remember that even though causes of overdoses are grouped by common effects, there are characteristics and toxicities unique to individual agents even within the same group.

   A. Anticholinergic agents. The anticholinergics cause delirium, choreoathetosis, hypertension, tachypnea, tachycardia, and hyperthermia. Other characteristic signs include dry mouth, reduced bowel sounds, flushing of skin, dilated pupils, and urinary retention. Examples are tricyclic antidepressants (also commonly cause arrhythmias), antihistamines, phenothiazines, cyclobenzaprine, and belladonna alkaloids.

   B. Sympathomimetic agents. These toxins cause hyperalert and delusional mental states. Hyperthermia, hypertension, tachypnea, and tachycardia are common. Other signs include tremor, dilated pupils, diaphoresis, hyperreflexia, and, on occasion, seizures. Examples are cocaine, amphetamines, methamphetamines, pseudoephedrine, and theophylline.

   C. Sedatives/hypnotics/opiates. These agents cause CNS depression and, in extreme cases, coma. Vital signs show hypothermia, bradycardia, bradypnea, and hypotension. Reflexes are depressed, and noncardiogenic pulmonary edema is common. Examples are opiates (morphine, oxycodone, heroin), benzodiazepines (diazepam, lorazepam, oxazepam, alprazolam), barbiturates and alcohols (ethanol, methanol, isopropyl alcohol, ethylene glycol).

   D. Cholinergic agents. The mnemonic **SLUDGE** describes the symptoms of cholinergic overdose. **S**alivation, **S**weating, **L**acrimation, **U**rination, **D**iarrhea, **G**I hypermotility and cramping, and **E**mesis are the common findings. Confusion, coma, and seizures can also occur. Pupils are constricted, bradycardia is present, and the respiratory rate and blood pressure can be elevated or decreased. Examples are organophosphates, insecticides, and nicotine.

E. Serotonin agents. These chemicals cause hyperthermia, confusion, and agitation. Neuromuscular findings include hyperreflexia, myoclonus, and ataxia. Diaphoresis, shivering, and dilated pupils are also seen. Vital signs show hypertension, tachycardia, and tachypnea. Examples are serotonin reuptake inhibitors including citalopram, fluoxetine, paroxetine, sertraline, and dextromethorphan.

F. Hallucinogens. These agents cause hallucination, agitation, perceptual distortion, and paranoia. Pupils are usually dilated and nystagmus is common. All vital signs are elevated. Examples are lysergic acid diethylamide (LSD), phencyclidine (PCP), mescaline, and "designer" amphetamines.

G. Other agents. The following causes do not fit any specific classification.

    1. Acetaminophen. The patient can initially be asymptomatic. Anorexia, nausea, emesis, diaphoresis, and lethargy are common. Acetominophen is primarily hepatotoxic. The hepatotoxicity is not manifested for 24–36 hours after ingestion.

    2. Salicylates. These cause vertigo, nausea, emesis, noncardiac pulmonary edema, and acid–base disturbances (most commonly a combined metabolic gap acidosis and respiratory alkalosis).

    3. Insulin/oral hypoglycemics. Cause hypoglycemia (see Section I, Chapter 37, Hypoglycemia, p 213). In the case of oral agents, this can be long lasting.

    4. Carbon monoxide (CO). Headache, nausea, confusion, dyspnea, syncope, and coma can occur. Suspect this in cold weather, often from faulty heating or improper ventilation of exhaust from car or some other machine or heating device.

    5. Heavy metals. Iron, mercury, lead.

    6. Digoxin. This causes nausea, emesis, fatigue, yellow-green halos; and ventricular arrhythmias, atrioventricular block, and junctional tachycardia.

    7. Antihypertensives. Beta-blockers, calcium channel blockers.

    8. Lithium. This causes tremor, fasciculation, ataxia, sluggishness, nausea, emesis, and hypotension.

H. New drugs of abuse. The following drugs have recently become popular and need to be considered in cases of overdose. They are predominantly used by adolescents and young adults and are associated with "raves" (dance parties involving young adults, with electronically synthesized music enhanced with psychedelic lights; drugs such as ecstasy are often used).

1. **Ecstasy (3,4-methylenedioxymethamphetamine, or MDMA).** Increases serotonin, dopamine, and norepinephrine release in the central nervous system (CNS) and prevents reuptake. Ecstasy also causes diaphoresis, mydriasis, tachycardia, hypertension, hallucinations, delirium, muscle spasms and rigidity, and arrhythmias. In severe cases, it can lead to death. It shares many similar features to those of serotonin syndromes and sympathomimetic syndromes.

2. **Gamma hydroxybutyrate (GHB).** Increases dopaminergic activity in the CNS and causes drowsiness, confusion, aggressive behavior, incontinence, ataxia, tremors, and seizures in some cases. GHB also can lead to bradycardia, respiratory depression, hypothermia, nausea, and vomiting. Gamma butyrolactone (GBL) and 1,4-butanediol (1,4-BD) are GHB prodrugs that are converted to GHB after ingestion. They are found in several health and fitness products.

3. **Ketamine.** A PCP (phenylcyclidine hydrochloride) derivative that causes agitation, nystagmus, mydriasis, hallucinations, hypertonicity, delirium, and a floating sensation. It can also cause seizures, tachycardia, hypertension, and palpitations.

I. **Alternative medicines.** With the increased interest in alternative medicine in this country, attention should be paid to possible overdoses of easily acquired herbal medications and dietary supplements. Agents such as ephedrine can lead to a sympathomimetic syndrome. Ginkgo, ginseng, and garlic can lead to bleeding. Kava overdose can cause hepatic failure.

IV. **Database**

A. **Physical examination key points**

1. **Vital signs.** The vital signs can often be used to help determine the cause of the overdose (eg, sinus tachycardia is commonly seen in tricyclic antidepressant overdoses, whereas bradycardia is seen with beta-blocker or cholinergic overdoses). Temperature should be checked because hyperthermia (cocaine) and hypothermia (alcohol) are common. For accuracy, respirations should be counted rather than estimated.

2. **Skin.** The entire body surface should be examined. Examination should include investigation for bruising or other trauma, pressure sores, and track marks, suggesting injection drug usage. Flushing and erythema suggest an anticholinergic or CO overdose. Even though the cherry-red appearance of the skin and mucous membranes is classic for CO overdoses, cyanosis is more common. Pale diaphoretic skin is seen in overdoses of sympathomimetics and hallucinogens. Desquamation is found in heavy metal poisonings. Cyanosis suggests hypoxia.

3. **HEENT.** Look for evidence of head trauma, which can be concurrent with an overdose. A cervical collar should be applied if there

is a question of trauma. Pupil size should be recorded accurately and may be one more clue in determining the cause of the overdose. Constricted pupils are seen with opiate, clonidine, and organophosphate overdoses, whereas dilated pupils are seen with cocaine, amphetamine, LSD, antihistamine, and tricyclic antidepressant overdoses. The oropharynx should also be evaluated to determine moistness of the mucous membranes, which can differentiate between cholinergic and anticholinergic poisonings, and determine the presence of injection marks under the tongue, a sign of IV drug abuse. Breath odors can also provide useful information. Alcohols cause a fruity breath odor; salicylates, an odor similar to wintergreen; and arsenic or organophosphates, the smell of garlic.

4. **Lungs.** Look for evidence of aspiration, a common complication. Also, check for pulmonary edema (a complication of overdoses with hydrocarbons, antihypertensives, heavy metals, and inhalants).

5. **Cardiovascular.** Look for peripheral and central cyanosis.

6. **Abdomen.** The abdomen should be auscultated for bowel sounds, which can be decreased or increased depending on the cause of the overdose. Look for organomegaly. Check for melena or hematochezia.

7. **Neurologic exam.** Assessment of the patient's mental status can provide invaluable evidence in determining the cause of the overdose. A depressed mental state suggests overdose with a sedative or alcohol. An agitated state would be more consistent with sympathomimetic agents and hallucinogens. A neurologic exam should be done to evaluate for trauma or intracranial injury. With mental status changes, the gag reflex should be assessed and if depressed or absent, intubation may be indicated.

8. **Musculoskeletal.** Lithium and sympathomimetics cause tremor and fasciculations. Alcohols, neuroleptics, and CO cause rigidity. Heavy metals can cause weakness. Tricyclic antidepressants and antiepileptics cause choreoathetotic movements.

B. **Laboratory data**

1. **Serum and urine drug screens.** Although these tests are commonly ordered and can be useful, it is important to remember the following: (1) they often take several hours to complete, which decreases their usefulness; (2) they test for only a limited number of agents, and even a positive result does not confirm that the discovered agent caused the symptoms; and (3) urine screens may be falsely negative if obtained too early. Although recommended for overdoses of unknown cause, these tests need not be ordered when the causative agent can be determined by history and examination or in overdoses of minor severity.

2. **Tests for specific agents.** Tests for common causes of overdoses such as acetaminophen; salicylate; alcohols; iron, lead,

and other metals; lithium; and digoxin can be easily obtained. They should be used any time overdose with the agent in question is suspected by history and physical examination. Tests for acetaminophen, salicylate, and alcohols are recommended in instances in which the causative agent is unknown or in suicide attempts in which ingestion of multiple substances is suspected.

3. **Glucose.** All overdose patients, especially those with altered mental status, should have serum glucose tested by finger-stick so that hypoglycemia can be discovered early and treated.

4. **Serum creatine kinase and urine myoglobin.** To rule out suspected rhabdomyolysis.

5. **Arterial blood gases.** Useful with respiratory compromise and inhalation exposure, and in patients in whom an acid–base disturbance is suspected.

6. **Serum electrolytes, liver function tests, blood urea nitrogen, and serum creatinine.** Mandatory in severe overdoses. In less severe cases, order testing based on suspected toxicity of a particular agent or on clinical judgment. The anion gap can be helpful in alcohol and salicylate overdoses where acid–base disturbances are common.

7. **Serum osmolarity.** The osmol gap can be helpful in diagnosing overdose with alcohols such as ethylene glycol and methanol.

C. **Radiologic and other studies**

1. **Electrocardiogram (ECG).** An ECG can be helpful in managing an overdose patient. It is mandatory in evaluating an overdose of a drug known to affect the heart (tricyclic antidepressants, antihypertensives, and digoxin). Look for arrhythmias or prolonged QT, QRS, or PR intervals. A QRS interval > 0.10 seconds places the tricyclic antidepressant overdose patient at risk for arrhythmias and seizures.

2. **Chest x-ray.** To look for evidence of aspiration, acute respiratory distress syndrome, or noncardiogenic pulmonary edema.

3. **Abdominal x-ray.** Helpful with ingestions in which the toxin is radiopaque. Examples of such substances include **C**hlorinated hydrocarbons, **C**alcium salts, **C**rack vials, **H**eavy metals, **I**odinated compounds such as thyroxin, **P**sychotropics, **P**ackets of drugs, **E**nteric-coated tablets such as aspirin, **S**alicylates, **S**odium salts, and **S**ustained-release tablets. The mnemonic **CHIPES** may be useful. Abdominal films should also be done anytime intestinal obstruction is suspected.

4. **Head CT scan.** If there are mental status changes and the cause is unclear, especially in patients who have evidence of trauma along with a suspected overdose.

5. **Cervical x-rays.** With suspected neck trauma to rule out cervical fracture.

V. Plan. There are four components in the treatment of overdose: stabilization and support, decontamination, antidotes, and enhanced elimination. In unconscious patients, consider immediate assessment of blood glucose and treatment with dextrose 50%, 50 mL IV if hypoglycemic. Also, give thiamine 100 mg IV, since the mental status changes associated with Wernicke's encephalopathy include coma and in an unconscious patient it is impossible to assess for ataxia or ophthalmoplegia. Furthermore, naloxone 0.4–2.0 mg should be administered, especially if the respiratory rate is depressed, even before opiate toxicity is confirmed.

A. Stabilization and support

1. **ABCs (airway, breathing, and circulation).** Should be addressed first.

2. **Intubation.** See Section III, Chapter 7, Endotracheal Intubation, p 434. Intubation should be performed when hypoxia, hypercapnia, or respiratory distress is not easily reversible. It should also be done in any instance in which there is airway compromise or risk of aspiration. Some patients with altered mental status and agitation may need to be sedated and intubated to prevent hyperthermia and rhabdomyolysis.

3. **Hypotension.** See Section I, Chapter 42, Hypotension, V, p 241. Hypotension should initially be managed with fluid resuscitation. Always use an isotonic fluid solution such as normal saline or lactated Ringer's solution. If there is no response to IV fluids, use vasopressor agents.

4. **Hypertension.** See Section I, Chapter 35, Hypertension, V, p 208. Agitated patients should be treated initially with sedatives such as lorazepam. If medication is necessary, nitroprusside or labetalol can be used. With hypertension from sympathomimetic drugs, beta-blockers should not be used.

5. **Arrhythmias.** See Section I, Chapter 9, Cardiopulmonary Arrest, V, p 49; Chapter 60, Tachycardia, V, p 351; and Chapter 8, Bradycardia, V, p 45. Ventricular arrhythmias with adequate blood pressure should be treated with lidocaine except in tricyclic antidepressant overdose, in which $NaHCO_3$ should be used first. Atropine can be used for severe bradycardia; however, transcutaneous or transvenous pacing may be needed. In instances of torsades de pointes or ventricular tachycardia secondary to a prolonged QT interval, overdrive pacing should be considered. Magnesium can be used for polymorphic ventricular tachycardia, especially torsades de pointes.

6. **Monitoring.** Overdoses causing potential respiratory or hemodynamic compromise or cardiac arrhythmias such as tricyclic antidepressant overdose require intensive care monitoring. Patients with altered mental status also have better outcomes if monitored closely. Pulse oximetry should be used with respiratory compromise. Suicidal patients must be continuously observed.

B. Decontamination. Decontamination should be performed as rapidly as possible, since the best outcomes have been associated with early treatment. The purpose of decontamination is to prevent further absorption of the toxic agent. The method of decontamination is determined by the type of exposure.

1. Ingestion. Methods of decontamination include induction of emesis, gastric lavage, activated charcoal, whole bowel irrigation, and surgical or endoscopic removal of the toxin. Best results are obtained if these are performed in the first hour after ingestion. Activated charcoal has been shown to be the most effective method and is recommended in all cases of overdose ingestion except where contraindicated. The appropriate dose is 1 g/kg given orally or by nasogastric tube. Doses of activated charcoal should be repeated as indicated for the specific substance ingested. Often water or sorbitol is given in conjunction with the activated charcoal. Activated charcoal binds ingested drugs, preventing absorption. Contraindications to use include bowel obstruction, ingestion of hydrocarbons, ingestion of acidic or alkali corrosives, ingestion of substances that do not bind to charcoal (such as lithium and metals such as iron), and any instances in which aspiration is a risk. Charcoal can be given to patients with aspiration risk after intubation. In special cases, consider other methods of decontamination, such as whole bowel irrigation or endoscopic removal of the toxin.

2. Ocular. Decontamination of eye exposures starts with saline irrigation for at least 15–20 minutes. Surface particulate matter can be removed with a cotton swab. Embedded material should be removed by an ophthalmologist. Alkali corneal burns require immediate attention by an ophthalmologist.

3. Topical. Aggressive saline or water irrigation of the exposed area for at least 15 minutes is the best immediate method to prevent dermal absorption of toxic chemicals. Remove all contaminated clothing, and protect personnel from exposure. Exposure to several chemicals requires special treatment.

C. Antidotes. Many agents that are commonly associated with overdoses have antidotes that can prevent toxic injury or mortality. Listed below are commonly overdosed substances and the antidotes available. Antidotes should be used when the cause of the overdose is known and the possible toxicity is determined to be severe enough that the benefits of therapy outweigh the risks of the antidote. If you are unsure of how to manage an overdose or ingestion of a specific toxin, the local poison-control hotline can be extremely helpful.

1. Opiates. Naloxone 0.4–2.0 mg IV, IM, or SC. The diagnosis should be questioned if there is no response after repeated doses to a total dose of 10 mg.

2. Tricyclic antidepressants. Bicarbonate 1–2 mEq/kg IV push, then a sodium bicarbonate drip (two or three 50-mL ampules of

NaHCO$_3$ [50 mEq] added to 1 L of D5W) at 150–200 mL/hr. Follow the arterial pH and serum bicarbonate. Alkalinization reverses the cardiac conduction abnormalities.

3. **Benzodiazepines.** Flumazenil 0.2 mg, followed by increasing doses every minute until effect is seen, generally to a total dose of 3 mg. Duration of reversal is dependent on the benzodiazepine dose, the half-life of the drug taken, and the flumazenil dose. Administration of flumazenil to patients receiving a benzodiazepine for seizure control may precipitate seizures. Rapid access to a benzodiazepine (eg, IV lorazepam) is recommended. CNS effects of benzodiazepines may be reversed; however, respiratory support still may be required. Flumazenil is not recommended for use in multiple-drug overdoses. The drug may reverse the CNS effects of benzodiazepines, **but it may precipitate seizures, arrhythmias, and withdrawal symptoms in patients who also ingested a tricyclic antidepressant**. ECG findings suggesting a tricyclic antidepressant overdose are a relative contraindication to the use of flumazenil.

4. **Calcium channel blockers.** Calcium chloride 1 g IV over 5 minutes and repeated every 10–20 minutes for 3–4 additional doses. Glucagon can also be used (5–10 mg hourly) following a bolus of 50–150 μg/kg.

5. **Beta-blockers.** Glucagon, 50–150 μg/kg, then 5–10 mg hourly. Atropine 0.5–1 mg and repeated every 3–5 minutes up to 0.04 mg/kg may be used.

6. **Anticholinergics.** Physostigmine 1–2 mg IV over 5 minutes.

7. **Methanol and ethylene glycol.** Ethanol 10%, 10 mL/kg load, then 0.15 mL/kg/hr. The goal is a serum ethanol concentration of 100–120 mg/dL. Double this rate during dialysis. In ethylene glycol overdose, pyridoxine 100 mg IV and thiamine 100 mg should be given daily. An alternative therapy to ethanol is fomepizole (4-methylpyrazole), 15 mg/kg IV loading dose, followed by 10 mg/kg every 12 hours for 4 doses, then 15 mg/kg every 12 hours until levels fall to target range.

8. **Organophosphates and carbamates.** Atropine 2–5 mg IV, which may be repeated every 0–30 minutes to maintain full atropinization—noted by dried secretions and clearing of rales. Pralidoxime may be necessary.

9. **Digoxin.** Digoxin-specific antibody. Dose is based on digoxin level.

10. **Acetaminophen.** *N*-acetylcysteine (Mucomyst), 140 mg/kg initially, then 70 mg/kg/day every 4 hours for a total of 17 doses. Activated charcoal should be used initially; treatment with Mucomyst is based on acetaminophen blood levels. Serum blood levels should be drawn at least 4 hours after ingestion and the blood level plotted against time since ingestion. Using a standard acetaminophen toxicity nomogram, the risk for hepatotoxicity is

classified as probable, possible, or no risk. Recently, it has been suggested that shorter courses of *N*-acetylcysteine may be equally effective in treating acetaminophen overdose, although this has not been proved in a randomized controlled trial.

11. **Iron.** Deferoxamine 15 mg/kg/hr IV, total daily dose usually up to 6 g.

12. **Lead.** EDTA (edetic acid) 50–75 mg/kg/day by deep IM injection or slow IV infusion in 3–6 divided doses for up to 5 days. Treatment course may be repeated.

D. **Enhanced elimination**

1. **Alkalinization of urine and forced diuresis.** Useful for renally excreted chemicals, especially weakly acidic substances. Examples include salicylates and phenobarbital. The goal is to infuse enough fluid and bicarbonate to increase urine output to > 3 mL/kg/hr and urine pH > 7.5.

2. **Hemodialysis.** Useful for clearing methanol, ethylene glycol, salicylates, lithium, and theophylline.

3. **Hemofiltration.** Useful in clearing aminoglycosides, vancomycin, and metal chelate complexes.

REFERENCES

Brent J, McMartin K, Phillips S et al: Fomepizole for the treatment of methanol poisoning. N Engl J Med 2001;344:424.

Burns M, Schwartzstein R: General approach to drug intoxications. In: Fletcher SW, Fletcher RH, Aronson MD, eds. UpToDate [CD-ROM]. Version 8.2. Wellesley, MA;2000. www.uptodate.com

Ellenhorn MJ, Schonwald S, Ordog G et al, eds: *Ellenhorn's Medical Toxicology.* 2nd ed. Williams & Wilkins;1997.

Graeme K: New drugs of abuse. Emerg Med Clin North Am 2000;18:625.

Kulig K: Initial management of ingestions of toxic substances. N Engl J Med 1992;326:1677.

Rosen P, ed: *Emergency Medicine Concepts and Clinical Practice.* 4th ed. Mosby-Year Book;1998.

Toll LL, Hurlbut KM, eds: POISINDEX System. Englewood, CO: MICROMEDEX, Inc.;2001.

Zimmerman J: Poisonings and overdoses in the intensive care unit: General and specific management issues. Crit Care Med 2003;31:2794.

53. PACEMAKER TROUBLESHOOTING

I. **Problem.** A 44-year-old man was admitted to the coronary care unit (CCU) for an acute myocardial infarction (MI) complicated by third-degree heart block, and a transvenous pacemaker was inserted. The CCU nurse calls later to report seeing pacemaker spikes but no capture from the ventricle.

II. **Immediate Questions**

A. **What is the patient's condition and what are his or her vital signs?** Bradycardia with hypotension warrants immediate attention, as does the development of symptoms of hypoperfusion (confusion, pre-syncope or syncope, chest pain, and dyspnea).

B. What were the circumstances surrounding pacemaker insertion? Prophylactic insertion of a temporary pacemaker wire in the setting of an acute MI and Mobitz type II second-degree heart block is a less urgent situation than the development of third-degree heart block and hypotension. The latter situation may rapidly deteriorate to cardiac arrest, whereas the former may require no intervention other than close observation.

III. Differential Diagnosis. Most problems encountered with pacemakers are generally classified into one of two categories: failure to capture a pacing impulse or failure to sense a cardiac depolarization. Temporary pacemaker output is programmed to be inhibited by cardiac depolarization.

A. Failure to capture. *Failure to capture* occurs when the temporary intravenous (or transcutaneous) pacemaker generates an impulse (as evidenced by a narrow, vertical pacemaker "spike"), but there is no evidence of ventricular depolarization. Keep in mind that a transvenous pacing wire placed appropriately in the apex of the right ventricle should produce a wide complex depolarization immediately after the pacemaker spike. A 12-lead electrocardiogram (ECG) will reveal a superior axis (~– 90°) with a left bundle branch block morphology. See Figure I-5 for an example of failure to capture. Failure to capture represents one of the most common problems encountered in temporary transvenous pacing.

   1. Problems intrinsic to the pacemaker

      a. Malposition of the catheter resulting in loss of contact between the catheter tip and the endocardium. This can occur when the patient is repositioned in bed. Malposition results in raising the pacing threshold and thus failure to capture.

      b. Inappropriate lead placement

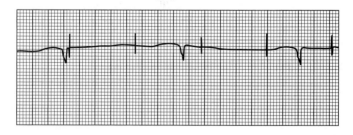

Figure I–5. Failure to capture. The rhythm is a nodal rhythm at 40 beats per minute. The pacemaker spikes occur at 72 beats per minute. The pacemaker spikes are not associated with the ventricular depolarizations.

  c. **Inappropriate generator settings.** Be sure that the heart rate and output settings have not been changed.
  d. **Malfunction of the generator.** This is an uncommon reason; however, generators run on alkaline batteries, which sometimes fail. Be sure to check the generator battery regularly.
  e. **Fractured pacing electrode**
  f. **Poor connection between the electrodes and the generator**
2. **Local factors**
  a. **Profound hypoxemia**
  b. **Severe acidemia**
  c. **Marked hyperkalemia**
  d. **Fibrosis at the electrode**
  e. **Myocardial infarction** that includes the right ventricular apex
  f. **Myocardial edema at the catheter tip**
  g. **Drugs.** Type IIC antiarrhythmic agents (eg, flecainide, encainide) can raise the myocardial threshold for depolarization.

B. **Failure to sense.** *Failure to sense* occurs when the pacemaker fails to recognize a native depolarization and subsequently generates a pacemaker spike without being inhibited by the native depolarization. See Figure I-6 for an example of failure to sense. Often, this inappropriate pacemaker spike falls somewhere between the QRS complex and the T wave of the native depolarization, and a ventricular depolarization does *not* follow this pacemaker spike. This is because the pacemaker spike is occurring during the refractory period of the ventricle (the native depolarization was not sensed by the pacemaker). Failure to sense should not be interpreted as failure to capture, even though failure to capture often accompanies failure to sense, especially when the problem results from pacing electrode displacement and poor endocardial contact. In essence, the same circumstances that cause failure to capture can also cause failure to sense. If the timing of the pacemaker spike is on top of the T wave, sustained ventricular tachycardia can occur.

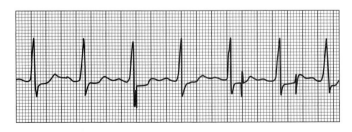

Figure I–6. Failure to sense. A pacemaker spike is seen immediately after the 3rd, 4th, 5th, and 6th QRS complexes. The pacemaker should have been inhibited by the QRS complexes. *(Photograph courtesy of Alberto Mazzoleni, MD.)*

C. **Other complications of transvenous pacemakers**
   1. **Oversensing of P waves and T waves**
   2. **Myocardial perforation** with pericardial effusion and tamponade (rare)
   3. **Ventricular ectopy**
   4. **Tricuspid valve dysfunction**
   5. **Line sepsis**
   6. **Venous thrombosis**

IV. Database

A. **Physical examination key points**
   1. **Vital signs.** Heart rate and blood pressure are essential to determine the need for immediate intervention.
   2. **Cardiopulmonary examination.** An elevated jugular venous pressure, inspiratory rales at the bases, and an S_3 indicate congestive heart failure, possibly secondary to hypoperfusion. An elevated jugular venous pressure, new pericardial friction rub, and loss of a palpable apical impulse could indicate a pericardial effusion from myocardial perforation by the pacemaker wire.
   3. **Neurologic exam.** A change in mental status or confusion may indicate hypoperfusion.

B. **Laboratory data**
   1. **Portable chest x-ray.** To check placement of the catheter tip. This is helpful if catheter displacement or myocardial perforation is a concern. In addition, comparison with postinsertion chest x-rays can be useful. Unfortunately, the most relevant information is obtained from the lateral projection, which often is not obtained after insertion and is often not feasible to obtain at the time of malfunction.
   2. **ECG and rhythm strip.** To rule out MI as a cause of the problem and to rule out myocardial ischemia as another indicator of hypoperfusion. Clues as to the current location of the catheter can be obtained from the surface ECG. For instance, a pacemaker in the right ventricular apex results in a QRS configuration with a left bundle branch morphology. If a right bundle branch morphology is present, the clinician should suspect interventricular septum rupture and subsequent pacing from the left ventricle.
   3. **Arterial blood gases.** To rule out acidemia or hypoxemia as a cause.
   4. **Electrolytes.** To rule out hyperkalemia as a cause of the pacemaker's failure to sense or capture.

V. Plan

A. **Electrode placement.** If there has been any decline in the patient's condition or significant change in vital signs, ask the nurse to place anterior and posterior transcutaneous pacing electrodes in preparation for possible use until the transvenous pacing wire problem can be resolved. In addition, have the "crash cart" readily available in case of cardiopulmonary arrest.

B. Obtain back-up. There are few problems in internal medicine more anxiety-provoking than a dysfunctional pacemaker in a pacemaker-dependent patient. If a senior resident or cardiology fellow supervises you in the CCU, give him or her a call.

C. Inspect the generator and connections to the pacing wire. Care must be taken to avoid "short-circuiting" the system. Be sure you are wearing rubber gloves. Empiric replacement of a new generator "box" is generally preferred over attempts to replace batteries. In addition, replace the generator if something appears to be wrong with it. The pacing wire can be tested for electrode fracture by connecting the distal cathode to the V lead on the ECG machine and then connecting the proximal anode to the V lead. If an ECG can be recorded from each electrode, the pacing wire has not fractured. When you cannot see a pacemaker spike, the problem usually lies with either the generator or the pacing wire. Pacemaker spikes are more easily seen with unipolar pacing (eg, the proximal anode is usually a subcutaneous wire). Also, a unipolar pacing configuration is more sensitive than a bipolar pacing configuration. Thus, changing from a bipolar to a unipolar configuration may help to restore both capture and sensing.

D. Adjust the pacemaker settings. Check the settings to be certain that the output, heart rate, and sensitivity settings are appropriate.

  1. Check the pacing threshold of the electrode. First, raise the pacing rate on the generator to a level at which the patient's rhythm is completely paced. Second, turn down the pacing output until paced beats no longer appear. This is the pacemaker's pacing threshold. Acceptable threshold values are usually < 2 mA. *Caution:* Be sure to raise the pacing output back to its original setting before leaving the patient's bedside.

  2. For failure to capture. Increase the output until capture reappears. A high pacing threshold may be related to electrode displacement or other problems as listed above.

  3. For failure to sense. Increase the sensitivity until it reliably detects and is inhibited by cardiac depolarization.

E. Consider repositioning the catheter if adjusting the pacemaker settings does not solve the problem. Pacemaker wires can be advanced and repositioned blindly by following the configuration of the ECG tracing recorded from the endocardium. *This should be done only by someone experienced in this technique.* It is much safer to use fluoroscopy, if available, or to rely temporarily on transcutaneous pacing until someone skilled in pacemaker insertion arrives. Many hospitals have fluoroscopy available in a CCU procedure room or have portable fluoroscopy on a "C-arm." If either is available, reposi-

tioning of transvenous pacing electrodes under fluoroscopic visualization is advised.

REFERENCES

Emergency cardiac pacing. In: Cummins RO, ed. *Textbook of Advanced Cardiac Life Support.* American Heart Association;1994:5.
Narula OS: Clinical concepts of spontaneous and induced atrioventricular block. In: Mandel WJ, ed. *Cardiac Arrhythmias: Their Mechanisms, Diagnosis and Management.* Lippincott;1995:441.
Watanabe Y, Dreifus LS, Mazyalev T: Atrioventricular block: Basic concepts. In: Mandel WJ, ed. *Cardiac Arrhythmias: Their Mechanisms, Diagnosis and Management.* Lippincott;1995:417.
Wood M: Temporary cardiac pacing. In: Ellenbogen KA, Kay GN, Wilkoff BL, eds. *Clinical Cardiac Pacing.* Saunders;1995:687.
Wood M, Ellenbogen KA: Temporary cardiac pacing. In: Ellenbogen KA, ed. *Cardiac Pacing.* 2nd ed. Blackwell Science;1996:168.

54. PAIN MANAGEMENT

I. **Problem.** A 72-year-old man admitted for treatment of metastatic prostate cancer cannot sleep because of persistent back pain.

II. **Immediate Questions**

   A. **Has the patient experienced this pain before?** If the pain is of recent onset, the patient will require a full evaluation to rule out causes
   other than malignancy. For example, the pain may be from herpes
   zoster, acute pyelonephritis, renal colic, abdominal aortic aneurysm,
   epidural abscess or pulmonary embolism.

   B. **What are the severity and character of the pain?** Accurate pain
   assessment is the basis for appropriate pain management. First, ascertain the severity of pain using a numeric rating scale of 0–10 with
   10 being the worst imaginable pain. Determine the other descriptors
   of pain including onset, location, duration, aggravating factors, and
   relieving factors. Certain characteristics may be helpful in distinguishing different types of pain. Neuropathic pain is described as
   sharp, burning, or electrical. Visceral pain is cramping, squeezing,
   and poorly localized. Somatic pain (eg, bone pain) is well localized
   and dull or aching.

   C. **Is the patient currently receiving pain medication, and, if so,
   what is the drug—its dosage and dosing interval?** If the patient
   has previously received narcotics, the pain may represent development of tolerance and therefore an inadequate dose of medication.
   Similarly, physicians frequently prescribe an inappropriately long interval between doses of narcotics. Analgesics should not be delayed
   while the initial assessment and evaluation are being completed.

III. **Differential Diagnosis.** The following discussion pertains chiefly to the
management of pain in terminally ill cancer patients. The management

of *chronic pain* (pain that has lasted longer than 3 months) is not discussed here. Pain in a patient with cancer may be caused by primary or metastatic disease, or it may occur as a complication of treatment (surgery, radiation, chemotherapy, immobility, or infections).

A. **Pain caused directly by tumors**
  1. **Tumor invasion of bone and pathologic fracture**
  2. **Infiltration/compression of nerves**
  3. **Obstruction of a hollow viscus**
  4. **Expansion of a viscus or its capsule.** For example, liver metastases.
  5. **Tissue ischemia after tumor invasion of lymphatics and blood vessels**
  6. **Paraneoplastic syndromes.** Hypertrophic osteoarthropathy and neuropathy.

B. **Iatrogenic causes of cancer pain**
  1. **Surgery.** Incisions; phantom limb pain.
  2. **Chemotherapy.** May cause infectious, gastrointestinal, and neurologic pain.
  3. **Radiation.** Colitis, esophagitis.

C. **Psychological pain.** Anxiety, depression, spiritual distress, and a feeling of loss of control are frequently associated with malignancy and may intensify the patient's perception of pain.

IV. **Database**

A. **Physical examination key points**
  1. **Vital signs.** Tachycardia occurs with a variety of causes of acute pain and therefore is too nonspecific to suggest a specific cause. Fever suggests an infectious cause or acute venous thrombosis.
  2. **Skin.** Chemotherapy and hematologic malignancies can predispose to herpes zoster infections; therefore, ascertain whether the pain is in the distribution of a specific dermatome. Look for vesicles on an erythematous base that would suggest shingles. Pain may precede the development of the typical vesicular rash by 2–3 days.
  3. **HEENT.** Papilledema suggests increased intracranial pressure from cerebral metastases.
  4. **Neck.** Nuchal rigidity could indicate infectious or carcinomatous meningitis causing back or neck pain.
  5. **Chest.** In addition to auscultating the lungs for evidence of pneumonia, palpate the ribs and sternum for evidence of bone pain suggesting metastases.
  6. **Abdomen.** In a patient with abdominal pain, examine for hepatomegaly, which could indicate liver metastases. Bowel obstruction could result from the underlying malignant process itself, or it could occur as a result of decreased bowel motility from the administration of narcotics. A pulsatile epigastric mass would suggest an abdominal aortic aneurysm.

7. **Extremities.** Examine for evidence of bone pain, arthropathy, or deep venous thrombosis, which may occur with underlying malignancy.

8. **Neurologic exam.** In a patient complaining of headache, perform a careful neurologic exam looking for localizing findings that could indicate the presence of cerebral metastases. Stocking-glove distribution of pain may result from a peripheral neuropathy caused by underlying cancer or chemotherapeutic agents such as vincristine.

B. **Laboratory data**

1. **Complete blood count.** Obtain if infection is suspected.

2. **Alkaline phosphatase and serum calcium.** Order if bone metastases are suspected. Remember to correct the total calcium in the face of hypoalbuminemia or check an ionized calcium. See Section I, Chapter 36, Hypocalcemia, p 210.

3. **Alkaline phosphatase, γ-glutamyl transpeptidase (GGT), and transaminases (AST and ALT).** Obtain liver function tests if hepatic metastases are suspected.

C. **Radiologic and other studies.** Specific radiographs should be directed by findings from history and physical examination. Keep in mind that bone scintigraphy is more sensitive for bony metastases than plain films. Bone scintigraphy may be falsely negative if there is bone destruction without accompanying osteoblastic response, such as in multiple myeloma.

V. **Plan.** The following discussion pertains to the management of cancer pain. However, the principles of pain management apply to patients with pain from other medical conditions as well. Nearly 80% of patients with advanced malignant disease will experience pain before death. Fear of uncontrolled pain is one of the greatest concerns of a patient with malignancy. The physician should reassure patients that every effort will be made to alleviate their pain. Physician fear of addiction, tolerance, and side effects frequently results in underprescribing opioid analgesics. This is an unfounded fear in treating patients with acute pain, especially those patients with pain related to malignancy. Most patients do *not* develop addiction or psychological dependence. Physical dependence and tolerance may occur after prolonged administration of narcotics. Sedation and nausea may occur in opioid-naive patients; however, tolerance to these side effects may develop over a few days. Remember that many patients with intractable pain suffer from sleep deprivation. The opportunity for restful sleep for the first time in weeks may result in somnolence that could be misinterpreted as excessive sedation. Tolerance to constipation does not develop, and all patients treated with opioid analgesics should be placed on a laxative and stool softener. Constipation is much easier to prevent than to treat. Respiratory depression is rare and usually preceded by sedation (an advantage of patient-controlled analgesia (PCA), since the sedated patient is less likely to self-administer medication). It most often occurs after the first dose in an opioid-naive patient. To prevent opioid withdrawal while reversing respiratory depression, 1 ampule of naloxone (Narcan) 0.4 mg can be diluted in 10 mL of sterile water or saline and administered in 1-mL increments until respiratory depression has been reversed. Finally, careful and frequent reassessment is necessary in all patients treated with opioids. Dehydration and renal insufficiency typically occur in the final days of life. Opioids and their metabolites can accumulate and result in opioid-induced neurotoxicity including hallucinations, myoclonus, and a hyperirritable state.

A. Mild pain (numeric rating 1–3). Nonnarcotic analgesics may be tried initially.

1. **Acetaminophen (Tylenol).** Give 650–1000 mg PO Q 4 hr (to a maximum of 4 g/day). Doses of 4 g/day can be toxic in patients with hepatic disease or with a history of alcohol abuse. Acetaminophen may also be used to supplement the analgesic effects of opioids.
2. **Nonsteroidal anti-inflammatory drugs (NSAIDs).** Ibuprofen (Motrin) 400–600 mg PO Q 6 hr or naproxen (Naprosyn) 250–500 mg PO Q 12 hr are particularly effective for patients with bone metastases because of the high prostaglandin content of periosteum. Use NSAIDs cautiously in patients with underlying renal insufficiency, congestive heart failure, or peptic ulcer disease. Patients at risk for gastrointestinal complications should be treated with a selective cyclooxygenase-2 inhibitor such as celecoxib (Celebrex) or rofecoxib (Vioxx).

B. Moderate pain (numeric rating 4–6). For patients whose pain persists despite the preceding measures, a weak narcotic-analgesic may be administered. Usually, these are administered in combination with either acetaminophen or aspirin, because the analgesic effect is greatly heightened by adding these agents.

1. **Tylenol #3.** Acetaminophen 300 mg with codeine phosphate 30 mg PO Q 4 hr.
2. **Percodan.** Aspirin 325 mg with oxycodone 5 mg PO Q 4 hr.
3. **Percocet.** Acetaminophen 325 mg with oxycodone 5 mg PO Q 4 hr.
4. **Vicodin.** Acetaminophen 500 mg with hydrocodone 5 mg PO Q 4hr.

C. Severe pain (numeric rating 7–10). Although a variety of drugs may be used for treating severe pain, morphine sulfate remains the gold standard for management; no other drug is more effective for analgesia. It is important to emphasize that narcotics should be administered on a round-the-clock basis rather than on an as-needed basis. This provides a more sustained effect, reduces the overall narcotic requirement, and lessens overall patient suffering. Avoid the intramuscular route of administration because erratic absorption can occur, dose titration may be difficult, and onset of action may be delayed.

1. **Morphine sulfate.** For most patients presenting with acute severe pain, parenteral administration of morphine is usually required. For an opioid-naive patient, 1–5 mg of morphine can be administered every 15 minutes (time to peak effect for intravenous dosing) until pain relief has been obtained. PCA can then be used for the next 12–24 hours. Once the patient's opioid requirement over 12–24 hours has been determined, a basal infusion rate can be estimated. Be sure to provide for breakthrough pain by administering a dose equivalent to 10–15% of the 24-hour requirement with a 15-minute lockout interval. Eventually, the patient will need to be converted to oral dosing. This can be accomplished by calculating the daily parenteral dose and converting to an equivalent long-acting oral form of morphine (MS Contin) using a narcotic conversion table (Table I–9). Stop the PCA morphine 6 hours after the first oral dose. Provide coverage for breakthrough pain using immediate-release morphine at a dose of 10% of the daily requirement every hour.

2. **Meperidine (Demerol).** The use of this agent is discouraged in the management of acute pain. Meperidine is metabolized in the liver to normeperidine, which can accumulate in patients with renal insufficiency and result in agitation, confusion, and seizures. It has a short half-life, necessitating every-3-hour dosing.

3. **Fentanyl (Duragesic).** Most patients with severe pain can eventually be adequately managed with oral medication. However, nearly 80% require an alternative route in the 1–2 weeks before death. Transcutaneous fentanyl allows an alternative to resumption of intravenous dosing. Again, using a narcotic conversion table (see Table I–9), the appropriate fentanyl patch (25 µg/hr, 50 µg/hr, 75 µg/hr, 100 µg/hr) can be chosen. Oral transmucosal fentanyl lozenges or 1–2 mL of immediate-release morphine elixir 20 mg/mL (Roxanol) placed between the cheek and gum can provide a route for treating breakthrough pain. The peak effect of the first fentanyl transcutaneous patch may not occur for 12–24 hours. Although the recommended dosing interval is 72 hours, some patients may require every-48-hour dosing. Finally, be aware that fever can enhance absorption of transcutaneous fentanyl.

D. **Adjunctive measures.** Most cancer patients (85–90%) obtain relief with one of the preceding regimens. For those with persistent pain, a variety of measures can be used.

1. **Spinal analgesia (epidural or intrathecal opioids).** These measures are costly and complicated by infections. They should be reserved for patients who cannot tolerate the side effects of systemic opioids.

TABLE I–9. APPROXIMATE DOSING EQUIVALENTS OF COMMONLY PRESCRIBED OPIOIDS

	Equivalent Dose IV	Equivalent Dose PO	Half-life (hours)	Duration (hours)
Morphine	10 mg	30 mg	2–3.5	4–6
Hydromorphone	1.5 mg	7.5 mg	2–3	4–5
Oxycodone	—	30 mg	2–3	4–6
Hydrocodone	—	30 mg	4	4–6
Codeine	120 mg	200 mg	2–3	4–6
Fentanyl[1]	0.1 mg	—	2–4	1–2
Methadone[2]	10 mg	20 mg	15	4–8
Meperidine[3]	75 mg	300 mg	3–4	2–4

[1]Transdermal fentanyl given every 72 hours is equivalent to 1/2 of daily oral morphine dose
[2]Important note: Equivalent doses for methadone and morphine may change at morphine doses greater than 300 mg per day.
[3]Not recommended for routine use

Reproduced with permission from Lawson AP, Smith LM. Are all opioids created equal? Orthopedics 2004;27:1.

2. **Corticosteroids.** Effective for neurologic compression syndromes due to tumor infiltration.
3. **Antidepressants.** Amitriptyline (Elavil), nortriptyline, and desipramine have some analgesic effect, especially for neuropathic pain. The selective serotonin reuptake inhibitors are less effective for neuropathic pain. However, depression can lower the pain threshold; therefore, do not ignore the importance of addressing the cognitive and emotional aspects of terminal malignancy.
4. **Anticonvulsants.** Both gabapentin and carbamazepine may be effective for neuropathic pain.

REFERENCES

Abramowicz M, ed: Drugs for pain. Med Lett Drugs Ther 2000;42:73.

Acute Pain Management Guideline Panel: *Acute Pain Management: Operative or Medical Procedures and Trauma.* Clinical Practice Guideline No. 1. US Dept of Health and Human Services, Public Health Service, Agency for Health Care Policy and Research;1992.

Bruera E, Kim HN: Cancer pain. JAMA 2003;290:2476.

Ducharne J: Acute pain and pain control: State of the art. Ann Emerg Med 2000;35:592.

Martin JJ, Moore GP: Pearls, pitfalls, and updates for pain management. Emerg Med Clin North Am 1997;15:399.

Moynihan TJ: Use of opioids in the treatment of severe pain in terminally ill patients. Mayo Clin Proc 2003;78:1397.

55. POLYCYTHEMIA

I. **Problem.** A 65-year-old man is admitted because of chest pain; his hematocrit is 62%.

II. **Immediate Question. Are there any medical conditions that require the prompt institution of therapy directed at the elevated hematocrit?** Usually, the finding of an elevated hematocrit is incidental, being discovered during the evaluation of a nonacute problem. You should determine that there is no evidence of decompensated congestive heart failure and cardiac or cerebral ischemia that might benefit acutely from phlebotomy. Evidence of profound intravascular volume depletion requiring fluid replacement should be noted.

III. **Differential Diagnosis.** When you are confronted with an elevated hematocrit (> 50% for men, > 45% for women), you can simplify the differential diagnosis by separating polycythemia into three broad diagnostic categories.

   A. **Relative (or apparent) polycythemia.** This condition is a consequence of a decrease in the plasma volume and is generally asymptomatic. Patients can, however, present with venous thrombosis, which can occur with severe volume depletion. Relative polycythemia is associated with obesity, hypertension, and smoking.

   B. **Polycythemia vera.** Onset is usually insidious, often found on routine blood counts for other reasons. Patients with polycythemia vera may present with major venous thrombosis or hemorrhage. Possible symptoms include headache, dizziness, vertigo, tinnitus, diplopia, blurred vision, claudication, angina, symptoms of peptic ulcer disease, pruritus, mucosal bleeding, epistaxis, ecchymoses, and symptoms of deep venous thrombosis, pulmonary embolism, or cerebral vascular thrombosis. Polycythemia vera is usually a disease of middle and later years of life with a peak incidence in the sixth and seventh decades. There is a slight male predominance.

      1. **Clinical criteria for diagnosis have been defined by the Polycythemia Vera Study Group (PVSG). The diagnosis is made by meeting three major criteria, or the first two major criteria and two minor criteria.**

         a. **Major criteria**
            • **Elevated red blood cell (RBC) mass** ($\geq$ 36 mL/kg in a male; $\geq$ 32 mL/kg in a female)
            • **Arterial oxygen saturation > than 92%** in the presence of erythrocytosis.
            • **Splenomegaly**

         b. **Minor criteria**
            • **Platelet count > 400,000/mL**
            • **Elevated leukocyte alkaline phosphatase (LAP) score**
            • **Elevated vitamin B_{12}**
            • **Leukocytosis > 12,000/mL**

    c. **Additional clinically useful criteria that are not part of the PVSG criteria:**
- **Bone marrow hypercellularity associated with megakaryocytic hyperplasia and absent iron stores**
- **Low serum erythropoietin levels (< 30 mU/mL) in the presence of an increased RBC mass**
- **Abnormal marrow proliferative capacity as manifested by formation of erythroid colonies in the absence of exogenous erythropoietin**

C. **Secondary polycythemia.** Typically, only the numbers of erythrocytes in the blood are increased. Secondary polycythemia is classified by whether the polycythemia is physiologically *appropriate* (response to tissue hypoxia) or physiologically *inappropriate* (inappropriate stimulation or secretion of erythropoietin).

  1. **Physiologically appropriate polycythemia**
    a. **High-altitude acclimatization**
    b. **Chronic obstructive pulmonary disease (COPD).** Caused by a pO_2 below 90% saturation. COPD may occur as a result of desaturation at night or with exercise.
    c. **Cardiovascular disease (right-to-left shunts).** Most commonly as a result of congenital heart disease.
    d. **Alveolar hypoventilation.** Sleep apnea.
    e. **High-oxygen-affinity hemoglobins.** The patient may have a positive family history for this condition.
    f. **Congenital deficiency of 2,3-diphosphoglyceric acid**
    g. **Carboxyhemoglobinemia**
    h. **Cobalt ingestion**
  2. **Physiologically inappropriate polycythemia**
    a. **Renal vascular disease**
    b. **Hepatic tumors**
    c. **Uterine leiomyomas**
    d. **Cerebellar hemangioblastomas**
    e. **Renal transplantation**
    f. **Renal cell carcinoma**
    g. **Ovarian carcinoma**
    h. **Renal cysts.** Flank pain or hematuria may be present.
    i. **Pheochromocytoma.** Familial erythrocytosis

IV. **Database**

A. **Physical examination key points**
  1. **Vital signs.** Hypertension is indicative of possible renal vascular disease or pheochromocytoma and may be present with polycythemia vera. Respiratory rate helps to assess the presence of cardiac or pulmonary disease. Fever may indicate underlying systemic illness that may have caused volume depletion or may be a sign of underlying malignancy.

2. **General appearance.** Plethora is not helpful in distinguishing polycythemia vera from secondary polycythemia. Clubbing should be noted as a sign of underlying pulmonary or cardiac disease. Cyanosis is usually an indicator of hypoxemia and might be more suggestive of a secondary polycythemia.

3. **HEENT.** Look for conjunctival injection and, on funduscopic exam, hemorrhages and engorged vessels. Congested mucous membranes are often present and are nonspecific. All these symptoms would be more in favor of polycythemia vera or secondary polycythemia.

4. **Heart.** The presence of any murmurs or an S_3 might either suggest a cardiac etiology or be a sign of cardiac dysfunction caused by polycythemia.

5. **Lungs.** Rales, barrel chest, or diminished breath sounds suggest COPD.

6. **Abdomen.** Hepatomegaly and abdominal masses suggest a secondary cause, whereas splenomegaly is one of the major criteria for diagnosing polycythemia vera.

7. **Extremities.** Clubbing, cyanosis, and edema point to secondary physiologically appropriate causes. Evidence of deep venous thrombosis may be a complication of polycythemia. Excessive marrow proliferation and turnover often lead to increased serum uric acid, and gout is a frequent complication.

8. **Neurologic exam.** Look for focal findings consistent with cerebrovascular accident or tumor. Global findings consistent with hypoxic encephalopathy suggest a secondary cause of polycythemia.

B. **Laboratory data.** If there are obvious clues from the history and/or physical exam, an extensive lab evaluation may not be indicated. For example, a patient with a history of vomiting and diarrhea, poor oral intake, and marked orthostasis and tachycardia with a hematocrit of 55% would be appropriately treated with fluid resuscitation and evaluation of the cause of the volume loss. Unfortunately, the diagnosis is often not obvious and further evaluation is indicated.

1. **Hematocrit.** Generally, a hematocrit > 60% predicts a true increase in the RBC mass; hematocrits < 60% may result from either true or relative increases in the RBC mass.

2. **Platelet count.** A count > 400,000/μL suggests polycythemia vera.

3. **White blood cell count.** Leukocytosis > 12,000/ μL suggests polycythemia vera.

4. **Arterial blood gases.** Oxygen saturation < 90% points to a physiologically appropriate secondary cause.

5. **LAP score.** An elevated LAP score is consistent with polycythemia vera.

6. **Vitamin B_{12}.** Elevated B_{12} or unbound B_{12} binding capacity is seen with polycythemia vera.

7. **p50 (Oxygen affinity of hemoglobin).** This test evaluates the presence of abnormal hemoglobins with high oxygen affinity.
8. **Carboxyhemoglobin level.** An elevated carboxyhemoglobin level points to a physiologically appropriate secondary cause.
9. **Erythropoietin level.** This value is elevated with physiologically inappropriate causes (eg, hepatoma) as well as with physiologically appropriate causes.

C. **Radiologic and other studies**
1. **RBC mass.** A nuclear medicine study to distinguish between relative and true polycythemia. A normal RBC mass with a diminished or low normal plasma volume is characteristic of relative (apparent) polycythemia. If this is found, no further evaluation of the elevated hematocrit is needed. An elevated RBC mass with a normal or increased plasma volume is found in true polycythemia. If this is the case, then further evaluation is indicated to determine whether this represents a primary (polycythemia vera) or secondary polycythemia.
2. **Abdominal and pelvic CT scan.** To look for benign or malignant neoplasms of the liver, kidney, adrenals, and endometrium, and also to look for splenomegaly.
3. **CT scan or MRI scan of the brain.** To rule out cerebellar tumor.
4. **Echocardiogram.** Look for right-to-left shunts. An echocardiogram may also show left ventricular dysfunction, a possible complication of polycythemia.
5. **Pulmonary function studies.** May reveal severe obstructive lung disease.

V. **Plan.** Treatment depends on the type of polycythemia.
A. **Relative (apparent) polycythemia.** This condition requires no therapeutic intervention directed specifically at reduction of the hematocrit, although the underlying disorder needs to be addressed (eg, volume depletion; or the impact of stress-related disorders such as obesity, hypertension, and nicotine addiction). Isovolemic phlebotomy can be used but has not been shown to affect morbidity or mortality.

B. **True polycythemia of secondary cause**
1. In physiologically appropriate secondary polycythemia, it may be difficult to determine whether symptoms are due to the underlying disease or to the elevated hematocrit. Remember that the elevated hematocrit is a physiologically important compensatory mechanism; you must prove that the erythrocytosis is detrimental before phlebotomy. In physiologically inappropriate polycythemia, therapy should be directed at the underlying cause.
2. **Therapeutic phlebotomy** is performed in physiologically appropriate polycythemia if the patient is clearly symptomatic from the elevated hematocrit. If phlebotomy is indicated, the goal should

be to reduce the hematocrit to normal levels. In patients with physiologically inappropriate polycythemia, phlebotomy is reasonable and can be done safely. The goal should be to maintain a hematocrit of 45%, especially if surgery is contemplated.

3. **Cytotoxic therapy** is contraindicated in any type of secondary polycythemia.

C. **Polycythemia vera.** Therapy is directed at overproduction of RBCs and the frequently accompanying platelet disorders.

1. **Phlebotomy.** This procedure is effective in lowering the hematocrit. It is essentially free of complications as long as the patient is monitored for signs of hypovolemia during the phlebotomy and treated appropriately with crystalloid infusion if hypotension occurs; or, the volume should be replaced prophylactically if there is risk that a brief period of hypotension would be detrimental. An expected long-term complication with frequent phlebotomy is iron deficiency. It has been debated whether or not to replace iron in this setting because this increases the phlebotomy requirements. At least two reasons are commonly cited for iron replacement therapy.

   a. As RBCs become progressively more microcytic, there is an actual increase in the whole blood viscosity, which is the reason for doing therapeutic phlebotomy in the first place.

   b. Iron is a cofactor in many enzyme systems; the effects of iron depletion at this level are uncertain.

2. **Cytotoxic therapy.** In patients with a history of thrombotic or bleeding problems, phlebotomy may be inadequate therapy. Cytotoxic therapy should also be considered in patients who require phlebotomy more than once every month or in patients with severe pruritus. These patients benefit from therapy with chemotherapeutic agents or radioactive phosphorus injections.

   a. **Hydroxyurea** has been shown to be effective, appearing to have much less potential for leukemic transformation than other myelosuppressive agents.

   b. **Alkylating agents** such as chlorambucil and busulfan have been associated with an increased risk of secondary leukemias, especially in younger patients.

   c. **^{32}P** is also associated with an increased risk of secondary leukemias. This historically has been touted as the simplest and most effective initial treatment, associated with a response rate of > 90% and a median remission of 2 years.

   d. **Interferon** is particularly useful for patients with severe pruritus. This more recent therapy is not associated with leukemogenesis.

3. **Antiplatelet agents** such as aspirin and dipyridamole (Persantine) are inadequate therapy for polycythemia vera. However, patients with thrombocytosis unresponsive to hydroxyurea may

benefit from either interferon or anagrelide (a platelet-aggregating agent).

4. **Recommendations for therapy by the PVSG:**

   a. Most newly diagnosed patients should undergo phlebotomy to obtain symptomatic control of polycythemia. The rate and volume of phlebotomy are dictated by the patient's clinical condition. The goal is to reduce the hematocrit to the upper normal range (45%).

   b. The therapy chosen to manage disease long term should be influenced by the patient's age, whether or not there is a history of thrombosis and/or severe thrombocytosis. Patients younger than 50 years without thrombosis or severe thrombocytosis may be managed by phlebotomy alone. The risk of thrombosis increases with age; therefore, patients between 50 and 70 years of age may be managed with phlebotomy alone or with myelosuppressive therapy. Patients older than 70 years and those with a history of thrombosis or severe thrombocytosis should receive myelosuppressive therapy. Hydroxyurea is the current myelosuppressive drug of choice.

   c. **Patients with other symptoms** such as pruritus, bone pain, and troublesome splenomegaly are best managed by a myelosuppressive agent.

REFERENCES

Berk PD et al: Therapeutic recommendations in polycythemia vera based on Polycythemia Vera Study Group Protocol. Semin Hematol 1986;23:132.

Berlin NI: Polycythemia vera. Hematol/Oncol Clin North Am 2003;17:1191.

Beutler E, Lichtman MA, Coller RS et al, eds. *Williams Hematology.* 6th ed. McGraw-Hill;2001.

Gruppo Italiano Studio Policitemia: Polycythemia vera: The natural history of 1213 patients followed for 20 years. Ann Intern Med 1995;123:656.

Hoffman R, Benz EJ, Shattil SJ et al, eds. *Hematology: Basic Principles and Practice.* 2nd ed. Churchill Livingstone;1995.

Means RT: Erythrocytosis. In: Greer JP, Foerster J, Lukens F et al, eds. *Wintrobe's Clinical Hematology.* 11th ed. Lippincott Williams & Wilkins;2004:1495.

Means RT: Polycythemia vera. In: Greer JP, Foerster J, Lukens F et al, eds. *Wintrobe's Clinical Hematology.* 11th ed. Lippincott Williams & Wilkins;2004:2259.

56. PRURITUS

I. **Problem.** A 25-year-old man is admitted for lethargy and a hematocrit of 21%. He also complains of severe generalized itching (*pruritus*).

II. **Immediate Questions**

   A. **Is there an associated rash or other skin lesions?** In determining the cause of pruritus, this is the initial question in helping to establish a differential diagnosis. See III. Differential Diagnosis.

B. **Is the pruritus localized or generalized?** The following are conditions causing localized pruritus.

1. **Scalp.** Atopic dermatitis, folliculitis, pediculosis (*Pediculus capitis*), psoriasis, and seborrheic dermatitis.

2. **Hands and arms.** Atopic dermatitis, contact dermatitis, dermatitis herpetiformis, eczema, lichen planus (especially wrists) and scabies (*Sarcoptes scabiei*).

3. **Trunk.** Contact dermatitis, pediculosis (*Pediculus corporis*), pityriasis rosea, scabies, seborrheic dermatitis, tinea corporis, and urticaria.

4. **Groin.** *Candida albicans,* contact dermatitis, erythrasma, lichen planus, pediculosis (*Phthirus pubis*), scabies (*S scabiei*), and tinea cruris.

5. **Anus.** Contact dermatitis, *Enterobius vermicularis, Trichuris trichiura, Neisseria gonorrhoeae,* hemorrhoids, psoriasis, and tinea cruris.

6. **Legs.** Atopic dermatitis, dermatitis herpetiformis, eczema, lichen planus, lichen simplex, stasis dermatitis.

7. **Feet.** Contact dermatitis, erythrasma, and tinea pedis. An erythematous vesicular rash with intense pruritus may be seen at the point of entry of hookworm (*Necator americanus*).

C. **What is the duration of the symptoms?** A recent and sudden onset of pruritus is more often related to an identifiable cause such as a new medication or a new laundry soap.

D. **Has the patient been exposed to any new medications, foods, clothing, detergents, or soaps?** These are common causes of pruritus in both the hospital and the ambulatory care setting.

E. **Are there any other symptoms?** Although uncommon, itching can be the first symptom of an anaphylactic reaction. See Section I, Chapter 4, Anaphylactic Reaction, p 25. Inquire about dyspnea, swelling in and around the mouth, and wheezing. Dyspnea may occur with systemic mastocytosis or Löffler's syndrome (cough, fever as well as dyspnea, eosinophilia, and transient pulmonary infiltrates) associated with *Ascaris lumbricoides, N americanus,* and *Strongyloides stercoralis* infestation. Gastrointestinal symptoms suggest a parasitic infection, carcinoid tumor, or systemic mastocytosis.

F. **Is there a history of chronic medical conditions?** AIDS, uremia, cholestatic liver disease, hypothyroidism, hyperthyroidism, hyperparathyroidism, polycythemia vera, and multiple sclerosis are but a few of the chronic medical conditions associated with pruritus.

G. **Is there a history of travel or residence in the southeastern United States or an area endemic for parasitic infection?** Many parasitic infections may present with pruritus. They may also cause diarrhea, weight loss, intestinal or biliary obstruction, anemia, or malnutrition.

III. Differential Diagnosis. Most cases of pruritus seen in hospitalized patients are related to contact dermatitis or medications. However, one must first rule out life-threatening conditions such as an anaphylactic reaction (see Section I, Chapter 4, Anaphylactic Reaction, p 25).

A. Skin disorders. Pruritus associated with visible skin lesions.

1. **Papulosquamous diseases.** Examples are carcinoid, dermatomyositis, erythrasma (*Corynebacterium minutissimum*), fungal infections (tinea cruris, tinea corporis, tinea pedis, *C albicans*), lichen planus and lichen simplex, lymphoma (cutaneous T-cell), pityriasis rosea, psoriasis, parasitic infections (*A lumbricoides, N americanus, S stercoralis,* and *Trichinella*), and seborrheic dermatitis. Carcinoid is associated with flushing (especially the upper body) and wheals with central clearing.

2. **Bullous diseases.** Includes bullous pemphigoid, dermatitis herpetiformis, pemphigus.

3. **Eczematous diseases.** Atopic dermatitis, contact dermatitis, eczema.

4. **Urticaria.** This can result from a variety of medications (see below), heat or cold, local irritation such as insect bites, or it can be a systemic reaction to foods, intestinal parasites (including *Giardia lamblia*), systemic mastocytosis, or cancer.

5. **Allergic reactions**
   a. **Contact dermatitis.** Most often caused by soaps, detergents, adhesive tapes, and antibacterial ointments (especially neomycin).
   b. **Urticaria.** In hospitalized patients, urticaria is often due to medications such as narcotics (oral and epidural); antibiotics (penicillin and sulfonamides), aspirin, intravenous contrast agents, and thiazide diuretics. If a patient is allergic to aspirin, other nonsteroidal anti-inflammatory drugs (NSAIDs) may cause urticaria, and aspirin is likely to exacerbate chronic urticaria.

6. **Infestation.** Pediculosis (lice) caused by *P capitis* (head louse), *P corporis* (body louse), and *P pubis* (pubic louse); scabies caused by *S scabiei.*

7. **Folliculitis.** *Pseudomonas aeruginosa* may cause "hot tub folliculitis," resulting in erythematous papules. "Hot tub folliculitis" also may be caused by *Staphylococcus aureus*, often involving the scalp or extremities. Also, *Pityrosporum* folliculitis presents with dome-shaped follicular papules and pustules.

8. **Fiberglass dermatitis.** Intense itching with macules and papules. Contact with fiberglass products such as insulation is likely.

9. **Xerosis (dry skin).** More common in the elderly and worse in the winter, colder climates, and dry humidity. Xerosis is aggravated by hot water and multiple baths each day.

10. **Neurotic excoriations.** Seen in patients with depression or obsessive-compulsive disorder.

B. Systemic pruritus. Can be caused by a variety of systemic conditions without an associated rash.

    1. Liver disease. Secondary to bile salts.

        a. Primary biliary cirrhosis. Often the earliest symptom is pruritus. It is usually seen in middle-aged women.

        b. Cholestasis of pregnancy. Usually seen in the third trimester. Pruritus is often the initial symptom. Fatigue is an accompanying symptom.

        c. Biliary obstruction

        d. Hepatitis

    2. Uremia. Seen in many patients with chronic renal failure who receive hemodialysis; may be secondary to associated hyperparathyroidism.

    3. Metabolic. Associated with hypothyroidism, hyperthyroidism, diabetes mellitus, hyperparathyroidism, and gout. Pruritus is infrequently the presenting symptom of diabetes mellitus.

    4. Hematologic

        a. Lymphoma. Pruritus occurs in up to 10% of patients with Hodgkin's lymphoma. Unlike other systemic symptoms (weight loss, fever, and night sweats), pruritus does not affect prognosis.

        b. Leukemia. Various leukemias, including hairy cell leukemia, may have associated pruritus.

        c. Multiple myeloma

        d. Polycythemia vera. Pruritus may be aggravated by hot baths or showers and occurs in about 50% of patients with polycythemia vera (see Section I, Chapter 55, Polycythemia, p 312).

        e. Iron deficiency anemia. Pruritus is seen with iron deficiency, with or without the anemia, and improves with repletion of iron stores.

        f. Systemic mastocytosis. Urticaria may be associated with diarrhea, abdominal cramping, flushing, palpitations, and headache. NSAIDs, penicillin, sulfa-containing medications, alcohol, and morphine may precipitate symptoms. Papules (that may urticate) and macules that are hyperpigmented may be present.

    5. Malignancy. Reported with breast, colon, gastric, lung, prostate, thyroid, and uterine cancer.

    6. Parasitic infections. Including *A lumbricoides, E vermicularis* (pinworm), *G lamblia, N americanus* (hookworm), *S stercoralis, Trichinella* (roundworm), and *T trichiura* (whipworm).

    7. Medications. Patients with pruritus secondary to medications usually present with a rash. Medications causing pruritus without a rash include allopurinol, birth control pills, captopril, cephalosporins, cimetidine, clonidine, diuretics (decrease extracellular fluid and exacerbate xerosis), HMG-CoA reductase in-

hibitors, ketoconazole, narcotics, niacin, penicillin, phenothiazines, and phenytoin.
8. **Rheumatologic.** Sjögren's syndrome.
9. **Neurologic and psychiatric disorders.** Several neurologic and psychiatric conditions may have pruritus as a symptom, including cerebral lesions (infarction, abscess, tumor), Creutzfeldt-Jakob disease, multiple sclerosis, depression, and psychosis.

IV. Database
A. Physical examination key points
1. **Skin.** Examination of the skin is the most important component of the physical exam in determining the cause of pruritus. Examine the entire patient, especially areas of localized pruritus. Be sure to examine areas the patient cannot scratch (mid-upper back). What appears to be a rash may be excoriations secondary to scratching. Chronic neurotic excoriations may appear hypo- or hyperpigmented, whereas areas difficult to reach are spared. Carefully record the distribution and appearance of the rash. Look for lice or nits (pediculosis) and mites, eggs, and burrows (scabies). In dermatophyte or candidal infections, look for fissuring, scaling, maceration between the toes, or irregular, well-demarcated, red-brown macules with fine scales in the intertriginous areas (groin, axillae, buttocks, and underneath the breasts). In dermatomyositis, a red to purple hue is present on the eyelids and extensor surfaces; violaceous flat papules are present over the knuckles.
2. **HEENT.** Stridor suggests a severe allergic reaction. Scleral icterus is seen with cholestasis, a common systemic cause of pruritus. Thyromegaly suggests hypothyroidism or hyperthyroidism as the cause of the pruritus.
3. **Chest.** Wheezing may indicate an anaphylactic reaction.
4. **Abdomen.** Hepatomegaly suggests hepatitis, lymphoma, metastatic disease, or systemic mastocytosis. An enlarged spleen is seen with lymphomas, polycythemia vera, and systemic mastocytosis.
5. **Rectal exam.** Pinworms (*Enterobius vermicularis*) can be seen without magnification and may resemble a fiber or a piece of thread. Adhesive clear tape pressed against the perianal area in the early morning for several days is highly sensitive for detecting pinworms.
6. **Neurologic exam.** A decrease (*fast return*) in the relaxation phase of the reflexes is seen in hyperthyroidism; an increase (*slow return*) in the relaxation phase of the reflexes is seen in hypothyroidism. Decreased proximal muscle strength is seen in dermatomyositis.
7. **Lymph nodes.** Lymphadenopathy suggests lymphoma, carcinoma, or systemic mastocytosis.

B. Laboratory data

1. **Hemogram and differential.** An elevated hematocrit/hemoglobin, white blood cell (WBC) count, and platelet count suggest polycythemia vera. A low mean cell volume and a low mean cellular hemoglobin indicate iron deficiency anemia. A low hematocrit/hemoglobin, WBC count, and platelet count may be seen with lymphoma or carcinoma. Eosinophilia occurs with occult parasitic infection. An elevated WBC count (or decreased WBC count) with blasts, monoclonal lymphocytosis, or granulocytes at all stages of development suggests leukemia as the cause.

2. **Liver function tests.** Total bilirubin, alkaline phosphatase, γ-glutamyltransferase, alanine aminotransferase, and aspartate aminotransferase should be obtained.

3. **Blood urea nitrogen and creatinine.** Uremia needs to be ruled out.

4. **Thyroid function tests.** Thyroid-stimulating hormone to assess for hypothyroidism or hyperthyroidism.

5. **Glucose.** To rule out diabetes mellitus.

6. **Calcium.** To rule out hyperparathyroidism.

7. **Uric acid.** If gout is considered. However, the diagnosis of gout is made by aspiration of joint fluid and examination of the fluid for crystals.

8. **Stool test for ova and parasites.** Consider especially with gastrointestinal symptoms and eosinophilia.

9. **Other tests.** Specific tests such as serum and urine histamine (systemic mastocytosis) and 24-hour urine for 5-HIAA (carcinoid) may be helpful. An arterial blood gas test, leukocyte alkaline phosphatase (LAP) score, and vitamin B_{12} level are helpful if polycythemia vera is considered (see Section I, Chapter 55, Polycythemia, p 312).

C. Radiologic and other studies

1. **Chest x-ray.** May reveal hilar adenopathy (lymphoma), a lung mass, or infiltrates (transient infiltrates seen with several parasitic infections).

2. **KOH (potassium hydroxide) preparation of skin scrapings.** Any rash suspected to be fungal in origin should be scraped with a #15 blade. Scrapings should fall on a microscopic slide recently wiped with an alcohol pad (which will help keep the scrapings on the slide). Add 1 drop of KOH (10–20%), place a coverslip over the scrapings and KOH, and view under the microscope at magnifications of 10× and 40×. Heating the slide under an alcohol flame may facilitate visualization of fungal elements.

3. **Wood's ultraviolet light.** Erythrasma has a coral-red or pink color.

4. **Skin biopsy.** May be very helpful in establishing the diagnosis in systemic mastocytosis and various dermatologic conditions. The

biopsy specimen should be sent for direct immunofluorescence if a primary blistering process is suspected (ie, bullous pemphigoid).

5. **Bone marrow biopsy.** May be needed if lymphoma, leukemia, multiple myeloma, or systematic mastocytosis is suspected.
6. **Red blood cell mass scan and spleen scan.** Helpful if polycythemia vera is considered.

V. Plan. Unless caused by a significant systemic disease or as an early sign of an anaphylactic reaction, pruritus usually does not require immediate treatment. However, pruritus may be a clue to a major illness. The patient's comfort during his or her hospitalization can be greatly enhanced by some simple measures until the underlying cause is established and specific therapy is instituted.

A. Specific causes
1. **Anaphylactic reaction.** See Section I, Chapter 4, Anaphylactic Reaction, V, p 27.
2. **Xerosis.** Patients should limit the amount of time in the bath or shower and the number of baths per week and use mild soaps. Immediately after bathing, they should apply an emollient. Patients should avoid any creams with an alcohol base. Humidifying the air and the use of petroleum and steroid ointment may also help.
3. **Uremia.** Cholestyramine, intravenous lidocaine, or ultraviolet B light may relieve the pruritus associated with uremia.
4. **Cholestasis.** Cholestyramine should be considered.
5. **Hematologic.** Aspirin, cyproheptadine, and ultraviolet B light are beneficial in treating pruritus secondary to polycythemia vera. Pruritus secondary to iron deficiency resolves with iron replacement.
6. **Contact dermatitis.** Removal of the offending agent is essential. Topical steroids can be used for mild or very localized cases. Systemic steroids (prednisone 0.5–1.0 mg/kg/day for 2–3 days and then a tapering dose schedule) can be used in more severe and generalized cases.
7. **Eczematous dermatitis.** Prescribe emollients and steroid ointment.

B. Symptomatic treatment
1. **Antihistamines (H_1 blockers).** May provide relief. Nonsedating antihistamines (in the morning) such as cetirizine (Zyrtec), fexofenadine (Allegra), and loratadine (Claritin) may be less effective in relieving pruritus than other H_1 blockers. Patients should use the sedating antihistamines in the evening.
2. **Diphenhydramine (Benadryl).** Give 25–50 mg PO or IV Q 6–8 hr.
3. **Cyproheptadine (Periactin).** Give 4 mg PO Q 8 hr.
4. **Hydroxyzine (Atarax or Vistaril).** Give 25–50 mg Q 6–8 hr.

5. **Topical agents.** Camphor, menthol, phenol, and pramoxine are commonly used. Camphor, phenol, and pramoxine provide relief through local anesthetic effect. Menthol cools the skin. Other topical agents often used are Eucerin cream and Sarna lotion. Menthol and phenol are contained in Sarna lotion.
6. **Other.** Additional agents that have been shown to be effective are opiate antagonists (naloxone), doxepin (a tricyclic antidepressant with greater efficacy as an H_1 blocker than diphenhydramine or hydroxyzine), and capsaicin.

REFERENCES

Greco PJ, Ende J: Pruritus: A practical approach. J Gen Intern Med 1992;7:340.
Fleisher AB: Pruritus in the elderly. Adv Dermatol 1995;10:41.
Kantor GR, Lookingbill DP: Pruritus. In: Sams WM, Lynch PJ, eds. *Principles and Practice of Dermatology.* Churchill Livingstone;1990:861.
Yosipovitch G, David M: The diagnostic and therapeutic approach to idiopathic generalized pruritus. Int J Dermatol 1999;38:881.

57. PULMONARY ARTERY CATHETER PROBLEMS

See also Section I, Chapter 10, Central Venous Line Problems, p 56; and Section III, Chapter 12, Pulmonary Artery Catheterization, p 449).

I. **Problem.** A 50-year-old man is admitted to the coronary care unit (CCU) with an anterior myocardial infarction (MI). A pulmonary artery (PA) catheter is placed. You are notified 24 hours later by the CCU nurse that he is having trouble interpreting the pressure tracings.

II. **Immediate Questions**

A. **What does the waveform look like?** The PA waveform varies with inspiration and expiration and has a characteristic systolic/diastolic waveform. (See Figure III–10, p 455; and Section III, Chapter 12, Pulmonary Artery Catheterization, p 449.)

B. **Is there a waveform when the catheter is tapped?** The absence of a waveform or a "dampened" tracing suggests that the catheter is not patent, or that there are technical difficulties including transducer malfunction, cracked hub, loose connections, incorrect stopcock positions, too-tight skin sutures, and too-tight plastic sleeve diaphragms.

C. **Can the catheter be flushed? Can blood be withdrawn?** If the catheter cannot be flushed or blood withdrawn, the catheter may not be patent. The catheter may be kinked, or a venous thrombus may be obstructing the catheter. (See Section I, Chapter 10, Central Venous Line Problems, p 56.)

D. **Is the catheter in permanent wedge?** After a period of time within the patient's circulation, PA catheters tend to become softer and more pliable and may migrate distally. With a decreasing pulmonary pressure, the same effect may occur as the pulmonary vascular bed shrinks relative to the catheter position. The catheter may end up wedged with its balloon deflated, a situation analogous to a pulmonary embolus. The catheter position must be corrected as soon as possible. Careful evaluation is needed to ensure that the problem is really a case of permanent wedge and not a kink or system malfunction. If all else fails to help distinguish the various causes of a flat tracing, wedge position can be confirmed with blood gas sampling, showing saturation in the arterial range, as opposed to the mixed venous range usually found when blood gases are sampled from the PA position.

E. Can a wedge tracing be obtained with the balloon inflated? If not, the balloon may have ruptured or the catheter may have been partially removed. *Do not continue to inject air if the balloon has ruptured,* because the air is injected directly into the PA.

F. Are there any associated symptoms? Chest pain may result from a PA catheter in permanent wedge, resulting in a pulmonary infarction. Hemoptysis can result from pulmonary infarction or from PA rupture or erosion. This is usually associated with inflation of the balloon in a vessel smaller than the balloon, rupturing the PA with entry of blood into the airways. Hemoptysis usually results and can sometimes be severe, but is rarely life-threatening. A fever may be secondary to catheter infection, catheter sepsis, or pulmonary infarction.

G. What is the relative necessity of the PA catheter? If critical measurements are being made, such as hourly PA wedge pressure readings, the situation is more serious than if the line has outlived its usefulness and can be removed.

III. **Differential Diagnosis.** Problems with PA catheters (Swan-Ganz) can be conveniently divided into problems occurring inside the patient and problems occurring outside the patient.

    A. Outside the patient

        1. Transducer error. This type of error often results in a "dampened" or flattened tracing and/or in an erratic nonlinear response to pressure changes. This has become an infrequent problem with the development of very reliable disposable transducers, but occasionally even these transducers can be defective or can become damaged by rough handling or exposure to extreme conditions of light and heat. Bubbles within the transducer setup and any improper mounting also result in low-quality pressure tracings.

        2. Cables. As with most electrical systems, particularly nondisposable systems, cables are a common source of problems. The best way to evaluate a cable is to simply use a different one, after first making sure that the transducer setup and its linear response are appropriate, that the system is properly zero-balanced, and that the monitor is set on the proper pressure scale for the measurements being made.

3. **Monitor-related problems.** Perhaps the most common monitor-related problems arise when the monitor is set on an improper scale or when the transducer/monitor setup is not properly zero-balanced.

B. **Inside the patient**
   1. **Catheter migration.** The catheter may have moved from its original insertion position, migrating either distally or proximally. Distal migration may result in a permanent wedge.
   2. **Thrombosis.** A blood clot in the pressure-monitoring lumen may preclude good-quality pressure recordings.
   3. **Kinks.** The most common sites for kinking are at the skin surface, under the clavicle, and at the proximal and distal ends of the sheath. Kinks are another cause of poor-quality tracings.
   4. **Malfunctioning balloon.** If the catheter does not wedge, the balloon may have ruptured or the catheter may have migrated proximally. *Do not continue to inject air into the catheter system if a wedge tracing does not appear,* because a ruptured balloon may be the cause.

IV. **Database**
   A. **Physical examination key points**
      1. **General exam.** As in most technical areas of medicine, be sure that the information provided by your technology correlates with your clinical assessment.
      2. **Vital signs.** The presence of fever suggests catheter infection or sepsis, especially if the catheter has been in place longer than 3 days.
   B. **Laboratory data**
      1. **Blood gases.** A blood gas sample obtained from the distal port of the catheter can be helpful in determining whether a PA catheter is in permanent wedge position. If the catheter is wedged, the oxygen saturation will approximate arterial oxygen saturation, whereas mixed venous saturation is found in pulmonary artery locations.
      2. **Blood cultures.** These should be obtained in the presence of a fever or elevated white cell count with an increase in segmented and banded neutrophils.
   C. **Radiologic and other studies**
      1. **Chest x-ray.** A chest x-ray is useful in determining whether the catheter is kinked or is in the correct position. Permanent wedge may be suggested by a markedly distal location of the catheter tip. After injection with air, a deflated balloon also points to balloon rupture.
      2. **Culture of PA catheter.** If catheter-related sepsis or infection is suspected, the PA catheter and the introducer sheath must be re-

moved, and at least the subcutaneous portion of the introducer sheath should be sent for culture. It is unlikely that routinely culturing the PA catheter itself would yield additional useful information in most cases.

V. Plan. For replacement of a PA catheter, see Section III, Chapter 12, Pulmonary Artery Catheterization, p 449.

  A. Problems outside the patient. If simple tapping on the catheter does not result in a waveform, the cause clearly resides outside the patient. Faulty line connections and stopcocks that are improperly set up, as well as transducer, cable, and monitor-related problems, should be addressed first.

  B. Problems inside the patient. When a good waveform is obtained by tapping the catheter, the problem most likely resides within the patient.

    1. Permanent wedge. This problem is reported much more frequently than actually exists. Often, a well-placed PA catheter is withdrawn when the position is fine.

      a. System inspection. Thoroughly inspect the PA catheter system before you attempt to move the catheter. The transducer should be evaluated for proper functioning. The system should be evaluated for leaks, loose connections, and similar mechanical problems, before any manipulation of the catheter.

      b. Chest x-ray. For PA catheter positioning and evaluation of the balloon. If the catheter is truly stuck in wedge, the chest x-ray will show the catheter to be in the distal pulmonary circulation. Less commonly, the balloon will not deflate because the catheter is kinked.

      c. Check the oxygen saturation. As mentioned earlier, the oxygen saturation will be close to arterial when obtained from a truly wedged catheter.

      d. Catheter withdrawal. If the catheter is really wedged and the waveform cannot be returned to the expected waveform by manual aspiration or flushing of the catheter, withdraw the catheter centimeter by centimeter while flushing between each withdrawal using a pressure-bag flush system. During catheter withdrawal, the balloon must always be completely deflated. When an appropriate waveform for PA position returns, the balloon should be reinflated to be certain that the catheter will wedge when desired. With most properly placed PA catheters, the balloon needs to be inflated with only 1–1.5 mL of air to obtain the wedge tracing. Once the balloon is deflated, the original PA pressure waveform should return within 3–5 heartbeats.

    2. A balloon that will not wedge. In most cases, the catheter has been pulled back too far, or the balloon is not functioning. The catheter should not be advanced unless a sterile sleeve protects the catheter portion lying outside the patient. If the balloon is malfunctioning, the catheter should be removed and a new one placed through the same introducer sheath if hemodynamic monitoring is still needed.

3. **Inaccurate or poorly reproducible cardiac outputs**
   a. In cases of apparently inappropriate cardiac outputs, be sure that the constant on the cardiac output computer is correct for the size/type of PA catheter used. The thermodilution technique is not accurate in patients with very low cardiac outputs (CO) or significant tricuspid regurgitation. Use the mixed venous oxygen saturation (should be below normal if CO is indeed low), and the Fick oxygen method to confirm the low CO. With the Fick method, the CO is calculated as the oxygen consumption (VO_2) divided by the difference between arterial O_2 content (CaO_2) and venous O_2 content (CvO_2).

   $$CO = VO_2 \div (CaO_2 - CvO_2)$$

   The oxygen content of blood is calculated as the hemoglobin concentration (in grams per deciliter) × 1.36 (amount of O_2 in milliliters contained by 1 g of hemoglobin that is 100% saturated; values of 1.34 and 1.39 have also been used) × measured O_2 saturation (SaO_2 or SvO_2, as appropriate).

   The amount of dissolved oxygen in the plasma is negligible and can be ignored. When a directly measured O_2 consumption is used, we call this the "direct Fick" method, but if an assumed normal O_2 consumption of 125 mL/min/m^2 is used instead, we call it "indirect Fick." **Caution:** Remember that to do these calculations correctly all volumes must be eventually expressed in the same units: mL, dL, or L.

   b. If no cardiac output is obtained, the catheter may not be properly connected to the computer, or the wire connecting the thermistor to the computer may be fractured. Most computers flash a code indicating that the catheter is at fault in this circumstance.

4. **PA rupture or erosion.** Treatment depends on the severity of the bleeding. It is prudent to remove the PA catheter; if it is crucial for managing the patient, it can be replaced. The new catheter should be directed toward the opposite lung. This procedure requires fluoroscopy. Careful attention to the adequacy of ventilation and blood pressure, serial chest x-rays, and a low threshold for requesting cardiothoracic surgery consultation are advisable in this situation. The complication of rupture or erosion can be avoided by always inflating the balloon slowly and carefully and by monitoring the pressure waveform so that the catheter is not overwedged or left in a "permanent" wedge position. For replace-

ment of central venous catheters, see Section III, Chapter 6, Central Venous Catheterization, p 426.

REFERENCES

Davidson CJ, Bonow RO: Cardiac catheterization. In: Braunwald E, Zipes DP, Libby P, eds. *Heart Disease: A Textbook of Cardiovascular Medicine.* 6th ed. Saunders;2001:359.

Sprung CL, ed: *The Pulmonary Artery Catheter: Methodology and Clinical Applications.* 2nd ed. Critical Care Research Associates;1993.

58. SEIZURES

I. **Problem.** A 65-year-old man experiences a seizure-like episode the day after being admitted for a fractured hip.

II. **Immediate Questions**

A. **Did the patient have an epileptic seizure, or could something else have happened to explain this behavioral change?** The most common cause of a loss or alteration of consciousness is not an epileptic seizure. Disorders that may be confused with an epileptic seizure include syncope (as a result of orthostatic hypotension, arrhythmia, valvular heart disease, or vasovagal syncope), transient ischemic attack, transient global amnesia, decorticate posturing from increased intracranial pressure, sleep disorder (REM sleep disorder, or somnambulism), confusional episode associated with migraine headache, hypoglycemia, panic attack or fugue state, neuroleptic malignant syndrome, and a psychogenic seizure. A detailed history from the patient and a reliable witness usually help to distinguish an epileptic seizure from other disorders.

B. **What type of epileptic seizure did the patient experience?** Seizures are classified according to whether they are generalized or focal in onset (Table I–10). Primary generalized seizures occur without warning and have nonlocalizing behavioral changes, whereas a warning, or aura, may precede partial seizures that exhibit localizing behavioral changes. Seizures that are localized in onset could be due to a focal, structural brain lesion.

C. **Was the seizure symptomatic or idiopathic?** Idiopathic seizures have no known cause and account for 50% of all cases. They often occur in younger patients who have a family history of idiopathic seizures. Symptomatic seizures indicate that the seizure is a symptom of another disorder that affects the central nervous system (CNS) (see III. Differential Diagnosis).

D. **Does the patient have a history of previous epileptic seizures?** If the patient were taking an anticonvulsant before admission, the drug may have been discontinued, taken irregularly or not at all, or other

TABLE I–10. CLASSIFICATION BY SEIZURE TYPE.

Primary generalized seizures
Primary generalized tonic-clonic seizures
Absence seizures
Myoclonic seizures
Tonic seizures
Clonic seizures
Atonic seizures
Partial seizures
Simple partial seizures
Complex partial seizures
Partial seizures evolving to $2°$ generalized seizures

medications may have altered the absorption or metabolism of the anticonvulsant, leading to subtherapeutic drug levels and breakthrough seizures. The most common cause of recurrent seizures in a patient previously well controlled is poor compliance. Other causes of uncontrolled seizures include severe CNS disease, incorrect diagnosis of epilepsy, wrong anticonvulsant for that seizure type, and prescribed anticonvulsant doses that are subtherapeutic.

   E. **Does the patient have a history of alcohol or drug abuse?** Alcohol or drug withdrawal may trigger an epileptic seizure. Alcohol withdrawal seizures commonly occur 12–24 hours after stopping alcohol intake in a person who drinks daily or binge drinks for 5 or more days. The seizures are usually generalized tonic-clonic and self-limited, but status epilepticus may occur and should be treated similarly to other episodes of status. Additional causes of epileptic seizures such as meningitis, head injury, electrolyte abnormalities, hypoglycemia, and thiamine deficiency should be considered when seizures occur in the setting of alcohol and drug abuse.

III. **Differential Diagnosis.** An epileptic seizure is the result of abnormal electrical activity of the cerebral cortex and may result in loss of consciousness or confusion, abnormal motor activity, or sensory sensations. Generalized tonic-clonic seizures are typified by loss of consciousness with severe, tonic stiffening of muscles followed by clonic jerking. The entire episode usually lasts 2–3 minutes, after which the patient may sleep for several hours and later awaken confused. Partial seizures that secondarily generalize and are symptomatic are more commonly the presenting seizure type in older adults, especially the elderly. Idiopathic primary generalized seizures are more likely seen in children and young adults.

   A. **Head trauma.** Recent or remote head trauma that is sufficient to produce loss of consciousness or prolonged amnesia, a depressed skull fracture, dural tear, intracranial hemorrhage, or focal neurologic deficits is associated with a high risk of later development of epileptic seizures.

B. Infections. Bacterial, fungal, or viral meningitis or encephalitis; cerebral abscess; mycotic aneurysm; or parasitic infestation by cysticercosis, toxoplasmosis, or paragonimiasis may cause epileptic seizures.

C. Stroke. A common cause of epileptic seizures in the elderly. Cortical vein thrombosis is especially epileptogenic, but other vascular causes include subarachnoid hemorrhage, arteriovenous malformation, CNS vasculitis, hypertensive encephalopathy, or eclampsia.

D. Carcinoma. Epileptic seizures may be the presenting symptom in a primary or metastatic brain tumor. Common cancers that metastasize to the brain are lung, breast, kidney, and gastrointestinal cancers and melanoma. Meningeal carcinomatosis, paraneoplastic disorders such as limbic encephalitis, and cancer-associated vascular disorders should be considered.

E. Drugs. Toxic or therapeutic doses of certain drugs may precipitate an epileptic seizure. They include psychotropic agents, isoniazid, high doses of penicillin, lidocaine, clozapine, theophylline, chemotherapeutic agents (etoposide, ifosfamide, and *cis*-platinum); and drugs of abuse such as amphetamines, cocaine, heroin, gamma hydroxybutyrate (GHB), and phencyclidine. Abrupt withdrawal of alcohol, benzodiazepines, or barbiturates also causes seizures. Certain medications such as bupropion and phenothiazines can decrease the seizure threshold.

F. Neurodegenerative disorders. Alzheimer's disease is associated with a high risk of seizures, which are usually myoclonic but can be generalized tonic-clonic seizures. Down's syndrome patients often develop Alzheimer's disease and may have epileptic seizures as a presenting feature of Alzheimer's dementia

G. Metabolic or toxic disorders. Hypoglycemia, hyponatremia, hypocalcemia, hypomagnesemia, hypophosphatemia, uremia, severe alkalosis or acidosis, hepatic failure, and possibly hyperkalemia may precipitate epileptic seizures. Osmolar changes with hemodialysis for acute or chronic renal failure can cause seizures with multifocal myoclonus sometimes preceding generalized tonic-clonic seizures. Myoclonic seizures may occur in the setting of severe hypoxic encephalopathy after cardiopulmonary arrest. Toxins including methanol, ethylene glycol, lead, or carbon monoxide (CO) poisoning (with CO levels > 50%) have been associated with seizures.

H. Nonepileptic psychogenic seizures. Caused by malingering or a conversion disorder, psychogenic seizures (or pseudoseizures) may be difficult to distinguish from an epileptic seizure. Prolonged complex movements, shaking side to side, pelvic thrusting, and failure to respond to therapeutic doses of anticonvulsants in a patient with a psychiatric history, no risk factors for epileptic seizures, and a normal exam without postictal confusion following the seizure are clues that the behavioral change is a nonepileptic psychogenic seizure.

I. **Other causes.** Mesial temporal sclerosis, systemic lupus erythematosus, acute intermittent porphyria, Whipple's disease, sickle cell anemia, sarcoidosis involving the CNS, or neurofibromatosis in adulthood may be associated with epileptic seizures. Porphyria should be considered as a cause if the seizure activity is exacerbated by standard anticonvulsants. Genetic disorders such as tuberous sclerosis, inherited inborn errors of amino acid metabolism (phenylketonuria), glycogen or lipid storage diseases, cerebral malformations, and prenatal or postnatal birth injuries usually present in childhood with epileptic seizures.

IV. **Database**

A. **Physical examination key points.** Although a detailed history and general physical examination are necessary for all patients who present with an epileptic seizure, key points include the following:

1. **Vital signs.** The blood pressure is often normal after a seizure, but hypotension in an elderly person may signal a recent myocardial infarction due to the profound muscular exertion accompanying a generalized tonic-clonic seizure. Hypertension may suggest a cause of the seizure, such as hypertensive encephalopathy, toxemia, or a recent stroke.

2. **Skin.** Skin changes of neurocutaneous syndromes including tuberous sclerosis, Sturge–Weber syndrome, ataxia-telangiectasia, von Hippel–Lindau syndrome, and neurofibromatosis can give clues regarding the cause of an epileptic seizure. Inspection of the skin for needle tracks might indicate illegal drug use, and a rash could suggest an underlying vasculitis or connective tissue disease. Enlarged lymph nodes could imply HIV or other infections, malignancy, sarcoidosis, or systemic lupus erythematosus.

3. **HEENT.** A deeply bitten and bleeding tongue is strongly associated with generalized tonic-clonic seizures and rarely if ever occurs in psychogenic seizures. Inspection of the skull for recent or remote head injuries, burr holes, or craniotomy scar can provide significant clues regarding the cause of the patient's seizure. Papilledema on funduscopic examination implies intracranial hypertension from a tumor, infection, hemorrhage, or brain edema. Measuring head circumference is important to detect microcephaly and an associated disorder of maldevelopment, which can cause epileptic seizures. Meningismus, or nuchal rigidity, could signify a neck injury, meningitis, or a subarachnoid hemorrhage.

4. **Heart and lungs.** A cardiac dysrhythmia or valvular abnormality could suggest syncope rather than an epileptic seizure. After a

seizure, aspiration pneumonia or noncardiogenic pulmonary edema may lead to respiratory insufficiency.

5. **Genitourinary system and rectum.** Urinary or stool incontinence may occur with an epileptic seizure, although some patients with psychogenic seizures may be incontinent, too.

6. **Back and extremities.** Severe muscle contraction with generalized tonic-clonic seizures can cause vertebral body fractures in osteoporotic patients, whereas falls may cause fractures of long bones.

B. **Neurologic exam.** A detailed neurologic examination is necessary to identify the location of the lesion within the CNS, which may be the source of the epileptic seizure.

1. **Mental status.** After an epileptic seizure, the patient may be confused for an hour or longer. After a brief syncopal event or psychogenic seizure, the patient is usually alert and lucid.

2. **Cranial nerves.** An asymmetric enlarged pupil could be an early sign of uncal herniation. Small pupils occur with metabolic disorders or narcotics; fixed and dilated pupils can accompany severe hypoxic encephalopathy or the use of drugs such as cocaine and atropine. Both upper and lower facial weakness on one side could suggest a basal skull fracture, but weakness limited to the lower face on one side occurs with a contralateral brain stem lesion or cerebral hemisphere lesion. An isolated visual field deficit may pinpoint a lesion in the occipital cortex.

3. **Motor and sensory.** Focal motor or sensory findings, asymmetric reflexes, and an abnormal Babinski reflex may occur subsequent to the epileptic seizure and aid in localizing the seizure focus. Transient hemiparesis after the seizure could represent a Todd's paralysis and point to a lesion or seizure focus in the contralateral motor cortex.

C. **Laboratory data**

1. **Serum glucose and electrolytes.** Rule out hypoglycemia, hypocalcemia, and hyponatremia or a hyperosmolar state due to hyperglycemia or hyponatremia. A high anion gap metabolic acidosis secondary to high lactate levels often occurs with a generalized tonic-clonic seizure. Methanol or ethylene glycol poisoning can also accompany a high anion gap metabolic acidosis.

2. **Renal profile and creatine phosphokinase.** Rule out acute or chronic renal failure. Rhabdomyolysis with myoglobinuria can complicate a generalized tonic-clonic seizure and precipitate acute renal failure.

3. **Drug screen.** Consider whether the clinical history suggests the use of cocaine, amphetamines, phencyclidine, barbiturates, benzodiazepines, alcohol, methanol, or ethylene glycol.

4. **Levels of prescribed anticonvulsants.** Perform immediately to determine whether the recent seizure is due to subtherapeutic an-

ticonvulsant levels, which could be due to poor patient compliance, prescribed subtherapeutic doses, or interference with absorption or metabolism of the anticonvulsant. If the level is within the therapeutic range, the dose can sometimes be increased. Or, if it is feared that increasing the dose will lead to drug toxicity, a new anticonvulsant may need to be started.

5. **Complete blood count with differential.** A high white blood cell count could indicate an underlying infection. However, after a generalized tonic-clonic seizure, a postictal leukocytosis may occur but can be distinguished from a leukemoid response to an infection by the presence of primarily mature granulocytes with few immature forms and a relative lymphocytopenia.

6. **Arterial blood gases.** To rule out hypoxemia or acidosis as a cause or complication of the epileptic seizure. After a generalized tonic-clonic seizure, the patient hyperventilates to correct the metabolic and respiratory acidosis that occurred during the seizure. A severe alkalosis can also cause seizures.

7. **Other tests.** Consider obtaining prothrombin time, partial thromboplastin time, and platelet count if a lumbar puncture is anticipated. Sedimentation rate or antinuclear antibody should be obtained if the clinical findings suggest a vasculitis or lupus.

D. Radiologic and other studies

1. **CT or MRI brain scan.** A neuroimaging study should be performed on all patients who present with new-onset seizures and in whom no other cause of seizure is apparent. A CT head scan is usually more convenient in the emergency situation and may provide adequate images when the patient is postictally confused and cannot lie quietly for an MRI scan. Later, if no cause of the seizure is discovered and an MRI was not initially obtained, an MRI with and without contrast should be completed.

2. **Lumbar puncture.** It should be done immediately if meningitis, encephalitis, or meningeal carcinomatosis is suspected, or if there is clinical suspicion for a subarachnoid hemorrhage not revealed by neuroimaging. A neuroimaging study should precede the lumbar puncture, especially if focal neurologic findings or papilledema suggest increased intracranial pressure. See Section III, Chapter 10, Lumbar Puncture, p 000.

3. **Electroencephalogram (EEG).** Usually not necessary as an emergency procedure. However, EEG is helpful in classifying epileptic seizures. An interictal recording may demonstrate focal epileptiform activity consistent with a partial seizure disorder, whereas generalized epileptiform activity indicates a primary generalized seizure disorder. Although an interictal EEG is usually abnormal, a normal interictal EEG recording does not exclude the diagnosis of an epileptic seizure disorder. An immediate EEG is essential for monitoring patients in a pentobarbital coma for status

epilepticus, or for monitoring a comatose patient with suspected subclinical epileptic seizures as a cause of the coma.

4. **Chest x-ray and electrocardiogram.** Helpful if aspiration pneumonia, noncardiogenic pulmonary edema, or an acute myocardial infarction is suspected as a complication of the epileptic seizure.

V. **Plan.** Support life functions with the ABCs (airway, breathing, and circulation) of cardiopulmonary resuscitation and protect the patient from self-inflicted injury during the seizure.

A. **Emergency management.** Place the patient in a lateral decubitus position with a suction device to prevent aspiration if vomiting occurs. Move objects away from the patient or place padding between the patient and the floor or other immovable items. Do not place objects in the patient's mouth or try to force the mouth open because these measures are unnecessary and may lead to injury to the patient or yourself.

B. **Seizure control.** See Section VII, Therapeutics, for a discussion of drugs listed here.

1. Most seizures are self-limited, last no more than 2–3 minutes, and may not need immediate treatment until a detailed evaluation is completed. *Status epilepticus* is recurrent seizures without complete recovery between seizures. Any seizure type can evolve into status epilepticus, but generalized tonic-clonic status epilepticus is a medical emergency requiring prompt treatment to prevent serious morbidity and mortality. In clinical practice, a generalized tonic-clonic seizure lasting more than 5–10 minutes or two generalized tonic-clonic seizures occurring in quick succession without the patient fully recovering between seizures should be treated as status epilepticus.

2. Immediately establish IV access and collect a serum specimen for laboratory tests. If hypoglycemia is a suspected cause, do not wait for the results of the laboratory tests. Promptly give 50 mL of 50% dextrose IV. If there is clinical suspicion of chronic alcohol abuse or another disorder associated with nutritional deprivation, give 50 mg thiamine IV with dextrose to prevent precipitation of Wernicke's encephalopathy.

3. For generalized tonic-clonic status epilepticus with the patient in an active seizure, give lorazepam 0.1 mg/kg at 1–2 mg/min IV, and repeat, if necessary, in 15 minutes (maximum dose 0.2 mg/kg or 5–10 mg total; doses > 0.2 mg/kg are usually unnecessary or ineffective). Diazepam may also be used at doses of 5–10 mg at 1–2 mg/min IV, and repeated, if necessary, in 15 minutes (maximum dose 20–40 mg). However, lorazepam may be preferred because of its longer effect. Both drugs may cause respiratory depression (especially if given with phenobarbital) and may require intubation and ventilatory support.

4. If the patient is in status epilepticus but not in an active seizure, fosphenytoin can be given to prevent further seizures by loading intravenously with 15–20 mg phenytoin equivalents (PE)/kg at 100–150 mg PE/min. PE may also be used intravenously with a loading dose of 15–20 mg/kg but must be given at slower rates of ≤50 mg/min to avoid significant hypotension. PE extravasation can cause severe skin sloughing. Another option would be to load with IV valproate at doses of 15–20 mg/kg at 1.5–3 mg/kg/min. Phenobarbital with a loading dose of 10–20 mg/kg at 50–100 mg/min IV (maximum dose of 1.5–2 g) may be added if seizures recur with maximal doses of fosphenytoin, PE, or valproate.

5. If you are unable to immediately secure an IV access and the patient is in an active seizure, diazepam rectal gel may be given at a dose of 0.2 mg/kg (maximum 20 mg). Midazolam may be given IM at a dose of 0.07–0.08 mg/kg (approximately 5 mg), or fosphenytoin can be given IM at doses of 15–20 mg/kg.

6. Generalized tonic-clonic status epilepticus refractory to the above measures may require general anesthesia with an agent such as pentobarbital (by this time neurologic consultation and emergency EEG are necessary to exclude psychogenic seizures or other disorders that may masquerade as refractory status epilepticus). The loading dose for pentobarbital is 15–20 mg/kg IV at 25–50 mg/min. Additional doses of 25–50 mg every 2–5 minutes may be given until a burst suppression pattern appears on EEG recording; then, a continuous infusion is maintained at 1–2 mg/kg/hr. The patient must be intubated, and a central venous pressure monitor is required to monitor volume status. Dopamine or dobutamine drips may be necessary to treat hypotension because of the cardiac depressant effects of pentobarbital. Other options for refractory status include IV midazolam 0.2 mg/kg bolus, maintained at 0.75–10 μg m/kg/min; or IV propofol 1–2 mg/kg bolus, maintained at 2–10 mg/kg/hr. Continuous EEG monitoring is maintained throughout the pentobarbital coma to identify development of subclinical status epilepticus.

7. Complications from generalized tonic-clonic status include acute myocardial infarction, rhabdomyolysis, acute renal failure, aspiration pneumonia, pulmonary edema, hyperkalemia, severe acidosis, compression fractures, and trauma. These complications should be anticipated, closely monitored, and treated early to minimize their effects.

8. Admit the patient for observation and treatment if he or she has had status epilepticus, first generalized tonic-clonic seizure, associated disorder requiring hospitalization (eg, acute stroke, brain edema, meningitis, drug toxicity). Patients with a history of epilepsy do not necessarily require admission if a source of their breakthrough seizure is found and corrected (eg, subtherapeutic anticonvulsant level due to incomplete compliance) or if the

seizure type would not predict serious harm to the patient if released from the hospital (eg, absence or brief myoclonic seizure, or some complex partial or simple partial seizures).

9. Not all isolated seizures need to be treated with an anticonvulsant. Epileptic seizures due to alcohol or drug withdrawal, drug abuse, severe sleep deprivation, or seizures associated with acute illness such as hypoglycemia do not need to be treated. If the patient has a history of brain injury, a structural lesion of the brain such as a tumor or arteriovenous malformation, or an abnormal EEG with epileptiform activity, or if the presentation with status epilepticus is at the onset, treatment with an anticonvulsant to prevent further seizures is recommended.

REFERENCES

Blum AS: Recurrent generalized and partial seizures. In: Johnson RT, Griffin JW, McArthur JC, eds. *Current Therapy in Neurologic Disease.* 6th ed. Mosby;2002:46.

Browne TR, Holmes GL: Epilepsy. N Engl J Med 2001;344:1145.

Delanty N, Vaughan CJ, French JA: Medical causes of seizures. Lancet 1998;352:383.

Leppik IE: *Contemporary Diagnosis and Management of the Patient with Epilepsy.* 5th ed. Handbooks in Health Care;2000.

Manno EM: New management strategies in the treatment of status epilepticus. Mayo Clin Proc 2003;78:509.

Pedley TA: The epilepsies. In: Goldman L, Ausiello D, eds. *Cecil Textbook of Medicine.* 22nd ed. Saunders;2004:2257.

59. SYNCOPE

I. **Problem.** A patient admitted for palpitations and chest pain loses consciousness while ambulating to the bathroom.

II. **Immediate Questions**

Definition: *Syncope* **is transient loss of consciousness with loss of postural tone.** True syncope must be differentiated from dizziness, "spells," or near syncope, which are not associated with loss of consciousness and are generally more benign.

A. **What was the patient's activity and position immediately before the incident?** Syncope in the recumbent position is almost always due to Stokes-Adams attacks (high-grade atrioventricular block). Vasovagal syncope or fainting from orthostatic hypotension requires the patient to have been in the seated or upright position. Exertional syncope is frequently cardiac in origin. Other key activities (situational syncope) to ask about include turning or twisting the head, coughing, getting up quickly, and micturition. A witness can provide key information as to loss of consciousness or abnormal limb movements.

B. **Is the patient still unconscious?** Vasovagal syncope rarely lasts more than a few seconds and resolves with recumbency. Persistent unconsciousness suggests a cardiac or neurologic cause (brain stem stroke or seizure [see Section I, Chapter 58, Seizures, p 329]).

C. **What were the vital signs during the episode? What are the vital signs now?** Vasovagal syncope is associated with bradycardia, but frequently a reflex tachycardia is noted after the episode. The blood pressure is usually normal after a vasovagal faint. Orthostatic changes in blood pressure and tachycardia are frequently evidence of volume depletion or blood loss as the cause. Neurologic causes are generally associated with a normal or elevated blood pressure. Cardiac syncope may occur when arrhythmias result in a pulse < 40 or > 180 bpm.

D. **Was there evidence of seizure activity?** Some clonic jerking of the limbs may occur with syncope, and, in some rare instances, a brief tonic-clonic seizure may occur (*convulsive syncope*). Fecal and urinary incontinence are more typical of seizures than of other causes of syncope. Seizures that occur in the absence of typical postictal symptoms may suggest hypotension from an arrhythmia or vasovagal episode as a cause of the syncope.

E. **How quickly was consciousness regained? Was the patient immediately oriented?** Cardiac causes and vasovagal episodes are associated with a rapid return to full consciousness. Seizures are characterized by postictal confusion and headache.

F. **How did the patient feel immediately before losing consciousness?** Vasovagal episodes are normally preceded by a symptom complex consisting of sweating, lightheadedness, and abdominal queasiness. Seizures often have an *aura* (frequently recurring visual or olfactory sensations). Postural or exertional symptoms may be present in cardiac and orthostatic syncope; however, symptoms are often not present, or may only be associated with sensations of the room closing in or going dark. Dizziness and vertigo in association with syncope have been associated with increased psychiatric causes of syncope. However, dizziness may also be a sign of an arrhythmia.

G. **What medical conditions does the patient have?** Several medical conditions predispose to syncope. Diabetics are at risk for hypoglycemia as well as orthostasis secondary to autonomic dysfunction. A history of atherosclerotic vascular disease suggests arrhythmias as well as cerebrovascular events. Other important illnesses to ask about include a history of a seizure disorder, valvular disorders, presence of a pacemaker, migraines, and any history of head trauma. Isolated episodes of syncope are more likely to be benign, whereas more frequent episodes are often associated with some underlying disorder.

H. **What medications is the patient receiving?** A variety of medications predispose to orthostatic hypotension, including diuretics, antihypertensives, and tricyclic antidepressants such as amitriptyline (Elavil).

Varying degrees of heart block can be induced by verapamil (Calan, Isoptin), diltiazem (Cardizem), digoxin (Lanoxin), and beta-blockers. Many class I antiarrhythmics can also induce ventricular arrhythmias leading to syncope ("quinidine syncope"). Antianginals, analgesics, and CNS depressants have been associated with syncope.

III. **Differential Diagnosis.** In five population-based studies, the most common causes of syncope were vasovagal causes, heart disease and arrhythmias, orthostatic hypotension, and seizures. No diagnosis was found in 34% of patients. The cause of syncope may be placed into one of five categories.

A. **Neural-mediated reflexes associated with vasodilatation or bradycardia**
1. **Vasovagal syncope.** Also called *neurocardiogenic syncope.* It is by far the most common cause of syncope and is associated with the symptom complex previously described (see II.F.). Generally, vasovagal syncope has a benign prognosis.
2. **Situational—sudden decrease in venous return**
a. **Micturition syncope**
b. **Cough syncope**
c. **Valsalva maneuver.** Increases vagal tone.
d. **Swallow syncope**
3. **Other**
a. **Carotid sinus.** Associated with head turning or neck pressure
b. **Glossopharyngeal neuralgia.** Intermittent tongue, larynx, or pharynx pain that can stimulate the vagus nerve, resulting in bradycardia.

B. **Orthostatic hypotension**
1. **Age-related physiologic changes**
2. **Volume depletion**
a. **Dehydration**
b. **Blood loss**
3. **Medications.** Diuretics, antihypertensives, and tricyclic antidepressants such as amitriptyline.
4. **Autonomic insufficiency**
a. **Shy-Drager syndrome.** Idiopathic autonomic dysfunction.
b. **Diabetes.** Autonomic dysfunction with long standing diabetes.
5. **Postprandial orthostasis in the elderly**

C. **Psychiatric causes.** Generally associated with frequent symptoms and lack of injury.
1. **Anxiety**
2. **Depression**
3. **Conversion disorder**

D. **Neurologic causes**
1. **Transient ischemic attack.** Most commonly vertebrobasilar area. Seldom does a cerebrovascular accident involving the ante-

rior circulation result in syncope except with bilateral disruption of the reticular activating system.

2. **Migraines.** Basilar artery ("drop attacks")
3. **Seizures.** See Section I, Chapter 58, Seizures, p 329.
4. **Carotid sinus syndrome.** Presents as syncope caused by turning head to one side or having too tight a collar.
5. **Subclavian steal syndrome**
6. **Subarachnoid hemorrhage.** May present as brief syncope followed by severe headache.

E. **Cardiac syncope**
   1. **Organic heart disease**
      a. **Atrial myxoma.** Intermittent obstruction of a valve.
      b. **Aortic stenosis.** Associated with left ventricular outflow obstruction. Syncope is a marker for significant mortality.
      c. **Acute myocardial infarction with cardiogenic shock**
      d. **Primary pulmonary hypertension.** Caused by decreased pulmonary flow and left-sided return.
      e. **Idiopathic hypertrophic subaortic stenosis.** Same cause as aortic stenosis.
      f. **Pulmonary embolism**
      g. **Aortic dissection**
      h. **Cardiac tamponade**
      i. **Pregnancy.** Aortocaval compression by an enlarged uterus.
   2. **Dysrhythmias**
      a. **Tachycardias.** See Section I, Chapter 60, Tachycardia, p 345.
         i. **Ventricular tachycardia**
         ii. **Paroxysmal atrial tachycardia**
         iii. **Atrial fibrillation with rapid ventricular response**
         iv. **Atrial flutter**
         v. **Wolff-Parkinson-White syndrome.** Look for short PR interval and delta wave.
         vi. **Torsades de pointes**
      b. **Bradycardias.** See Section I, Chapter 8, Bradycardia, p 42.
         i. **Sinus bradycardia**
         ii. **Second- and third-degree atrioventricular block**
         iii. **Sinus node disease**
         iv. **Pacemaker syncope.** If the patient has a pacemaker, malfunction must be considered as a possible cause of syncope (see Section I, Chapter 53, Pacemaker Troubleshooting, p 301).

F. **Miscellaneous causes**
   1. **Hypoxemia**
   2. **Hyperventilation**
   3. **Hypoglycemia.** Often occurs in patients on insulin or oral hypoglycemic agents who miss a meal or receive the wrong dose.

G. **Unknown**

IV. Database. History and physical examination identify approximately 45% of patients whose syncope has an identifiable cause.

A. Physical examination key points

1. **Vital signs.** (See II.C). Vitals should be rechecked frequently during the evaluation. Check for orthostatic changes in blood pressure and pulse.

2. **HEENT.** Look for evidence of trauma, and palpate for bony abnormalities. Look for subhyaloid hemorrhages as evidence of subarachnoid hemorrhage. Tongue or cheek lacerations suggest seizure activity. Meningitis and subarachnoid hemorrhage have associated neck stiffness. Carotid bruits suggest diffuse atherosclerosis.

3. **Chest.** Auscultate for crackles and wheezes that may accompany aspiration during the syncopal episode. Palpate for rib injury caused by a fall.

4. **Heart.** Assess rate and rhythm, especially during or immediately after the episode. Auscultate for murmurs, listening for characteristic changes with position that would differentiate aortic stenosis and idiopathic hypertrophic subaortic stenosis from other systolic murmurs. Assess the jugular venous pulse as an indicator of volume status.

5. **Genitourinary system.** Look for evidence of urinary and/or fecal incontinence.

6. **Neurologic exam.** Slow resolution of mental status to normal points to a postictal state. Focal deficits suggest a cerebrovascular event. Persistent mental obtundation suggests hypoglycemia, hypoxemia, or other metabolic derangement.

7. **Reproduction of event.** Perform maneuvers intended to reproduce the event. *Caution:* **Do this only with appropriate monitoring and resuscitation equipment available (including venous access). Have the patient cough, turn his or her head, and hyperventilate; or perform carotid massage as appropriate.**

B. Laboratory data. The American College of Physicians (ACP) suggests a workup based on the algorithm in Figure I–7.

1. **Routine blood testing.** Testing for complete blood cell count, electrolytes, blood urea nitrogen, and glucose is *not* recommended in the ACP Syncope Guideline because they rarely lead to diagnostically useful information. However, these tests are recommended to confirm a cause suggested by history or physical exam.

2. **Electrocardiogram (ECG) with a rhythm strip.** Look for tachyarrhythmias or bradyarrhythmias. A short PR interval and delta wave suggest Wolff-Parkinson-White syndrome. Also, look for evidence of ischemia or myocardial damage and new conduction abnormalities. Approximately 5% of patients with syncope have an identifiable cause on ECG. Despite the low yield, the ECG is

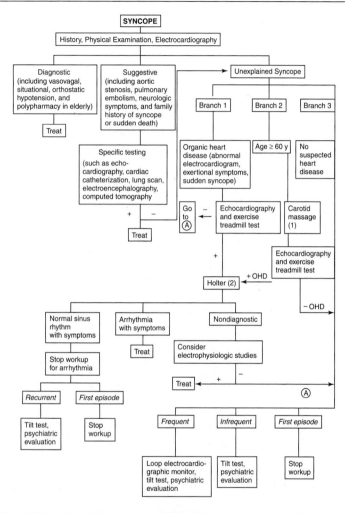

Figure I–7. Algorithm for diagnosing syncope (1) Carotid massage can be performed in an office setting only in the absence of bruits, ventricular tachycardia, recent stroke, and myocardial infarction. (2) Holter monitoring may be replaced by inpatient telemetry if there is a concern about arrhythmias. OHD, organic heart disease. *(Reprinted, with permission, from Linzer M, Yang EH, Estes M et al: Diagnosing syncope: Part I. Value of history physical examination, and electrocardiography. Ann Intern Med 1997;126:989.)*

risk-free and inexpensive, and abnormalities can guide further testing.

Based on history, physical exam, and ECG, the remainder of the evaluation may be divided into one of three categories:

3. **Diagnostic** (ie, vasovagal, medication, orthostasis, situational). Treat the patient.

4. **Suggestive** (ie, aortic stenosis, neurologic symptoms, trauma, family history of sudden death). Perform specific testing such as echocardiography, CT scan, V̇/Q̇ scan, or electroencephalography. If workup is unrevealing, then go to 5.

5. **Unexplained syncope**
   a. **Unexplained syncope with clinical organic heart disease or abnormal ECG**
      i. **Echocardiography.** Look for valvular lesion, thrombi, new wall motion abnormalities, or myxoma. Unsuspected findings are found in 5–10% of patients.
      ii. **Exercise testing.** With exertional symptoms, exercise testing may lead to a diagnosis of ischemia or an exercise-induced arrhythmia. Echocardiography should be performed first to exclude hypertrophic cardiomyopathy.
      iii. **24-hour Holter monitor.** Useful if an arrhythmia is suspected, particularly in patients with frequent attacks. An event recorder may be more useful if the attacks are infrequent and the evaluation is in the outpatient setting.
      iv. **Electrophysiologic (EP) testing.** Patients with normal hearts (ie, normal ECG and no evidence of underlying structural heart disease) should rarely undergo EP testing. EP studies are most revealing with organic, structural, or conduction abnormalities.
      v. **Signal-averaged ECG.** In patients with coronary artery disease (CAD) and those in whom ventricular tachycardia is suspected, signal-averaged ECG has a high sensitivity and specificity for inducible tachycardia.
   b. **Unexplained syncope in the elderly (> 60 years).** Carotid sinus massage may be performed when no bruits are present and when there is no history of recent myocardial infarction, stroke, or ventricular tachycardia. It is advised to have intravenous access, cardiac monitoring, and atropine readily available before carotid sinus massage. If a cardioinhibitory response (asystole > 3 seconds) occurs, the patient may be treated with a pacemaker.

C. **Unexplained syncope with no CAD and no suspected CAD**
   1. **Long-term loop ECG.** A noninvasive event monitor is most beneficial with frequent symptoms. The monitor constantly records and is activated after an episode saving the last several minutes before and after an event.

    2. Head-up tilt-table. Most helpful with a negative cardiac and arrhythmia evaluation. Passive tilt-table at 65 degrees for 45 minutes may be followed by the use of isoproterenol in patients who have a high pretest probability for neurally mediated syncope. The test is positive only if typical symptoms are reproduced.

V. Plan. This is dictated by your initial impression based on the preceding evaluation. The causes of syncope range from a relatively benign vasovagal episode to life-threatening complete heart block. The treatment plan should reflect the severity of the underlying cause. Remember that injuries from a fall secondary to syncope can result in significant morbidity, especially in the elderly, so a thorough evaluation for injury should be performed.

A. Vasovagal syncope
1. Instruct the patient to assume a recumbent position at the onset of presyncopal symptoms. If unable to lie down, the patient should be seated with his or her head down.
2. The patient should be made aware of situations that bring on the episodes, such as prolonged standing, and should avoid these situations.
3. For patients with suspected recurrent neurocardiogenic syncope, consider head-up tilt-table testing to confirm diagnosis and direct further treatment (beta-blockers, disopyramide).

B. Orthostatic hypotension
1. Assess for signs of volume contraction and correct as indicated. Review medications to eliminate, if possible, those that could cause volume depletion or cause vasodilatation.
2. If gastrointestinal bleeding is diagnosed, see Section I, Chapter 27, Hematemesis, Melena, V, p 169, and/or Chapter 28, Hematochezia, V, p 174.
3. Instruct the patient to rise and change positions slowly, with adequate support available.

C. Cardiac syncope
1. Treat arrhythmias. See Section I, Chapter 8, Bradycardia, V, p 45, Chapter 45, Irregular Pulse V, p 254 and Chapter 60, Tachycardia, V, p 351.
2. If an arrhythmia is suspected but cannot be confirmed with Holter monitoring, consider EP testing, especially if ischemic heart disease is present.
3. If ischemia is suspected, treat as possible myocardial infarction, and institute a rule-out myocardial infarction protocol.

D. Miscellaneous disorders
1. **Carotid sinus syndrome (carotid sinus hypersensitivity).** Instruct the patient to avoid sudden turning of the head, tight collars, and vigorous rubbing with electric shavers.

2. **Micturition.** Instruct the patient to sit when voiding and to remain seated for several minutes after voiding.
3. **Cough and hyperventilation.** Informing the patient of the cause is frequently the only thing that can be done; however, if hyperventilation is due to anxiety, the anxiety should be addressed and treated appropriately.

REFERENCES

Kapoor WN: Evaluation and management of the patient with syncope. JAMA 1992;268:2553.

Linzer M, Yang EH, Estes M et al: Diagnosing syncope part 1: Value of history, physical examination, and electrocardiography. Ann Intern Med 1997;126:989.

Linzer M, Yang EH, Estes M et al: Diagnosing syncope part 2: Unexplained syncope. Ann Intern Med 1997;127:76.

60. TACHYCARDIA

I. **Problem.** You are asked to evaluate an 18-year-old woman with sudden onset of chest pain, palpitations, and dizziness. Cardiac monitoring reveals a rapid, regular, narrow-complex tachycardia at a rate of 180 beats per minute (bpm).

II. **Immediate Questions**

A. **What are the patient's other vital signs?** Hypotension accompanying a tachyarrhythmia demands immediate action. Tachypnea and tachycardia may be present with acute pulmonary embolism (PE); a severe pneumonia; exacerbation of chronic obstructive pulmonary disease (COPD); and acute pulmonary edema. Tachycardia accompanied by a fever may suggest an infection or thyrotoxicosis. The presence of *pulsus paradoxus* (a variation in the systolic blood pressure of more than 10 mm Hg between inspiration and expiration) suggests pericardial tamponade or an exacerbation of COPD.

B. **What has been the patient's heart rate previously?** A sudden change in heart rate may signify a change in cardiac rhythm, such as the sudden onset of atrial fibrillation.

C. **Does the patient have any symptoms related to the tachycardia?** Ask about dyspnea, chest pain, dizziness, syncope, agitation, and confusion.

D. **What medication is the patient currently taking?** Drugs that can cause tachyarrhythmias include diuretics, theophylline, sympathomimetic drugs, catecholamine infusions, digoxin, and thyroid supplements. Diuretics can lead to intravascular volume loss as well as hypokalemia and hypomagnesemia that can result in tachyarrhythmias. Theophylline, even in therapeutic doses, may cause sinus tachycardia; in toxic doses (serum levels > 20 μg/mL) it can lead to ventricular tachyarrhythmias.

III. Differential Diagnosis

A. Sinus tachycardia. This condition is defined as a sinus node controlled rhythm > 100 bpm. The extensive list of its causes includes varying states of emotion and pain; fever; anemia; hypoxemia; hemorrhage; infection; thyrotoxicosis; myocardial infarction; pneumothorax; pericarditis; use of drugs or medications that include caffeine, nicotine, and atropine; and ingestion or overdoses of amyl nitrite, quinidine, cocaine, antihistamines, decongestants, or tricyclic antidepressants. Sinus tachycardia is typically gradual in onset and termination. Vagal maneuvers and carotid sinus massage may slow the heart rate temporarily, but the tachycardia returns when these maneuvers are stopped. Sinus tachycardia rarely occurs in quiet patients at rates greater than 140 bpm. Fever can be expected to raise the sinus rate about 10 bpm for every degree above normal core body temperature.

B. Supraventricular tachyarrhythmias (SVT). When you are examining the electrocardiogram (ECG) or rhythm strip of a suspected SVT for the first time, check the tracing for the following features:

1. **Regularity.** Atrial fibrillation, multifocal atrial tachycardia, and on occasion atrial flutter are irregular rhythms, whereas most other SVTs are regular.

2. **Baseline.** The *baseline* is that portion of the ECG between the end of the T wave and the beginning of either the P wave or the next QRS complex. If this section is flat, then the atria are either quiescent or fibrillating, or their activity is hidden in another section of the ECG.

3. **QRS complex.** SVTs generally have QRS complexes with axes and widths that are similar to those found during sinus rhythm, but not always. Wide QRS complexes can result from a rate-dependent bundle branch block, or antegrade conduction across an accessory atrioventricular (AV) pathway.

4. **P waves.** Determine whether the P-wave morphology and axis during the tachycardia is similar to or different from normal sinus rhythm. If different, then atrial activation is initiated somewhere other than the sinoatrial node.

5. **P-wave–QRS complex relationship.** A constant timing relationship between P waves and the QRS complexes is found in most regular SVTs. Atrial flutter may demonstrate a variable relationship, depending on the degree of AV conduction. The presence of AV dissociation indicates a ventricular tachyarrhythmia.

6. After you examine the characteristics of a particular SVT, it is then helpful to classify the arrhythmia based on the mechanisms used to sustain it.

a. **Atrial flutter.** Atrial flutter involves a reentry circuit localized entirely within the atrial myocardium. The atrial rate is typically 250–400 bpm. Coarse, saw-toothed "flutter waves" are usually visible in the inferior leads. The ventricular rate depends on conduction in the AV node and is usually 1:2 or 1:3 of the atrial rate. If AV conduction is rapid and the atrial flutter waves are therefore hard to see, carotid sinus massage transiently decreases AV node conduction and allows a better view of the baseline or the saw-toothed pattern of the ECG. Atrial flutter can be irregular or regular, depending on whether the conduction through the AV node is variable or constant. Atrial flutter can be seen with rheumatic heart disease or ischemic heart disease; with recent cardiac surgery, as part of the postpericardiotomy syndrome; in cardiomyopathy of various causes; and in atrial septal defect, acute PE, mitral or tricuspid valve disease, thyrotoxicosis, ethanol abuse, and pericarditis.

b. **Atrial fibrillation.** Atrial fibrillation is a rhythm that involves many disorganized atrial electrical circuits leading to chaotic atrial depolarizations. It is characterized by an atrial rate of 350–600 bpm. Distinct P waves are not visible. The ventricular rate is classically described as "irregularly irregular" and is controlled by the rate of conduction of the atrial impulses through the AV node. Ventricular rates are commonly 100–160 bpm in the untreated patient. Carotid sinus massage temporarily decreases AV node conduction and slows the ventricular rate to allow the baseline to be better seen. Predisposing conditions are similar to those for atrial flutter.

c. **Automatic AVTs.** These tachycardias develop because of abnormally enhanced automaticity in the atrial myocardium or bundle of His.

   i. **Paroxysmal atrial tachycardia with block.** This tachycardia is usually related to digoxin toxicity and therefore occurs in patients with some type of organic heart disease. Enhanced automaticity in the atrial myocardium is the most likely mechanism. Hypokalemia may cause this arrhythmia. There is organized, visible atrial activity, although the P-wave axis is different from normal P-wave axis in sinus rhythm. The atrial rate is typically 180–240 bpm. Conduction of the rapid atrial discharges through the AV node is partially suppressed by digitalis, resulting in the intermittent AV block.

   ii. **Automatic AV junctional tachycardia.** The mechanism of this tachycardia is incompletely understood. It is generally attributed to increased automaticity of the pacemaker cells in the AV node. This tachycardia rarely occurs without underlying cardiac disease. It can be seen in digitalis intoxication, in acute inferior or posterior myocardial infarctions, after cardiac surgery, or with viral or rheumatic myocarditis. This arrhythmia is usually benign and self-limited. The QRS complex is usually narrow and resembles that of sinus rhythm. The rate rarely exceeds 130 bpm. AV dissociation is commonly visible; P waves are visible between QRS complexes. This arrhythmia has a gradual onset and termination.

d. Reentrant SVT. Reentry circuits are the most common mechanism sustaining regular SVTs. Reentry requires myocardium with differing degrees of refractoriness to maintain the electrical circuit. These reentry circuits are located within the AV node, the atrial myocardium, or the sinus node; or they involve both the atria and the ventricles in the case of accessory conduction pathways.

    i. **AV nodal reentry tachycardia.** This is the most common type of reentrant tachycardia, accounting for up to 30% of all SVTs. The reentry circuit usually consists of a slowly conducting antegrade AV nodal pathway and a rapidly conducting retrograde AV nodal pathway. This arrhythmia is characterized by the presence of normal QRS complexes at a regular rate between 150 and 250 bpm. P waves are usually not visible. The onset and termination of the tachycardia are generally abrupt. Carotid sinus massage or vagal maneuvers may result in the abrupt termination of the tachyarrhythmia.

    ii. **AV reciprocating tachycardia.** This tachyarrhythmia, also known by the eponym Wolff-Parkinson-White syndrome, involves an accessory conduction pathway between the atria and the ventricles. The QRS complex is usually narrow during tachycardia because antegrade conduction moves through the AV node, and the accessory pathway is conducting the ventricular electrical activity retrograde to the atria. Heart rates may exceed 200 bpm. During sinus rhythm, a "delta" wave, representing ventricular preexcitation, may be visible as a slurring of the upstroke of the QRS complex. This also results in an abnormally short PR interval (< 0.12 seconds). This tachyarrhythmia may account for up to 20% of all SVTs. P waves may be present inside the QRS complex or in the QT interval. The P waves have an abnormal axis reflective of the retrograde atrial depolarization.

e. SVTs of uncertain mechanism. *Multifocal atrial tachycardia* is an arrhythmia characterized by the presence of multiple foci of atrial depolarization, resulting in more than one P-wave morphology. This arrhythmia is found most commonly with chronic pulmonary disease and pulmonary hypertension. The ventricular rhythm is usually irregular as a result of variable conduction through the AV node. The QRS complexes are generally normal. The ventricular rate can range from 100 to 140 bpm.

C. Ventricular arrhythmias

1. **Accelerated idioventricular rhythm (AIVR).** This is a rhythm of ventricular origin with a rate of 50–100 bpm. It can be seen in patients with digitalis intoxication or acute myocardial infarction, as well as in otherwise healthy individuals. It is a common arrhythmia seen in patients given reperfusion therapy for acute myocardial infarction. Most AIVRs are benign, except those associated with digitalis intoxication. Onset and termination are gradual. AIVRs do not usually result in hemodynamic collapse. The QRS complexes are wide, consistent with the ventricular origin of the arrhythmia. AIVRs can be recognized by the appearance of a monomorphic ventricular rhythm that appears to overtake a slower sinus rhythm; P waves and fusion beats are frequently visible. No specific therapy is necessary unless digitalis intoxication is present. If hypotension does result from the AIVR, use of atropine to raise the sinus node rate usually terminates this arrhythmia and restores hemodynamic stability.

2. **Ventricular tachycardia (VT).** These arrhythmias are characterized by a cardiac rhythm with wide QRS complexes and heart rates of 100–250 bpm. They usually compromise blood pressure and are a common cause of sudden cardiac death. Electrocardiographic criteria suggesting a ventricular arrhythmia, as opposed to a wide-complex supraventricular arrhythmia, include the following: (1) a QRS duration > 0.14 seconds; (2) the presence of fusion and capture beats; (3) identification of P waves in the baseline of the ECG, suggesting AV dissociation; and (4) a QRS morphology that appears similar to isolated premature ventricular contractions seen before the initiation of sustained VT. A *fusion beat* is a hybrid beat, in which a beat originating in the atrium fuses with one originating in the ventricle. VT is invariably associated with organic heart disease, especially coronary artery disease following myocardial infarction, and cardiomyopathies with impaired left ventricular function. The mechanism behind most ventricular tachyarrhythmias involves a reentry circuit located within the ventricular myocardium. There is usually an abnormality of impulse conduction, with a region of normally conducting myocardium located adjacent to a region of slowly conducting myocardium, frequently involving a section of scarred or fibrotic tissue. These areas of slow conduction are the myocardial substrate needed to maintain a reentry electrical circuit. This region of slowly conducting myocardium produces low-amplitude, high-frequency after-depolarizations that help to maintain the reentry circuit. These after-depolarizations are visible on signal-averaged electrocardiograms.

3. **Ventricular fibrillation (VF).** This is the most common arrhythmia in cardiac arrest patients. Coronary artery disease is the major underlying cause. Death is certain unless rapid and immediate electrical defibrillation is instituted. If resuscitation efforts are successful, further investigation is indicated, since recurrence rates are as high as 30% during the first year. Invasive electrophysiologic studies are helpful in finding the patients who are at highest risk for recurrence of VT or VF. These studies have proved to be useful in guiding long-term therapy.

4. **Torsades de pointes.** This is a distinctive form of polymorphic VT. This arrhythmia is uniquely characterized by a basic variation in the electrical polarity of the QRS complex, such that the QRS complexes appear to be twisting around an isoelectric baseline. Multiple leads may be necessary to accurately visualize the changes in the electrical polarity. The rate of the tachyarrhythmia can range from 150 to 280 bpm. Variation in the R–R interval is commonly seen. Spontaneous termination and recurrences are common. Torsades de pointes can occasionally progress to a sustained ventricular arrhythmia. The electrocardiographic abnormality that is the hallmark of this tachyarrhythmia is a prolonged corrected QT interval during sinus rhythm > 0.50 seconds. This tachyarrhythmia is seen in quinidine and procainamide toxicity.

IV. **Database**
   A. **Physical examination key points**
      1. **Vital signs.** Hypotension requires rapid action. Palpation of carotid, brachial, or femoral pulses can give the examiner a rapid estimate of the adequacy of systolic pressure.
      2. **Neck.** Distended jugular veins are present with acute decompensation of congestive heart failure, exacerbations of chronic pulmonary disease, pneumothorax, and pericardial tamponade. The presence of cannon "A" waves in the jugular venous pulsations suggests the presence of AV dissociation.
      3. **Chest.** Rales and wheezes can be present in many of the associated cardiopulmonary diseases that predispose to tachyarrhythmias.
      4. **Heart.** Listen in particular for S_3 or S_4 heart sounds or a murmur that might suggest mitral valve disease.
      5. **Abdomen.** Localized or rebound tenderness pinpoint a source of infection as the cause of the tachyarrhythmia.
      6. **Extremities.** Examine for signs of peripheral perfusion as an assessment of the adequacy of cardiac output.
   B. **Laboratory data**
      1. **Serum electrolytes.** Hypokalemia and hypomagnesemia can be responsible for sustained arrhythmias, particularly in patients taking digoxin. Both supraventricular and ventricular arrhythmias can result from potassium and magnesium deficiencies.

2. **Arterial blood gases.** Severe disturbances of acid–base status can be responsible for the initiation of tachyarrhythmias.

3. **Hemogram.** An elevated white blood cell count with a left shift suggests the presence of an infection.

4. **Thyroid function studies.** Check to exclude hyperthyroidism as a cause of an SVT.

5. **Serum drug levels.** In particular, digoxin, theophylline, and antiarrhythmic drug levels should be checked in patients with new onset of a sustained tachyarrhythmia.

C. **ECG and rhythm strip**. A 12-lead ECG is the most important piece of diagnostic information in a patient with acute onset of sustained ventricular tachyarrhythmia. It should be obtained before initiating therapy as long as the patient's condition allows the extra time. Otherwise, you will have to rely on a single-lead rhythm strip recorded from the cardiac monitor to direct therapy. Examine the ECG for visible P waves, fusion or capture beats and their relationship to the QRS complexes, the rate and regularity of the rhythm, and the width of the QRS complexes. If a baseline ECG is available, look for prolongation of the QT interval.

V. **Plan.** A discussion of definitive or long-term therapy of tachyarrhythmias is not within the scope of this book. The reader is referred to the reference edited by Horowitz for an in-depth explanation of the use of antiarrhythmic medications, radiofrequency ablative procedures, automatic implantable cardioverter defibrillators, and antitachycardia pacemakers. The present discussion deals primarily with the use of medications for acute treatment of sustained tachyarrhythmias.

A. **Treat any underlying predisposing conditions.** Correction of serum electrolyte imbalances is essential. Therefore, treatment with IV potassium and magnesium when appropriate may help prevent further episodes of sustained tachyarrhythmias related to these electrolyte disturbances. Administration of supplemental oxygen may be helpful in the hypoxic patient. If acute digitalis intoxication is responsible for a life-threatening recurrent tachyarrhythmia, consider treating the patient with digoxin immune Fab fragments (Digibind). The dose is based on the amount of digoxin acutely ingested or the serum digoxin concentration and body weight. See dosing charts provided with the drug.

B. **Synchronized electrical cardioversion.** If a tachyarrhythmia is responsible for causing an acute unstable episode of congestive heart failure, acute myocardial ischemia, or hemodynamic collapse, the quickest and most appropriate therapy for the termination of the tachyarrhythmia is synchronized electrical cardioversion. If the patient remains conscious during the tachycardia, it is appropriate to administer an intravenous sedative such as midazolam (Versed) before electrical cardioversion. Ventricular fibrillation may result if the electrical shock is not synchronized to the R wave in cases of SVT and VT. Most SVTs can be terminated using 50–100 joules, and most ventricular tachyarrhythmias respond to 100–200 joules. ***Caution:*** Electrical cardioversion is contraindicated in cases of digitalis toxicity, and is not helpful if used for sinus tachycardia.

C. **Carotid sinus massage.** This maneuver can be very helpful in establishing the diagnosis of many SVTs and can result in the termination of some tachycardias, such as AV nodal reentry tachycardia. Carotid sinus massage or other maneuvers that raise vagal tone, such as Valsalva's and Mueller's maneuver, should be tried first when you are treating an episode of SVT as long as the patient's condition will allow the time. Vagal maneuvers should be repeated after each pharmacologic agent is administered until the arrhythmia stops. Carotid sinus massage should be done in a monitored setting because of the potential of inducing symptomatic bradycardia or sinus arrest in the case of hypersensitive carotid sinus syndrome.

D. **Medications**
   1. **Adenosine (Adenocard).** The electrophysiologic effects of adenosine include a negative chronotropic action on the sinus node and a negative dromotropic effect on the AV node. Adenosine is helpful in the management of paroxysmal SVTs caused by a reentry circuit involving the AV node. Adenosine has also been used to diagnose the mechanism of a particular tachycardia and occasionally to differentiate SVTs from aberrant conduction from ventricular tachyarrhythmias. Adenosine (6 mg) is administered as a rapid intravenous dose. The onset of action is 10–30 seconds, and its therapeutic effect lasts for only 60–90 seconds. If the initial dose does not terminate the tachycardia, a second bolus of 12 mg is given. Conduction over accessory AV pathways is not affected. Patients with unstable bronchial asthma should not receive intravenous adenosine. Patients with AV reciprocating tachycardias (Wolff-Parkinson-White syndrome) should be watched closely, because adenosine may induce atrial fibrillation, which could lead to acceleration of the tachyarrhythmia and subsequent cardiac arrest. Dipyridamole, cardiac glycosides, verapamil, and benzodiazepines can potentiate the electrophysiologic effects of adenosine. Therefore, the initial dose should be reduced for patients taking these medications. Aminophylline antagonizes the actions of adenosine, and therefore higher doses may be required.
   2. **Amiodarone (Cordarone).** Indicated for ventricular tachycardia, cardiac arrest (pulseless ventricular tachycardia or ventricular fibrillation), paroxysmal SVT, atrial fibrillation, atrial flutter, and junctional tachycardia. The drug of choice by most experts for cardiac arrest due to pulseless ventricular tachycardia or ventricular fibrillation. The dose for arrhythmias other than cardiac arrest is 150

mg IV over 10 minutes, followed by 1 mg/min IV over 6 hours, then 0.5 mg/min. For cardiac arrest, the dose is 300 mg IV push; may follow with a second dose of 150 mg. Follow the initial bolus(es) with a continuous infusion as above. The maximum dose is 2.2 g over 24 hours. Dilute the bolus in 20–30 mL normal saline or 5% dextrose in water.

3. **Beta-blockers (propranolol, metoprolol, esmolol).** Beta-blockers are helpful in controlling a rapid heart rate with sinus tachycardia, atrial flutter and fibrillation, automatic atrial tachycardia, and SVTs associated with digitalis intoxication. Beta-blockers should be used with caution in impaired left ventricular function or COPD. The usual intravenous dose for propranolol (Inderal) is 1–3 mg (not to exceed 1 mg/min); may repeat if necessary in 2 minutes. No additional doses should be given in less than 4 hours. Metoprolol (Lopressor) 5–15 mg is given in divided doses (administered in doses of 5 mg given at about 2-minute intervals). Esmolol (Brevibloc) 500 μg/kg is given over 1 minute followed by a continuous infusion of 50 μg/kg/min.

4. **Digoxin (Lanoxin).** Digoxin is useful in the treatment of many SVTs to control the ventricular response. It is an established drug in the treatment of atrial fibrillation or flutter. An initial dose of 0.25–0.50 mg is given IV followed by additional doses of 0.25 mg every 4–6 hours (carefully assess clinical response and signs of toxicity before each additional dose), for a total loading dose of 1.0 mg. Daily maintenance doses of 0.125–0.25 mg are required to sustain adequate serum levels with normal renal function. If digoxin alone does not adequately control the ventricular rate of an SVT, addition of a calcium channel blocker such as verapamil or diltiazem may be helpful.

5. **Diltiazem (Cardizem, Dilacor).** Diltiazem comes in an injectable form for the acute management of new-onset atrial fibrillation or flutter, and the treatment of acute episodes of paroxysmal SVT. The initial dose is 0.25 mg/kg IV administered over 2 minutes (maximum dose 20 mg), to be repeated 0.35 mg/kg in 15 minutes if needed. The patient can then be maintained on an IV infusion of 10 mg/hr, or started on oral maintenance doses of 60–90 mg given Q 6 hr. The dose can be changed to a long-acting preparation after 24 hours. Precautions are similar to those for verapamil.

6. **Lidocaine.** Lidocaine can be used for the treatment of ventricular tachyarrhythmias that are not associated with hemodynamic collapse; however, evidence for the use of lidocaine is poor and methodologically weak. Amiodarone and procainamide are recommended before lidocaine for the initial treatment of hemodynamically stable wide-complex tachycardia. A loading dose of 1 mg/kg is given as an IV bolus followed by a continuous infusion of 1–4 mg/min. A second loading dose of 0.5 mg/kg is recommended and should be given 5–10 minutes after the initial bolus.

Lidocaine may also be helpful in arrhythmias associated with digoxin intoxication.

7. **Magnesium.** Indicated for polymorphic ventricular tachycardia (torsades de pointes) and suspected hypomagnesemia. The dose is 1–2 g IV over 15 minutes (for hypomagnesemia) and 2 g IV over 1–2 minutes followed by 0.5–1.0 g/hr (for torsades de pointes). Dilute the bolus in 50–100 mL of 5% dextrose in water.

8. **Procainamide (Pronestyl).** Procainamide can be used to convert ventricular tachyarrhythmias. A loading dose of 15–18 mg/kg is given IV at a rate of 25 mg/min, followed by a continuous infusion of 1–4 mg/min. Hypotension can develop during loading infusions if the drug is administered at rates > 25 mg/min.

9. **Verapamil (Calan).** Verapamil IV converts approximately 90% of episodes of AV nodal reentry tachycardia to sinus rhythm. It is also helpful in the acute management of atrial flutter and fibrillation. Give an initial bolus of 2.5–10 mg IV over 2 minutes, then start an oral maintenance dose of 80- to 120-mg tablets Q 8 hr. Verapamil is not the drug of choice for patients with congestive heart failure, poor left ventricular function, or acute myocardial infarction. It should *never* be used in the treatment of wide-complex tachyarrhythmias because it frequently worsens the patient's condition.

   Special Note: Treatment of AV reciprocating tachyarrhythmias, or Wolff-Parkinson-White syndrome, should focus on drugs that prolong the refractory period of the accessory AV pathway or of the AV node. An acute-onset tachyarrhythmia suspicious for an accessory AV pathway (normal QRS width, regular R–R interval, rate around 200 bpm, and retrograde P waves visible in ST segment) can be approached with drugs that prolong conduction in the AV node, such as adenosine, verapamil, diltiazem, or beta-blockers, or with procainamide. Procainamide is the preferred drug of choice for initial management, because it prolongs the effective refractory period of the accessory bypass pathway and other involved myocardium and has less chance of accelerating the rate of tachycardia. Procainamide's electrophysiologic properties make this drug an excellent choice for the initial pharmacologic therapy of AV reciprocating tachycardias. Digitalis may shorten the refractory period of the accessory pathway and accelerate ventricular response in some patients with AV reciprocating tachyarrhythmias.

REFERENCES

Falk RH: Atrial fibrillation. N Engl J Med 2001;344:1067.

Horowitz LN, ed: *Current Management of Arrhythmias.* Decker;1991.

Miller JM, Zipes DP: Management of patient with cardiac arrhythmias. In: Braunwald E, Zipes DP, Libby P, eds. *Heart Disease: A Textbook of Cardiovascular Medicine.* 6th ed. Saunders;2001:700.

Wagner GS, ed: *Marriott's Practical Electrocardiography.* 9th ed. Williams & Wilkins;1994.

Wellens HJJ, Bar FWH, Lie K: The value of the electrocardiogram in the differential diagnosis of tachycardia with widened QRS complex. Am J Med 1978;64:27.

61. THROMBOCYTOPENIA

I. **Problem.** You are called to see a 73-year-old patient admitted to the cardiology service with unstable angina. His admission laboratory data reveal a platelet count of 32,000/µL.

II. **Immediate Questions**

A. **Is the patient bleeding?** The risk of bleeding from trauma increases with a platelet count < 50,000/µL; the risk of spontaneous bleeding increases with a platelet count < 20,000/µL.

B. **Is the count real? Could the results be due to laboratory error (clotted specimen or wrong patient)? Recheck the lab.** Rule out the phenomenon of platelet clumping. Review the peripheral smear if available. Recheck the platelet count using a different anticoagulant such as citrate or heparin. Clumping can occur in some patients using the more common anticoagulant, EDTA (edetic acid).

C. **Is there an obvious cause of thrombocytopenia?** Recent chemotherapy or radiation can result in decreased production of platelets. Also, an enlarged spleen can result in sequestration of platelets.

D. **Does the patient have a history of low platelet count?** Does this appear to be an acute problem such as idiopathic thrombocytopenic purpura (ITP); or is there an underlying disorder contributing to the low platelet count, such as cirrhosis with hypersplenism, chronic ITP, or perhaps an inherited disorder such as Fanconi's syndrome or Wiskott-Aldrich syndrome?

E. **Is the patient on any medicines that might cause thrombocytopenia?** Drug-induced thrombocytopenia is one of the most common causes. Many drugs can cause thrombocytopenia. Quinidine and quinine together account for the largest number of cases. Other commonly associated drugs are ethanol, antibiotics, sulfonamides, heparin, gold, thiazide diuretics, cimetidine (Tagamet), and captopril (Capoten).

F. **Is there a history of a recent viral infection?** A viral infection days to weeks before the onset of thrombocytopenia suggests a chronic form of ITP or acute interference with normal megakaryocyte maturation.

III. **Differential Diagnosis.** Quantitative platelet disorders are usually divided into two categories: decreased production and peripheral destruction or sequestration.

A. **Pseudothrombocytopenia.** Thrombocytopenia may be artifactual, particularly when you are relying on an automated counter. Platelet autoagglutinins may cause clumping in the presence of EDTA or may cause adherence to neutrophils. This can occur in 1/1000 normal adults and requires no further workup.

B. **Decreased production**
1. **Infiltrative processes.** Leukemias (acute or chronic), carcinoma, or lymphomas crowd out the normal marrow elements, resulting in a decreased number of megakaryocytes. Infection (granulomatous disease) such as tuberculosis can cause a similar picture.
2. **Myelodysplasia (preleukemic syndrome).** This condition frequently leads to morphologically abnormal megakaryocytes and results in low platelet levels.
3. **Drugs.** Virtually any drug can be associated with thrombocytopenia either by decreasing platelet production or by causing an immune mechanism. Some known myelosuppressive drugs are particularly toxic to platelet production, For example, cytosine arabinoside (ARA-C), cyclophosphamide (Cytoxan), busulfan (Myleran), methotrexate (MTX), carboplatin (Paraplatin), and interferon. Thiazide diuretics have been associated with a decreased number of megakaryocytes leading to thrombocytopenia. Thiazides may also induce platelet-directed antibodies that can lead to peripheral destruction. Thrombocytopenia is common in those with chronic alcoholism. Ethanol has been shown to decrease the number of megakaryocytes.
4. **Radiation.** Ionizing radiation can affect all marrow elements—frequently megakaryocytes to a lesser extent. Patients who have had therapeutic radiation to large areas of marrow can have transient thrombocytopenia, and recovery to preradiation levels may not occur.
5. **Nutrition.** Malnutritional states, such as vitamin B_{12} and folate deficiency, and occasionally iron deficiency, can lead to depressed numbers of megakaryocytes.
6. **Virus infection.** Viral illnesses such as hepatitis B, rubella, and infectious mononucleosis may cause an acute interference with normal megakaryocyte maturation.
7. **Paroxysmal nocturnal hemoglobinuria.** This can be associated with insufficient platelet production. Episodic red-brown urine occurs most often with the first morning urine. There is associated thrombosis, especially of the hepatic and mesenteric veins.

C. **Peripheral destruction**
1. **Immune-mediated disorders**
   a. **ITP.** This is an autoimmune disorder and a frequent cause of thrombocytopenia. ITP is a diagnosis of exclusion made by history, physicial exam, and review of blood work. The diagnosis can be made definitively if antiplatelet antibodies can be

demonstrated; however, this test is not available in all clinical labs and is not necessary for the diagnosis. There are two forms of ITP:

    i. **Chronic.** Usually seen in adults. Abnormal platelet count is present for more than 6 months.

    ii. **Acute.** More frequently seen in children but also in adults. Patients usually are asymptomatic at time of presentation.

  b. Drugs. May also cause immune destruction; quinidine is the best known. In addition to exerting a toxic effect on megakaryocytes, quinidine may act as a hapten with antibody complex adhering to the platelet, followed by complement-mediated platelet destruction. Sulfa drugs work in a similar fashion. Antibiotics are often a common cause of decreased platelets. Heparin-induced thrombocytopenia should not be overlooked and can be associated with minimal heparin use, even heparin flushes (see III.C.8).

  c. Systemic lupus erythematosus. Can cause autoimmune thrombocytopenia.

  d. Human immunodeficiency virus (HIV). An ITP-like syndrome has been associated with HIV. The thrombocytopenia is caused by an IgG antibody; platelet counts may fall below $10,000/\mu L$. The incidence increases with the severity of the disease.

2. Infection. Direct platelet toxicity may occur from viruses, gram-positive organisms, or the lipopolysaccharides of gram-negative bacteria. Complement, immunoglobulins, and fibrinogen may also play a role. Disseminated intravascular coagulation (DIC), frequently caused by infection, can lead to a consumptive platelet loss. Thrombocytopenia may also be seen in the absence of DIC in septicemia, as with Rocky Mountain spotted fever and malaria.

3. Snake bite. Thrombocytopenia may be related to DIC or direct platelet destruction.

4. Burns. Thrombocytopenia may be secondary to sequestration within damaged tissue and can be further aggravated by concomitant sepsis.

5. Glomerulonephritis. Thrombocytopenia presumably secondary to immune-mediated mechanisms.

6. Aortic valvular stenosis. Occasional cause of thrombocytopenia. Presumed mechanism is direct platelet injury secondary to turbulent flow.

7. Thrombotic thrombocytopenic purpura (TTP, Moschcowitz's disease). TTP is a pentad of microangiopathic hemolytic anemia, thrombocytopenia, fluctuating neurologic findings, fever, and renal dysfunction.

8. Direct toxins to platelets. Heparin appears to cause a direct antiplatelet factor causing aggregation (type II heparin-induced thrombocytopenia) and can induce aggregation in the absence of antibody (type I heparin-induced thrombocytopenia). The incidence of heparin-induced thrombocytopenia is about 5%. Heparin-induced thrombocytopenia can occur with IV or SC delivery, and with bovine or porcine heparin, but it is more common with bovine heparin. This entity is infrequently associated with thromboembolism.

D. Sequestration. Normally, the spleen contains 30% of the circulating platelet pool. When the spleen is enlarged and hypersplenism ensues, up to 90% of circulating platelets may be pooled within the spleen. Hypersplenism is often seen in patients with chronic liver disease with associated portal hypertension. Typically, platelet counts range between 50,000 and 100,000.

E. Pregnancy-related thrombocytopenia. Gestional thrombocytopenia is usually mild and can be seen in about 5% of pregnant women. The cause is unknown and resolves after delivery. Thrombocytopenia may occur at delivery or shortly after delivery and may be related to pre-eclampsia; HELLP syndrome (hemolysis, increased liver enzymes and low platelets); or DIC, which may occur secondary to placental abnormalities.

IV. Database

A. History key points. Is there a history of abnormal blood work or hematologic disease? Take a thorough medication history including medications started since admission, recent antibiotics, and any medication changes within the last month. Inquire about nutritonal status and alcohol history. Also, determine whether there is any family history of bleeding or thrombocytopenia.

B. Physical examination key points. Look for evidence of bleeding and peripheral sequestration.

1. **Vital signs.** Fever requires consideration of infectious causes as well as TTP.

2. **Eyes.** Examine ocular fundus for evidence of bleeding.

3. **Skin and mucous membranes. Are there petechiae or purpura?** The lower extremities frequently reveal petechiae when petechiae may not be easily seen elsewhere. Multiple bruises out of proportion to the degree of trauma may give further evidence of quantitative or qualitative platelet defects. Look for gingival hyperplasia or skin nodules, which suggest leukemia.

4. **Heart.** Severe aortic stenosis can cause thrombocytopenia. A new murmur may indicate bacterial endocarditis.

5. **Lymph Nodes.** Examine lymph nodes to look for enlargment that could indicate underlying hematologic abnormality.

6. **Abdomen.** Splenomegaly may be associated with thrombocytopenia resulting from sequestration. Chronic alcoholics may have evidence of portal hypertension such as dilated abdominal and

chest wall veins, ascites, and splenomegaly. Splenomegaly is also seen with lymphoproliferative and myeloproliferative disorders, as well as infectious causes (eg, infectious mononucleosis and endocarditis). The lack of splenomegaly is also important to note. The presence of palpable splenomegaly makes ITP much less likely.

7. **Neurologic exam.** Fluctuating neurologic findings are frequently seen in TTP.

B. **Laboratory data**

1. **Peripheral blood smear.** Extremely important to review to rule out pseudothrombocytopenia. Pseudothrombocytopenia can be confirmed by obtaining a normal platelet count from heparin-anticoagulated blood. Large platelets (megathrombocytes) are frequently seen with ITP and may indicate peripheral destruction. Morphology of red blood cells may indicate DIC or TTP if a microangiopathic picture is present. Look for blasts as a sign of acute leukemia. The presence of left-shifted granulocytes, nucleated red blood cells, and teardrops may indicate marrow infiltration. Left-shifted granulocytes and toxic granulation are consistent with a bacterial infection.

2. **Coagulation studies.** Elevated prothrombin time, partial thromboplastin time, and thrombin time may be seen in patients with DIC and liver disease. They are normal in those with ITP and TTP. A bleeding time is always abnormal in the face of a low platelet count and is never indicated in the evaluation for thrombocytopenia.

3. **Fibrinogen and D-dimers.** A decrease in fibrinogen and an increase in D-dimers are suggestive of DIC.

4. **Antinuclear antibodies (ANA).** To help rule out a collagen vascular disease as a cause.

5. **Blood urea nitrogen and creatinine.** Renal failure can cause marrow suppression of megakaryocytes and may coexist with other causes such as sepsis, DIC, and TTP.

6. **Bone marrow.** Investigation of bone marrow is essential in the evaluation if there is no obvious reason for thrombocytopenia. An adequate or increased number of megakaryocytes implies peripheral destruction. Marrow infiltration or primary marrow disease can be identified with a bone marrow aspirate and biopsy (often results in decreased megakaryocytes). Megaloblastic changes in the marrow suggest the possibility of vitamin B_{12} or folate deficiency. See Section III, Chapter 5, Bone Marrow Aspiration & Biopsy, p 423.

7. **Liver function tests.** Total bilirubin, alkaline phosphatase, and transaminases (AST and ALT) may support viral hepatitis, alcoholic liver disease, or sepsis from a biliary source as the cause.

C. **Radiologic and other studies**

1. **CT scan of the abdomen.** May demonstrate hepatosplenomegaly or lymphadenopathy in indicated situations.

2. **Liver/spleen scan.** Demonstrates splenomegaly in questionable cases and also indicates hepatic dysfunction and findings consistent with portal hypertension.

3. **Platelet antibodies.** Much variability exists among the techniques for various assays. A negative antiplatelet antibody study does not rule out the presence of antiplatelet antibodies.

V. Plan

A. **Bleeding.** Initially, it is important to determine whether there is life-threatening bleeding, in which case platelet transfusion is indicated. (See Section V, Blood Component Therapy, p 465.) If there is no active bleeding and the thrombocytopenia is immunologic, platelet transfusions are to be avoided. In this situation, transfusions are frequently ineffective and may actually worsen the thrombocytopenia with further immunologic challenge.

B. **Immune-mediated destruction.** If this situation is suspected, all nonessential medicines should be stopped. Do not overlook heparin flush from catheters and Hep-Locks, as well as heparin-banded central venous catheters.

C. **Treatment of underlying cause.** Especially important for leukemias, lymphomas, infections, and DIC.

D. **ITP**

1. **High-dose steroids (1–2 mg/kg prednisone) daily is the initial treatment for ITP.** IV immunoglobulins can also be used in steroid-unresponsive ITP or when steroids are contraindicated.

2. **Splenectomy** may be required in chronic ITP or acute ITP that is unresponsive to steroids or immunoglobulins. If the platelet count is consistently > 50,000/μL, close observation may be best, depending on the underlying medical condition(s). Before splenectomy, be sure the patient receives appropriate vaccinations, including pneumococcal vaccine (if possible, at 2 weeks before splenectomy).

E. **TTP**

1. **Plasmapheresis.** Considered standard treatment, although the mechanism of action is unknown. It may be related to removal of an offending agent or replacement of missing factor(s).

2. **High-dose prednisone.** Frequently used treatment; however, there is no proven benefit.

F. **Prophylactic platelet transfusion.** This may be indicated with myeloproliferative disorders or bone marrow suppression from myelotoxic drugs. Frequently, transfusions are given for platelet counts < 20,000/μL. Three units per meter squared, or approximately 6 units, should give an adequate increment in most adults. Pheresed or single-donor platelets are often given to those who require repeated transfusion to decrease donor exposure and risk of developing antibodies. Repeated transfusion may cause alloimmunization, with resultant smaller incremental increases in the platelet count after transfusion. Human leukocyte antigen–matched platelets increase platelet survival and are indicated in patients receiving multiple platelet transfusions who have a suboptimal response.

G. **Chemotherapy-related thrombocytopenia.** Oprelvekin (Neumega), a recombinant human interleukin-2, may be used for prevention of severe thrombocytopenia, and may decrease the need for platelet transfusion after myelosuppressive chemotherapy in nonmyeloid malignancies. The usual dose is 50 µg/kg SC every day and is initiated 6–24 hours after completion of chemotherapy and continued 14–21 days or until the postnadir platelet count is at least 50,000/µL. Discontinue at least 2 days before the next chemotherapy cycle. Severe thrombocytopenia related to chemotherapy requires platelet transfusion.

REFERENCES

Beutler E: Platelet transfusions: The 20,000/microliter trigger. Blood 1993;81:1411.

George JN: Drug-induced thrombocytopenia: A systemic review of published case reports. Ann Intern Med 1998;129:886.

George JN, Rizvi MA: Thrombocytopenia. In: Beutler E, Lichtman MA, Coller BS et al, eds. *William's Hematology.* 6th ed. McGraw-Hill;2001:1495.

George JN, Vesely SK. Immune thrombocytopenia purpura—let the treatment fit the patient. N Engl J Med 2003;349:903.

Rizvi MA, Kojouri K, George JN. Drug-induced thrombocytopenia: An updated systematic review. Ann Intern Med 2001;134:346.

Rodgers G: Thrombocytopenia. In: Kjeldsberg C, ed. *Practical Diagnosis of Hematologic Disorders.* 3rd ed. ASCP Press;2000:739.

62. TRANSFUSION REACTION

See also Section V, Blood Component Therapy, p 465.

I. **Problem.** During a transfusion of packed red blood cells (PRBCs), the patient's temperature rises to 38.5 °C (101.3 °F).

II. **Immediate Questions.** Fever is a common complication of transfusion of PRBCs and may result from infusion of a bacterially contaminated unit, mistransfusion of an ABO-incompatible unit, or a self-limited febrile-associated transfusion reaction. The first two conditions are life-threatening, and your initial evaluation is directed at differentiating among these.

A. **What are the patient's vital signs?** Presenting signs and symptoms of fever and chills, tachycardia, and tachypnea are nonspecific and do not allow you to differentiate reliably between a self-limited and a life-threatening transfusion reaction. Hypotension suggests a severe hemolytic transfusion reaction.

B. **Does the patient have any complaints?** Fever, frequently accompanied by shaking chills, may be the only clinical symptom of a febrile nonhemolytic transfusion reaction. However, severe acute hemolytic reactions are often accompanied by other symptoms, including nausea, vomiting, headache, and back pain. Often patients experience bronchospasm and pulmonary edema.

C. **Is there any evidence of generalized bleeding from mucosal membranes, previous venipuncture sites, or the present IV site?** Diffuse bleeding would be consistent with disseminated intravascular coagulation (DIC); it suggests a severe, life-threatening hemolytic reaction.

D. **Has the patient ever had a transfusion? If so, has she or he ever reacted to blood products in the past?** Patients who have histories of transfusion are likely to have become alloimmunized to blood group antigens. Patients with a history of febrile reactions to transfusion likely have cytotoxic or agglutinating antibodies to HLA antigens present on granulocytes, lymphocytes, and platelets. Although these reactions are troublesome, they are typically self-limited.

E. **Most important, does the name on the unit of PRBCs match that on the patient's armband?** Most fatal acute hemolytic transfusion reactions result from transfusion of ABO-incompatible blood. This is frequently the result of human error in patient or specimen identification occurring during situations of high stress.

III. **Differential Diagnosis**

A. **Hemolytic transfusion reaction**
1. **Severe sequelae from a hemolytic transfusion reaction.** These occur even when a small volume of incompatible blood is transfused. If there is concern that a patient may be experiencing a severe reaction, the transfusion must be stopped immediately. If the label on the transfusion unit of blood does not match that on the patient's armband, the blood bank should be notified immediately for assistance.
2. **Transfusion of ABO-incompatible blood results in intravascular hemolysis.** The naturally occurring anti-A or anti-B antibodies activate the classic complement pathway, resulting in membrane lysis and a liberation of free hemoglobin within the bloodstream. Fever, hypotension, shock, and renal failure may result. Approximately 10% of all transfusion reactions associated with infusion of an ABO-incompatible unit of PRBCs are fatal.

B. **Self-limiting febrile transfusion reaction.** This reaction is not hemolytic. It often occurs in patients who have had numerous transfusions or in multiparous women. Although this type of reaction often results in interruption of the transfusion, if no further symptoms develop the transfusion may be restarted.

C. Transfusion of blood contaminated with bacteria. This is an infrequent transfusion reaction (in the United States the estimated contamination rate is less than 1 per million red blood cell units). The most commonly implicated bacterial organism is *Yersinia enterocolitica*. The onset of symptoms frequently occurs during transfusion. The mortality rate is high (approximately 60%).

D. Delayed hemolytic reaction. This type of reaction should be suspected if a post-transfusion hemoglobin level cannot be maintained several days after the transfusion. Mild jaundice and fever with or without chills should alert the clinician to the possibility of a delayed hemolytic transfusion reaction. Many of these reactions are not detected because patients have been discharged from the hospital. The serologic findings of a delayed hemolytic transfusion reaction include a positive direct Coombs' test. The previously alloimmunized patient may not have had detectable antibody levels in his or her routine pre-transfusion antibody screening study. However, after reexposure to the relevant antigen, an amnestic response to the transfused red blood cells occurs. IgG antibody alone or IgG with complement may then be detected. A single antibody or multiple antibodies may be involved. The antibodies most often implicated are directed against Rh, Kidd, Duffy, or Kell antigens. Because the antibody titer may again drop to undetectable levels, a chart notation or Medic Alert card may prevent future reactions with known antibodies. Delayed hemolytic transfusion reactions are generally regarded as mild.

IV. Database

A. Physical examination key points

1. **Vital signs.** If the constellation of hypotension, fever, and tachycardia is present, the transfusion reaction must be considered to be a severe hemolytic reaction.
2. **Skin and mucous membranes.** Generalized bleeding may be part of a severe hemolytic reaction.
3. **Chest.** Wheezing or rales is consistent with a life-threatening reaction.

B. Laboratory data

1. **Hemogram.** May point to contaminated blood or show evidence of hemolysis.
2. **Prothrombin time, partial thromboplastin time, thrombin time, fibrinogen, and fibrin split products.** To rule out DIC.
3. **Peripheral smear.** Look for schistocytes as evidence of DIC.
4. **Urine for hemoglobinuria.** Supports the diagnosis of a severe transfusion reaction.
5. **Serum for free hemoglobin.** If positive, indicates hemolysis.
6. **Post-transfusion direct antiglobulin testing.** A negative study in the absence of serum-free hemoglobin supports that an acute hemolytic transfusion has not occurred.

7. **Gram's stain of remaining untransfused blood.** To rule out bacterial contamination of the unit.

V. Plan. The treatment plan depends on the type of reaction.

A. **Severe hemolytic reaction**
   1. If a serious transfusion reaction is suspected, the transfusion should be stopped immediately.
   2. **Supportive care** including IV fluids. The patient should be closely monitored for hypotension and decreasing urine output. If oliguria occurs, diuretics and mannitol may be required. If physical signs and laboratory findings indicate DIC, administration of platelets and cryoprecipitate is recommended.

B. **Self-limiting febrile transfusion reactions.** The findings of isolated fever and chills with a history of a febrile reaction support the diagnosis of a self-limiting febrile transfusion reaction. Antihistamines and antipruritics may be administered. Meperidine (Demerol) may be used for patients experiencing severe shaking chills. After premedication, transfusion may be safely resumed. Steps to prevent this type of reaction in the future include decreasing the granulocytes in the transfused unit. Leukofiltration and premedication are indicated for future transfusions.

C. **Transfusion of blood contaminated with microorganisms.** If this is suspected, broad-spectrum antibiotics should be instituted.

REFERENCES

Cookson ST, Arduino MJ, Aguero SM et al: *Yersinia enterocolitica*-contaminated red blood cells: An emerging threat to blood safety. 1996 Interscience Conference on Antimicrobial Agents and Chemotherapy. ABS:2352.
Goodnough LT. Risks of blood transfusion. Crit Care Med 2003;31:S678.
Jeter EK, Spivey MA. Noninfectious complications of blood transfusion. Hematol Oncol Clin North Am 1995;9:187.
Linden JV, Wagner K, Voytovich AE et al: Transfusion errors in New York State: An analysis of 10 years' experience. Transfusion 2001;40:1207.
Red blood cell transfusions contaminated with *Yersinia enterocolitica*—United States, 1991-1996, and initiation of a national study to detect bacteria-associated transfusion reactions. MMWR 1997;46:553.

63. WHEEZING

I. Problem. You are asked to evaluate a recently admitted patient who develops respiratory distress and wheezing.

II. Immediate Questions
   A. **What are the vital signs?** A respiratory rate greater than 30/min may indicate the need for immediate treatment. Associated hypotension may suggest an anaphylactic reaction, an acute myocardial in-

farction (MI) with pulmonary edema, or a pulmonary embolism (PE). Fever may point to an underlying infection, PE, or MI.

B. **Were any diagnostic tests recently performed or medicines administered?** A beta-blocker may precipitate an acute attack of bronchospasm when given to a patient with stable or undiagnosed asthma. Wheezing after the administration of a drug such as penicillin or radiocontrast dye suggests an anaphylactic reaction.

C. **Why was the patient admitted?** Acute pulmonary edema may accompany an MI, and aspiration can result from gastric outlet obstruction secondary to a gastric ulcer. Pulmonary edema is one of the more common nonasthmatic causes of wheezing. Similarly, aspiration can lead to stridor or wheezing.

D. **Is there a history of asthma?** Childhood asthma may reactivate at any age, given the right stimuli.

E. **Does the patient have any allergies to medications or other substances such as shellfish?** It is prudent to inquire about known allergies.

III. **Differential Diagnosis**

A. **Diffuse wheezing**
   1. **Acute bronchospasm.** May be caused by asthma, exacerbation of chronic obstructive pulmonary disease (COPD), anaphylactic reaction, or carcinoid syndrome.
   2. **Aspiration.** May trigger bronchospasm from mucosal irritation or from impacted foreign bodies.
   3. **Cardiogenic pulmonary edema.** The primary finding in "cardiac asthma" may be wheezing. Other findings of pulmonary edema should be present, and the chest x-ray will be diagnostic.
   4. **PE.** Mediators may be released in PE that cause not only hypoxemia but also transient bronchospasm.

B. **Stridor (upper airway wheezing)**
   1. **Laryngospasm.** This may be part of an anaphylactic reaction or secondary to aspiration.
   2. **Laryngeal or tracheal tumor.** A history of dysphagia, hoarseness, cough, or weight loss and anorexia may be present.
   3. **Epiglottitis.** The patient is often unable to speak or to swallow secretions. The mouth is held open and there may be drooling. (Similar presentation may occur with Ludwig's angina or an abscess involving the floor of the mouth.)
   4. **Foreign body aspiration**
   5. **Vocal cord dysfunction.** Bilaterally paralyzed vocal cords may result in severe stridor and dyspnea. A subgroup of patients has recently been recognized to have "factitious asthma" or laryngeal dyskinesia. These patients adduct their vocal cords when they should be holding them open (abducting them).

C. Localized wheezing

1. **Tumors.** May obstruct one bronchus, leading to localized wheezing.
2. **Mucous plugging**
3. **Aspirated foreign body**

IV. Database

A. Physical examination key points. Localization of wheezing allows categorization, as outlined in the differential diagnosis (see III).

1. **Vital signs.** A fever may indicate an infectious cause. A pulsus paradoxus > 16 mm Hg indicates severe respiratory distress. Hypotension requires immediate assessment and action.
2. **HEENT.** Check the mouth carefully. Examine the neck and tongue for angioedema, which may be precipitated by angiotensin-converting enzyme (ACE) inhibitors. Palpate the sternocleidomastoid muscles to assess accessory muscle use in obstructive lung diseases. Auscultate over the mouth and larynx in an effort to identify upper airway wheezing (stridor).
3. **Chest.** Carefully auscultate for localized wheezing. Listen for bibasilar rales, which may be present in pulmonary edema. Rales, increased fremitus, and egophony suggest pneumonia.
4. **Heart.** Check carefully for evidence of an S_3 gallop or jugular venous distention, which points to cardiogenic pulmonary edema.
5. **Extremities.** Clubbing may indicate underlying lung cancer. Cyanosis indicates underlying hypoxemia. Edema may signify chronic congestive heart failure.
6. **Skin.** Urticaria suggests an acute allergic reaction.

B. Laboratory data

1. **Arterial blood gases.** An elevated $paCO_2$ indicates significant ventilatory failure. Hypoxemia is commonly present during bronchospasm because of $\dot{V}/\dot{Q}$ mismatch. It may worsen after beta-agonist aerosols.
2. **Complete blood count.** An increased white blood cell (WBC) count may indicate an underlying infection; however, an increase in WBCs without a left shift can be seen with an acute MI or PE. Eosinophilia suggests an allergic or asthmatic cause of the wheezing.

C. Radiologic and other studies

1. **Electrocardiogram (ECG).** An ECG may show an acute MI or ischemia. Occasionally, it is suggestive of a PE, showing an S wave in lead I, a Q wave in III, T-wave inversion in lead III $(S_1Q_3T_3)$, new right bundle branch block, and right-axis shift. It may also show a change in rhythm.
2. **Chest radiograph.** A PE (with infarction) severe enough to cause wheezing may be evident on the chest film. Look for a pleural-

based, wedge-shaped lesion (Hampton's hump) or localized oligemia of the pulmonary arteries. Kerley B lines, bilateral pleural effusions, vascular redistribution, and cardiomegaly may suggest congestive heart failure. Look for localized infiltrates or masses suggesting other causes.

V. Plan. Treatment depends on the diagnosis. The preceding differential diagnoses and studies should enable you to form a tentative categorization on which to base initial therapy.

A. Bronchospasm (asthma, COPD, allergic reaction)
1. **Methylprednisolone (Solu-Medrol).** Give 60–125 mg IV Q 6 hr.
2. **Nebulized albuterol.** Give 0.5 mL of 0.5% solution (2.5 mg) in 2.5 mL normal saline stat and every 20 minutes for 3 doses, then every 1–4 hours as needed. Alternatively, four puffs albuterol metered-dose inhaler via spacer device may be given every 20 minutes up to 4 hours (12 doses), then every 1–4 hours as needed.

B. Stridor
1. **Methylprednisolone 40 mg IV stat dose**
2. **Nebulized racemic epinephrine.** Give 0.5 mL in 3 mL normal saline.
3. **Continuous positive airway pressure (CPAP).** Give 10–15 cm H_2O applied continuously; if ventilatory failure is suspected, consider bilevel positive airway pressure (BiPAP) instead at 15/10 cm H_2O.
4. **Intubation or tracheostomy.** If there is no response to the above measures.

C. Pulmonary edema
1. **Furosemide (Lasix) 20–80 mg IV**
2. **Nitroglycerin.** Give 0.4 mg sublingually, or paste ½ inch on skin, or nitroglycerin drip 10–20 μg/min and increase by 5–10 μg every 10 minutes.
3. **Afterload reduction.** Use agents such as IV nitroprusside (Nipride), or oral agents such as captopril (Capoten) or enalapril (Vasotec), or any other ACE inhibitor.
4. **Intravenous morphine.** For venodilation and to relieve anxiety. Morphine may suppress respiratory drive and cause further respiratory compromise, necessitating intubation.
5. **Oxygen.** Start with 100% oxygen by nonrebreather mask, as long as the patient is not a carbon dioxide retainer.
6. **CPAP (10 cm) or BiPAP (12/8 cm).** Recently proven efficacious in acute pulmonary edema.

D. Miscellaneous disorders. Treatment varies with the disease. PE should be treated with anticoagulants (see Section I, Chapter 11, Chest Pain, V, p 66). Suspected tumors require additional tests such as bronchoscopy before reasonable treatment can be initiated.

REFERENCES

Aboussouan LS, Stoller JK: Diagnosis and management of upper airway obstruction. Clin Chest Med 1994;15:35.

Leatherman J: Life-threatening asthma. Clin Chest Med 1994;15:453.

NHLBI Expert Panel Report 2: *Guidelines for the Diagnosis and Management of Asthma.* NIH Publication # 97-4051; April 1997.

II. Laboratory Diagnosis

Notes: The ranges of normal values are given below each test, first in conventional units such as metric (eg, milligrams per liter) and then in international units if there is a difference. Reference ranges for each laboratory may vary from the values given; therefore, you should interpret the results of a patient's laboratory value in light of an individual facility's range.

■ ACID-FAST STAIN

Positive: *Mycobacterium* species (tuberculosis and atypical mycobacteria such as *M avium-intracellulare*) and *Nocardia*.

■ ACTH (ADRENOCORTICOTROPIC HORMONE)

8 AM: 20–100 pg/mL or 20–100 ng/L; midnight value: ~ 50% of AM value.

Increased: Addison's disease; ectopic ACTH production (small cell carcinoma, pancreatic islet cell tumors, thymic tumors, renal cell carcinoma).

Decreased: Adrenal adenoma or carcinoma, nodular adrenal hyperplasia, pituitary insufficiency.

■ ACTH STIMULATION TEST

Used to help diagnose adrenal insufficiency. Cosyntropin (Cortrosyn), an ACTH analogue, is given at a dose of 0.25 mg IM or IV. Collect blood at times 0, 30, and 60 minutes for cortisol.

Normal response: Basal cortisol of at least 5 µg/dL, an increase of at least 7 µg/dL, and a final cortisol of 16 µg/dL at 30 minutes or 18 µg/dL at 60 minutes.

Subnormal/abnormal response: Addison's disease (primary adrenal insufficiency) and secondary adrenal insufficiency: Secondary insufficiency is caused by pituitary insufficiency or suppression by exogenous steroids. An ACTH level and pituitary stimulation tests can be used to differentiate primary from secondary adrenal insufficiency.

■ ALBUMIN, SERUM

3.5–5.0 g/dL or 35–50 g/L.

Decreased: Malnutrition, nephrotic syndrome, cystic fibrosis, multiple myeloma, Hodgkin's disease, leukemia, protein-losing enteropathies, chronic glomerulonephritis, cirrhosis, inflammatory bowel disease, collagen-vascular diseases, hyperthyroidism.

■ ALBUMIN, URINE

Normal = < 30 mg/day.

Microalbuminuria 30–300 mg/day (a sign of early renal damage in diabetes mellitus, hypertension, and other diseases affecting the kidney. Its presence helps identify patients at risk for renal failure, neuropathy, retinopathy, and coronary artery disease. Renal function may be preserved with the use of an angiotensin-converting enzyme [ACE] inhibitor or angiotensin-receptor blocker [ARB]). Microalbuminuria can be detected by determining the albumin to creatinine ratio by obtaining a spot urine for albumin and creatinine. Normal is < 30 μg of albumin per milligram of creatinine, and microalbuminuria is defined as 30–300 μg of albumin per milligram of creatinine.

Note: Microalbuminuria can be seen with prolonged exercise, hematuria, fever, or prolonged upright posture.

Nephrotic proteinuria > 3.5 g/day.

■ ALDOSTERONE

Serum—supine: 3–10 g/dL or 0.083–0.28 nmol/L early AM, normal sodium intake; upright: 5–30 g/dL or 0.138–0.83 nmol/L.

Urinary—2–16 μg/24 hr or 5.4–44.3 nmol/day.

Increased: Hyperaldosteronism (primary or secondary). Should confirm after oral or IV salt loading.

Decreased: Adrenal insufficiency.

■ ALKALINE PHOSPHATASE

Adults: 20–70 U/L.

A γ-glutamyltransferase (GGT) is often useful to differentiate whether an elevated alkaline phosphatase originates from bone or liver. A normal GGT suggests bone origin.

Increased: Increased calcium deposition in bone (hyperparathyroidism), Paget's disease, osteoblastic bone tumors, osteomalacia, pregnancy, childhood, liver disease, and hyperthyroidism.

Decreased: Malnutrition, excess vitamin D ingestion.

■ ALPHA-FETOPROTEIN (AFP)

< 30 ng/mL or < 30 μg/L.

Increased: Hepatoma, testicular tumor (embryonal carcinoma, malignant teratoma), spina bifida (in mother's serum).

■ ALT (ALANINE AMINOTRANSFERASE) (SGPT: SERUM GLUTAMIC-PYRUVIC TRANSFERASE)

8–20 U/L.

Increased: Liver disease–liver metastases, biliary obstruction, liver congestion, hepatitis (ALT is more elevated than AST in viral hepatitis; AST is more elevated than ALT in alcoholic hepatitis.)

■ AMMONIA

Arterial: 15–45 μg/dL or 11–32 μmol N/L.

Increased: Hepatic encephalopathy, Reye's syndrome.

■ AMYLASE

25–125 U/L.

Increased: Acute pancreatitis, pancreatic duct obstruction (stones, stricture, tumor, sphincter of Oddi spasm), alcohol ingestion, mumps, parotiditis, renal disease, macroamylasemia, cholecystitis, peptic ulcers, intestinal obstruction, mesenteric thrombosis, after surgery (upper abdominal), ovarian cancer, ruptured ectopic pregnancy, and diabetic ketoacidosis.

Decreased: Pancreatic destruction (pancreatitis, cystic fibrosis), liver disease (hepatitis, cirrhosis).

■ ANION GAP

8–12 mmol/L.
   Note: The anion gap is a calculated estimate of unmeasured anions and is used to help differentiate the cause of metabolic acidosis.

$$\text{Anion gap} = (Na^+) - (Cl^- + HCO_3^-)$$

Increased (high): (> 12 mmol/L): Lactic acidosis, ketoacidosis (diabetic, alcoholic, starvation); uremia; toxins (salicylates, methanol, ethylene glycol, paraldehyde). In addition, dehydration, alkalosis, use of certain penicillins (carbenicillin), and salts of strong acids such as sodium citrate (used as a preservative in packed red blood cells) can cause a mild increase in the anion gap.

Decreased (low): (< 8 mmol/L): Seen with bromide ingestion, hypercalcemia, hypermagnesemia, multiple myeloma, and hypoalbuminemia.

■ ANTICARDIOLIPIN ANTIBODIES

See Antiphospholipid Antibodies, p 373.

■ ANTINEUTROPHIL CYTOPLASMIC ANTIBODIES (ANCAS)

Negative = < 10 U/mL.
Equivocal = 10–20 U/mL.
Positive = > 20 U/mL.

Antibodies to cytoplasmic components of neutrophils, seen in vasculitides. Two types:

1. **C-ANCA (cytoplasmic-staining ANCA).** Present in ~ 90% of patients with generalized Wegener's granulomatosis; also seen in rapidly progressive glomerulonephritis and a type of polyarteritis nodosa (microscopic). C-ANCA may be used to follow disease activity; it is also especially useful in distinguishing active disease from an infectious complication. C-ANCA is not present in other collagen-vascular diseases.

2. **P-ANCA (perinuclear-staining ANCA).** Seen in a variety of collagen-vascular diseases such as limited Wegener's granulomatosis, polyarteritis nodosa, Goodpasture's syndrome, other vasculitides, and inflammatory bowel disease (Crohn's disease). It is also seen in several types of glomerulonephritides.

■ ANTINUCLEAR ANTIBODIES (ANA)

Negative: A useful screening test in patients with symptoms suggesting collagen-vascular disease, especially if titer is > 1:160.

Positive: Systemic lupus erythematosus (SLE), drug-induced lupus (procainamide, hydralazine, isoniazid, etc), scleroderma, mixed connective tissue disease (MCTD), rheumatoid arthritis, polymyositis, juvenile rheumatoid arthritis (JRA) (5–20%). Low titers are also seen in patients with non–collagen-vascular disease and in those without any disease.

Specific Immunofluorescent ANA Patterns

1. ANA patterns
   - **Homogeneous:** Nonspecific, from antibodies to deoxyribonucleoproteins (DNP) and native double-stranded deoxyribonucleic acid (DNA). Seen in SLE and a variety of other diseases. Antihistone is consistent with drug-induced lupus.
   - **Speckled:** Pattern seen in many connective tissue disorders. From antibodies to extractable nuclear antigens (ENA) including antiribonucleoproteins (anti-RNP), anti-Sm, anti-PM-1, and anti-SS. Anti-RNP is positive in MCTD and SLE. Anti-Sm is found in SLE. Anti-SS-A and anti-SS-B are seen in Sjögren's syndrome and subacute cutaneous lupus. The speckled pattern is also seen with scleroderma.

- **Peripheral RIM pattern:** From antibodies to native double-stranded DNA and DNP. Seen in SLE.
- **Nucleolar pattern:** From antibodies to nucleolar ribonucleic acid (RNA). Positive in Sjögren's syndrome and scleroderma.
2. Other autoantibodies
   - **Antimitochondrial:** Primary biliary cirrhosis.
   - **Anti–smooth muscle:** Low titers are seen in a variety of illnesses; high titers (> 1:100) are suggestive of chronic active hepatitis.
   - **Antimicrosomal:** Hashimoto's thyroiditis.

■ ANTIPHOSPHOLIPID ANTIBODIES

Note: There are two basic categories of antiphospholipid antibody—anticardiolipin and lupus anticoagulant. Both are associated with recurrent arterial or venous thrombosis or fetal demise.

Anticardiolipin antibody. Two forms: IgG, IgM.
   IgG normal < 23 U.
   IgM normal < 11 U.

Lupus anticoagulant\eh4
   Negative = normal.
   Positive = presence.
   Should be suspected with an isolated elevated partial thromboplastin time (PTT) with no other likely cause.

■ AST (ASPARTATE AMINOTRANSFERASE) (SGOT: SERUM GLUTAMIC-OXALOACETIC TRANSFERASE)

8–20 U/L.
   Generally parallels changes in ALT in liver disease.

Increased: Liver disease, acute myocardial infarction, Reye's syndrome, muscle trauma and injection, pancreatitis, intestinal injury or surgery, factitious increase (erythromycin, opiates), burns, brain damage.

Decreased: Beri-beri, diabetes mellitus with ketoacidosis, chronic liver disease.

■ B$_{12}$ (VITAMIN B$_{12}$)

140–700 pg/mL or 189–516 pmol/L.

Increased: Leukemia, polycythemia vera.

Decreased: Pernicious anemia, bacterial overgrowth, dietary deficiency (rare—humans normally have 2–3 years of stores), malabsorption, pregnancy.

■ BASE EXCESS/DEFICIT

See Table II–1, p 374. A decrease in base (bicarbonate) is termed *base deficit*; an increase in base is termed *base excess*.

Excess: Metabolic alkalosis (see Section I, Chapter 3, Alkalosis, p 19), respiratory acidosis (see Section I, Chapter 2, Acidosis, p 10).

Deficit: Metabolic acidosis (see Section I, Chapter 2, Acidosis, p 10), respiratory alkalosis (see Section I, Chapter 3, Alkalosis, p 19).

■ BENCE–JONES PROTEINS—URINE

Negative: Normal.

Positive: Multiple myeloma, idiopathic Bence–Jones proteinuria.

■ BICARBONATE (SERUM HCO_3^-)

22–29 mmol/L.
See Tables II–1 and II–2. Also see Carbon Dioxide, Arterial, p 377, for pCO_2 values.

Increased: Metabolic alkalosis, compensation for respiratory acidosis. See Section I, Chapter 2, Acidosis, p 10; and Section I, Chapter 3, Alkalosis, p 19.

TABLE II–1. NORMAL BLOOD GAS VALUES.

Measurement	Arterial	Mixed Venous[1]	Venous
pH	7.40	7.36	7.36
(range)	(7.36–7.44)	(7.31–7.41)	(7.31–7.41)
pO_2 (decreases with age)	80–100 mm Hg	35–40 mm Hg	30–50 mm Hg
pCO_2	36–44 mm Hg	41–51 mm Hg	40–52 mm Hg
O_2 saturation (decreases with age)	>95%	60–80%	60–80%
HCO_3^-	22–26 mmol/L	22–26 mmol/L	22–29 mmol/L
Base difference (deficit/excess)	–2 to +2	–2 to +2	–2 to +2

[1]From right atrium.
Modified and reproduced with permission from Gomella LG, ed. *Clinician's Pocket Reference.* 10th ed. McGraw-Hill; 2004.

TABLE II–2. ACID–BASE DISORDERS WITH APPROPRIATE COMPENSATION.

Disorder	Changes in Normal Values		
	pH	HCO$_3^-$	pCO$_2$
Metabolic acidosis	↓	↓↓	↓
Metabolic alkalosis	↑	↑↑	↑
Acute respiratory acidosis	↓	slight↑	↑↑
Chronic respiratory acidosis	slight↓	↑	↑↑
Acute respiratory alkalosis	↑	slight↓	↓↓
Chronic respiratory alkalosis	slight↑	↓	↓↓

Decreased: Metabolic acidosis, compensation for respiratory alkalosis. See Section I, Chapter 2, Acidosis, p 10; and Section I, Chapter 3, Alkalosis, p 19.

■ BILIRUBIN

Total: < 0.2–1.0 mg/dL or 3.4–17.1 µmol/L;

Direct: < 0.2 mg/dL or < 3.4 µmol/L;

Indirect: < 0.8 mg/dL or < 13.7 µmol/L.

Increased total: Hepatic damage (hepatitis, toxins, cirrhosis), biliary obstruction (gallstone or tumor), hemolysis, fasting.

Increased direct (conjugated): Biliary obstruction (gallstone, tumor, stricture), drug-induced cholestasis, Dubin-Johnson syndrome, and Rotor's syndrome.

Increased indirect (unconjugated): Hemolytic anemia (transfusion reaction, sickle cell, collagen-vascular disease), Gilbert's disease, Crigler-Najjar syndrome.

■ BLEEDING TIME

Duke, Ivy: < 6 min; Template: < 10 min.

Increased: Thrombocytopenia, thrombocytopenic purpura, von Willebrand's disease, defective platelet function (aspirin, nonsteroidal anti-inflammatory drugs, uremia).

■ BLOOD GAS, ARTERIAL

See Tables II–1 and II–2, p 375. For acid–base disorders, see Section I, Chapter 2, Acidosis, p 10; and Chapter 3, Alkalosis, p 19.

■ BLOOD GAS, VENOUS

See Table II–1, p 374. **Note:** There is little difference between arterial and venous pH and bicarbonate (except with congestive heart failure [CHF] and shock). Therefore, the venous blood gas may be occasionally used to assess acid–base status, but venous oxygen levels are significantly lower than arterial levels.

■ BLOOD UREA NITROGEN (BUN)

7–18 mg/dL or 1.2–3.0 mmol urea/L.

Increased: Renal failure, prerenal azotemia (decreased renal perfusion secondary to CHF, shock, volume depletion), postrenal obstruction, gastrointestinal bleeding, hypercatabolic states.

Decreased: Starvation, malnutrition, liver failure (hepatitis, drugs), pregnancy, infancy, nephrotic syndrome, overhydration.

■ BLOOD UREA NITROGEN/CREATININE RATIO

Between 10 and 20:1.

Elevated ratio (> 20:1): CHF, dehydration, gastrointestinal bleeding, increased protein intake, drugs such as tetracycline and steroids, infection (sepsis), high fevers, burns, and cachexia.

Decreased ratio (< 10:1): Acute tubular necrosis, low-protein diet, starvation, malnutrition, liver disease, syndrome of inappropriate antidiuretic hormone, pregnancy, and rhabdomyolysis.
   Note: The ratio may not be appropriate if the patient is in diabetic ketoacidosis or receiving drugs such as cephalosporin.
   The ratio can be altered by interferences in the chemical methods used to measure the creatinine or the BUN, resulting in spurious results. The presence of ketones may seriously elevate the serum creatinine level. Drugs such as cephalosporins, ascorbic acid, and barbiturates may also interfere with the serum creatinine measurement.

■ CALCITONIN

< 100 pg/mL or < 100 g/L.

Increased: Medullary carcinoma of the thyroid, pregnancy, chronic renal insufficiency, Zollinger-Ellison syndrome, pernicious anemia.

■ CALCIUM, SERUM

8.4–10.2 mg/dL (4.2–5.1 mEq/L) or 2.10–2.55 mmol/L;
   Ionized: 4.5–4.9 mg/dL (2.2–2.5 mEq/L) or 1.1–1.2 mmol/L.

Note: To interpret a total calcium value, you must know the albumin level. If the albumin is not within normal limits, a corrected calcium can be roughly calculated with the following formula. Values for ionized calcium need no special correction.

Corrected total Ca = 0.8 (normal albumin − measured
albumin) + reported Ca

Increased: See Section I, Chapter 31, Hypercalcemia, p 185.

Decreased: See Section I, Chapter 36, Hypocalcemia, p 210.

■ CALCIUM, URINE

Average calcium diet: 100–300 mg per 24-hour urine.

Increased: Hyperparathyroidism, hyperhyroidism, hypervitaminosis D, distal renal tubular acidosis (type I), sarcoidosis, immobilization, osteolytic lesions (bony metastasis, multiple myeloma), Paget's disease, glucocorticoid excess (either endogenous or exogenous), furosemide.

Decreased: Thiazide diuretics, hypothyroidism, renal failure, steatorrhea, rickets, osteomalacia.

■ CARBON DIOXIDE, ARTERIAL (PCO₂)

36–44 mm Hg. See Tables II–1 and II–2, p 374, 375.

Increased: Respiratory acidosis, compensation for metabolic alkalosis. See Section I, Chapter 2, Acidosis, p 10; and Chapter 3, Alkalosis, p 19.

Decreased: Respiratory alkalosis, compensation for metabolic acidosis. See Section I, Chapter 2, Acidosis, p 10; and Chapter 3, Alkalosis, p 19.

■ CARBOXYHEMOGLOBIN

Nonsmoker: < 2%.
  Smoker: < 6%.
  Toxic: > 15%.

Increased: Smoking, smoke inhalation; exposure to automobile exhaust, faulty heating units with inadequate ventilation.

■ CARCINOMA MARKERS

CA 125.
  0–35 m/L.

Elevated level is abnormal. CA 125 is a glycoprotein that is used to evaluate response to chemotherapy in serous carcinoma of the ovary. It is not associated with mucinous carcinoma of the ovary. It can also be elevated in other gynecologic conditions such as endometrial adenocarcinoma and neoplasms of the cervix and vulva. CA 125 may be elevated in pancreatic carcinoma as well as in carcinomas of the lung and liver. Trophoblastic neoplasms can be related to elevated levels, as can some benign conditions such as menstruation and pregnancy.

BRCA-1 and BRCA-2 (Breast Cancer Gene 1 and Gene 2)

An expensive test that looks for genetic mutations that have been associated with development of breast carcinoma and ovarian carcinoma. It may be useful in a person who has a strong family history of either breast cancer or ovarian cancer. If ordered, this test should be discussed with patient in light of family history and in the setting of genetic counseling, since the implications go beyond the individual patient and may affect siblings, children, and other relatives. It may not be covered by insurance plans. This test could be used to rate an individual's health and life insurability.

Her2/neu-

Positive result is abnormal. This means that the gene is overexpressed in the breast carcinoma, suggesting an aggressive breast carcinoma that tends to be resistant to hormonal therapy and chemotherapy. Some patients may respond to Herceptin.

Carcinoembryonic Antigen (CEA)

Nonsmoker: < 3.0 g/mL or < 3.0 μg/L.
  Smoker: < 5.0 g/mL or < 5.0 μg/L.

Increased: Carcinoma (colon, pancreas, lung, stomach), smokers, nonneoplastic liver disease, Crohn's disease, and ulcerative colitis. Test used predominantly to monitor patients for recurrence of carcinoma, especially after colon carcinoma resection.

■ CATECHOLAMINES, FRACTIONATED

Note: Values are variable and depend on the lab and method of assay used. Normal levels listed in Table II–3 are based on high-performance liquid chromatography technique.

Increased: Pheochromocytoma, neural crest tumors (neuroblastoma). In extra-adrenal pheochromocytoma, norepinephrine may be markedly elevated compared with epinephrine.

TABLE II–3. FRACTIONATED CATECHOLAMINES.

Catecholamine	Plasma (Supine)	Urine
Norepinephrine	70–750 pg/mL 414–4435 pmol/L	14–80 µg/24-hr 82.7–473 nmol/d
Epinephrine	0–100 pg/mL 0–100 pg/mL	0.5–20 µg/24-hr 2.73–109 nmol/d
Dopamine	<30 pg/mL <196 pmol/L	65–400 µg/24-hr 424–2612 nmol/d

■ CATECHOLAMINES, URINE, UNCONJUGATED

> 15 years old: < 100 µg/24 hr.
   Measures free (unconjugated) epinephrine, norepinephrine, and dopamine.

Increased: Pheochromocytoma, neural crest tumors (neuroblastoma).

■ CBC (COMPLETE BLOOD COUNT, HEMOGRAM)

Note: For normal values, see Table II–4. For differential, see specific tests.

■ CHLORIDE, SERUM

98–106 mEq/L.

Increased: Metabolic nongap acidosis such as diarrhea, renal tubular acidosis, mineralocorticoid deficiency, hyperalimentation, medications (acetazolamide, ammonium chloride).

Decreased: Vomiting, diabetes mellitus with ketoacidosis, mineralocorticoid excess, renal disease with sodium loss.

■ CHLORIDE, URINE

110–250 mmol per 24-hour urine.
   See Urinary Electrolytes, p 411.

■ CHOLESTEROL (TOTAL)

140–240 mg/dL or 3.63–6.22 mmol/L.
   Desired level: < 200 mg/dL or 5.18 mmol/L.

Increased: Primary hypercholesterolemia (types IIA, IIB, III), elevated triglycerides (types I, IV, V), biliary obstruction, nephrosis, hypothyroidism, diabetes mellitus, pregnancy.

TABLE II–4. NORMAL CBC VALUES—ADULTS.[1]

WBC	4800–10,800 cells/μL
RBCs	M: 4.7–6.1 × 10^6 cells/μL
	F: 4.2–5.4 × 10^6 cells/μL
Hemoglobin	M: 14–18 g/dL
	F:12–16 g/dL
Hematocrit	M: 40–54%
	F: 37–47%
MCV	M: 80–94 fL
	F: 81–99 fL
MCH	27–31 pg
MCHC (%)	33–37%
RDW	11.5–14.5
Platelets	150,000–450,000/μL
■ **Differential**	
Segmented neutrophils	41–71%
Banded (stab) neutrophils	5–10%
Lymphocytes	24–44%
Monocytes	3–7%
Eosinophils	1–3%
Basophils	0–1%

[1]Refer to hospital reference values.
Modified and reproduced with permission from Gomella LG, ed. *Clinician's Pocket Reference.* 10th ed. McGraw-Hill; 2004.

Decreased: Chronic liver disease, hyperthyroidism, malnutrition (cancer, starvation), myeloproliferative disorders, steroid therapy, lipoproteinemias.

High-Density Lipoprotein (HDL) Cholesterol

Fasting male: 40–60 mg/dL or 0.78–1.81 mmol/L.
   Fasting female: 40–60 mg/dL or 0.78–2.07 mmol/L.
   Note: HDL highly correlates with the development of coronary artery disease; a decreased HDL (< 40 mg/dL) leads to an increased risk, and an increased HDL (> 60 mg/dL) is associated with a decreased risk.

Increased: Estrogen (females), exercise, ethanol.

Decreased: Male gender, beta-blockers, anabolic steroids, uremia, obesity, diabetes, liver disease, Tangier's disease.

Low-Density Lipoprotein (LDL) Cholesterol

Desired: < 130–160 mg/dL or 3.36–4.14 mmol/L. In the presence of coronary artery disease or diabetes mellitus or with an increased risk of myocardial infarction in the next 10 years (> 10 %), desired LDL is < 100 mg/dL or 2.58 mmol/L (optimal < 70 mg/dL).

Increased: Excess dietary saturated fats, myocardial infarction, hyperlipoproteinemia, biliary cirrhosis, endocrine disease (diabetes, hypothyroidism).

Decreased: Malabsorption, severe liver disease, abetalipoproteinemia.

Triglycerides

See Triglycerides, p 407.

■ COLD AGGLUTININS

Normal = < 1:32.

Increased: *Mycoplasma* pneumonia; viral infections (especially mononucleosis, measles, mumps); cirrhosis; some parasitic infections.

■ COMPLEMENT C3

80–155 mg/dL or 800–1550 ng/L.
> 60 years: 80–170 mg/dL or 80–1700 ng/L.
Note: Normal values may vary greatly depending on the assay used.

Increased: Rheumatic fever, neoplasms (gastrointestinal, prostate, others).

Decreased: SLE, glomerulonephritis (poststreptococcal and membranoproliferative), vasculitis, severe hepatic failure.

Variable: Rheumatoid arthritis.

■ COMPLEMENT C4

20–50 mg/dL or 200–500 ng/L.

Increased: Neoplasia (gastrointestinal, lung, others).

Decreased: SLE, chronic active hepatitis, cirrhosis, glomerulonephritis, hereditary angioedema.

Variable: Rheumatoid arthritis.

■ COMPLEMENT CH50 (TOTAL)

33–61 mg/mL or 330–610 ng/L. Tests for complement deficiency in the classic pathway.

Increased: Acute-phase reactants (eg, tissue injury, infections).

Decreased: Hereditary complement deficiencies, any cause of deficiency of individual complement components. See Complement C3 and Complement C4.

■ COOMBS' TEST, DIRECT

Uses patient's erythrocytes; tests for the presence of antibody or complement on the patient's red blood cells.

Positive: Autoimmune hemolytic anemia (leukemia, lymphoma, collagen-vascular diseases, eg, SLE); hemolytic transfusion reaction; sensitization to some drugs (methyldopa, levodopa, penicillins, cephalosporins).

■ COOMBS' TEST, INDIRECT

More useful for red blood cell typing. Uses serum that contains antibody from the patient.

Positive: Isoimmunization from previous transfusion; incompatible blood as a result of improper cross-matching.

■ CORTISOL

Serum—8 AM: 5.0–23.0 µg/dL or 138–635 nmol/L; 4 PM: 3.0–15.0 µg/dL or 83–414 nmol/L.
   Urine (24-hour): 10–100 µg/day or 27.6–276 nmol/day.

Increased: Adrenal adenoma, adrenal carcinoma, Cushing's disease, non-pituitary ACTH-producing tumor, steroid therapy, oral contraceptives.

Decreased: Primary adrenal Insufficiency (Addison's disease), Water-house-Friderichsen syndrome, ACTH deficiency.

■ CORTROSYN STIMULATION TEST

See ACTH Stimulation Test, p 369.

■ COUNTERIMMUNOELECTROPHORESIS (CIE)

Normal = negative.
   CIE is an immunologic technique that allows rapid identification of infectious organisms from body fluids, including serum, urine, cerebrospinal fluid, and others. Organisms that can be identified include *Neisseria meningitidis, Streptococcus pneumoniae, Haemophilus influenzae,* and group B streptococcus.

■ C-PEPTIDE

Fasting: ≤ 4.0 g/mL or = 4.0 µg/L;
   Males > 60 years: 1.5–5.0 g/mL or 1.5–5.0 µg/L;
   Females: 1.4–5.5 g/mL or 1.4–5.5 µg/L.

Decreased: Diabetes (insulin-dependent diabetes mellitus), insulin administration, hypoglycemia.

Increased: Insulinoma. Test is useful to differentiate insulinoma from surreptitious use of insulin as a cause of hypoglycemia.

■ C-REACTIVE PROTEIN (CRP)

Normal: < 8 mg/L.
   An acute-phase reactant with a relatively short half-life.

Increased: Infections (increase in bacterial infections > increase in viral infections); tissue injury or necrosis (acute myocardial infarction, malignant disease [especially lung, breast, and gastrointestinal] and organ rejection following transplantation); and some inflammatory disorders (rheumatoid arthritis). With certain inflammatory disorders such as SLE, scleroderma, and Crohn's disease, the CRP will not be elevated as much as one would expect for the degree of inflammation; therefore, the sedimentation rate may be a better marker of inflammation in these disorders.

High-sensitivity C-reactive protein: Not widely used but several labs are now performing. Check your lab for reference ranges. Elevated levels are associated with increased risk of cardiovascular disease such as myocardial infarction and possibly unstable atherosclerotic plaques of carotid arteries. This is an important predictor at all levels of LDL.
   This test is used to predict a *healthy person's risk* for cardiovascular conditions such as heart attack. Since it measures CRP, people with inflammatory diseases such as rheumatoid arthritis should not be evaluated based on this test.

■ CREATINE PHOSPHOKINASE (CK)

25–145 mU/mL or 25–145 U/L.

Increased: Cardiac muscle (acute myocardial infarction, myocarditis, defibrillation); skeletal muscle (intramuscular injection, hypothyroidism, rhabdomyolysis, polymyositis, muscular dystrophy); cerebral infarction.

CK isoenzymes MM, MB, BB: MB (normal < 6%) increased in acute myocardial infarction (increases in 4–8 hours, peaks at 24 hours), cardiac surgery; BB not useful.

■ CREATININE CLEARANCE

Males: 100–135 mL/min or 0.963–1.300 mL/s/m^2.
  Females: 85–125 mL/min or 0.819–1.204 mL/s/m^2.
  A concurrent serum creatinine and a 24-hour urine creatinine are needed. A shorter time interval can be used and corrected for in the formula. A quick formula for estimation is also found in Table VII–18, Aminoglycoside Dosing, p 630.

$$\text{Creatinine clearance} = \frac{(\text{urine creatinine} \times \text{total urine volume})}{(\text{plasma creatinine} \times \text{time in minutes})}$$

  To verify if the urine sample is a complete 24-hour collection, determine whether the sample contains at least 14–26 mg/kg/24 hr or 124–230 mmol/kg/day creatinine for adult males; or 11–20 mg/kg/24 hr or 97–177 mmol/kg/day for adult females. This test is not a requirement.

Decreased: A decreased creatinine clearance results in an increase in serum creatinine, usually secondary to renal insufficiency. Clearance normally decreases with age. See Creatinine, Serum, Increased, which follows..

Increased: Pregnancy, prediabetic renal failure.

■ CREATININE, SERUM

Males: 0.7–1.3 mg/dL.
  Females: 0.6–1.1 mg/dL.

Increased: Renal failure (prerenal, renal, or postrenal), acromegaly, ingestion of roasted meat, large body mass. Falsely elevated with ketones and certain cephalosporins, depending on assay.

■ CREATININE, URINE

Male total creatinine: 14–26 mg/kg/24 hr or 124–230 μmol/kg/day.
  Females: 11–20 mg/kg/24 hr or 97–177 μmol/kg/day. See Creatinine Clearance, p 384.

■ CRYOCRIT

≤ 0.4%. (Negative if qualitative.) Cryocrit, a quantitative measure, is preferred over the qualitative method. It should be collected in nonanticoagulated tubes and transported at body temperature. Positive samples can be analyzed for immunoglobulin class, and light-chain type on request.
  > 0.4%. (Positive if qualitative.) *Monoclonal*—Multiple myeloma, Waldenström's macroglobulinemia, lymphoma, chronic lymphocytic leukemia.
  Mixed polyclonal or mixed monoclonal—Infectious diseases (viral, bacterial, parasitic) such as subacute bacterial endocarditis and malaria, SLE,

rheumatoid arthritis, essential cryoglobulinemia, lymphoproliferative diseases, sarcoidosis, chronic liver disease (cirrhosis).

■ DEXAMETHASONE SUPPRESSION TEST

Used in the differential diagnosis of Cushing's syndrome.

Overnight Dexamethasone Suppression Test

In the rapid version of this test, the patient takes dexamethasone 1 mg PO at 11 PM; a fasting 8 AM plasma cortisol is obtained. Normally, the cortisol level should be < 5 μg/dL or < 138 nmol/L. A value > 5 μg/dL or > 138 nmol/L suggests Cushing's syndrome; however, suppression may not occur with obesity, alcoholism, or depression. In these patients, the best screening test is a 24-hour urine for free cortisol.

Low-Dose Dexamethasone Suppression Test

After collection of baseline serum cortisol and 24-hour urine free cortisol levels, dexamethasone 0.5 mg PO is administered Q 6 hr for eight doses. Serum cortisol and 24-hour urine for free cortisol are repeated on the second day. Failure to suppress to a serum cortisol of < 5 μg/dL (138 nmol/L) and a urine free cortisol < 30 μg/dL (82 nmol/L) confirms the diagnosis of Cushing's syndrome.

High-Dose Dexamethasone Suppression Test

If the low-dose test is positive, dexamethasone 2 mg PO Q 6 hr for eight doses is administered. A fall in urinary free cortisol to 50% of the baseline value occurs in patients with Cushing's disease, but not in patients with adrenal tumors or ectopic ACTH production.

■ ERYTHROPOIETIN (EPO)

Normal = 5–30 mU/mL.
   There is an inverse relationship between erythropoietin and hematocrit.

Decreased or normal levels: Myelodysplastic syndrome, polycythemia vera, chronic renal disease, early pregnancy; also in preterm infants.

Increased: Zidovudine (AZT)-treated HIV infection, normocytic anemia, and microcytic anemia.
   Radioimmunoassay measurement detects EPO in both the active and inactive forms while the mouse bioassay assesses functional hormones.

■ ETHANOL LEVEL

See Drug Levels, Table VII–16, p 629.

■ FERRITIN

Males: 15–200 ng/mL or 15–220 µg/L.
  Females: 12–150 ng/mL or 12–150 µg/L.

Decreased: Iron deficiency, severe liver disease.

Increased: Hemochromatosis, hemosiderosis, sideroblastic anemia, any inflammatory process (acute-phase reactant).

■ FIBRIN DEGRADATION PRODUCTS (FDP)

< 10 µg/mL.

Increased: Any thromboembolic condition (deep venous thrombosis, myocardial infarction, pulmonary embolus); disseminated intravascular coagulation; hepatic dysfunction.

■ FIBRINOGEN

150–450 mg/dL or 150–450 g/L.

Decreased: Congenital; disseminated intravascular coagulation (sepsis, amniotic fluid embolism, abruptio placentae, prostatic or cardiac surgery); burns; neoplastic and hematologic malignancies; acute severe bleeding; snake bite.

Increased: Inflammatory processes (acute-phase reactant).

■ FOLATE RED BLOOD CELL

160–640 ng or 360–1450 nmol/mL RBC.
  More sensitive for detecting folate deficiency from malnourishment if the patient has started proper nutrition before the serum folate is measured (even one well-balanced hospital meal can increase the serum folate to normal levels).

Increased: See Folic Acid (Serum Folate).

Decreased: See Folic Acid (Serum Folate).

■ FOLIC ACID (SERUM FOLATE)

2–14 ng/mL or 4.5–31.7 nmol/L.

Increased: Folic acid administration.

Decreased: Malnutrition, malabsorption, massive cellular growth (cancer), hemolytic anemia, pregnancy.

■ FTA-ABS (FLUORESCENT TREPONEMAL ANTIBODY ABSORBED)

Nonreactive.

Positive: Syphilis (test of choice to confirm diagnosis). Test may be negative in early primary syphilis; may remain positive after adequate treatment.

■ FUNGAL SEROLOGIES

Negative (< 1:8). Complement-fixation fungal antibody screen that usually detects antibodies to *Histoplasma, Blastomyces, Aspergillus,* and *Coccidioides.*

■ γ-GLUTAMYLTRANSFERASE (GGT)

Males: 9–50 U/L.
  Females: 8–40 U/L. Generally parallels changes in serum alkaline phosphatase and 5′-nucleotidase in liver disease.

Increased: Liver disease (hepatitis, cirrhosis, obstructive jaundice); pancreatitis.

■ GASTRIN

Males: < 100 pg/mL or < 100 ng/L.
  Females: < 75 pg/mL or < 100 ng/L.

Increased: Zollinger-Ellison syndrome, pyloric stenosis, pernicious anemia, atrophic gastritis, ulcerative colitis, renal insufficiency, steroid and calcium administration.

■ GLUCOSE

Fasting: 70–105 mg/dL or 3.89–5.83 nmol/L.
  2 hours postprandial: 70–120 mg/dL or 3.89–6.67 mmol/L.

Increased: See Section I, Chapter 32, Hyperglycemia, p 190.

Decreased: See Section I, Chapter 37, Hypoglycemia, p 213.

■ GLYCOHEMOGLOBIN (HEMOGLOBIN A$_{1C}$)

4.0–6.0%.

Increased: Poorly controlled diabetes mellitus.

■ GRAM'S STAIN

Rapid Technique

Spread a thin layer of specimen onto a glass slide and allow it to dry. Fix with heat. Apply Gentian violet (15–20 seconds); follow with iodine (15–20 seconds), then alcohol (just a few seconds until effluent is barely decolorized). Rinse with water and counterstain with safranin (15–20 seconds). Examine under oil immersion lens: gram-positive bacteria are dark blue and gram-negatives are red.

Gram-Positive Cocci: *Staphylococcus, Streptococcus, Enterococcus, Micrococcus, Peptococcus* (anaerobic), and *Peptostreptococcus* (anaerobic) species.

Gram-Positive Rods: *Clostridium* (anaerobic), *Corynebacterium, Listeria,* and *Bacillus.*

Gram-Negative Cocci: *Neisseria, Branhamella, Moraxella, Acinetobacter* species.

Gram-Negative Coccoid Rods: *Haemophilus, Pasteurella, Brucella, Francisella, Yersinia,* and *Bordetella* species.

Gram-Negative Straight Rods: *Acinetobacter* (*Mima, Herellea*), *Aeromonas, Bacteroides* (anaerobic), *Campylobacter* (comma-shaped) species, *Eikenella, Enterobacter, Escherichia, Fusobacterium* (anaerobic), *Helicobacter, Klebsiella, Legionella* (small, pleomorphic; weakly staining), *Proteus, Providencia, Pseudomonas, Salmonella, Serratia, Shigella, Vibrio, Yersinia.*

■ HAPTOGLOBIN

26–185 mg/mL.

Increased: Obstructive liver disease; any inflammatory process.

Decreased: Hemolysis (eg, transfusion reaction); severe liver disease.

■ *HELICOBACTER* ANTIBODIES

Normal = negative.

Serologic test to detect antibodies to *Helicobacter pylori* in patients with peptic ulcer disease. High titers of IgG to *Helicobacter* are indicative of *H pylori* infection (sensitivity > 95% and specificity > 95%). More sensitive than biopsy for detecting presence of *H pylori*. It may take 6 months or longer for antibodies to decline appreciably after treatment.

■ HEMATOCRIT

See Table II–4, p 380, for normal values.

Increased: See Section I, Chapter 55, Polycythemia, p 312.

Decreased: See Section I, Chapter 5, Anemia, p 28.

■ HEMOGLOBIN

See Table II–4, p 380, for normal values.

Increased: See Section I, Chapter 55, Polycythemia, p 312.

Decreased: See Section I, Chapter 5, Anemia, p 28.

■ HEPATITIS TESTS

See Table II–5, p 390.

- **Anti-HAV Tot:** Total antibody to hepatitis A virus, both IgG and IgM. Confirms previous exposure to hepatitis A virus and is also positive with acute infection.
- **Anti-HAV IgM:** IgM antibody to hepatitis A virus. Indicates acute infection with hepatitis A virus.
- **HBsAg:** Hepatitis B surface antigen. Indicates either chronic or acute infection with hepatitis B. Used by blood banks to screen donors and part of routine hepatitis panel for evaluation of liver injury.
- **Total Anti-HBc:** IgG and IgM antibody to hepatitis B core antigen. Confirms either previous exposure to hepatitis B virus (HBV) or ongoing infection. Used by blood banks to screen donors.
- **Anti-HBc IgM:** IgM antibody to hepatitis B core antigen. Early and best indicator of acute infection with hepatitis B.
- **HBeAg:** Hepatitis B_e antigen. When present, indicates high degree of infectiousness. Order only when evaluating a patient with chronic HBV infection.
- **Anti-HBe:** Antibody to hepatitis B_e antigen. Order with HbeAg. Presence is associated with resolution of active viral proliferation, but often means virus is integrated into host DNA, especially if host remains HbsAg-positive.
- **Anti-HBs:** Antibody to hepatitis B surface antigen. Typically indicates immunity associated with clinical recovery from an HBV infection or previous immunization with hepatitis B vaccine. Order only to assess effectiveness of vaccine, and results will often be reported as a titer.
- **HBV-DNA:** Detects presence of viral DNA in serum (pg/mL) quantitatively to confirm infection and assess therapy with antivirals such as lamivudine and adefovir. Relatively expensive assay.
- **Anti-HDV:** Antibody to delta-agent hepatitis. Order only in patients with known chronic HBV infection who have flare of transaminase elevation.
- **Anti-HCV:** Antibody against hepatitis C. Order to evaluate both acute and chronic hepatitis. Has a low false-positive rate. Used by blood

TABLE II–5. HEPATITIS PANEL TESTING.

Profile Name	Tests	Purpose
■ Screening		
Admission: High-risk patients (homosexuals, IV drug users, dialysis patients)	HBsAg Anti-HCV	To screen for chronic or active infection.
All pregnant women	HBsAg	To screen for chronic or active infection.
Percutaneous inoculation	HBsAg Anti-HCV	Test serum of patient (if known) for possible infectivity. Start Hep B vaccination if health care worker not previously immunized.
	Anti-HBs	Determine if vaccinated health care worker is immune and protected.
Pre-HBV vaccine in high-risk patients	HBsAg Anti-HBc	To determine if an individual is infected or already has antibodies and is immune.
■ Diagnosis		
Differential diagnosis of acute hepatitis	Anti-HAV IgM HBsAg Anti-HBc IgM Anti-HCV	To differentiate between hepatitis A, hepatitis B, and hepatitis C (Anti-HCV may take 4–8 weeks to become positive)
Differential diagnosis of chronic hepatitis (Abnormal Liver Function Tests [LFTs])	HBsAg Anti-HCV (and RIBA or HCV RNA if Anti-HCV is positive)	To rule out chronic hepatitis B or C as a cause of chronically elevated LFTs.
■ Monitoring		
Chronic hepatitis B	LFTs HBsAg HBeAg/Anti-HBe Anti-HDV IgM α-fetoprotein HBV DNA	To test for activity, late seroconversion, or disease latency in known hepatitis B carrier, superinfection with HDV, development of hepatoma, or resolution of infection after therapy or spontaneously.
Chronic hepatitis C	LFTs HCV RNA α-fetoprotein	To test for activity of hepatitis likelihood of response to interferon, or development of hepatoma
Postvaccination screening	Anti-HBs	To ensure immunity after vaccination
Sexual contact	HBsAg	To monitor sexual partners with acute or chronic hepatitis B

banks to screen donors and part of routine hepatitis panel for evaluation of liver injury.

- **Anti-HCV RIBA:** Measures antibody to four separate HCV antigens. However, no longer used to confirm positive anti-HCV test.
- **HCV-RNA:** Detects presence of virus either qualitatively by sensitive RT-PCR or quantitatively by one of a number of tests with varying sensitivities and dynamic ranges. The qualitative test is used to confirm that the HCV-Ab represents an active infection; it is also used to assess the end-of-treatment response and the "sustained viral response" (RNA negative at 24 weeks after therapy and likely cured) to interferon and ribavirin antiviral therapies. The quantitative test (viral load, in International Units) is obtained only before instituting antiviral therapy and at 12 weeks into therapy. This is to determine whether there has been an "early viral response" to therapy defined as ≥ 100-fold drop in IU or undetectable virus. Therapy is not continued beyond 12 weeks without an early viral response. The HCV viral load does NOT correlate with amount of liver injury.
- **HCV-Genotype:** Important for determining likelihood of the HCV infection responding to antiviral therapy with interferon and ribavirin. Genotype 1 patients with quantitative RNA values > 850,000 IU are less likely to respond to therapy than genotypes 2 and 3 patients. Genotype 1 patients usually require 48 weeks of therapy to achieve a 40–50% chance of cure; genotypes 2 and 3 patients require only 24 weeks of therapy to achieve a 70–80% chance of cure.

■ 5-HIAA (5-HYDROXYINDOLEACETIC ACID)

2–8 mg or 10.4–41.6 μmol/24-hr urine collection. 5-HIAA is a serotonin metabolite.

Increased: Carcinoid tumors; certain foods (banana, pineapple, tomato).

■ *HISTOPLASMA CAPSULATUM* ANTIGEN, URINE

< 1.0 units/mL.

Elevated in disseminated histoplasmosis, less commonly elevated in localized pulmonary *Histoplasma* infections. The most sensitive and rapid diagnostic test available for disseminated histoplasmosis in AIDS patients. After amphotericin B treatment, levels fall to low or nondetectable range. If measurement increases, it is an indication of relapse.

■ HOMOCYSTEINE

5–12 mmol/mL.

Increased: Arteriosclerotic vascular disease, deep venous thrombosis, pregnancy complicated by neural tube defects.

Increases with aging, smoking, and many drugs.

■ HUMAN CHORIONIC GONADOTROPIN, SERUM (HCG BETA SUBUNIT)

< 3.0 mIU/mL;
    7–10 days postconception: > 3 mIU/mL; 30 days: 100–5000 mIU/mL;
    10 weeks: 50,000–140,000 mIU/mL; > 16 weeks: 10,000–50,000 mIU/mL;
thereafter: levels slowly decline.

Increased: Pregnancy, testicular tumors, trophoblastic disease (hydatidiform mole, choriocarcinoma levels usually > 100,000 mIU/mL).

■ HUMAN IMMUNODEFICIENCY VIRUS (HIV) ANTIBODY TEST

Negative: Used in the diagnosis of acquired immunodeficiency syndrome (AIDS) and HIV infection and to screen blood for use in transfusion. May be negative in early HIV infection.
    ELISA (Enzyme-Linked Immunosorbent Assay)
    Used to detect HIV antibody. A positive test is usually repeated and then confirmed by Western blot analysis.

Positive: AIDS, asymptomatic HIV infection, false-positive test.

Western Blot

The technique is used as the reference procedure for confirming the presence or absence of HIV antibody, usually after a positive HIV antibody by ELISA determination.

Positive: AIDS, asymptomatic HIV infection.
    Note: Polymerase chain reaction is a very useful tool for detection of the HIV virus. It is especially useful in very early infection, when antibody may not be present.

■ INTERNATIONAL NORMALIZED RATIO (INR)

See also Prothrombin Time, p 402.
    Normal = 1.0.
    The INR is used to standardize prothrombin results in patients taking anticoagulants.

- **INR 2–3:** Therapeutic range for most indications, including atrial fibrillation, deep venous thrombosis, pulmonary embolus, and transient ischemic attacks.
- **INR 2.5–3.5:** Prevention of arterial thromboembolism with mechanical valves. This range may also be required in hypercoagulable states, or in recurrent arterial or venous thromboembolic disease.

■ IRON

Males: 65–175 µg/dL or 11.64–31.33 µmol/L.
Females: 50–170 µg/dL or 8.95–30.43 µmol/L.

Increased: Hemochromatosis, hemosiderosis caused by excessive iron intake, excess destruction or decreased production of erythrocytes, liver necrosis.

Decreased: Iron deficiency anemia, nephrosis (loss of iron-binding proteins), anemia of chronic disease.

■ IRON BINDING CAPACITY, TOTAL (TIBC)

250–450 µg/dL or 44.75–80.55 µmol/L.
The normal iron/TIBC ratio is 20–50%; < 15% is characteristic of iron deficiency anemia. An increased ratio is seen with hemochromatosis.

Increased: Acute and chronic blood loss, iron deficiency anemia, hepatitis, oral contraceptives.

Decreased: Anemia of chronic disease, cirrhosis, nephrosis, hemochromatosis.

■ 17-KETOGENIC STEROIDS (17-KGS)

Males: 5–23 mg or 17–80 µmol/24-hr urine.
Females: 3–15 mg or 10–52 µmol/24-hr urine.

Increased: Adrenal hyperplasia.

Decreased: Panhypopituitarism, Addison's disease, acute steroid withdrawal.

■ 17-KETOSTEROIDS (17-KS)

Males: 9–22 mg or 31–76 µmol/24-hr urine.
Females: 6–15 mg or 21–52 µmol/24-hr urine.

Increased: Cushing's syndrome, 11- and 21-hydroxylase deficiency, severe stress, exogenous steroids, excess ACTH or androgens.

Decreased: Addison's disease, anorexia nervosa, panhypopituitarism.

■ KOH PREP

Negative: Normal.

Positive: Superficial mycoses (*Candida, Trichophyton, Microsporum, Epidermophyton, Keratinomyces*).

■ LACTATE DEHYDROGENASE (LDH)

45–100 U/L.

Increased: Acute myocardial infarction, cardiac surgery, hepatitis, pernicious anemia, malignant tumors, pulmonary embolus, hemolysis, renal infarction, prognostic factor in hiv patients with *pneumocystis carinii* pneumonia.

■ LACTIC ACID (LACTATE)

4.5–19.8 mg/dL or 0.5–2.2 mmol/L.

Increased: In hypoxia, hemorrhage, circulatory collapse, sepsis, cirrhosis, with exercise.

■ LEUKOCYTE ALKALINE PHOSPHATASE SCORE (LAP SCORE)

70–140.

Increased: Leukemoid reaction, Hodgkin's disease, polycythemia vera, myeloproliferative disorders, pregnancy, liver disease, acute inflammation.

Decreased: Chronic myelogenous leukemia, pernicious anemia, paroxysmal nocturnal hemoglobinuria, nephrotic syndrome.

■ LIGASE CHAIN REACTION FOR *NEISSERIA GONORRHOEAE* AND *CHLAMYDIA TRACHOMATIS* FOR URINE

Normal: Not detected.
    This is a useful screening test for infections by these agents in populations in which there is high prevalence. The patient should not have voided 2 hours before providing specimen.

■ LIPASE

Variable depending on the method; 10–150 U/L by turbidimetric method.

Increased: Acute pancreatitis; pancreatic duct obstruction (stone, stricture, tumor, drug-induced spasm); fat emboli. Usually normal in mumps.

■ LUPUS ANTICOAGULANT

See Antiphospholipid Antibodies, p 373.

■ LYMPHOCYTES, TOTAL

1800–3000/mL.
    Used to assess nutritional status. Calculated by multiplying the white blood cell count by the percentage of lymphocytes: < 900, severe;

900–1400, moderate; 1400–1800, minimal nutritional deficit. Lymphopenia is also seen with certain viral infections, including HIV.

■ MAGNESIUM

1.6–2.4 mg/dL or 0.80–1.20 mmol/L.

Increased: Renal failure, hypothyroidism, magnesium-containing antacids, Addison's disease, severe dehydration.

Decreased: See Section I, Chapter 39, Hypomagnesemia, p 222.

■ MAGNESIUM, URINE

6.0–10.0 mEq/day or 3.00–5.00 mmol/day.

Increased: Hypermagnesemia, diuretics, hypercalcemia, metabolic acidosis, hypophosphatemia.

Decreased: Hypomagnesemia, hypocalcemia, hypoparathyroidism, metabolic alkalosis.

■ METANEPHRINES, URINE

Total: < 1.0 mg or 0.574 mmol/24-hr urine;
    Fractionated metanephrines-normetanephrines: < 0.9 mg or 0.517 mmol/24-hr urine;
    Fractionated metanephrines: < 0.4 mg or 0.230 mg/24-hr urine.

Increased: Pheochromocytoma, neural crest tumors (neuroblastoma), false-positives with drugs (phenobarbital, hydrocortisone, others).

■ MONOSPOT

Negative: Normal.

Positive: Mononucleosis.

■ MYOGLOBIN, URINE

Qualitative negative.

Positive: Disorders affecting skeletal muscle (crush injury, rhabdomyolysis, electrical burns, delirium tremens, surgery), acute myocardial infarction.

■ 5'-NUCLEOTIDASE

2–15 U/L.

Increased: Obstructive liver disease.

■ OSMOLALITY, SERUM

275–295 mOsm/kg.

A rough estimation of osmolality is [2(Na) + BUN/2.8 + glucose/18]). The calculation will not be accurate if foreign substances that increase the osmolality (eg, mannitol) are present. If foreign substances are suspected, osmolality should be measured directly.

Increased: Hyperglycemia; alcohol or ethylene glycol ingestion; increased sodium resulting from water loss (diabetes insipidus, hypercalcemia, diuresis); mannitol.

Decreased: Low serum sodium, diuretics, Addison's disease, hypothyroidism, syndrome of inappropriate antidiuretic hormone (SIADH), iatrogenic causes (poor fluid balance).

■ OSMOLALITY, URINE

Spot 50–1400 mOsm/kg; > 850 mOsm/kg after 12 hours of fluid restriction.

Loss of the ability to concentrate urine, especially during fluid restriction, is an early indicator of impaired renal function.

■ OXYGEN, ARTERIAL (PO$_2$)

See Table II–1, p 374; see also Section VI, Ventilator Management, p 470.

Decreased:
- **Ventilation-perfusion (V̇/Q̇) abnormalities:** Chronic obstructive pulmonary disease, asthma, atelectasis, pneumonia, pulmonary embolus, adult respiratory distress syndrome, pneumothorax, cystic fibrosis, obstructed airway.
- **Alveolar hypoventilation:** Skeletal abnormalities, neuromuscular disorders, Pickwickian syndrome.
- **Decreased pulmonary diffusing capacity:** Pneumoconiosis, pulmonary edema, pulmonary fibrosis.
- **Right-to-left shunt:** Congenital heart disease (tetralogy of Fallot, transposition, others).

■ PARATHYROID HORMONE (PTH)

Normal based on relation to serum calcium, usually provided on the lab report. Also, reference values vary depending on the laboratory and whether N-terminal, C-terminal, or midmolecule is measured.

PTH midmolecule: 0.29–0.85 ng/mL or 29–85 pmol/L with calcium 8.4–10.2 mg/dL or 2.1–2.55 mmol/L.

Increased: Primary hyperparathyroidism, secondary hyperparathyroidism (hypocalcemic states such as chronic renal failure, others).

Decreased: Hypercalcemia not resulting from hyperparathyroidism and hypoparathyroidism.

■ PARTIAL THROMBOPLASTIN TIME (PTT)

27–38 seconds.

Prolonged: Heparin and any defect in the intrinsic clotting mechanism, such as severe liver disease or disseminated intravascular coagulation (includes factors I, II, V, VIII, IX, X, XI, and XII); prolonged use of a tourniquet before drawing a blood sample; hemophilia A and B; lupus anticoagulant; liver disease. Also, elevated in the presence of lupus anticoagulant. See Section I, Chapter 12, Coagulopathy, p 70.

■ PH, ARTERIAL

See Tables II–1 and II–2, pp 374, 375.

Increased: Metabolic and respiratory alkalosis. See Section I, Chapter 3, Alkalosis, p 19.

Decreased: Metabolic and respiratory acidosis. See Section I, Chapter 2, Acidosis, p 10.

■ PHOSPHORUS

2.7–4.5 mg/dL or 0.87–1.45 mmol/L.

Increased: Hypoparathyroidism, pseudohypoparathyroidism, excess vitamin D, secondary hypoparathyroidism, acute and chronic renal failure, acromegaly, tumor lysis (lymphoma or leukemia treated with chemotherapy), alkalosis, factitious increase (hemolysis of specimen).

Decreased: See Section I, Chapter 41, Hypophosphatemia, p 233.

■ PLASMINOGEN

7–17 mg/dL.
   Plasminogen activity: 75–140%.

Decreased: Uncommon cause of inherited thrombosis, primary and secondary fibrinolysis, liver disease, after fibrinolytic therapy.

■ PLATELETS

See Table II–4, p 380.
   Platelet counts may be normal in number, but abnormal in function (eg, aspirin therapy); platelet function with a normal platelet count can be assessed by measuring bleeding time.

Increased: Primary thrombocytosis (idiopathic myelofibrosis, agnogenic myeloid metaplasia, polycythemia vera, primary thrombocythemia, chronic myelogenous leukemia). Secondary thrombocytosis (collagen-vascular diseases, chronic infection [osteomyelitis, tuberculosis], sarcoidosis, hemolytic anemia, iron deficiency anemia, recovery from B_{12} deficiency or iron deficiency or heavy ethanol ingestion, solid tumors and lymphomas; after surgery, especially postsplenectomy; response to drugs such as epinephrine, or withdrawal of myelosuppressive drugs).

Decreased: See Section I, Chapter 61, Thrombocytopenia, p 355.

■ POTASSIUM, SERUM

3.5–5.1 mmol/L.

Increased: See Section I, Chapter 33, Hyperkalemia, p 197.

Decreased: See Section I, Chapter 38, Hypokalemia, p 217.

■ POTASSIUM, URINE

25–125 mmol/24-hr urine; varies with diet. See Urinary Electrolytes, p 411.

■ PROLACTIN

Females: 1–25 ng/mL.
  Males: 1–20 ng/mL.

Increased: Pregnancy, nursing after pregnancy, prolactinoma, hypothalamic tumors, sarcoidosis or granulomatous disease of the hypothalamus, hypothyroidism, renal failure, Addison's disease, phenothiazines, butyrophenones (eg, haloperidol [Haldol]).

Decreased: Sheehan's syndrome.

■ PROSTATE-SPECIFIC ANTIGEN (PSA)

< 4 ng/dL.
  Most useful as a measure of response to therapy for prostate cancer. Also used for screening for prostate carcinoma. Values > 8.0 ng/dL are associated with carcinoma at the 90% confidence level.

Increased: Prostate cancer, some cases of benign prostatic hypertrophy, prostatic infarction, postejaculation (returns to normal level in 48 hours), vigorous exercise (returns to normal in 48–72 hours).

Decreased: Total prostatectomy, response to therapy for prostatic carcinoma.

■ PROTEIN ELECTROPHORESIS, SERUM AND URINE (SERUM PROTEIN ELECTROPHORESIS [SPEP]; URINE PROTEIN ELECTROPHORESIS [UPEP])

Quantitative analysis of the serum proteins is often used in the evaluation of hypoglobulinemia, macroglobulinemia, α_1-antitrypsin deficiency, collagen disease, liver disease, and myeloma; occasionally used in nutritional assessment. Serum electrophoresis yields five different bands (see Figure II–1, p 400; and Table II–6, p 401). If a monoclonal gammopathy or a low globulin fraction is detected, quantitative immunoglobulins should be checked.

Urine protein electrophoresis can be used to evaluate proteinuria and can detect Bence–Jones (light-chain) protein that is associated with myeloma, Waldenström's macroglobulinemia, and Fanconi's syndrome.

■ PROTEIN, SERUM

6.0–7.8 g/dL or 60–78 g/L.

Increased: Multiple myeloma, Waldenström's macroglobulinemia, benign monoclonal gammopathy, lymphoma, sarcoidosis, chronic inflammatory disease.

Decreased: Any cause of decreased albumin or any cause of hypogammaglobulinemia such as common variable hypogammaglobulinemia.

■ PROTEIN, URINE

See also Albumin, Urine, p 370.
   < 100 mg/24-hr urine;
   Spot: < 10 mg/dL (< 20 mg/dL if early-morning collection);
   Dipstick: negative.

Increased: Nephrotic syndrome, glomerulonephritis, lupus nephritis, amyloidosis, renal vein thrombosis, severe CHF, multiple myeloma, pre-eclampsia, postural proteinuria, polycystic kidney disease, diabetic nephropathy, radiation nephritis, malignant hypertension.

False-positive: Gross hematuria, very concentrated urine, phenazopyridine hydrochloride (Pyridium), very alkaline urine.

■ PROTEIN C, PLASMA

Normal = 60–130%.

Decreased: Hypercoagulable states resulting in recurrent venous thrombosis; chronic liver disease; disseminated intravascular coagulation; postoperatively; neoplastic disease and autosomal recessive deficiency.

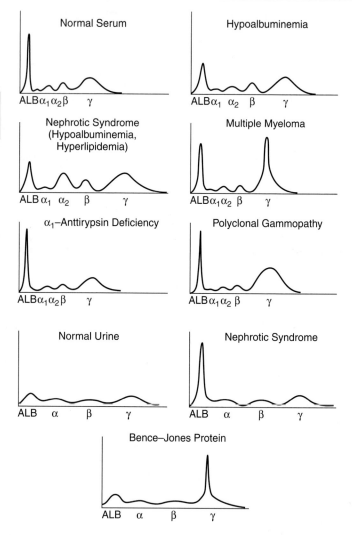

Figure II-1. Protein electrophoresis patterns. Examples of (**A**) serum and (**B**) urine protein electrophoresis patterns.

TABLE II–6. NORMAL SERUM PROTEIN COMPONENTS AND FRACTIONS AS DETERMINED BY ELECTROPHORESIS ALONG WITH ASSOCIATED CONDITIONS.

Protein Fraction	Percentage of Total Protein	Constituents	Increased	Decreased
Albumin	52–68	Albumin	Dehydration (only known cause)	Nephrosis, malnutrition, chronic liver disease
α_1-Globulin	2.4–4.4	Thyroxine-binding globulin, antitrypsin, lipoproteins, glycoprotein, transcortin	Inflammation, neoplasia	Nephrosis, α_1-antitrypsin deficiency (emphysema-related)
α_2-Globulin	6.1–10.1	Haptoglobin, glycoprotein, macroglobulin, ceruloplasmin	Inflammation, infection, neoplasia, cirrhosis	Severe liver disease, acute hemolytic anemia
β-Globulin	3.5–14.5	Transferrin, glycoprotein, lipoprotein	Cirrhosis, obstructive jaundice	Nephrosis
γ-Globulins (immunoglobulins)	10–21	IgA, IgG, IgM, IgD, IgE	Infections, collagen-vascular diseases, leukemia, myeloma	Agammaglobulinemia, hypogammaglobulinemia, nephrosis

Reproduced with permission from Gomella LG, ed. *Clinician's Pocket Reference.* 10th ed.: McGraw-Hill; 2004.

■ PROTEIN S, PLASMA

Normal = 60–140%.

Decreased: See Protein C, Plasma. Protein S is a cofactor of protein C; should be ordered along with protein C.

■ PROTHROMBIN TIME (PT)

See International Normalized Ratio (INR), p 392.
   11.5–13.5 seconds.

EVALUATES EXTRINSIC CLOTTING MECHANISM (FACTORS I, II, V, VII, AND X).

Prolonged: Drugs such as sodium warfarin (Coumadin), decreased vitamin K, fat malabsorption, liver disease, prolonged use of a tourniquet before drawing a blood sample, disseminated intravascular coagulation, lupus anticoagulant (usually selectively increased PTT). See Section I, Chapter 12, Coagulopathy, p 70.

■ QUANTITATIVE IMMUNOGLOBULINS

IgG: 650–1500 mg/dL or 6.5–15 g/L;
IgM: 40–345 mg/dL or 0.4–3.45 g/L;
IgA: 76–390 mg/dL or 0.76–3.90 g/L;
IgE: 0–380 IU/mL or KIU/L;
IgD: 0–8 mg/dL or 0–80 mg/L.

Increased: Multiple myeloma (myeloma immunoglobulin increased, other immunoglobulins decreased), Waldenström's macroglobulinemia (IgM increased, others decreased), lymphoma, carcinoma, bacterial and viral infections, liver disease, sarcoidosis, amyloidosis, myeloproliferative disorders.

Decreased: Hereditary immunodeficiency, leukemia, lymphoma, nephrotic syndrome, protein-losing enteropathy, malnutrition.

■ RAPID PLASMA REAGIN (RPR)

See VDRL, p 412.

■ RED BLOOD CELL COUNT (RBC)

See Table II–4, p 380. Also see Hematocrit, p 388.

■ RED BLOOD CELL INDICES

See Table II–4, p 380.

MCV (Mean Cell Volume)

Increased: Megaloblastic anemia (B_{12}, folate deficiency), reticulocytosis, chronic liver disease, alcoholism, hypothyroidism, aplastic anemia.

Decreased: Iron deficiency, sideroblastic anemia, thalassemia, some cases of lead poisoning, hereditary spherocytosis.

MCH (Mean Cellular Hemoglobin)

Increased: Macrocytosis (megaloblastic anemias, high reticulocyte counts).

Decreased: Microcytosis (iron deficiency).

MCHC (Mean Cellular Hemoglobin Concentration)

Increased: Severe and prolonged dehydration; spherocytosis.

Decreased: Iron deficiency anemia, overhydration, thalassemia, sideroblastic anemia.

RDW (Red Cell Distribution Width)

Measure of the degree of homogeneity of RBC size.

Increased: An increase in the RDW suggests two different populations of RBCs, such as a combination of macrocytic and microcytic anemia or recovery from iron deficiency anemia (microcytosis plus reticulocytosis).

■ RED BLOOD CELL MORPHOLOGY

Poikilocytosis: Irregular RBC shape (sickle, burr).
  Anisocytosis: Irregular RBC size (microcytes, macrocytes).
  Basophilic stippling: Lead, heavy metal poisoning, thalassemia.
  Howell-Jolly bodies: Seen after a splenectomy and in some severe anemias.
  Sickling: Sickle cell disease and trait.
  Nucleated RBCs: Severe bone marrow stress (hemorrhage, hemolysis), marrow replacement by tumor, extramedullary hematopoiesis.
  Target cells: Thalassemia, hemoglobinopathies (sickle cell disease), obstructive jaundice, any hypochromic anemia, after splenectomy.
  Spherocytes: Hereditary spherocytosis, immune or microangiopathic hemolysis.
  Helmet cells (schistocytes): Microangiopathic hemolysis, hemolytic transfusion reaction, other hemolytic anemias.
  Burr cells (acanthocytes): Severe liver disease; high levels of bile, fatty acids, or toxins.

Polychromasia: Appearance of a bluish-gray RBC on routine Wright's stain suggests reticulocytes.

■ RETICULOCYTE COUNT

0.5–1.5%.

If the patient's hematocrit is abnormal, a corrected reticulocyte count should be calculated as follows:

$$\text{Corrected reticulocyte count} = \%\ \text{reticulocytes} \times \frac{\text{patient's hematocrit}}{45\%}$$

Increased: Hemolysis, acute hemorrhage, therapeutic response to treatment for iron, vitamin B_{12}, or folate deficiency.

Decreased: Infiltration of bone marrow by carcinoma, lymphoma, or leukemia, marrow aplasia, chronic infections such as osteomyelitis, toxins, drugs (> 100 reported), many anemias.

■ RHEUMATOID FACTOR (RA LATEX TEST)

< 15 IU by microscan kit or < 1:40.

Increased: Rheumatoid arthritis, SLE, Sjögren's syndrome, scleroderma, dermatomyositis, polymyositis, syphilis, chronic inflammation, subacute bacterial endocarditis, hepatitis, sarcoidosis, interstitial pulmonary fibrosis.

■ SEDIMENTATION RATE (ESR)

- **Wintrobe Scale:** Males: 0–9 mm/hr; females: 0–20 mm/hr.
- **ZETA Scale:** 40–54%, normal; 55–59%, mildly elevated; 60–64%, moderately elevated; > 65%, markedly elevated.
- **Westergren Scale:** Males < 50 years: 15 mm/hr; males > 50 years: 20 mm/hr; females < 50 years, 25 mm/hr; females > 50 years: 30 mm/hr. This is a very nonspecific test. The ZETA method is not affected by anemia. The Westergren scale remains the preferred method.

Increased: Infection, inflammation, rheumatic fever, endocarditis, neoplasm, acute myocardial infarction.

■ SGGT (SERUM γ-GLUTAMYLTRANSFERASE)

See γ-Glutamyltransferase (GGT), p 387.

■ SGOT (SERUM GLUTAMIC-OXALOACETIC TRANSFERASE) OR AST (SERUM ASPARTATE AMINOTRANSFERASE)

See AST, p 373.

■ SGPT (SERUM GLUTAMIC-PYRUVIC TRANSFERASE) OR ALT (SERUM ALANINE AMINOTRANSFERASE)

See ALT, p 371.

■ SODIUM, SERUM

136–145 mmol/L.

Increased: See Section I, Chapter 34, Hypernatremia, p 201.

Decreased: See Section I, Chapter 40, Hyponatremia, p 226.

■ SODIUM, URINE

40–210 mmol/24-hr urine. See Urinary Electrolytes, p 411.

■ STOOL FOR OCCULT BLOOD (HEMOCCULT TEST)

Negative: Normal.

Positive: Swallowed blood; ingestion of red meat; any gastrointestinal tract lesion (ulcer, carcinoma, polyp); large doses of vitamin C (> 500 mg/day). See also Section I, Chapter 28, Hematochezia, p 171; and Chapter 27, Hematemesis, Melena, p 166.

■ STOOL FOR WHITE BLOOD CELLS (WBCS)

Occasional WBCs, usually polymorphonuclear neutrophils.

Increased: *Shigella, Salmonella,* enteropathogenic *Escherichia coli,* pseudomembranous colitis (*Clostridium difficile*), ulcerative colitis.

■ T$_3$ (TRIIODOTHYRONINE) RADIOIMMUNOASSAY

120–195 ng/dL or 1.85–3.00 nmol/L.

Increased: Hyperthyroidism; T$_3$ thyrotoxicosis; exogenous T$_4$; any cause of increased thyroid-binding globulin such as oral estrogens, pregnancy, or hepatitis.

Decreased: Hypothyroidism, euthyroid sick state, any cause of decreased thyroid-binding globulin (eg, malnutrition).

■ T_3 RU (RESIN UPTAKE)

24–34%.

Increased: Hyperthyroidism; medications (phenytoin, anabolic steroids, corticosteroids, heparin, aspirin, others); nephrotic syndrome.

Decreased: Hypothyroidism, pregnancy, medications (estrogens, iodine, propylthiouracil, others).

■ T_4 TOTAL (THYROXINE)

5–12 µg/dL or 65–155 nmol/L.
  Males: 5–10 µg/dL: 5–10 µg/dL or 65–129 nmol.
  Females: 5.5–10.5 µg/dL or 71–135 nmol/L.

Increased: Hyperthyroidism; exogenous thyroid hormone; any cause of increased thyroid-binding globulin (eg, estrogens, pregnancy, or hepatitis); euthyroid sick state.

Decreased: Hypothyroidism, euthyroid sick state, any cause of decreased thyroid-binding globulin (eg, malnutrition).

■ THROMBIN TIME

10–14 seconds.

Increased: Heparin, disseminated intravascular coagulation, elevated fibrin degradation products, fibrinogen deficiency, congenitally abnormal fibrinogen molecules. See Section I, Chapter 12, Coagulopathy, p 70.

■ THYROGLOBULIN

0–60 ng/mL or < 60 µg/L.
  Used primarily to detect recurrence of nonmedullary thyroid carcinoma after resection.

Increased: Differentiated thyroid carcinomas (papillary, follicular), thyroid adenoma, Graves' disease, toxic goiter, nontoxic goiter, thyroiditis.

Decreased: Hypothyroidism, testosterone, steroids, phenytoin.

■ THYROID-BINDING GLOBULIN (TBG)

1.5–3.4 mg/dL or 15–34 mg/L.

Increased: Hypothyroidism, pregnancy, medications (oral contraceptives, estrogens), hepatitis, acute porphyria, familial.

Decreased: Hyperthyroidism, medications (androgens, anabolic steroids, corticosteroids, phenytoin), nephrotic syndrome, severe illness, liver failure, malnutrition.

■ THYROID-STIMULATING HORMONE (TSH)

0.7–5.3 mU/mL.
 Newer sensitive assays are excellent screening tests for hyperthyroidism as well as hypothyroidism; they allow you to distinguish between a low normal and a decreased TSH.

Increased: Hypothyroidism.

Decreased: Hyperthyroidism. Fewer than 1% of cases of hypothyroidism are from pituitary or hypothalamic disease resulting in a decreased TSH.

■ TRANSFERRIN

220–400 mg/dL or 2.20–4.00 g/L.

Increased: Acute and chronic blood loss, iron deficiency anemia, hepatitis, oral contraceptives.

Decreased: Anemia of chronic disease, cirrhosis, malnutrition nephrosis, hemochromatosis.

■ TRIGLYCERIDES

Males: 40–160 mg/dL or 0.45–1.81 mmol/L.
 Females: 35–135 mg/dL or 0.40–1.53 mmol/L; may vary with age.

Increased: Hyperlipoproteinemias (types I, IIb, III, IV, V), hypothyroidism, liver diseases, diabetes mellitus, alcoholism, pancreatitis, acute myocardial infarction, nephrotic syndrome.

Decreased: Malnutrition, congenital abetalipoproteinemia.

■ TROPONIN I

< 0.6 ng/mL or < 0.6 µg/L.

Increased: In myocardial injury levels > 1.5 ng/mL (1.5 µg/L) is consistent with myocardial infarction. Sensitivity is similar to CK-MB (creatine kinase MB fraction) but more specific. Does not tend to be elevated with skeletal muscle injury nor chronic renal disease as much as the CK-MB. False-positives can be seen in clotted specimens and in the presence of heterophil antibodies. Elevated within 4–8 hours of myocardial injury with peak at 12–16 hours, but remains elevated for 5–9 days unlike CK-MB, which begins to decrease after 24–36 hours.

■ TROPONIN T

< 0.1 ng/mL or < 0.1 μg/L.

Increased: In myocardial injury but also in muscle diseases such as muscular dystrophy. Not as valuable in assessing acute myocardial injury, although it parallels troponin I. Its importance may be in risk stratification of cardiac patients (determining those patients with unstable angina who are more likely to have a cardiac-related death).

■ TRYPTASE

5.6–13.5 μg/L.

Increased: Diseases of mast cell activation such as anaphylaxis or mastocytosis.
   Released in a slower manner than histamine and more stable so that it can be detected for a longer period of time than histamine. In anaphylaxis, histamine peaks in 5 minutes and returns to normal in less than 1 hour. Tryptase peaks in 1–2 hours and returns to normal after a few hours.

■ URIC ACID

Males: 4.5–8.2 mg/dL or 0.27–0.48 mmol/L.
   Females: 3.0–6.5 mg/dL or 0.18–0.38 mmol/L.

Increased: Gout; renal failure; destruction of massive amounts of nucleoproteins (tumor lysis after chemotherapy, leukemia or lymphoma); toxemia of pregnancy; drugs (especially diuretics); hypothyroidism; polycystic kidney disease; parathyroid diseases.

Decreased: Uricosuric drugs (salicylates, probenecid, allopurinol), Wilson's disease, Fanconi's syndrome, pregnancy.

■ URINALYSIS, ROUTINE

Appearance

- **Normal:** Yellow, clear, straw-colored
- **Pink/red:** Blood, hemoglobin, myoglobin, food coloring, beets
- **Orange:** Pyridium, rifampin, bile pigments
- **Brown/black:** Myoglobin, bile pigments, melanin, cascara bark, iron, nitrofurantoin, metronidazole, sickle cell crisis
- **Blue:** Methylene blue, *Pseudomonas* urinary tract infection (rare), hereditary tryptophan metabolic disorders
- **Cloudy:** Urinary tract infection (pyuria), blood, myoglobin, chyluria, mucus (normal in ileal loop specimens), phosphate salts (normal in alkaline urine), urates (normal in acidic urine), hyperoxaluria
- **Foamy:** Proteinuria, bile salts

pH

(4.6–8.0)

Acidic: High-protein diet; methenamine mandelate; acidosis; ketoacidosis (starvation, diabetic); diarrhea; dehydration.

Basic: Urinary tract infection, involving *Proteus;* renal tubular acidosis; diet (high vegetable, milk, immediately postprandial); sodium bicarbonate or acetazolamide therapy; vomiting; metabolic alkalosis; chronic renal failure.

Specific Gravity

Normal: 1.001–1.035.

Increased: Volume depletion, CHF, adrenal insufficiency, diabetes mellitus, SIADH, increased proteins (nephrosis). If markedly increased (1.040–1.050), suspect artifact, excretion of radiographic contrast medium, or some other osmotic agent.

Decreased: Diabetes insipidus, pyelonephritis, glomerulonephritis, water load with normal renal function.

Bilirubin

Negative dipstick.

Positive: Obstructive jaundice, hepatitis, cirrhosis, CHF with hepatic congestion, congenital hyperbilirubinemia (Dubin-Johnson syndrome).

Blood (Hemoglobin)

Negative dipstick.

Positive: Hematuria (See Section I, Chapter 29, Hematuria, p 175); free hemoglobin (from trauma, transfusion reaction, or lysis of red blood cells); or myoglobin (crush injury, burn, or tissue ischemia).

Glucose

Negative dipstick.

Positive: Diabetes mellitus; other endocrine disorders (pheochromocytoma, hyperthyroidism, Cushing's syndrome, hyperadrenalism); stress states (sepsis, burns); pancreatitis; renal tubular disease; medications (corticosteroids, thiazides, birth control pills); false-positive with vitamin C ingestion.

Ketones

Negative dipstick.

Positive: Starvation, high-fat diet, alcoholic and diabetic ketoacidosis, vomiting, diarrhea, hyperthyroidism, pregnancy, febrile states.

Leukocyte Esterase

Negative dipstick.

Positive: Infection (test detects 5 or more WBC/HPF or lysed WBCs).

Microscopy

Note: Many laboratories no longer perform urine microscopy on a routine basis when the dipstick is negative and the gross appearance is normal.

- **RBCs:** (Normal: 0–2/HPF.) Trauma, urinary tract infection, prostatic hypertrophy, genitourinary tuberculosis, nephrolithiasis, malignant and benign tumors, glomerulonephritis.
- **WBCs:** (Normal: 0–4/HPF.) Infection anywhere in the urinary tract, genitourinary tuberculosis, renal tumors, acute glomerulonephritis, radiation damage, interstitial nephritis (analgesic abuse). (Glitter cells represent WBCs lysed in hypotonic solution.)
- **Epithelial cells:** (Normal: occasional.) Acute tubular necrosis, necrotizing papillitis.
- **Parasites:** (Normal: none.) *Trichomonas vaginalis, Schistosoma haematobium.*
- **Yeast:** (Normal: none.) *Candida albicans* (especially in diabetics and immunosuppressed patients, or if a vaginal infection is present).
- **Spermatozoa:** (Normal: after intercourse or nocturnal emission.)
- **Crystals:**
    Normal:
        Acid urine: Calcium oxalate (small square crystals with a central cross), uric acid.
        Alkaline urine: Calcium carbonate, triple phosphate (resemble coffin lids).
    Abnormal:
        Cystine, sulfonamide, leucine, tyrosine, cholesterol, or excessive amounts of the crystals noted earlier.
- **Contaminants:** Cotton threads, hair, wood fibers, amorphous substances (all usually unimportant).
- **Mucus:** (Normal: small amounts.) Large amounts suggest urethral disease. Ileal loop urine normally has large amounts.
- **Hyaline cast:** (Normal: occasional.) Benign hypertension, nephrotic syndrome.
- **RBC cast:** (Normal: none.) Acute glomerulonephritis, lupus nephritis, subacute bacterial endocarditis, Goodpasture's disease, vasculitis, malignant hypertension.
- **WBC cast:** (Normal: none.) Pyelonephritis or interstitial nephritis.
- **Epithelial cast:** (Normal: occasional.) Tubular damage, nephrotoxin, viral infections.

- **Granular cast:** (Normal: none.) Results from breakdown of cellular casts, leads to waxy casts.
- **Waxy cast:** (Normal: none.) End stage of a granular cast; evidence of severe chronic renal disease, amyloidosis.
- **Fatty cast:** (Normal: none.) Nephrotic syndrome, diabetes mellitus, damaged renal tubular epithelial cells.
- **Broad cast:** (Normal: none.) Chronic renal disease.

Nitrite

Negative dipstick.

Positive: Bacterial infection (a negative test does not rule out infection).

Protein

See also Albumin, Urine, p 370.
Negative dipstick.

Positive: See Protein, Urine, p 399.

Reducing Substance

Negative dipstick.

Positive: Glucose, fructose, galactose.

False-positives: Vitamin C, antibiotics.

Urobilinogen

Negative dipstick.

Positive: Bile duct obstruction, suppression of gut flora with antibiotics.

■ URINARY ELECTROLYTES

These "spot urines" are of limited value because of large variations in daily fluid and salt intake. Results are usually indeterminate if a diuretic has been given. Sodium is most useful in the differentiation of volume depletion, oliguria, or hyponatremia. Chloride is useful in the diagnosis and treatment of metabolic alkalosis. Urinary potassium levels are often used in the evaluation of hypokalemia.

- **Chloride < 10 mmol/L:** Chloride-sensitive metabolic alkalosis. See Section I, Chapter 3, Alkalosis, p 19.
- **Chloride > 20 mmol/L:** Chloride-resistant metabolic alkalosis. See Section I, Chapter 3, Alkalosis, p 19.
- **Potassium < 10 mmol/L:** Hypokalemia, from extrarenal losses.

- **Potassium > 10 mmol/L:** Renal potassium wasting (diuretics, brisk urinary output).
- **Sodium < 20 mmol/L:** Volume depletion, hyponatremic states, prerenal azotemia (CHF, shock, others), hepatorenal syndrome, edematous states.
- **Sodium > 40 mmol/L:** Acute tubular necrosis, adrenal insufficiency, renal salt wasting, SIADH.
- **Sodium > 20–40 mmol/L:** Indeterminate.

■ URINARY INDICES

The indices in Table II–7 are used in determining the cause of oliguria. See Section I, Chapter 51, Oliguria/Anuria, p 283.

■ VANILLYLMANDELIC ACID (VMA), URINE

2–7 mg/dL or 10.1–35.4 mmol/day.
    VMA is urinary metabolite of both epinephrine and norepinephrine.

Increased: Pheochromocytoma; neural crest tumors (neuroblastoma, ganglioneuroma). False-positive with methyldopa, chocolate, vanilla, others.

■ VDRL TEST (VENEREAL DISEASE RESEARCH LABORATORY) OR RAPID PLASMA REAGIN (RPR)

Normal: Nonreactive.
    Good for screening syphilis. Almost always positive in secondary syphilis, but frequently becomes negative in late syphilis. Also, in some patients with HIV infection, the VDRL can be negative in primary and secondary syphilis.

TABLE II–7. URINARY INDICES IN ACUTE RENAL FAILURE ACCOMPANIED BY OLIGURIA: DIFFERENTIAL DIAGNOSIS OF OLIGURIA.

Index	Prerenal	Renal (ATN)
Urine osmolality	> 500	< 350
Urinary sodium	< 10–20	> 30–40
Urine/serum creatinine	> 40	< 20
Fractional excreted sodium[1]	< 1	> 1
Renal failure index[2]	< 1	> 1

[1] Fractional excreted sodium $= \dfrac{\text{(urine / serum sodium)}}{\text{(urine / serum creatinine)}} \times 100$.

[2] Renal failure index $= \dfrac{\text{(urine sodium} \times \text{serum creatinine)}}{\text{(urine creatinine)}}$

Modified and reproduced with permission from Gomella LG, ed. *Clinician's Pocket Reference.* 10th ed. McGraw-Hill; 2004.

Positive (reactive): Syphilis, SLE, pregnancy, and drug addiction. If reactive, confirm with FTA-ABS (False-positives may occur with bacterial or viral illnesses.

■ WHITE BLOOD CELL COUNT

See Table II–3, p 379

Increased: See Section I, Chapter 48, Leukocytosis, p 266.

Decreased: See Section I, Chapter 49, Leukopenia, p 270.

■ WHITE BLOOD CELL DIFFERENTIAL

See Table II–4, p 380. Many hospitals now perform differentials on automated machines. The newer automated differentials can differentiate neutrophils, lymphocytes, monocytes, eosinophils, and basophils. A manual differential must be done to differentiate segmented and banded neutrophils.

Neutrophils

40–70% segmented neutrophils, 5–10% banded neutrophils.

Increased: Exercise, pain, stress, infection, burns, drugs, thyrotoxicosis, steroids, malignancy, chronic inflammatory disease (vasculitis, collagen-vascular disease, colitis), lithium, epinephrine, asplenia, idiopathic.

Decreased: Congenital, immune-mediated, drug-induced, infectious (viral, rickettsial, parasitic).

Lymphocytes

Normal: 24–44%.

Increased: Measles; German measles (rubeola); mumps, whooping cough (*Bordetella pertussis*); smallpox; chickenpox (Varicella); influenza; viral hepatitis; infectious mononucleosis (Epstein-Barr virus); virtually any viral infection; acute and chronic lymphocytic leukemias.

Decreased: Following stress, burns, trauma; normal finding in 22% of population; uremia; some viral infections (including HIV).

Lymphocytes, Atypical

Normal: 0–3%.
     > 20%: Infectious mononucleosis (Epstein-Barr virus), cytomegalovirus infection, viral hepatitis, toxoplasmosis.
     3–20%: Viral infections (mumps, rubeola, varicella), rickettsial infections, tuberculosis.

Monocytes

Normal: 3–7%.

Increased: Subacute bacterial endocarditis, brucellosis (*Brucella*), typhoid fever (*Salmonella typhi*), kala-azar (visceral leishmaniasis), trypanosomiasis (*Trypanosoma*), rickettsial infection, ulcerative colitis, sarcoidosis, Hodgkin's disease, monocytic leukemias, collagen-vascular diseases.

Decreased: Myelodysplasia, aplastic anemia, hairy cell leukemia, cyclic neutropenia, thermal injuries, collagen-vascular diseases.

Eosinophils

Normal: 0–3%.

Increased: Allergies, parasites, skin diseases, malignancy, drugs, asthma, Addison's disease, collagen-vascular diseases. (A handy mnemonic is **NAACP: N**eoplasm, **A**llergy, **A**ddison's disease, **C**ollagen-vascular diseases, **P**arasites).

Decreased: After steroids; ACTH; after stress (infection, trauma, burns); Cushing's syndrome.

Basophils

Normal: 0–1%.

Increased: Chronic myeloid leukemia; rarely, in recovery from infection and from hypothyroidism.

Decreased: Acute rheumatic fever, lobar pneumonia, after steroid therapy, thyrotoxicosis, stress.

■ WHITE BLOOD CELL MORPHOLOGY

- **Auer rod:** Acute myelogenous leukemias.
- **Döhle bodies:** Severe infection, burns, malignancy, pregnancy.
- **Hypersegmentation:** Megaloblastic anemias, iron deficiency, myeloproliferative disorders, drug induced.
- **Toxic granulation:** Severe illness (sepsis, burns, high temperature).

■ ZINC

60–130 µg/dL or 9–20 µmol/L.

Increased: Atherosclerosis, coronary artery disease.

Decreased: Inadequate dietary intake (parenteral nutrition, alcoholism); malabsorption; increased needs such as pregnancy or wound healing; acrodermatitis enteropathica.

REFERENCES

Burtis CA, Ashwood ER: *Tietz's Textbook of Clinical Chemistry*. 3rd ed. Saunders;1999.

Coudrey L: The troponins. Arch Intern Med 1998;158:1173.

Jurado R, Mattix H: The decreased serum urea nitrogen-creatinine ratio. Arch Intern Med 1998;115:2509.

Henry JB, ed. Clinical Diagnosis and Management by Laboratory Methods. 20th ed. WB Saunders;2001.

Pettijohn TL, Doyle T, Spiekerman AM et al: Usefulness of positive troponin-T and negative creatine kinase levels in identifying high-risk patients with unstable angina pectoris. Am J Cardiol 1997;80:510.

Tchetgen M-B, Song JT, Strawderman M et al: Ejaculation increases the serum prostate-specific antigen concentration. Urology 1996;47:511.

III. Procedures

1. ARTERIAL LINE PLACEMENT

See also Section I, Chapter 6, Arterial Line Problems, p 36.

Indications: Frequent sampling of arterial blood; hemodynamic monitoring when continuous blood pressure readings are needed, such as in a patient with malignant hypertension or a patient in shock, where indirect cuff pressures may be inaccurate.

Contraindications: Poor collateral circulation. Avoid the femoral artery if severe aortoiliac atherosclerosis is present. Coagulopathy is a relative contraindication. See Section I, Chapter 12, Coagulopathy, p 70.

Materials: 20-gauge (or smaller) 1.5- to 2-in. catheter-over-needle assembly (Angiocath), arterial line setup per ICU routine (transducer, tubing, and pressure bag with heparinized saline), armboard, sterile dressing, lidocaine.

Procedure

1. The radial artery is most frequently used; this approach is described here. Other sites, in decreasing order of preference, are the dorsalis pedis, femoral, brachial, and axillary arteries. Axillary arteries are infrequently used; catheters in these arteries should be placed by an intensivist or anesthesiologist.
2. Verify the patency of the collateral circulation between the radial and ulnar arteries using the **Allen test.** See Section III, Chapter 2, Arterial Puncture, p 417.
3. Place the extremity on an armboard with a roll of gauze behind the wrist to hyperextend the joint. Prep with povidone-iodine and drape with sterile towels. The operator should wear gloves and a mask.
4. Raise a very small skin wheal at the puncture site with 1% lidocaine using a 25-gauge needle. Carefully palpate the artery and choose the puncture site where it appears most superficial.
5. While palpating the path of the artery with your nondominant hand, advance the 20-gauge catheter-over-needle assembly into the artery at a 30-degree angle to the skin with the needle bevel up. Once a "flash" of blood is seen in the hub, hold the needle steady and advance the entire unit 1–2 mm so that the needle and catheter are in the artery. Advance the catheter over the needle into the artery. Remove the needle while briefly occluding the artery with manual pressure and connect the pressure tubing. Penetration of both sides of the vessel may occur; therefore, withdraw the catheter slowly while observing for blood return. Never reinsert the needle into a plastic

catheter that lies beneath the skin. Finally, no more than three attempts at cannulation should be performed at a single site.

6. Suture in place with 3-0 silk and apply a sterile dressing.

7. Splint the dorsum of the wrist to limit mobility and provide catheter stability.

8. Kits are available with a needle and guidewire that allow the Seldinger technique to be used. This is especially useful for femoral artery cannulation.

9. Arterial lines should be replaced using a different site every 4 days to decrease risk of infection.

Complications: Thrombosis, hematoma, arterial embolism, arterial spasm, infection, hemorrhage, pseudoaneurysm formation.

2. ARTERIAL PUNCTURE

Indications: Blood gas determination; need for arterial blood in certain chemistry determinations.

Contraindications: Systemic fibrinolytic states, such as after thrombolytic therapy, are relative contraindications to arterial puncture.

Materials: Blood gas sampling kit *or* 3- to 5-mL syringe, 23- to 25-gauge needle (20- to 22-gauge for femoral artery), 1 mL heparin (1000 U/mL), alcohol or povidone-iodine swabs, and a cup of ice.

Procedure

1. Use a heparinized syringe for blood gas and a nonheparinized syringe for chemistry determinations. Obtain a blood gas kit (contains a preheparinized syringe), or a small syringe (3–5 mL) with a small-gauge needle (23- to 25-gauge for radial artery; 20- to 22-gauge is acceptable for femoral artery). Heparinize the syringe (if not preheparinized) by drawing up about 0.5–1 mL of heparin, pulling the plunger all the way back, and discarding the heparin.

2. Arteries, in order of preference, are radial, femoral, and brachial. If using the radial artery, perform the **Allen test** to verify collateral flow from the ulnar artery (15–20% of patients have inadequate collateral circulation to the hand). Have the patient make a tight fist. Occlude both the radial and ulnar arteries at the wrist and have the patient make a fist and release several times. Then have the patient open the hand. The hand should appear pale. While maintaining pressure on the radial artery, release the ulnar artery. If the ulnar–brachial arterial arch is patent, the entire hand should flush red within 10 seconds. If the Allen test is positive (the radial distribution remains white beyond 10 seconds), the artery should not be used.

3. Hyperextension of the wrist joint or elbow often brings the radial and brachial arteries closer to the surface.

4. If you are using the femoral artery, the mnemonic **NAVEL** can aid in locating the important structures in the groin. Palpate the femoral artery just two fingerbreadths below the inguinal ligament. From lateral to medial, the structures are **n**erve, **a**rtery, **v**ein, **e**mpty space, **l**ymphatic. You may wish to inject 1% lidocaine subcutaneously for anesthesia. Palpate the artery proximally and distally with two fingers, or trap the artery between two fingers placed on either side of the vessel.

5. Prep the area with either a povidone-iodine solution or an alcohol swab. Hold the syringe like a pencil with the needle bevel up and enter the skin at a 60- to 90-degree angle. Maintain slight negative pressure on the syringe.

6. Obtain blood on the downstroke or on slow withdrawal. Aspirate very slowly. A good arterial sample should require only minimal backpressure. If a glass or blood-gas syringe is used, the barrel usually rises spontaneously. You should obtain 2–3 mL.

7. If the vessel cannot be located, redirect the needle without taking it out of the skin.

8. Withdraw the needle quickly and apply *firm* pressure at the site for at least 5–10 minutes, even if the sample was not obtained, to avoid a hematoma.

9. If the sample is for a blood gas, expel any air from the syringe, mix the contents thoroughly by twirling the syringe between your fingers, and make the syringe airtight with a cap. Place the syringe on ice before the sample is taken to the laboratory.

Complications: Localized bleeding; thrombosis of the artery, which may lead to arterial insufficiency; infection.

3. ARTHROCENTESIS (DIAGNOSTIC & THERAPEUTIC)

Indications

Diagnostic. Arthrocentesis is helpful in the diagnosis of new-onset arthritis and to rule out infection in acute or chronic unremitting joint effusion.

Therapeutic. The procedure is used to instill steroids and maintain drainage of septic arthritis.

Contraindications: None. Care must be taken, however, not to cause excessive trauma if a coagulopathy or thrombocytopenia is present or if the patient is taking anticoagulant medications.

Materials: Povidone-iodine, alcohol swabs, sterile gloves, 1% lidocaine or ethyl chloride spray, an 18- or 20-gauge needle (a smaller-gauge needle if aspirating finger or toe joints), a large syringe (size depends on the amount of fluid present), a 3-mL syringe with a 25-gauge needle, and two heparinized tubes for cell count and crystal examination.

Discuss with your microbiology laboratory staff their preference for transporting fluid for bacterial, fungal, and acid-fast bacillus (AFB) cultures, and Gram's stain. A Thayer-Martin plate is needed if you suspect *Neisseria gonorrhoeae* (GC). A small syringe containing a long-acting corticosteroid such as Depo-Medrol or triamcinolone is optional for therapeutic arthrocentesis.

Procedure
General

1. Obtain consent. Describe the procedure and complications including bleeding, pain, infection. If injecting steroids, also include skin atrophy, tendon rupture, and systemic side effects of elevated blood pressure and elevated serum glucose. Postinjection flare-ups of joint pain and swelling can occur after steroid injection and can persist up to 48 hours. This complicatioon is thought to be a crystal-induced synovitis from the crystalline suspension used in long-acting steroids.
2. Determine the optimal site for aspiration and mark with indelible ink. Alternatively, make an indentation in the skin with the retracted tip of a ballpoint pen.
3. Wear gloves (universal precautions) to protect yourself against hepatitis and HIV. When aspiration is to be followed by corticosteroid injection, maintaining a sterile field with sterile implements minimizes the risk of infection to the patient.
4. Clean the area with povidone-iodine, and dry and wipe over the aspiration site with alcohol. Povidone-iodine can render cultures negative. Let the alcohol dry before beginning the procedure.
5. Anesthetize the area with lidocaine using a 25-gauge needle, taking care not to inject the solution into the joint space. Lidocaine is bactericidal. Avoid preparations containing epinephrine, especially in a digit. Alternatively, spray the area with ethyl chloride just before needle aspiration.
6. Insert the aspirating needle, applying a small amount of vacuum to the syringe. Remove as much fluid as possible, repositioning the syringe if necessary.
7. If a corticosteroid is to be injected, remove the aspirating syringe from the needle, which is still in the joint space. It is helpful to ensure that the syringe can easily be removed from the needle before undertaking step 6. Attach the syringe containing the corticosteroid, pull back on the plunger to ensure that the needle is not in a vein, and inject contents. ***Caution:*** Never inject steroids when there is a possibility that the joint is infected. Remove the needle and syringe, and apply pressure to the area. Generally, the equivalent of 40 mg of methylprednisolone is injected into large joints such as the knee and 20 mg into medium-sized joints such as the ankle or wrist. Preparations of intraarticular steroids are equivalent in potency. Injections of 0.5 mL into

the knee or shoulder and 0.25 mL into the ankle or wrist are recommended dosages.

8. Joint fluid is sent for cell count and differential, crystal exam, Gram's stain, and cultures for bacteria, fungi, and AFB as indicated. See Section I, Chapter 47, Joint Swelling, p 260.

Arthrocentesis of the Knee

1. **With the patient in the supine position,** the knee should be slightly bent with a small towel under it to help with relaxation. Wait until the patient's quadriceps muscle has relaxed, because its contraction plants the patella against the femur, making aspiration painful.
2. Insert the needle posterior to the lateral portion of the patella into the patellar-femoral groove. Direct the advancing needle slightly posteriorly and superiorly (Figure III–1).

Arthrocentesis of the Wrist. The easiest site for aspiration lies between the navicular bone and the radius on the dorsal wrist.

1. Locate the distal radius between the tendons of the extensor pollicis longus and the extensor carpi radialis longus of the second finger. This site is just ulnar to the anatomic snuff box.
2. Direct the needle perpendicular to the mark (Figure III–2).

Arthrocentesis of the Ankle

1. The most accessible site lies between the tibia and the talus. The angle of foot to leg is positioned at 90 degrees. Make a mark lateral

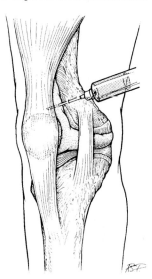

Figure III–1. Arthrocentesis of the knee.

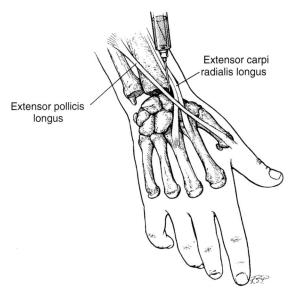

Extensor carpi
radialis longus

Extensor pollicis
longus

Figure III–2. Arthrocentesis of the wrist.

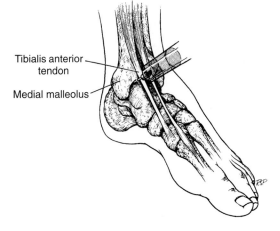

Tibialis anterior
tendon

Medial malleolus

Figure III–3. Arthrocentesis of the ankle.

and anterior to the medial malleolus and medial and posterior to the tibialis anterior tendon. Direct the advancing needle posteriorly toward the heel.

2. The subtalar ankle joint does not communicate with the ankle joint and is difficult to aspirate even by an expert. Keep in mind that "ankle pain" may originate in the subtalar joint rather than in the ankle (Figure III–3).

4. BLADDER CATHETERIZATION

See also Section I, Chapter 24, Foley Catheter Problems, p 148).

Indications: Relieve urinary retention; collect an uncontaminated urine sample; monitor urinary output; and perform bladder tests (cystogram, cystometrogram; determine postvoid residual urine volume).

Contraindications: Urethral disruption is associated with pelvic fracture, acute prostatitis (relative).

Materials: Prepackaged Foley catheter insertion tray (usually may need to add a catheter and collection bag), catheter of choice (16–20 F Foley with 5–10 mL balloon in adults, latex or silicone. The coudé catheter has a curved tip that is useful in men with known significant prostatic hypertrophy).

Procedure

1. Have the patient in a well-lit area in a supine position. With females, knees should be flexed, hips internally rotated, and heels placed together to adequately expose the meatus.

2. Open the kit and put on the gloves. Prepare all the materials before you attempt to insert the catheter. Open the prep solution and soak the cotton balls; apply the sterile drapes.

3. Inflate and deflate the balloon of the Foley catheter with 5–10 mL of sterile water to ensure proper functioning. Coat the end of the catheter with sterile lubricant jelly.

4. In females, use one gloved hand to prep the urethral meatus in a pubis-toward-anus direction; hold the labia apart with the other gloved hand. With uncircumcised males, retract the foreskin to prep the glans; use a gloved hand to hold the penis still.

5. The hand used to hold the penis or labia should not touch the catheter while you are inserting it. You can use disposable forceps in the kit to insert the catheter, or use the forceps to prep. You can then insert the catheter with your gloved hand.

6. In males, stretch the penis upward perpendicular to the body to eliminate any folds in the urethra that might create a false passage. Use *gentle* pressure to slowly advance the catheter. Any significant resistance that is encountered may represent a stricture and requires uro-

logic consultation. In males with benign prostatic hypertrophy, a coudé-tip catheter may facilitate passage. Other means of facilitating catheter passage are ensuring that the penis is well stretched and instilling 30–50 mL of sterile surgical lubricant into the urethra with a catheter-tipped syringe.

7. In both males and females, insert the catheter to the hilt of the drainage end. Compress the penis toward the pubis. These maneuvers ensure that the balloon will be inflated in the bladder and not in the urethra. Inflate the balloon with 5–10 mL of sterile water. After inflation, pull the catheter back so that the balloon will come to rest against the bladder neck. There should be good urine return when the catheter is in place. ***Caution:*** Any male who is uncircumcised should have the foreskin repositioned to prevent massive edema of the glans after the catheter is inserted.

8. If no urine returns, attempt to irrigate with 25–50 mL of sterile saline via a catheter-tipped syringe. ***Note:*** A catheter that will not irrigate is in the urethra, not the bladder.

9. Catheters in females can be taped to the leg. In males, the catheter should be taped to the abdominal wall to decrease urethral stricture formation (prevents the catheter from damaging the urethra at the penoscrotal junction).

Complications: Infection, bleeding, bladder spasm, false passage.

5. BONE MARROW ASPIRATION & BIOPSY

Indications: For diagnostic purposes in patients with splenomegaly, dysproteinemias, unexplained deficiency or excess of white blood cells, platelets, or red blood cells. It is also indicated to evaluate immature or morphologically atypical cells in the peripheral blood. Bone marrow aspiration and biopsy are performed to obtain material for culture or to examine for infectious organisms, neoplasms, or granulomatous changes in patients with fever of unknown origin. It is performed as a staging procedure in patients with lymphoproliferative diseases and to assess therapeutic effect in patients undergoing treatment for hematopoietic neoplasms.

Contraindications: Infection near the puncture site. Relative contraindications include severe uncorrected coagulopathy or thrombocytopenia. The posterior superior iliac crest is the preferred site for the procedure. However, sites that have been previously irradiated are relatively contraindicated. The aspirate and the biopsy provide complementary information, and both specimens should be obtained. However, a bone marrow biopsy should never be obtained from the sternum.

Materials: Commercial kits containing all necessary materials are presently available. If you do not have such a kit, you will need the following items: bone marrow biopsy needle (Jamshidi, Westerman, or similar type); sterile gloves and surgical drapes; iodine prep solution and alcohol; 22- and 26-gauge needles; at least two 10-mL syringes; 1% lidocaine solution; no. 11 scalpel blade, 4 × 4 gauze pads; and several microscope slides for staining.

Procedure

1. Explain the procedure in detail to the patient or to the legally responsible person and obtain an informed consent.
2. Local anesthesia is usually all that is required; however, it is reasonable to premedicate extremely anxious patients with an anxiolytic or sedative such as diazepam (Valium) or lorazepam (Ativan) or with an analgesic.
3. To obtain a bone marrow aspirate and biopsy from the posterior iliac crest (safest and easiest location), position the patient either on the abdomen or on the side opposite the biopsy site.
4. Identify the posterior iliac crest with palpation, and mark the desired biopsy site with indelible ink. In most patients, the upper posterior superior iliac spine can be identified by a dimple in the skin at the lateral edge of the Michaelis' rhomboid.
5. Use sterile gloves and follow strict aseptic technique for the remainder of the procedure.
6. Prep the biopsy site with sterile iodine solution and allow the skin to dry. Then wipe the site free of iodine with sterile alcohol. Next, cover the surrounding areas with surgical drapes.
7. Using a 26-gauge needle, administer 1% lidocaine solution subcutaneously to raise a skin wheal. (The lidocaine may be buffered by 8.4% sodium bicarbonate solution (1 mEq/mL) to decrease the burning associated with this part of the procedure (2 mL sodium bicarbonate with 8 mL lidocaine). Then, with the 22-gauge needle, infiltrate the deeper tissues with lidocaine until you reach the periosteum. At this point, advance the needle just through the periosteum and infiltrate lidocaine subperiosteally. An area approximately 2 cm in diameter should be infiltrated, using repeated periosteal punctures.
8. Once local anesthesia has been obtained, use a no. 11 scalpel blade to make a 2- to 3-mm skin incision over the biopsy site.
9. Insert the bone marrow needle through the skin incision; then advance it with a rotating motion that alternates between clockwise and counterclockwise rotation and with gentle pressure until you reach the periosteum. After the needle is firmly seated on the periosteum, advance it through the outer table of bone into the marrow cavity with the same rotating motion and gentle pressure. Generally, a slight change in the resistance to needle advancement signals entry into the marrow cavity. At this point, advance the needle 2–3 mm.
10. Remove the stylet from the biopsy needle and attach a 10-mL syringe to the hub of the biopsy needle. Withdraw the plunger on the syringe briskly and aspirate 1–2 mL of marrow into the syringe. The patient

may experience severe, instantaneous pain with aspiration. Slow withdrawal of the plunger or collection of more than 1–2 mL of marrow with each aspiration results in excessive contamination of the specimen with peripheral blood.

11. The marrow aspiration specimen can be used to prepare coverslips for viewing under the microscope and for special studies such as cytogenetics and cell markers, or for culture. Repeat aspirations may be required to obtain enough marrow to perform all the preceding tests. Also, note that certain studies may require heparin or EDTA for collection. Contact the appropriate laboratory before the procedure to be sure that you collect the specimens in the appropriate solution.

12. To perform the biopsy, replace the stylet and withdraw the needle. Reinsert the needle at a slightly different angle and location, still within the area of periosteum previously anesthetized. Once you have reentered the marrow cavity, remove the stylet again. Advance the needle 5–10 mm using the same alternating rotating motion with gentle pressure. Withdraw the needle several millimeters (but not outside of the marrow cavity) and redirect it at a slightly different angle; then advance it again. Repeat this maneuver several times. About 2 or 3 cm of core material should enter the needle. Rotate the needle rapidly on its long axis in a clockwise and then counterclockwise direction. This will sever the biopsy specimen from the marrow cavity. Withdraw the needle completely without replacing the stylet. Some operators prefer to hold their thumb over the open end of the needle to create a negative pressure in the needle as it is withdrawn. This may help to prevent loss of the core biopsy specimen.

13. Remove the core biopsy specimen from the needle by inserting a probe (provided with the biopsy needle) into the distal end of the needle and then gently pushing the specimen the full length of the needle and finally out through the needle hub. The direction is important, because an attempt to push the specimen out the distal end may damage the biopsy specimen.

14. The core biopsy specimen is usually collected in formalin solution. Again, plans for special studies should be made before the procedure to allow for any special handling of the biopsy material.

15. Observe the biopsy site for excess bleeding and apply local pressure for several minutes. Clean the area thoroughly with alcohol and apply an adhesive strip or gauze patch. Instruct the patient to assume a supine position and to place their weight over the wound for 30 minutes to decrease the risk of further bleeding.

Complications: Local bleeding and hematoma, pain, possible infection. Rare patients may experience unilateral lower extremity numbness, presumably from infiltration of the sacral nerve plexus. This is usually self-limited and resolves without intervention.

6. CENTRAL VENOUS CATHETERIZATION

See also Section I, Chapter 10, Central Venous Line Problems, p 56.

Indications: Administration of fluids and medications when peripheral administration is impossible, inappropriate, or unreliable; hemodynamic monitoring; transvenous pacemaker placement.

Contraindications: A coagulopathy dictates the use of the femoral or median basilic vein approach to avoid bleeding complications.

Materials: The commonly used Seldinger technique involves puncturing the vein with a relatively small needle through which a thin guidewire is placed in the vein. After the needle has been withdrawn, the intravascular appliance—or a sheath through which a smaller catheter will be placed—is introduced into the vein over the guidewire. Disposable trays commercially available that provide all necessary needles, wires, sheaths, dilators, suture materials, and topical anesthetics. Some hospitals insist that these materials be assembled when central line placement becomes necessary. If needles, guidewires, and sheaths are collected from different places, it is very important to make sure that the needle will accept the guidewire, that the sheath and dilator will pass over the guidewire, and that the appliance to be passed through the sheath will indeed fit the inside lumen of the sheath. Supplies should include the following items:

1. Small needle (16- to 18-gauge)
2. Guidewire
3. 5- to 10-mL syringe
4. Scalpel
5. Intravascular appliance (triple-lumen catheter or a sheath through which a Swan-Ganz pulmonary artery catheter could be placed)
6. Heparinized flush solution: 1 mL of 1:100 U heparin in 10 mL of normal saline (to be used to fill all lumens prior to placement, to prevent clotting of the catheter during placement)
7. Lidocaine 1% with or without epinephrine
8. Chlorhexidine prep solution
9. Alcohol pads
10. Sterile towels
11. 4 × 4 gauze sponges
12. 21-gauge needle to draw up the lidocaine

Also, complete sterile procedure is highly recommended (mask, sterile gown, and gloves).

There seems to be little rationale for placement of a single-lumen catheter when multiple lumens can be installed for potential use at virtually the same risk.

Right Internal Jugular Vein Approach

Actually, three different sites are described and used in accessing the right internal jugular vein: (1) anterior (medial to the sternocleidomastoid muscle belly); (2) middle (between the two heads of the sternocleidomastoid muscle belly); and (3) posterior (lateral to the sternocleidomastoid muscle belly). The middle approach is most commonly used and has the advantage of well-defined landmarks.

Procedure

1. Sterilize the site with chlorhexidine and drape with sterile towels.
2. Administer local anesthesia with lidocaine in the area to be explored.
3. Place the patient in Trendelenburg (head-down) position.
4. Use a small-bore thin-walled needle with syringe attached to locate the internal jugular vein. It may be helpful to have a small amount of anesthetic (1% lidocaine) in the syringe to inject during exploration for the vein, if the patient notes some discomfort. Some operators find the vein with a long 21-gauge needle, leave the needle in place off the syringe, and pass the 19-gauge needle directly behind it, following the same course to the deep vein puncture site.
5. The internal diameter of the needle used to locate the internal jugular vein should be large enough to accommodate the passage of the guidewire. Some operators prefer a "micro-puncture" kit, which utilizes a smaller puncture needle, followed by a smaller-diameter guidewire, followed by a small-caliber dilator. The dilator actually then allows passage of the same guidewire usually passed via a 19-gauge needle. Less trauma is felt to occur because of the smaller puncture needle.
6. Percutaneous entry should be made at the apex of the triangle formed by the two heads of the sternocleidomastoid muscle and the clavicle.
7. The needle should be directed slightly laterally toward the ipsilateral breast and kept as superficial as possible.
8. Often a notch can be palpated on the posterior surface of the clavicle. This actually can help locate the vein in the lateral/medial plane, as the vein lies deep to this shallow notch.
9. Successful puncture of the vein is usually accomplished at a depth of needle insertion of 2–4 cm and is heralded by sudden aspiration of nonpulsatile venous blood.
10. After the needle is detached from the syringe, the guidewire should pass with ease all the way to the right atrium. Once the wire is passed, remove the needle.
11. Leave enough wire outside the patient to accommodate the length of the intravascular catheter, sheath, etc, **with an adequate amount to allow control over the distal end of the guidewire at all times.**
12. Nick the skin with a no. 11 scalpel blade just adjacent to the guidewire.

13. The catheter or sheath should be introduced over the guidewire, while the depth of the guidewire is kept relatively constant to avoid irritation of the right atrium or ventricle and possible ventricular ectopy.

14. When the sheath or catheter is placed over the guidewire, the proximal end of the guidewire should be held until the catheter or sheath completely passes over the distal end of the guidewire.

15. Then the distal end of the guidewire is controlled while the catheter or sheath is advanced through the incised skin and into the vein.

16. Once the catheter or sheath is in place, the guidewire is removed.

17. An occlusive sterile dressing should be applied.

18. A chest x-ray should be obtained to verify position of the line and to assess for a pneumothorax. The tip of the catheter should be positioned above the right atrium.

Complications

1. Central venous catheterization is relatively safe, with a low risk of pneumothorax.

2. Errant attempts at internal jugular puncture are likely to end up in the mediastinum. It is possible to perforate endotracheal tube cuffs by this approach. This is usually not a subtle event and generally requires prompt replacement of the now-faulty endotracheal tube before safe deep line placement can proceed.

3. The other procedural miscue is inadvertent puncture of the carotid artery. This commonly occurs if the needle is inserted medial to where it should be on the middle approach; it is also common with the anterior approach. With arterial puncture, the syringe fills without negative pressure because of arterial pressure, and bright red blood pulsates from the needle after the syringe is removed. The needle should be removed and manual pressure applied for 10–15 minutes to ensure adequate hemostasis.

Advantages: Central venous access from this site allows virtually every potential use of the deep line, including hemodynamic assessment (both central venous pressure and pulmonary artery measurements); temporary pacemaker placement; endomyocardial biopsy; and administration of fluids, drugs, and parenteral nutrition.

Disadvantages

1. The major disadvantage of this site is patient discomfort. The site is difficult to dress and is uncomfortable for patients who have the capacity to turn their heads.

2. The risk of infectious contamination for this line is intermediate between that for femoral lines and that for subclavian lines and is probably related to the difficulty in keeping the site occlusively dressed. Reports from centers in Europe have shown a markedly reduced incidence of catheter infection by including at least an 8-cm subcuta-

neous tunnel from the percutaneous venipuncture site to the skin exit site of the catheter. The procedure is more demanding by virtue of having to construct the tunnel (not described here).

Left Internal Jugular Vein Approach

The left internal jugular vein is not commonly used for central line placement. Better options exist and should be exhausted before resorting to this approach.

Procedure: Similar to right internal jugular vein approach.

Complications: In addition to the usual procedural complications common to central lines, this approach has some unique complications.

1. There are case reports of inadvertent left brachiocephalic vein and superior vena cava puncture with intravascular wires, catheters, and sheaths.
2. Laceration of the thoracic duct.

Advantages: None over right internal jugular vein approach.

Disadvantages: See Complications for Right Internal Jugular Vein Approach. Laceration of the thoracic duct and puncture of the left brachiocephalic vein and superior vena cava are also possible.

Subclavian Approach (Left or Right)

Procedure

1. A small rolled-up towel placed between the shoulder blades facilitates this approach.
2. Place the patient in Trendelenburg position (15–30 degrees).
3. Use sterile preparation and appropriate draping.
4. Anesthetize the skin with local anesthetic.
5. Percutaneous entry is then made caudal to the midclavicle and directed toward the suprasternal notch.
6. The needle is "marched" down the clavicle, keeping near the clavicle to avoid the pleura.
7. A small amount of topical anesthetic in the syringe can be used to anesthetize periosteal surfaces while the vein is located, but it is hoped that only one puncture is needed.
8. The guidewire should fit inside the lumen of the needle used to find the vein. As with internal jugular cannulation, some operators prefer the "micro puncture" approach. Some interventional radiologists use Doppler flow to mark the course of the subclavian vein, and some radiologists have contrast injected through an arm vein under fluoroscopy to help direct the puncture. These techniques are either not

available for bedside use or have not been associated with benefit in trials evaluating patient safety.

9. Direct the needle under the clavicle, above the first rib and toward the suprasternal notch (Figure III–4).
10. Apply constant negative pressure while the needle is advanced.
11. Successful entry is marked by free flow of nonpulsatile venous blood.
12. The patient's head should be directed to face the operator while the guidewire is inserted. This facilitates guidewire placement down the superior vena cava as opposed to up the internal jugular vein.
13. Remove the syringe.
14. Advance the guidewire through the needle.
15. The guidewire should slide easily through the needle, essentially to the hub of the needle.
16. If there is resistance to passage of the guidewire, it is important to reattach the syringe and reposition the needle so that the blood flows freely.
17. If the resistance is more distal than the tip of the needle, the guidewire is likely coursing cephalad at the internal jugular vein (an awake patient may remark that the ipsilateral ear hurts). Another pass of the guidewire with the entry needle pulled back slightly is appropriate.
18. Once the guidewire is passed, remove the needle.

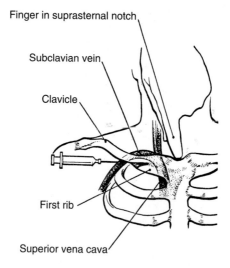

Figure III–4. Technique for catheterization of the subclavian vein. (Reproduced, with permission, from Gomella L, ed: *Clinician's Pocket Reference*. 10th ed. McGraw-Hill;2004.)

19. Follow steps 11 through 18 for placement via the right internal jugular vein approach.

Complications

1. Arterial puncture is usually obvious because bright red blood spurts from the needle when the syringe is detached or the syringe spontaneously fills without negative pressure. The needle is then withdrawn and manual pressure applied to stop arterial bleeding. Significant bleeding deep to the clavicle may occur and is heavily dependent on the patient's coagulation system and the size of the puncture. This underscores the importance of knowing the patient's coagulation profile before making the decision on which approach to use for central line placement.
2. Pneumothorax can be detected when a sudden gush of air is aspirated instead of blood. A postprocedure chest x-ray should always be done to rule out pneumothorax and check for line placement. A pneumothorax requires chest tube placement in virtually all cases, especially when the patient is being supported on a ventilator. The left-sided approach is associated with higher risk for pneumothorax because of the higher dome of the left pleura compared with the right.
3. Hemothorax
4. Air embolus

Advantages

1. The left subclavian approach affords a gentle, sweeping curve to the apex of the right ventricle and is the preferred entry site for placement of a temporary transvenous pacemaker without fluoroscopic assistance.
2. Hemodynamic measurements are often easier to record from the left subclavian approach.
3. From the left subclavian vein approach, the catheter does not have to negotiate an acute angle, as is commonly the case at the junction of the right subclavian with the right brachiocephalic vein en route to the superior vena cava. This is also a common site for kinking of the deep line.
4. Lowest risk of infection of various central line sites.

Disadvantages: Risk of pneumothorax.

Femoral Vein Approach

The femoral line is an option that is probably underutilized in critical care settings.

Procedure

1. Place the patient in the supine position.
2. Use sterile preparation and appropriate draping. Administer local anesthesia in the area to be explored.

3. Palpate the femoral artery.
4. Guard the artery with the fingers of one hand.
5. Explore for the vein just medial to the operator's fingers with a needle and syringe.
6. With exploration, it may be helpful to have a small amount of anesthetic in the syringe to inject.
7. The needle is directed cephalad at about a 30-degree angle and should be inserted below the femoral crease.
8. Puncture is heralded by the return of venous, nonpulsatile blood on application of negative pressure to the syringe.
9. Advance the guidewire through the needle.
10. The guidewire should pass with ease into the vein to a depth at which the distal tip of the guidewire is always under the operator's control. The operator should maintain control of the guidewire at its entry point through the skin while passing the sheath/dilator or catheter over the distal end of the wire.
11. Remove the needle once the guidewire has advanced into the femoral vein.
12. If the catheter is 6F or larger, a skin incision with a scalpel blade is generally needed. The catheter can then be advanced along with the guidewire in unison into the femoral vein. **Be sure always to control the distal end of the guidewire.**
13. Follow steps 14 through 17 for the right internal jugular vein approach.

Complications

1. The femoral deep line has the highest incidence of contamination and sepsis. If an occlusive dressing can remain in place and remain free from contamination, this is a safe option. Recent randomized series from centers in Europe testify to the benefit of a 10-cm long subcutaneous tunnel between the vein puncture site to the skin exit site of the catheter. A fourfold decrease in catheter-related infections was noted. The procedure is still done at bedside but is more involved in that the tunneling subcutaneously must be added to the percutaneous venipuncture.
2. Deep venous thrombosis (DVT) has occurred from femoral vein catheterization as well as with other sites. The risk for DVT increases if the catheter remains in place for prolonged periods.

Advantages

1. The procedure is safe, in that arterial and venous sites are compressible. This route or the median basilic vein approach is preferred in the presence of a coagulopathy or severe lung disease.
2. It is impossible to cause pneumothorax from this site.
3. Placement can be accomplished without interrupting cardiopulmonary resuscitation.

4. This site can be used to place a variety of intravascular appliances, including temporary pacemakers, pulmonary artery catheters (expertise with fluoroscopy is needed), and triple-lumen catheters.

Disadvantages

1. This approach has the highest rate of infection.
2. Fluoroscopy is required for placement of pulmonary artery catheters or transvenous pacemakers.

Median Basilic Vein Approach

It is possible in some patients, particularly men with well-developed upper extremities, to place an 8F-sized introducer into the median basilic vein. The median basilic vein is directed medially at the antecubital fossa. The cephalic vein should be avoided. It runs laterally at the antecubital fossa and should not be relied on to pass a deep line because the line will commonly hang up at the origin of the axillary vein. Passage to the central circulation may occur via the cephalic vein, but should be tested using a long, thin guidewire and fluoroscopy before this approach is counted on for central access.

Procedure

1. Use sterile preparation with appropriate draping.
2. Administer local anesthesia with lidocaine.
3. Place an Intracath needle into the vein through which the guidewire will pass. Alternatively, the "micro-puncture" technique described above is also applicable for use in the upper extremities as well.
4. Advance the guidewire through the Intracath/intermediate dilator.
5. Once the guidewire has passed into the median vein, remove the Intracath/intermediate dilator.
6. Incise the skin with a no. 11 scalpel. Advance the sheath/dilator system or triple-lumen catheter over the wire and into the vein **while controlling either the proximal or distal end of the guidewire at all times.**
7. Follow steps 14 through 17 for the right internal jugular vein approach.

Complications: Thrombophlebitis (line should be removed in 48–72 hours).

Advantages

1. Noncompressible bleeding is avoided. This route or the femoral route is preferred in the presence of coagulopathy or severe lung disease.
2. No risk of pneumothorax.

Disadvantages

1. Cannot be used in all patients.
2. Fluoroscopy is required for placement of pulmonary artery catheters or temporary pacemakers.
3. Uncomfortable and immobilizing.

REFERENCES

Maki DG, Stolz SM, Wheeler S et al: Prevention of central venous catheter-related bloodstream infection by use of an antiseptic-impregnated catheter. Ann Intern Med 1997;127:257.

Raad I, Darouiche R, Dupuis J et al: Central venous catheters coated with minocycline and rifampin for the prevention of catheter-related colonization and bloodstream infections. Ann Intern Med 1997;127:267.

Timsit J-F, Bruneel F, Cheval C et al: Use of tunneled femoral catheters to prevent catheter-related infection. Ann Intern Med 1999;130:729.

Timsit J-F, Sebille V, Farkas J-C et al: Effect of subcutaneous tunneling on internal jugular catheter-related sepsis in critically ill patients. JAMA 1996;276:1416.

7. ENDOTRACHEAL INTUBATION

See also Section VI, Ventilator Management, p 470.

Indications: These include cardiac arrest, acute hypoxemic respiratory failure, ventilatory failure, and the poorly responsive patient at risk for aspiration. Endotracheal intubation is also needed to ensure a patent airway in the presence of neurologic or mechanical impairment and to provide pulmonary toilet in the presence of overwhelming secretions or massive hemoptysis.

Contraindications: Massive (relative) maxillofacial trauma, fractured larynx, suspected cervical spinal cord injury. Nasotracheal intubation is contraindicated in suspected basilar skull fractures. Fiberoptic intubation or tracheostomy may be indicated in these instances.

Materials: Endotracheal tube (ETT), usually 7.0- to 9.0-mm internal diameter for most adults; laryngoscope handle and blade (no. 3 straight or curved); 10-mL syringe; adhesive tape; suction equipment; lubricant; malleable stylet (optional); gloves; protective eye wear; oximeter and end tidal CO_2 monitoring (if available).

Procedure: Orotracheal intubation is most commonly used and is described here.

1. If the patient is hypoxic or apneic, use a bag and mask with 100% oxygen before and during the intubation procedure. The risk of hypoxemia during intubation can be minimized by preoxygenation with 100% oxygen at high flow rates for 3–4 minutes and by avoiding prolonged periods without ventilation. Monitor oxygen saturation throughout the procedure, if possible.
2. Prepare the equipment. Don gloves and protective eyewear. Extend the laryngoscope blade to 90 degrees to verify that the light is working. Inflate the cuff to ensure competency. Apply a water-soluble lubricant to the tube. Enlist a respiratory therapist to maintain oxygenation and assist in airway control during the procedure.

3. **Position the patient.** This is likely the most important component of the procedure. Place folded towels under the patient's head to achieve the "sniffing position" (neck flexed and head slightly extended). Adjust the bed to a comfortable height. Remove the headboard and lock the wheels.

4. Intravenous sedation may be required in patients who are agitated, uncooperative, or combative. Consider using midazolam 1–2 mg IV every 5 minutes, fentanyl 25–50 mg IV, or etomidate 0.3 mg/kg IV.

5. Open the mouth by placing the thumb and index finger of the right hand on the lower and upper incisors, respectively, and spreading the thumb and finger with a scissorlike motion.

6. Grip the laryngoscope with the left hand. Insert the extended blade into the right side of the mouth. Use the blade to push the tongue to the left while keeping the tongue anterior to the blade. Advance carefully toward the midline until the epiglottis is seen (Figure III–5).

7. Pass the straight (Miller) laryngoscope blade posterior and inferior to the epiglottis. When using the curved (MacIntosh) blade, pass it ante-

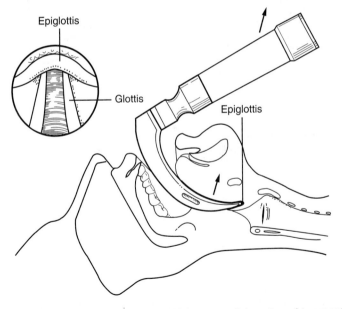

Figure III–5. Endotracheal intubation. Advance blade to groove between base of tongue and epiglottis. (Reproduced, with permission, from Vander Salm TJ, ed. *Atlas of Bedside Procedures.* 2nd ed. Little, Brown;1988:21.)

rior and superior to the epiglottis. Thrust the left arm upward at a 45-degree angle from the horizontal and visualize the vocal cords or the arytenoid cartilage. Avoid using the maxillary teeth as a fulcrum by keeping the wrist rigid and lifting only with the arm and shoulder. If the cords are not visualized, the straight blade may have progressed too posterior and inferior into the esophagus. In that case, slowly retract the laryngoscope while watching for the cords to appear. With either type of blade, application of cricoid pressure by an assistant may be a useful adjunct while attempting cord visualization.

8. While maintaining visualization of the cords, grasp the ETT in the right hand, pass it into the right corner of the mouth, and advance the cuff beyond the cords. With more difficult intubations, a malleable stylet can be used to direct the tube. In average-sized individuals, the incisors should be at the 23-cm mark for males and 21-cm mark for females.

9. Gently inflate the cuff with air until an adequate seal is obtained (about 5 mL). Auscultate over the epigastrium (with ventilation; loud gurgling over the epigastrium suggests a gastric intubation). Then auscultate over the left and right anterior and midaxillary chest. If the left side lacks breath sounds, a right mainstem bronchus intubation is likely. In that case, deflate the cuff, retract the ETT 1–2 cm, reinflate the cuff, and reassess breath sounds. End-tidal CO_2 monitoring will confirm tracheal intubation. Confirm the positioning with a stat chest x-ray. The end of the ETT should be 3–4 cm superior to the carina.

10. Secure tube position with tape. Record the centimeter mark at the incisors. Insert an oropharyngeal airway to prevent the patient from biting the ETT.

Complications: Oropharyngeal trauma, aspiration, improper tube positioning (esophageal or right mainstem bronchus intubation). Complications associated with a prolonged intubation attempt include cardiac arrest, seizures, and gastric distention. Right mainstem bronchus intubation has adverse consequences including pneumothorax and left lung atelectasis. Prolonged intubation (more than 10–14 days) can lead to tracheal stenosis.

REFERENCES

Einarsson O, Rochester CL, Rosenbaum SH: Airway management in respiratory emergencies. Clin Chest Med 1994;15:13.

Kaur S, Heard SO: Airway management and endotracheal intubation. In: Irwin RS, Rippe JM, Cerra FB et al, eds. *Procedures and Techniques in Intensive Care Medicine.* 2nd ed. Lippincott Williams & Wilkins;1999:3.

Pingleton SK: Management of complications of acute respiratory failure. In: Bone RC, ed. *Pulmonary and Critical Care Medicine.* 6th ed. Mosby;1998:R11-6.

8. GASTROINTESTINAL TUBES

Indications: Gastrointestinal (GI) decompression (paralytic ileus, obstruction, postoperatively); lavage of the stomach for GI bleeding or drug overdose; prevention of aspiration in an obtunded patient (protect the airway by endotracheal intubation first); feeding a patient who is unable to swallow.

Contraindications: Nasal fractures, basilar skull fracture.

Materials: GI tube of choice, lubricant jelly, catheter-tipped syringe, glass of water with straw, stethoscope.

1. **Gastric tubes primarily for lavage or decompression**
   a. **Levine:** Single-lumen tube that must be placed on intermittent suction to evacuate gastric contents.
   b. **Salem sump:** The best tube for continuous suction. The Salem sump is a double-lumen tube, with the smaller tube acting as an air intake vent. Use 14–18F size in adults.
   c. **Ewald:** Large (18–36F) single-lumen tube, especially suited for gastric lavage of drug overdoses. It is more often inserted by the orogastric route.
2. **Feeding tubes.** Although any small-bore nasogastric tube can be used as a feeding tube, certain weighted tubes are designed to pass into the duodenum and decrease the risk of aspiration of gastric contents.
   a. **Dobbhoff, Entriflex, Keogh:** These have a weighted mercury tip with stylet.
   b. **Vivonex:** Tungsten-tipped.
3. **Sengstaken-Blakemore tube:** A triple-lumen tube used exclusively for tamponade of esophageal varices to control bleeding. One lumen is for aspiration, one is for the gastric balloon, and the third is for the esophageal balloon.

Procedure

1. Inform the patient of the nature of the procedure and encourage the patient to cooperate. Choose the nasal passage that appears most patent by occluding one nostril and having the patient sniff.
2. Lubricate the distal 3–4 inches of the tube with a water-soluble jelly (K-Y Jelly or viscous 2% lidocaine), and insert the tube gently along the floor of the nasal passageway. Maintain gentle pressure that will allow the tube to pass into the nasopharynx. Running the tube under warm water before lubrication makes it more pliable and may help facilitate its placement. Flexing the head also helps facilitate passage of the tube.
3. When the patient can feel the tube in the back of the throat, ask him or her to swallow small amounts of water through a straw as you advance the tube 2–3 inches at a time.
4. To be sure that the tube is in the stomach, aspirate gastric contents or blow air into the tube and listen over the stomach with your stethoscope for a "pop" or "gurgle."

5. Attach sump tubes (Salem sump) to "continuous low wall suction" and the single-lumen tube (Levine) to "intermittent suction."
6. Feeding tubes are more difficult to insert because they are more flexible. You can use a stylet or guidewire or attach the smaller tube to a larger, stiffer tube by wedging both into a gelatin capsule. Pass the tube in the usual fashion and allow it to remain in the stomach for 10–15 minutes. After this time, the capsule will dissolve and the larger tube can be removed.
7. **Always** verify the position of feeding tubes by chest x-ray before beginning feedings.
8. Tape the tube securely in place but do not allow it to apply pressure to the nasal ala. Patients have been disfigured by ischemic necrosis of the nose caused by a poorly positioned tube.

Complications: Inadvertent passage into the trachea; coiling of the tube in the mouth or pharynx; bleeding from the nose, pharynx, or stomach; and sinusitis.

9. INTRAVENOUS TECHNIQUES

Indications: To establish intravenous (IV) access for the administration of fluids, blood, or medications.

Materials: IV fluid, connecting tubing, tourniquet, alcohol swab, IV cannulas (a catheter over a needle, such as Intracath, Angiocath, and Jelco or a butterfly needle), antiseptic ointment, dressing, and tape. You will find it helpful to rip the tape into strips and to flush the air out of the tubing with the IV fluid before you begin the procedure.

Procedure

1. An upper, nondominant extremity is the site of choice for an IV. Choose a distal vein so that if the vein is damaged, you can reposition the IV more proximally. Avoid veins that cross joint spaces. Also avoid the leg, since there is a high incidence of superficial thrombophlebitis. If no extremity vein can be found, try the external jugular vein. If all these fail, the only alternative is a central line or a cutdown.
2. Apply a tourniquet above the proposed IV site. Techniques to help expose difficult-to-locate veins include (1) wrapping the extremity in a warm towel; (2) leaving the arm in a dependent position for a few minutes after the tourniquet is applied; or (3) using a blood pressure cuff as a tourniquet, inflated so that the arterial flow is still maintained. Carefully clean the site with an alcohol or povidone-iodine swab. If a large-bore IV is to be used (16F or 14F), local anesthesia with 1% lidocaine may be helpful.
3. Stabilize the vein distally with the thumb of your free hand. Using the catheter-over-needle assembly (Intracath or Angiocath), enter the skin alongside the vein first, and then stick the vein along the side at

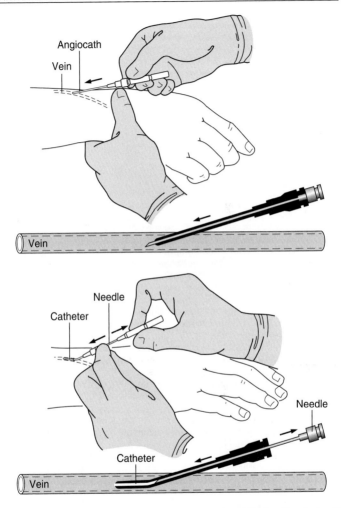

Figure III–6. To insert a catheter-over-needle assembly into a vein, stabilize the skin and vein with gentle traction. Enter the vein and advance the catheter while holding the needle steady; then remove the needle. (Reproduced, with permission, from Gomella LG, ed: *Clinician's Pocket Reference.* 10th ed. McGraw-Hill;2004.)

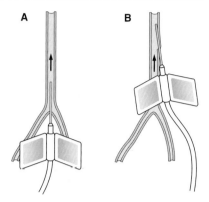

Figure III–7. Two techniques for entering the vein for intravenous access. (**A**) Direct puncture. (**B**) Side entry. (Reproduced, with permission, from Gomella TL, ed: *Neonatology: Management, Procedures, On-Call Problems, Diseases and Drugs.* 4th ed Originally published by Appleton & Lange. Copyright 1999 by the McGraw-Hill Companies, Inc.)

about a 20-degree angle. Once the vein is punctured, blood should appear in the "flash" chamber. Advance 4–5 mm to be sure that BOTH the needle AND the tip of the catheter have entered the vein. Carefully withdraw the needle as you advance the catheter into the vein (Figure III–6). *Never withdraw the catheter over the needle because this procedure can shear off the plastic tip and cause a catheter embolus.* Apply pressure with your thumb over the vein just proximal to the site, to prevent significant blood loss while you connect the IV line to the catheter.

4. Observe the site with the IV fluid running for signs of induration or swelling that indicate improper placement or damage to the vein.

5. Tape the IV securely in place; apply a drop of povidone-iodine or antibiotic ointment and a sterile dressing at the puncture site over the needle. Ideally, the dressing should be changed every 24–48 hours to help reduce infections. Armboards are also useful to help maintain an IV site, especially near a joint.

6. If the veins are deep and difficult to locate, a small 3- to 5-mL syringe can be mounted on the catheter assembly. Proper position inside the vein is determined by aspiration of blood.

7. If venous access is limited, a "butterfly" needle can be used (Figure III–7); or the external jugular vein may be considered as an alternative site.

8. All IV lines should be changed every 72 hours to decrease the risk of infection.

Complications: Thrombophlebitis; localized infection or sepsis.

10. LUMBAR PUNCTURE

Indications: For the diagnosis of central nervous system (CNS) infectious , postinfectious, or inflammatory disorders (eg, Guillain-Barré syndrome); intracranial hypotension or hypertension (eg, pseudotumor cerebri); meningeal carcinomatosis; subarachnoid hemorrhage; or demyelinating disorders (eg, multiple sclerosis). Lumbar puncture (LP) may also be necessary for the injection of diagnostic or therapeutic agents (contrast media, antibiotics, or chemotherapy).

Contraindications: Evidence of infection near the planned puncture site, bleeding disorder, or intracranial hypertension with focal neurologic signs and/or a mass lesion on neuroimaging. The presence of papilledema or a focal neurologic deficit is a contraindication unless a computed tomography or magnetic resonance imaging brain scan can exclude a focal or mass lesion (which may be evidenced by obstruction or displacement of the lateral, third, or fourth ventricles; obliteration of the suprachiasmatic, basilar, or quadrigeminal cisterns; or midline shift of the brain). If the patient is on heparin, the heparin should be discontinued at least 4–6 hours before LP. Patients on coumadin should not undergo LP with the international normalized ratio (INR) > 1.3, until anticoagulation has been reversed with fresh-frozen plasma and/or vitamin K. The platelet count should normally be > 50,000 before attempting the procedure. If a myelogram is anticipated, an elective LP should be delayed and cerebrospinal fluid (CSF) collected instead at the time of the myelogram.

Procedure

1. **Before** the procedure, a detailed evaluation of the patient and careful consideration of the potential risks and benefits must be made. A neuroimaging procedure should precede a LP if the patient has evidence of increased intracranial pressure (papilledema or headache) or focal neurologic findings.
2. The most important detail in the performance of a successful LP is to place the patient in a comfortable and accessible position. A lateral decubitus position with the back close to the edge of the bed or table and with the neck, back, knees, and hips maximally flexed to facilitate an open, clear approach to the vertebral interspaces is most effective. The hips and shoulders must be absolutely perpendicular to the bed. Padding placed between the iliac crest and inferior costal margin helps prevent sagging and keeps the spinal column straight and parallel with the bed. A pillow between the legs prevents the pelvis from rotating forward out of the perpendicular plane with the bed. It is often useful for an assistant to keep the patient in the optimal position. Alternatively, the LP may be performed with the patient sitting, leaning forward over the backrest of the chair or bed stand. However, in this position, accurate interpretation of the opening and closing pressures and comparison to standard pressures (which can only be done with the patient in a lateral decubitus position) are impossible.
3. The spinal needle should be inserted through the L_4-L_5 interspace. The tip of the spinal cord descends to L_2 in 94% of adults, whereas in another 6% it descends as low as the mid vertebral body of L_3. In

neonates, the lower margin of the spinal cord descends to the lower border of the L_3 vertebral body. An imaginary line drawn across the top of the iliac crests usually crosses the spine at about the L_4 vertebral body. Marking the skin overlying the L_4-L_5 interspace with an indentation of the fingernail is helpful in finding the spot later when the patient is prepped and draped.

4. Open the LP kit and put on sterile gloves. Prep the area with povidone-iodine solution in a circular fashion starting in the center and gradually working outward so that a circular area of skin measuring at least 6 inches in diameter has been sterilized. In the same fashion, repeat the process of sterilizing the patch of skin two more times. Next, drape the patient.

5. Anesthetize the overlying skin by raising a small wheal using a 25-gauge needle and 1% lidocaine. Avoid injecting too much solution, because too large a wheal may obscure palpable landmarks. With a 1½-inch 22-gauge needle, infiltrate deeper tissues with 1% lidocaine. Always attempt to aspirate the syringe before injecting to ensure that the needle has not entered the subarachnoid space or vessel.

6. Inspect the spinal needle, stylet, manometer, 3-way stopcock, and collection tubes for defects. Loosen the caps of the collection tubes and make certain that they are properly marked and that you are familiar with the sequence in which they will be used to collect serial specimens of CSF.

7. Using a 20-gauge spinal needle (Quinke needle) with a well-fitting stylet, insert the needle into the subcutaneous tissues. The beveled tip should be parallel with the long axis of the spine to minimize injury to the longitudinal dural fibers and reduce the chances of a postspinal headache. Guide the needle just caudal to the L_4 spinous process, keeping the needle parallel with the floor and perpendicular to the spine but directed slightly cephalad, targeting the tip of the needle toward the umbilicus. Keep pressure on the hub of the stylet to avoid having it displaced from the needle. One useful technique to help avoid misdirecting the needle is to hold the needle between the index fingers of both hands with the thumbs holding the hub of the needle and stylet while guiding the needle into the subarachnoid space (Figure III–8).

8. Continue to advance the needle slowly until a "give" or "pop" is felt, indicating that the tip has passed the resistance of the longitudinal ligament and has entered the subarachnoid space. Remove the stylet and check for CSF flow. Replacing the stylet and rotating the needle 90–180 degrees may facilitate flow if it is absent or slow. If this fails, replace the stylet and advance the needle a few millimeters, stopping each time to remove the stylet and check for CSF flow. Never advance the needle without first replacing the stylet. The hollow barrel of the needle may become occluded with epidermis, which can be introduced into the subarachnoid space, leading to an epidermoid tumor later. Pressing on the abdomen or having the patient undergo Valsalva's maneuver can improve flow when very low CSF pressure is

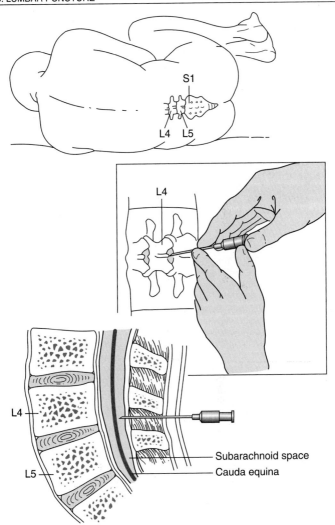

Figure III–8. When performing a lumbar puncture, place the patient in the lateral decubitus position and locate the L_4-L_4 interspace. Control the spinal needle with two hands and enter the subarachnoid space. (Reproduced, with permission, from Gomella LG, ed: *Clinician's Pocket Reference.* 10th ed. McGraw-Hill;2004.)

encountered. Lastly, applying minimal suction with a syringe attached to the hub of the needle may be necessary in obtaining a sample.

9. If you are unsuccessful at the L_4-L_5 interspace, attempt the procedure one interspace above or below this location.

10. Once the subarachnoid space is penetrated and CSF flow is obtained, attach the stopcock with the manometer to the needle hub and carefully measure the opening pressure. Be careful because unintentional movements during manipulation of the stopcock or manometer may displace the needle tip from the spinal canal. Some LP trays contain a short piece of flexible tubing that can be attached between the needle hub and stopcock, which dampens these movements and makes displacement of the needle less likely. Normal opening CSF pressure, with the patient lying comfortably in a lateral decubitus position, is 70–180 mm H_2O, but may be as high as 250 mm H_2O in the severely obese patient. Straining may falsely elevate the CSF pressure, as will positive pressure devices attached to mechanical ventilators. Before measuring the pressure, allow the patient to relax and slightly extend the legs. An elevated pressure may be due to cerebral edema, mass lesions, pseudotumor cerebri, or infectious or noninfectious CNS inflammatory disorders. Hyperventilation, chronic CSF leak, or subarachnoid block from a spinal tumor or meningitis can lower the CSF pressure. However, a low pressure is more often caused by incomplete needle penetration of the subarachnoid space, a needle with too small a bore, or other faulty technique.

11. Serially collect the CSF in four labeled containers. The quantity depends on the tests to be performed, plus a small extra amount for additional tests, which may only be thought of later. Usually, 20 mL is adequate, but repeating an LP because insufficient fluid was collected with the first procedure should rarely occur and subjects the patient to unnecessary risks. The collection tubes should be numbered in the order they were collected and taken immediately to the laboratory for processing. Do not allow the specimen to linger at the nursing station before being transported by routine carrier service. It is better to personally transport the CSF to guarantee it does not become lost or mishandled. It is often helpful to specify what laboratory studies are to be obtained from each tube; an example would be as follows:

- Tube 1 for cell count and differential
- Tube 2 for glucose and protein
- Tube 3 for bacterial culture and Gram's stain
- Tube 4 for cell count and differential

Although there may be an advantage to requesting fungal and AFB smears and cultures, or cytology from the last tube collected, special studies may be obtained from any of the other tubes. Other studies include VDRL, counterimmune electrophoresis (CIE) or latex agglutination for common bacterial antigens, multiple sclerosis profile, angiotensin-converting enzyme, viral cultures, and others. Table III–1 demonstrates typical CSF results for various disorders.

TABLE III–1. DIFFERENTIAL DIAGNOSIS OF CEREBROSPINAL FLUID.

Condition	Color	Opening Pressure (mm H$_2$O)	Protein (mg/100 mL)	Glucose (mg/100 mL)	Cells (per mL)
Adult (normal)	Clear	70–180	15–45	45–80	0–5 lymphs
Bacterial meningitis	Cloudy	Increased	50–1500	Decreased, may be < 20	25–10,000 polys
Granulomatous (TB, fungal)	Clear or cloudy	Increased	Increased, usually < 500	Decreased, may be 20–40	10–500 lymphs
Viral	Clear or slightly cloudy	Normal, or slightly increased	Normal, or slightly increased	Normal	10–500 lymphs (polys early)

Modified and reproduced with permission from Gomella LG, ed. *Clinician's Pocket Reference*. 10th ed. McGraw-Hill; 2004. WBC, white blood cell; RBC, red blood cell; lymphs, lymphocytes; polys, polymorphonuclear leukocytes; TB, tuberculosis.

12. Blood in the CSF may be due to a traumatic LP or subarachnoid hemorrhage (SAH). Clues that help to differentiate a traumatic LP from a SAH include the following: visualized clearing of blood from one tube to the next, higher red blood cell (RBC) count in the first tube than in the last, the ratio of white blood cell (WBC) count to RBC count from the CSF being similar to that of peripheral blood, the proportion of protein to RBC count in the CSF being similar to that of peripheral blood, centrifuged CSF showing a clear supernatant, and a normal opening pressure. A SAH that has been present for at least 2–4 hours shows the supernatant to be pigmented or xanthochromic, there is no visual clearing of the blood from one tube to the next, the RBC count is about the same from the first tube to the last, and the proportion of WBC count or protein to the RBC count from the CSF may be higher than found in the peripheral blood. The opening pressure with SAH may be elevated or normal. Remember that in the face of a SAH a traumatic LP may lead to misinterpretation of the results; therefore, a high index of suspicion is necessary so that a SAH is not erroneously discounted.

13. Replace the stylet, withdraw the needle, and place a sterile dressing over the puncture site. To minimize chances for a post-LP headache, have the patient avoid strenuous activities and remain mostly prone for the next 12–24 hours.

14. Carefully document the procedure in the patient's medical record, making sure to include the type and size of spinal needle that was used, opening and closing pressures, amount of CSF removed and its general appearance, the patient's position for the procedure, the vertebral interspace that was punctured, and any complications that were encountered.

Complications: The most common complication is a post-LP headache, which is improved by recumbency and aggravated by an upright position. It may occur within 1–2 days or as long as a week after the procedure. Using a needle smaller than 20-gauge may reduce the risk, but resistance of a very small gauge needle to CSF flow prolongs the procedure and may falsely lower the measured pressures. A persistent post-LP headache that does not respond to strict bed rest may need treatment with an autologous blood patch by an anesthesiologist. Other early complications from an LP procedure include local back pain, nerve root irritation and transient radicular symptoms, vasovagal syncope, nausea and vomiting, brain stem herniation, cranial subdural hematoma, SAH, spinal subdural or epidural hematoma, spinal cord hematoma, and nerve filament transection. Late complications include diplopia due usually to abducens nerve palsy (but also can occur with oculomotor or trochlear nerve palsy), trigeminal sensory loss, facial nerve palsy, hearing loss, discitis, osteomyelitis, epidural or spinal cord abscess, disc herniation, spinal arachnoid cyst, vertebral collapse, CSF cutaneous fistula, or epidermoid tumor.

REFERENCES

Evans RW: Complications of lumbar puncture. Neurol Clin 1998;16:83.

Fishman RA, ed: *Cerebrospinal Fluid in Diseases of the Nervous System.* 2nd ed. Saunders;1992.

Lumbar puncture and the examination of the cerebrospinal fluid. In: Haerer AF, ed. De-Jong's *The Neurologic Examination.* 5th ed. Lippincott;1992:755.

Roos KL: Lumbar puncture. Semin Neurol 2003;23:105.

11. PARACENTESIS

Indications: Determination of the cause of new-onset ascites; ruling out spontaneous bacterial peritonitis in patients with known ascites; therapeutic removal of fluid in patients with tense ascites for symptomatic relief (early satiety, abdominal discomfort, dyspnea).

Contraindications: Coagulopathy is a relative contraindication; only when there is evident fibrinolysis or disseminated intravascular coagulation should paracentesis be avoided. Data do not support the routine administration of platelets or fresh-frozen plasma in cirrhotic patients with coagulopathy. Because the bowel may be adherent to the peritoneal surface near a surgical scar, the needle should be inserted several centimeters from the scar. A midline paracentesis should be avoided in patients with a long midline scar.

Materials: Minor procedure tray; 20- to 60-mL syringe; sterile specimen containers; 1.5-inch steel needle or blunt steel cannula with removable steel stylet, 22-gauge for diagnostic taps and 16-gauge for therapeutic taps. A 3.5-inch needle may be required for obese patients. The use of steel needles rather than plastic-sheathed cannulas prevents the possibility of shearing off the plastic sheath into the peritoneal cavity and the tendency of the plastic sheath to kink and obstruct the flow of fluid.

Procedure

1. The patient's bladder needs to be empty. Patients with tense ascites can be placed supine with the head of the bed slightly elevated. Patients with less ascites can be placed in either lateral decubitus position and tapped in the midline or can be tapped in either lower quadrant while supine.

2. If there is any doubt about the presence of ascites, confirmation should be made by abdominal ultrasound. If the amount of ascites is small, ultrasound can be used to help locate the fluid during the procedure.

3. The entry site is usually the midline, 3–4 cm below the umbilicus. However, if a midline surgical scar is present, you can locate an alternative entry site in the left or right lower quadrant 4–5 cm above and medial to the anterior superior iliac spine (lateral to the rectus sheath). Note that in obese patients the abdominal wall in the midline is signifi-

cantly thicker than in the lower quadrants and may even exceed the length of a 3.5-inch needle.

4. Prep the patient's skin with povidone-iodine solution and apply sterile drapes. Raise a skin wheal with 1% lidocaine over the proposed entry site.

5. Use the Z tract technique to avoid postprocedure leakage of fluid. With the paracentesis needle mounted on a syringe in one hand, use the other gloved hand to displace the skin approximately 2 cm. Do not release the skin until the peritoneum has been penetrated. The needle should be advanced slowly in 5-mm increments aspirating intermittently rather than continuously; this prevents drawing bowel or omentum to the end of the needle.

6. Aspirate the amount of fluid needed for tests (30–50 mL). For a therapeutic tap, a 16- to 18-gauge steel needle can be connected to vacuum bottles with phlebotomy tubing. Large-volume paracentesis (5–10 L) can be safely performed in patients with tense ascites if the fluid is removed over 60–90 minutes.

7. Remove the needle quickly, apply a sterile 4 × 4 gauze, and apply pressure to the site with tape.

8. Routine ascitic fluid tests include cell count, albumin, and bedside inoculation of blood culture bottles, which significantly increases the sensitivity of cultures. Depending on the clinical picture, other tests may include total protein, glucose, lactate dehydrogenase, amylase, acid-fast bacilli smear and culture, and cytology. See Table III-2 (p 448) for differential diagnosis of the fluid obtained.

Complications: Peritonitis, perforated bowel, intra-abdominal hemorrhage, perforated bladder, abdominal wall hematoma, and abdominal wall abscess.

TABLE III–2. TESTING OF ASCITIC FLUID.

1) Albumin Gradient
   $ALB_{serum} - ALB_{ascites} = X$
     if $X > 1.1$ g/dL, then portal hypertension
     If $X < 1.1$ g/dL, then not from portal hypertension
2) Total Protein < 1.0 g/dL, high risk for spontaneous bacterial peritonitis
3) Cell Count—absolute neutrophil count > 250/μL, presume infected
4) Bacterial Culture: Blood culture bottles 85% sensitivity
                       Routine cultures 50% sensitivity
5) Bacterial Peritonitis—Spontaneous versus secondary
     Secondary: A) polymicrobial; B) total protein > 1.0 g/dL; C) LDH > normal serum
               value; D) glucose < 50 mg/dL
6) Food Fibers: Found in most cases of perforated viscus.
7) Cytology: Bizarre cells with large nuclei may represent reactive mesothelial cells and *not* a malignancy. Malignant cells suggest tumor.

LDH, lactate dehydrogenese.

REFERENCES

Marx JA: Peritoneal procedures. In: Roberts JR, Hedges JR, eds. *Clinical Procedures in Emergency Medicine*. 3rd ed. Saunders;1998:733.

Runyon BA: Ascites and spontaneous bacterial peritonitis. In: Feldman M, Scharschmidt B, Sleisenger M, eds. *Gastrointestinal and Liver Disease*. 7th ed. Saunders;2002:1517.

Runyon BA: Care of patients with ascites. N Engl J Med 1994;330:337.

Runyon BA: Diagnosis and evaluation of patients with ascites. In: Rose BD, ed. UpToDate. UpToDate, Wellesley, MA;2003.

Runyon BA, Montano AA, Akriviadis EA et al: The serum-ascites albumin gradient is superior to the exudate-transudate concept in the differential diagnosis of ascites. Ann Intern Med 1992;117:215.

12. PULMONARY ARTERY CATHETERIZATION

See also Section I, Chapter 57, Pulmonary Artery Catheter Problems, p 324.

Production: Controversy about the "value" of pulmonary artery catheters, or PACs (also called Swan-Ganz catheters), has been going on for over a decade, probably starting with Dr. Robin's editorials in 1985 and 1987. Debate regarding the proper use of pulmonary artery catheters nearly reached the level of public hysteria with the publication of the article by Dr. Connors and colleagues in 1996 (see references at the end of this chapter). The PAC is only a diagnostic tool, with no intrinsic therapeutic value. Thus, its ability to have a favorable impact on outcome in the clinical setting is entirely dependent on three basic conditions being met:

1. The PAC can provide, with a reasonable degree of safety, specific diagnostic information that is not otherwise readily available, and this information is germane to the management of the patient.
2. The physicians using this device know how to use it safely and how to obtain accurate information from it.
3. The therapy chosen in response to the diagnostic data obtained from the PAC is appropriate and timely for the specific clinical problem being addressed.

Published evidence has clearly suggested that many physicians and nurses who routinely use PACs are less than proficient in using them (Iberti et al 1990, 1994). Also, there is growing concern that management of shock and hemodynamic compromise may be done in a suboptimal manner by physicians without appropriate critical care expertise. Reynolds and colleagues (1988) at a single hospital showed that after going to full-time critical care physicians, there was nearly a 20% increase in the rate of PAC use for managing septic shock, accompanied by a 17% decrease in mortality and an 11% shift in overall ICU costs from nonsurvivors to survivors. Similarly, Knaus and colleagues (1982) reported that for critically ill patients with severe gastrointestinal illnesses (eg, acute gastrointestinal bleeding, pancreatitis), mortality in American ICUs was statistically significantly better than in comparable

French ICUs and that US physicians used PACs in these patients much more often than did their French counterparts. In both of these studies, claiming that the improved results were due to the increased rate of PAC use would be as misleading as it would be to blame the PAC for the lack of improvement or worse outcome associated with its use that was found in some retrospective observational studies (Robin 1987; Connors et al 1996).

The issues of when and by whom a PAC should be used, and also whether similar diagnostic information could be better obtained in the ICU by other means (eg, "continuous" echocardiography or bioimpedance studies), remain legitimate areas of research. Likewise, studying different therapeutic approaches for a specific type of hemodynamic derangement also remains a high priority. In any case, only experienced personnel should use PACs. Similarly, proper PAC use requires clearly defined diagnostic and/or therapeutic goals that can be achieved using the data obtained from this device.

Indications: Pulmonary artery catheterization is generally undertaken in acutely ill patients *as a diagnostic intervention* when a question exists regarding the patient's volume status, cardiac output, or peripheral vascular resistance. Some specific examples include (1) establishing the cause of hypotension or shock when this is not immediately apparent; (2) differentiating between congestive heart failure, acute respiratory distress syndrome (ARDS), or pneumonia as the cause of pulmonary infiltrates; (3) determining whether poor urine output is due to volume depletion, acute renal failure, or poor forward cardiac output; and (4) determining whether a patient with acute myocardial infarction and tachycardia has volume depletion, pain, anxiety, or left ventricular failure. Table III-3 outlines the various types of PAC data in different types of shock. Please note that critically ill patients often have more than one disease process going on simultaneously, and hemodynamic data may become somewhat confusing without careful correlation with the whole clinical context and all other available data.

Contraindications: If PAC is needed to manage a patient in a critical care setting, there are no absolute contraindications. For patients who are candidates for PACs and who have received thrombolytic therapy, jugular and subclavian vein approaches should be avoided. As with all indwelling catheters that involve frequent manipulation, maintaining strict sterile conditions at all times, particularly at the time of placement, is essential to avoid infections. There are no convincing data showing that routine site changes at 3- or 4-day intervals are clearly beneficial and cost-effective, but like all indwelling catheters, the PAC should be removed immediately as soon as it is no longer needed.

Materials: In most institutions, a single brand of a flow-directed balloon-tipped PAC is available. Use an insertion kit that provides the catheter as well as a sheath and the various syringes, needles, preparation material, local anesthetic, and other items that will be used to insert the catheter.

The PAC has four or five ports: air inflation or balloon port, thermistor, distal port, right atrial or proximal port, and (in some) a port for fluid or medica-

TABLE III–3. PULMONARY ARTERY CATHETER: DIAGNOSIS OF SHOCK.

Type of Shock	Central Venous Pressure (CVP)	Pulmonary Artery Pressure (PAP)	Pulmonary Wedge Pressure (PWP)	Cardiac Output (CO)	Systemic Vascular Resistance (SVR)	Mixed Venous Oxygen Saturation (SvO₂)
Oligemic[1]	↓	Normal to ↓	↓↓↓	↓	↑	↓
Cardiac[2]	Often ↓, may be normal or even ↑	Usually ↑	↑	↓↓↓	↑	↓
Distributive or "low SVR"[3]		Usually normal, may be ↓ or ↑	Usually ↓, may be normal or even ↑	Usually ↑, may become ↓	↓↓↓	Usually ↓, rarely can be normal or even ↑[4]
Obstructive, extra-cardiac[5]	Usually ↑	Usually ↑	Can be ↑ (eg, in tamponade), or ↓ (eg, with thromboembolism)	↓↓↓	↑	↓

[1] Oligemic shock refers to intravascular volume depletion, whether caused by true blood loss, by water loss (diarrhea, sweating, fever, burns, etc), or by venodilation and massive third-spacing (eg, SIRS or sepsis).

[2] Cardiac (or cardiogenic) shock can be subdivided into myopathic and valvular causes.

[3] Septic shock is the classic model of distributive (low SVR) shock, but this group includes other entities: anaphylaxis, toxic shock, drug-induced (eg, IL-2 given for bladder cancer therapy), and neurogenic. In all these scenarios, increased venous capacitance (venodilation) and/or massive third-spacing often initially add a hypovolemic picture, while specifically in sepsis myocardial depression may add a feature of myocardial failure. Thus the increased CO "classically" described in distributive shock is dependent on adequate fluid resuscitation, and may not be seen at all in septic patients with profound myocardial depression.

[4] Although oxygen uptake by the tissues is impaired in sepsis, in the presence of shock this results in an above-normal SvO₂ only in very rare instances. Initially the SvO₂ is usually below 60% (reflecting the decreased O₂ delivery to the tissues at a time when O₂ requirements are increased), even if it may not be as low as it would have been with normal peripheral extraction of O₂.

[5] The main examples of extracardiac obstructive shock are tamponade (where pressures tend to "equalize"), tension pneumothorax, and massive pulmonary thromboembolism.

tion administration (Figure III–9). The air inflation port is used to inflate the balloon to facilitate passage of the catheter from the right cardiac chambers to the pulmonary artery. The thermistor can be used to measure cardiac outputs by thermal dilution when connected to a cardiac output computer. The distal port is used to measure pulmonary artery pressure and pulmonary capillary wedge pressure (PCWP) with the catheter in the pulmonary artery. The right atrial port is used to administer fluids, to measure right atrial pressure, or to inject fluid to measure cardiac output in conjunction with the thermistor and the cardiac output computer (see Figure III–9). The catheter is often marked so that the clinician can determine how far the distal tip lies from the entry site. This information may help in catheter placement without fluoroscopy.

Procedure

1. The patient's informed consent is usually required.
2. Choose the site of operation; prep and drape the area. The choice of site is dictated by patient variables and operator experience. The eas-

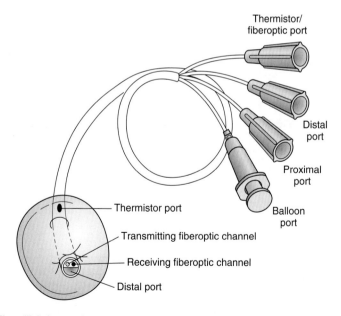

Figure III–9. An example of a pulmonary artery catheter. This one features an oximetric measuring feature. (Reproduced, with permission, from Gomella LG, ed. *Clinician's Pocket Reference.* 10th ed. McGraw-Hill;2004.)

iest sites to place a PAC without fluoroscopic guidance are the right internal jugular vein and the left subclavian vein. In a patient receiving thrombolytic therapy, femoral and median basilic veins are preferable routes when/if it is felt that placement of the PAC cannot be safely delayed for a few hours (the preferred option).

3. **Always** use a strict sterile approach with a properly large sterile field, and wear gown, gloves, and mask.

4. Prepare the PAC by flushing the lumens with heparinized saline solution (1 mL of 1:100 U heparin in 10 mL of normal saline). Check the balloon function, and tap the catheter to be sure that a waveform is generated. You should set the pressure transducer level to the middle of the patient's chest.

5. Cannulate the central vein. (See Section III, Chapter 6, Central Venous Catheterization, p 426, for details.) In general, *never* push a guide wire when there is resistance; *always* keep one hand on the guidewire, either proximal or distal to the dilator, needle, etc.

6. When the sheath is in place, you can advance the prepared catheter into the sheath. After it has been advanced approximately 15 cm, the balloon will have cleared the tip of the sheath. You can then gently inflate the balloon with about 1.0–1.5 cm^3 of air. The maximum amount of air for use with smaller catheters (5F) is $\leq$ 1.0 cm^3. If there is resistance to full inflation, check to see that the balloon has cleared the sheath or that it is not in an extravascular location (with an x-ray, or with fluoroscopy if available).

7. Once the balloon is inflated, advance the catheter to the level of the right atrium under the guidance of the pressure waveform and the electrocardiogram. Monitor the waveform and electrocardiogram at all times while advancing the balloon catheter. Remember to always advance the catheter with the balloon inflated and withdraw it with the balloon deflated. PACs usually come with a preformed curve on the tip. Insert the catheter with its tip pointing anteriorly and to the left. Positioning in the right atrium is probably best determined by watching for the characteristic waveform. The right atrium is generally located approximately 20 cm from the right internal jugular or subclavian vein insertion sites and approximately 25–30 cm from the left subclavian vein insertion site. The catheter should be advanced steadily. An abrupt change in the pressure tracing will occur as the catheter enters the right ventricle. There is generally little ectopy on entry into the right ventricle; however, as you advance the catheter into the right ventricular outflow tract, premature ventricular contractions (PVCs) may occur. Keep advancing the catheter until the ectopy disappears and the pulmonary artery tracing is obtained. If this does not occur, deflate the balloon, withdraw the catheter, and try again with the balloon inflated after slightly rotating the catheter. The PCWP will then be obtained by advancing the catheter another 10–15 cm. The catheter's final position should be such that the PCWP is obtained with full balloon inflation and the pulmonary artery pressure (PAP) tracing is pre-

sent with the balloon deflated. In the "ideal position," transition from PAP to PCWP (and vice versa) occurs within three or fewer heartbeats. ***Caution:*** Never withdraw the catheter with the balloon inflated. See Figure III–10, p 455, for normal waveforms. See Table III–4, p 456, for normal PAC measurements.

8. Suture the catheter in place and dress the site according to your institution's practice. A chest x-ray should be obtained to document the catheter's present position as well as to rule out a pneumothorax or other complication from central venous catheterization.

9. Common problems: Catheter placement is much more difficult if severe pulmonary artery hypertension is present. If there is significant cardiac enlargement, particularly dilation of the right heart structures, the catheter may have a propensity to coil and get lost in its path to the right ventricular outflow tract. Fluoroscopy may be required to get the catheter into the correct position; moreover, it will hold this position poorly. Placement of the catheter in the pulmonary artery may also be difficult in the setting of a low cardiac output because the balloon-tipped catheter is dependent on blood flow to carry it through the right heart chambers.

10. Cardiac output can be measured by thermal dilution. First, connect the thermistor port of the PAC to a cardiac output computer into which the correct catheter's constant and the proper volume and temperature of the injectate have been entered. After this is done, rapidly inject fluid (usually 10 mL of normal saline at room temperature) through the right atrial port. If feasible, it is preferred to time the injection to occur at the same point of the respiratory cycle in all trials, usually at the end of inspiration. The computer will display the cardiac output. Repeat this procedure **at least** two more times. The variability of serial thermodilution cardiac output measurements should not exceed 20%, and usually is 15% or less. For normal cardiac output and index, consult Table III–4, p 456.

11. You can often differentiate various clinical entities by measuring the blood pressure, PCWP, and cardiac output, and calculating the systemic vascular resistance. (See Table III–3, p 451.) Abnormalities in various pressures obtained from pulmonary artery catheterization can often help diagnose various disease states (see Table III–5, p 457) and may be helpful in directing fluid administration and inotropic and vasopressor therapy in certain patients.

Complications

1. Most complications that occur in the course of pulmonary artery catheterization are related to central vein cannulation and include arterial puncture and pneumothorax, as well as inadvertent placement of the catheter outside the vascular tree, most often in the pleural space.

2. Arrhythmias are another common complication. The most common of these are transient PVCs that occur when the catheter is advanced

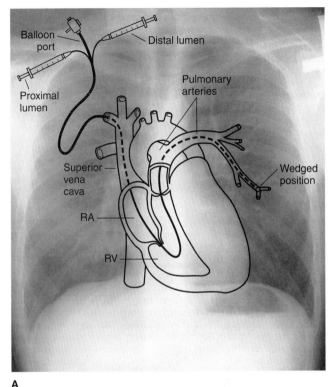

A

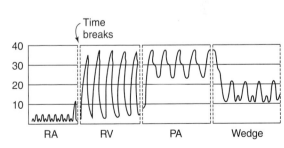

B

Figure III–10. (**A**) Positioning and (**B**) pressure waveforms seen as the pulmonary artery catheter is advanced. PA, pulmonary artery; RA, right atrium; RV, right ventricle. (Reproduced, with permission, from Stillman RM, ed. *Surgery Diagnosis & Therapy*. Originally published by Appleton & Lange. Copyright 1989 by The McGraw-Hill companies, Inc.)

TABLE III–4. NORMAL PULMONARY ARTERY CATHETER MEASUREMENTS.

Parameter	Range
Right artery pressure (RAP)	1–7 mm Hg
Right ventricular systolic pressure	15–25 mm Hg
Right ventricular diastolic pressure	0–8 mm Hg
Pulmonary artery systolic pressure	15–25 mm Hg
Pulmonary artery diastolic pressure	8–15 mm Hg
Pulmonary artery mean pressure	10–20 mm Hg
Pulmonary capillary wedge pressure (PCWP) (wedge)	6–12 mm Hg
Cardiac output (CO)	3.5–5.5 L/min
Cardiac index (CI)	2.8–3.2 l /min/m^2
Mixed venous O_2 saturation	> 60%
Systemic vascular resistance (SVR)	900–1200 dynes/sec/cm^5

$$SVR = \frac{(\text{mean arterial pressure } - \text{ central venous pressure (or RAP)})}{CO} \times 80$$

into the right ventricular outflow tract. If a patient with a PAC suddenly develops frequent PVCs, displacement of the catheter should be suspected. Sustained ventricular tachycardia and ventricular fibrillation are both very rare occurrences.

3. Transient right bundle branch block occurs occasionally as the catheter passes through the right ventricular outflow tract. In a patient with preexisting left bundle branch block, this can result in complete heart block. In this setting, some form of backup pacing should be readily available. Complete heart block has been reported but is a rare occurrence.

4. Significant pulmonary infarcts and pulmonary artery rupture are potentially very serious but infrequent complications of PACs caused by "permanent" wedge or peripheral placement of the catheter. Fortunately, these complications can be easily avoided with careful monitoring of the wave tracing to make sure that the PAC is not continuously or intermittently showing "spontaneous" PCWP position or "wedge."

5. Most complications and problems related to PACs tend to increase with the length of time that the catheter is left in place. Particularly relevant among them is the high risk of bacteremia and even subacute bacterial endocarditis that is seen in severely ill patients with chronic catheter placement. Thus, in the setting of unexplained fever, the PAC and introducer sheath should always be removed and cultured. It is essential to always culture the introducer sheath, but whether the PAC itself should also be routinely cultured is not well established. A new catheter and sheath can be placed at a different site if use of a PAC is still indicated.

TABLE III–5. DIFFERENTIAL DIAGNOSIS OF COMMON PULMONARY ARTERY CATHETER READINGS.

Low right atrial pressure	Volume depletion
High right atrial pressure	Volume overload; congestive heart failure; cardiogenic shock; increased pulmonary vascular resistance (hypoxia, ventilator effect of PEEP, pulmonary disease, primary pulmonary hypertension)
Low right ventricular pressure	Volume depletion
High right ventricular pressure	Volume overload; congestive heart failure; cardiogenic shock; increased pulmonary vascular resistance (hypoxia, ventilator effect of PEEP, pulmonary disease, primary pulmonary hypertension)
High pulmonary artery pressure	Congestive heart failure; increased pulmonary vascular resistance (hypoxia, ventilator effect of PEEP, pulmonary disease, primary pulmonary hypertension); cardiac tamponade
Low wedge pressure	Volume depletion
High wedge pressure	Cardiogenic shock, left ventricular failure, ventricular septal defect, mitral regurgitation and stenosis, severe hypertension, volume overload, cardiac tamponade

PEEP, Positive end-expiratory pressure.
Modified and reproduced with permission from Gomella LG, Lefor AT. eds. *Surgery On Call Reference.* 3rd ed. McGraw-Hill; 2001.

REFERENCES

Connors AF, Speroff T, Dawson NV et al: The effectiveness of right heart catheterization in the initial care of critically ill patients. JAMA 1996;276:889.

Iberti TJ, Daily EK, Leibowitz AB et al: Assessment of critical care nurses' knowledge of the pulmonary artery catheter. Crit Care Med 1994;22:1674.

Iberti TJ, Fisher EP, Leibowitz AB et al: A multicenter study of physician's knowledge of the pulmonary artery catheter. JAMA 1990;264:2928.

Knaus WA, LeGall JR, Wagner DP et al: A comparison of intensive care in the USA and France. Lancet 1982;2:642.

Reynolds HN, Haupt MT, Thill-Baharozian MC et al: Impact of critical care physician staffing on patients with septic shock in a university hospital medical intensive care unit. JAMA 1988;260:3446.

Robin ED: The cult of the Swan-Ganz catheter: Overuse and abuse of pulmonary flow catheters. Ann Intern Med 1985;103:445.

Robin ED: Death by pulmonary artery flow-directed catheter: Time for a moratorium? Chest 1987;92:721.

13. SKIN BIOPSY

Indications: To confirm or establish a diagnosis of any skin lesion or eruption.

Contraindications: Any skin lesion that is suspected of being a melanoma should be referred to a dermatologist or surgeon for an excisional biopsy when possible. Punch biopsies are not preferred in this setting as they may not provide adequate tissue for the measurement of tumor thickness. A platelet count < 10,000/mm^3 is a relative contraindication for skin biopsy.

Materials: A skin punch between 2 and 5 mm; 3 mL buffered lidocaine 1% with epinephrine; 3-mL syringe; 30-gauge needle; gloves; 4 × 4 gauze pads; alcohol pad; pair of curved iris scissors and fine-tooth forceps; a specimen bottle containing 10% formalin; 4-0 or 5-0 nonabsorbable suture; skin-marking pen. For biopsies of the penis or tips of digits, lidocaine without epinephrine should be used.

Procedure

1. If more than one lesion is present, it is important to choose a representative site. For patients with vesiculobullous disease or suspected vasculitis, an early intact lesion not older than 24–48 hours is preferable. For bullous or vesicular lesions, biopsy the edge of the blister or include the entire lesion if possible. For eruptions involving the trunk and extremities, choose a well-developed lesion on the trunk, avoiding a biopsy of the lower leg when possible.
2. Note the orientation of the resting skin tension lines. Wipe the area to be biopsied with the alcohol pad. Mark the area with a skin-marking pen. Apply gloves. Inject the lidocaine slowly, infiltrating an area slightly larger than the biopsy site.
3. Immobilize the skin with one hand, pulling the skin perpendicular to the resting skin tension lines. With the other hand, hold the skin punch vertical to the skin surface and apply firm pressure. Rotate the punch, alternating between clockwise and counterclockwise rotation while continuing to apply firm pressure. As the punch enters the subcutaneous fat, resistance will lessen. Remove the punch. The core of tissue can be elevated slightly by applying downward pressure on either side of the biopsy site. The tissue can then be snipped at the level of the subcutaneous fat with the scissors. If the tissue cannot be elevated, the core can be speared using the 30-gauge needle and lifted outward, allowing it to be snipped with the scissors.
4. The biopsy specimen should be immediately placed in the specimen container. If a primary blistering process (ie, bullous pemphigoid) is suspected, specimens should be sent for direct immunofluorescence as well as hematoxylin & eosin staining. A 3- to 4-mm biopsy for direct immunofluorescence should be performed from perilesional nonbullous skin. This specimen should be sent in a separate container in Michel's solution.
5. Hemostasis is achieved by applying pressure with the gauze pads.
6. Defects from 2-mm punches generally do not require suture placement. Punch defects larger than 2 mm should be closed with one or two sutures and placed perpendicular to skin tension lines to minimize the appearance of scarring.

7. Lubricant jelly (Vaseline) and an appropriately sized bandage should be applied. The dressing can be removed the following day, but the wound should be kept moist with lubricant jelly until completely healed.
8. Sutures can be removed as early as 3 days after the procedure from the face and 7–10 days from other areas.

Complications: Infection (unusual); hemorrhage (usually controlled with pressure, rare even in patients taking warfarin or aspirin); scarring and keloid formation.

REFERENCES

Robinson J, LeBoit P: Biopsy techniques: Description and proper use. In: Arndt KA, ed. *Cutaneous Medicine and Surgery.* Saunders;1996:120.

Dermatologic Surgery. In: Odom R, James W, Berger T: *Andrews' Diseases of the Skin.* Saunders;2000:1074.

Ng PC, Barzilai DA, Ismail SA et al: Evaluating invasive cutaneous melanoma: Is the initial biopsy representative of the final depth? J Am Acad Dermatol 2003;48:420.

14. THORACENTESIS

Indications: Establish the cause of a newly discovered pleural effusion, especially in a febrile patient; therapeutic removal of pleural fluid in patients with dyspnea.

Contraindications: Presence of pneumothorax, hemothorax, or other respiratory impairment on the contralateral side; coagulopathy (Protime more than twice normal or platelet count > 25,000/mm^3); very small pleural effusions (> 1 cm fluid stripe on a lateral decubitus film). Patients receiving mechanical ventilation do not have a higher risk of pneumothorax compared with nonventilated patients; however, they have an increased risk of tension physiology or persistent air leak if pneumothorax does occur.

Materials: Prepackaged thoracentesis kit; or minor procedure tray plus 20- to 60-mL syringe, 20- or 22-gauge 1.5-in. needle, three-way stopcock, specimen containers.

Procedure
1. Discuss the procedure with the patient and obtain informed consent. Teach the patient the Valsalva maneuver; or make sure the patient can hum (to increase intrathoracic pressure at a later point in the procedure). Position the patient so that he or she is sitting on the side of the bed with head and arms supported by pillows on a bedside table. (The back must be vertical; leaning too far forward causes the effusion to move anteriorly away from the thoracentesis needle.) For the debilitated patient unable to assume a sitting position, thoracentesis can be performed in the midaxillary line with the patient supine and the upper body elevated at a slight angle.

2. The usual site for a thoracentesis is midway between the spine and posterior axillary line. Percuss out the fluid level, or use the chest x-ray and count ribs. The entry site should be one to two interspaces below the level where the percussion note becomes dull or tactile fremitus is absent. Enter just above the rib to avoid the neurovascular bundle that traverses below the rib. Do not attempt thoracentesis below the eighth intercostal space to avoid injury to the spleen or liver. For high-risk patients (with mechanical ventilation, coagulopathy, small effusions), ultrasound guidance can be used to locate the optimal entry site. Be certain that during thoracentesis the patient is positioned in the same manner as during the ultrasound localization.

3. Prep the area with chlorhexidine and drape. Make a skin wheal over the proposed site with a 25-gauge needle and 1% lidocaine. Change to a 22-gauge 1.5-in. needle, and infiltrate up and over the rib; anesthetize the periosteum of the rib and parietal pleura. During this time, you should be aspirating (Figure III-11).

4. Attach the 20- to 22-gauge thoracentesis needle to a 50-mL syringe with a three-way stopcock. Open the stopcock to the syringe. Penetrate through the anesthetized area with the thoracentesis needle entering over the top of the rib to avoid the neuromuscular bundle that runs below the rib (see Figure III-11). After entering the pleural space, aspirate the amount of fluid needed. For a therapeutic thoracentesis, an 8F catheter over 18-gauge needle with self-sealing valve can be used. This prevents air from entering the pleural space when

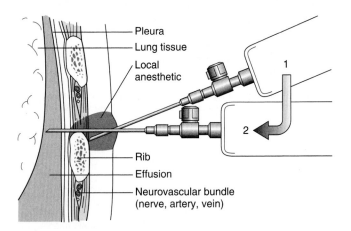

Figure III–11. In a thoracentesis, the needle is passed over the top of the rib to avoid the neurovascular bundle. (Reproduced, with permission, from Gomella LG, ed. *Clinician's Pocket Reference.* 10th ed. McGraw-Hill;2004.)

the needle is withdrawn. Do not use a sharp steel needle for therapeutic thoracentesis because as the lung expands after removal of fluid, it can be easily lacerated. After entering the pleural space, the catheter is advanced over the needle, which is then removed. One end of the drainage tubing is attached to the catheter, the other to a drainage bag system. To prevent reexpansion pulmonary edema, *do not remove more than 1000–1500 mL per tap!*

5. Have the patient hum or do the Valsalva maneuver as you withdraw the needle. These actions increase intrathoracic pressure and decrease the chance of a pneumothorax. Bandage the site.

6. Routine performance of a chest x-ray is not indicated after diagnostic thoracentesis in asymptomatic patients, but should be obtained in symptomatic patients (with new chest pain or dyspnea) and after therapeutic thoracentesis.

TABLE III–6. DIFFERENTIAL DIAGNOSIS OF PLEURAL FLUID.

Transudate: Nephrosis, congestive heart failure, cirrhosis.

Exudate: Infection (parapneumonic, empyema, tuberculosis, viral, fungal, parasitic), malignancy, peritoneal dialysis, pancreatitis, chylothorax.

Lab Value	Transudate	Exudate
Specific gravity	<1.016	>1.016
Protein (pleural fluid)	<2.5 g/100 mL	>3 g/100 mL
Protein ratio (pleural fluid-to-serum ratio)	<0.5	>0.5
LDH ratio (pleural fluid-to-serum ratio)	<0.6	>0.6
Pleural fluid LDH	<200 IU	>200 IU
Fibrinogen (clot)	No	Yes
Cell count and differential	Low WBC count	WBC count > 2500/mL; suspect an inflammatory exudate (early polys, later monos)

Grossly bloody tap: Trauma, pulmonary infarction, tumor, and iatrogenic causes.

pH: The pH of pleural fluid is usually > 7.3. If between 7.2 and 7.3, suspect tuberculosis or malignancy or both. If < 7.2, suspect an empyema.

Glucose: Normal pleural fluid glucose is two-thirds serum glucose. If the pleural fluid glucose is *much, much* lower than the serum glucose, then consider empyema or rheumatoid arthritis (0–16 mg/100 mL) as the cause of the effusion.

Triglycerides and positive Sudan stain: Chylothorax.

LDH, lactate dehydrogenase; WBC, white blood cells; polys, polymorphonuclear leukocytes; monos, monocytes.
Modified and reproduced with permission from Gomella LG, Lefor AT, eds. *Surgery On Call Reference.* 3rd ed. McGraw-Hill; 2002.

7. Measurement of pleural fluid protein, lactate dehydrogenase (LDH), white blood cell count and red blood cell count should be routinely performed. If initial results are consistent with a transudate (pleural fluid protein/serum protein ratio less than 0.5, pleural fluid LDH/serum LDH ratio less than 0.6, or pleural fluid LDH less than 60% of the upper limit of normal serum value), then no further testing is required. If the initial results are consistent with an exudate, other tests that may be ordered include glucose, pH, cytology, amylase, bacterial culture and acid-fast bacilli smear and culture (Table III–6).

Complications: Pneumothorax (5–10% incidence, of which 20% will require a chest tube), hemothorax, soft tissue infection, empyema, pulmonary laceration, hypoxemia, vasovagal response reexpansion pulmonary edema, laceration of spleen or liver, and cough (excessive coughing, usually toward the end of a therapeutic thoracentesis, is an indication to stop the procedure).

REFERENCES

Aleman C, Alegre J, Armadans L et al: The value of chest roentgenography in the diagnosis of pneumothorax after thoracentesis. Am J Med 1999;107:340.

Light RW: *Pleural Diseases.* 3rd ed. Williams & Wilkins;1995.

Ruhl TS: Thoracentesis. In: Pfenninger JL, Fowler GC, eds. *Procedures for Primary Care Physicians.* Mosby;1994:477.

Sahn S: Diagnostic thoracentesis. In: UpToDate, Rose BD, ed. UpToDate, Wellesley, MA;2003.

Sahn S. Diagnostic evaluation of a pleural effusion. In: UpToDate, Rose, BD, ed. UpToDate, Wellesley, MA;2003.

IV. Fluids & Electrolytes

Daily maintenance requirements for the average 70-kg male are as follows:

Fluid	2000–2500 mL
Dextrose	100–200 g
Sodium	60–100 mEq
Potassium	40–60 mEq

These requirements can be met with an infusion of D5¼ NS with 20–30 mEq of potassium chloride per liter infused at 100 mL/hr. The preceding combination of fluid and electrolytes may differ depending on other clinical parameters such as congestive heart failure, cirrhosis, hyponatremia, hypernatremia, hyperkalemia, and renal insufficiency. Maintenance fluids should be used for only 48–72 hours, at which time more effective measures of nutritional support (enteral tube feedings) should be instituted. For patients with severe volume depletion, normal saline can be administered as rapidly as 500–1000 mL/hr until the patient is stabilized. For patients undergoing nasogastric suction, measured losses can be replaced every 4 hours with an equal volume of normal saline. Additional potassium may have to be added to the maintenance fluids to replace that lost with gastric suction. (See Tables IV–1 and IV–2.)

TABLE IV–1. COMPOSITION OF COMMONLY USED CRYSTALLOID SOLUTIONS.

Fluid	Glucose (g/L)	Electrolytes (mEq/L)					kcal/L
		Na	Cl	K	Ca	HCO₃	
D5W (5% dextrose in water)	50	—	—	—	—	—	170
D10W (10% dextrose in water)	100	—	—	—	—	—	340
D20W (20% dextrose in water)	200	—	—	—	—	—	680
D50W (50% dextrose in water)	500	—	—	—	—	—	1700
½ NS (0.45% NaCl)	—	77	77	—	—	—	—
NS (0.9% NaCl)	—	154	154	—	—	—	—
3% NS (0.25% NaCl)	—	513	513	—	—	—	—
D5¼ NS	50	38	38	—	—	—	170
D5½ NS (0.45% NaCl)	50	77	77	—	—	—	170
D5% NS (0.9% NaCl)	50	154	154	—	—	—	170
D5LR (5% dextrose in lactated Ringer's)	50	130	110	4	3	27	180
Lactated Ringer's	—	130	110	4	3	27	<10

NS, normal saline.
Modified and reproduced with permission from Gomella LG, ed. *Clinician's Pocket Reference.* 10th ed.: McGraw-Hill; 2004.

TABLE IV–2. COMPOSITION AND DAILY PRODUCTION OF BODY FLUIDS.

Fluid	Electrolytes (mEq/L)				Average Daily Production (mL)
	Na	**Cl**	**K**	**HCO₃**	
Sweat	50	40	5	0	Varies
Saliva	60	15	26	50	1500
Gastric juices	60–100	100	10	0	1500–2500
Duodenum	130	90	5	0–10	300–2000
Bile	145	100	5	15	100–300
Pancreatic juice	140	75	5	115	100–800
Ileum	140	100	2–8	30	100–9000
Diarrhea	120	90	25	45	—

Modified and reproduced with permission from Gomella LG, ed. *Clinician's Pocket Reference. 10th ed.:* McGraw-Hill; 2004.

V. Blood Component Therapy

Whole blood contains red blood cells (RBCs), white blood cells (WBCs), plasma, antibodies, electrolytes, and an anticoagulate. Most patients who require replacement therapy require only one of these components. Transfusion with whole blood is rarely performed. It is used for volume expansion in a patient with an acute massive blood loss.

■ RED BLOOD CELL TRANSFUSIONS

The blood supply in the United States has never been safer; however, transfusion with blood should be carefully considered and avoided whenever possible. Transfusion packed red blood cells (PRBCs) are indicated when:

1. Symptoms from acute blood loss have failed to respond to crystalloid infusions.
2. Symptoms from a chronic anemia have not improved with other therapeutic interventions.

Clinicians should not establish empiric, automatic transfusion thresholds. A young, healthy person may tolerate a hemoglobin (Hgb) as low as 7.5 g, whereas an older patient with limited cardiorespiratory reserve may benefit from transfusion despite a Hgb of 10 g.

■ ANEMIA

See also Section I, Chapter 5, Anemia, p 28.

When confronted with a chronic anemia, the clinician must consider whether the Hgb and hematocrit (HCT) accurately reflect the RBC mass. The RBC mass is more important with respect to oxygen transport than the measured HCT or Hgb; however, low Hgb or HCT usually reflects a low RBC mass. An increased plasma volume may result in a dilutional change in Hgb and make an anemia appear more severe. Increased plasma volume may occur in congestive heart failure, pregnancy, and paraproteinemia.

Acute blood loss: In the setting of acute blood loss and hypotension, restoration of blood volume and tissue perfusion as well as improvement of oxygen-carrying capacity must be accomplished. Use electrolyte solutions or colloids initially. Blood losses of 500–1000 mL in an adult do not usually require blood transfusion unless there is an underlying anemia or another medical condition requiring added oxygen-carrying capacity.

RBC Products—availability and indications

1. **Whole blood.** There are few indications for transfusion of whole blood today, except for transfusion of the massively bleeding patient when volume and oxygen-carrying capacity can be supplied in one

product. Stored whole blood is not adequate replacement for platelets or labile coagulation factors.

2. **Packed RBCs.** Basically, PRBCs constitute a unit of whole blood with two-thirds of the plasma removed. This has become the standard RBC product for most transfusions. A number of modified PRBC components are available. These include the following:

3. **Leukocyte-poor RBCs.** In this product, 70–90% of the leukocytes have been removed by a variety of techniques (washing, centrifugation, or filtration). Leukocyte-poor RBCs are used in patients with a history of repeated febrile reactions to standard PRBC transfusions. These reactions are usually due to leukocyte antigens. Leukocyte-poor RBCs are indicated for patients expected to require extensive blood product support to decrease allo-sensitization (the formation of allo-antibodies directed against antigens expressed on other blood components, most often platelets).

4. **Washed RBCs.** Virtually all plasma and nonerythrocyte cellular elements are removed. Washed cells are indicated for patients with febrile reactions to leukocyte-poor RBCs, for patients with allergic reactions to plasma components (IgA deficiency), and for patients with paroxysmal nocturnal hemoglobinuria when exposure to complement may exacerbate the hemolytic process.

5. **Frozen stored RBCs.** Blood may be frozen to extend its shelf life. Glycerol is added before freezing to prevent dehydration and damage of the cells. When the unit is used, it is thawed and the glyerol is removed.

6. **Cytomegalovirus (CMV)-negative products.** Patients undergoing organ and bone marrow transplantation require aggressive immunosuppressive therapy to ensure engraftment and avoid graft rejection. If these patients or candidates for organ or bone marrow transplantation are CMV-negative before their transplantation, CMV-negative blood products will minimize the risk of CMV infection complicating their transplantation course.

Complications: See Section I, Chapter 62, Transfusion Reaction, p 361.

■ PLATELET TRANSFUSIONS

See also Section I, Chapter 61, Thrombocytopenia, p 355.

Indications: Platelet transfusions are indicated for any patient with a major bleeding event involving a qualitative or quantitative platelet disorder. Prophylactic platelet transfusions are most commonly indicated in settings of decreased platelet production, such as aplastic anemia, acute leukemia, or chemotherapy- or radiation-induced bone marrow suppression. In these settings, many institutions empirically give transfusions to patients with platelet counts < 10,000. Individuals with fever, mucosal ulcerations, and planned invasive procedures are frequently supported with platelets to maintain counts > 20,000. Individuals with thrombocytopenia on the basis of platelet destruction (either via antibodies or consumption) rarely benefit from prophylactic transfusion. In general, transfusion with ongoing platelet destruction is indicated only when bleeding of a microvascular nature is greater than that expected. The efficacy of platelet transfusion in the setting of platelet dysfunction is not well documented. Desmopressin (DDAVP) should be considered in this circumstance. Patients with lifelong quantitative or qualitative platelet disorders should not receive transfusion prophylactically solely on the basis of platelet count, bleeding time, or other platelet function studies. Overutilization of platelets increases the risk of alloimmunization and subsequent inadequate response to platelet transfusions. Likewise, patients with idiopathic thrombocytopenic purpura should not be prophylactically transfused.

Two types of platelet products are available, both may be infused via leukofiltration filters to remove most of the WBCs.

1. **Random donor platelets** are pooled concentrates from whole blood donations from several donors.
2. **Pheresis or single-donor platelets** are prepared by apheresis of a single donor. The donor selected may be HLA-matched to the intended recepient.

Complications

1. **Transmission of infectious agents.** The institution of polymerase chain reaction (PCR) screening has dramatically decreased the risk of transmission of a viral infection with transfusion. However, transfusion of bacterially contaminated platelets continues to be a rare but potentially lethal risk. Platelets are stored at 20 ° to 24 °C, and bacterial contamination is estimated to occur in 1 in 2000 units. Coagulase-negative *Staphylococcus* is the most frequently cultured bacteria.
2. **Reactions to plasma components, RBCs, and WBCs.** Reactions to RBC antigens rarely cause a hemolytic transfusion reaction. They can cause alloimmunity and a potential for problems such as the use of Rh-positive platelets in an Rh-negative female. The patient should receive intravenous anti-D globulin (RhoGAM) if she is of childbearing age.
3. **Possible transmission of bacterial infections.** A potential problem because of the storage time and storage temperature of platelet concentrates.
4. **Alloimmunization.** This problem eventually develops in two-thirds of patients receiving multiple transfusions of platelets. It may necessitate the use of HLA-matched platelets to achieve adequate post-transfusion counts.

■ PLASMA COMPONENT THERAPY

The following is a list of commonly available plasma products and selected remarks about indications and complications.

1. **Fresh-frozen plasma (FFP)** is prepared by removing the plasma from a whole unit of blood and freezing it. FFP is a source of all clotting factors, including factors V, VIII, and fibrinogen. However, titers of factors VIII and V decline with long-term storage. FFP is primarily indicated for patients with disseminated intravascular coagulation (DIC), liver disease, and the need for warfarin reversal. It is also used in therapeutic plasma exhange. FFP is not the optimal product for replacement in patients with congential single factor deficiencies (II, V, VII, X, or XI, or deficiencies of protein C or S).

2. **Cryoprecipitate** is the protein precipitate left after FFP is thawed at 4°C and most of the supernatant liquid plasma is removed. It is most commonly used to replace fibrinogen (either for acquired deficiencies due to DIC or thrombolytic therapy or for congential hypofibrinogenemia or dysfibrinogenemla). Cryoprecipitate may also be used to treat deficiencies of factor XIII. Although it contains factor VIII and von Willebrand factor, it is not the optimal replacement product for these deficiencies. Recombinant or virally inactivated factor VIII concentrates are preferred.

3. **Plasma-derived factor concentrates** are prepared by fractionation of large pools of thousands of units of donor plasma. The products are then processed to inactivate viruses using pasteurization, solvent, or detergent treatment of immunoaffinity column treatment. Despite these measures, these concentrates may still transmit hepatitis A and parvovirus 19.

    Products include intermediate purity factor VIII, immunoaffinity high purity factor VIII concentrate, porcine factor VIII, immunoaffinity high purity factor IX concentrate, prothrombin complex concentrate, and activated prothrombin complex concentrates. Factor concentrates produced by recombinant technology have the highest purity and level of safety.

4. **Albumin** is used for volume expansion when crystalloid solutions are not adequate. It comes in two concentrates: 5% and 25%.

5. **Intravenous immunoglobulin (IVIG)** is made from large pools of donor plasma. It is a polyclonal preparation that is used to provide passive immune protection (in primary immunodeficiency disorders or for chronic lymphocytic leukemia). It is also used in a variety of diseases for its immunomodulatory effect. Specific immune serum globulins are available, for example, hepatitis B immune globulin (HBIG), Rh immune globulin (RhIG), and varicella-zoster immune globulin (VZIG).

6. **Gamma globulin.** There are many different forms of intravenous and intramuscular gamma globulins available with a wide variety of indications and reactions. The following are adverse effects that might result from the administration of gamma globulin.

    a. **Anaphylactoid reaction.** An immediate reaction attributed to complement activation. Symptoms and signs may include flushing, chest tightness, dyspnea, fever, chills, nausea, vomiting, hypotension, and back pain. These are uncommon reactions with the currently available preparations but can occur with both intravenous and intramuscular administration. Therapy consists of discontinuation of the infusion and use of diphenhydramine (Benadryl), steroids, epinephrine, and vasopressors if necessary.

b. Inflammatory reaction. This is characteristically a delayed reaction. Signs and symptoms may include headache, malaise, fever, chills, and nausea. The reaction disappears with discontinuation of gamma globulin therapy.

REFERENCES

Ceccherini-Nelli L, Filipponi F, Mosca F, Campa M: The risk of contracting an infectious disease from blood. Transplant Proc 2004;36:680.

Fritsma MG: Use of blood products and factor concentrates for coagulation therapy. Clin Lab Sci 2003;16:115.

Goodnough LT, Brecher ME, Kanter MH et al: Transfusion medicine—blood transfusion. N Engl J Med 1999;340:438.

Miller R: Blood component therapy. Orthop Nurs 2001;20:57.

Wright-Kanuth MS, Smith LA: Developments in component therapy: Novel components and new uses for familiar preparations. Clin Lab Sci 2002;15:116.

VI. Ventilator Management

1. INDICATIONS & SETUP

I. Indications

A. Ventilatory failure. A $paCO_2$ > 50 Torr indicates ventilatory failure; however, many patients have chronic ventilatory failure with renal compensation (retaining HCO_3^-). The absolute pH is often a better guide than $paCO_2$ for determining the need for ventilatory assistance. The patient's mental status is actually the best indicator for this. Some chronically ill but compensated patients may have a normal mental status despite a $paCO_2$ of 70! A significant acidemia suggests an acute respiratory acidosis or acute decompensation of a chronic respiratory acidosis. A respiratory acidosis with a rapidly falling pH or an absolute pH < 7.24 is an indication for ventilatory support.

The prototype of pure ventilatory failure is the drug overdose patient who has a sudden loss of central respiratory drive with uncontrolled hypercarbia. Patients with sepsis, neuromuscular disease, and chronic obstructive pulmonary disease (COPD) may have hypercarbic ventilatory failure.

B. Hypoxemic respiratory failure. Inability to oxygenate is an important indication for ventilatory support. A paO_2 < 60 Torr on > 50% inspired fraction of oxygen (FiO_2) constitutes hypoxemic respiratory failure. Newer nomenclature uses the paO_2/FiO_2 (P/F) ratio to characterize hypoxemia. A P/F ratio < 200 is consistent with acute respiratory distress syndrome (ARDS), whereas a ratio between 200 and 300 is termed acute lung injury. Although these patients can sometimes be managed with higher FiO_2 delivery systems, such as partial or nonrebreather masks, or continuous positive airway pressure (CPAP) delivered by mask, they are at high risk for cardiopulmonary arrest. They should be closely monitored in an intensive care unit (ICU) if they are not intubated. Worsening of the respiratory status necessitates prompt intubation and ventilatory support.

The prototype disease for hypoxemic respiratory failure is ARDS, in which the high shunt fraction leads to refractory hypoxemia.

C. Mixed respiratory failure. Most patients have failure of both ventilation and oxygenation. The indications for ventilatory support remain the same as listed earlier.

An example of mixed respiratory failure is the COPD patient with an acute exacerbation. Bronchospasm alters the ventilation-perfusion ratio ($\dot{V}/\dot{Q}$) relationships, leading to worsening hypoxemia. Bronchospasm and accumulated secretions lead to a high work of breathing and consequent hypercarbia.

D. **Neuromuscular disease with respiratory failure.** This is actually a subcategory of ventilatory failure but deserves separate mention because of differing management. Hypercarbia occurs just before arrest; thus, criteria other than arterial blood gases (ABGs) are needed. Patients with myasthenia gravis, Guillain-Barré syndrome, and muscular dystrophy are at risk of respiratory failure.

   1. Respiratory rates > 24/min are an early sign of respiratory failure. A progressive rise in the respiratory rate, or sustained respiratory rates > 35/min, are indications for ventilatory support.

   2. Abdominal paradox indicates dyssynergy of chest wall muscles and diaphragms and impending respiratory failure. It is manifested by inward movement of the abdominal wall during inspiration rather than the normal outward motion.

   3. A vital capacity < 15 mL/kg or 1 liter in the normal-sized adult is associated with acute respiratory arrest as well as an inability to clear secretions. Similarly, a negative inspiratory force < –25 cm H_2O implies impending respiratory arrest.

   Guillain-Barré syndrome is the prototypic neuromuscular disease in which the preceding criteria require strict attention. A patient with Guillain-Barré syndrome should be closely observed and followed up with frequent vital capacity (VC) measurements. A rapidly falling VC, or VC < 1000 mL, requires respirator support.

II. Partial Ventilatory Assistance

A. **CPAP (continuous positive airway pressure)** may be administered by full face mask or nasal mask. Pressures of 5–15 cm H_2O may be used to recruit alveoli and improve oxygenation for refractory hypoxemia. CPAP has proven efficacy in respiratory failure due to pulmonary edema as well as in acute exacerbations of COPD. (CPAP is thought to decrease the work of breathing by splinting airways open, thus counteracting intrinsic positive end-expiratory pressure [PEEP].)

B. **BiPAP (bidirectional positive airway pressure)** may provide significant ventilatory assistance for patients with chronic neuromuscular diseases, COPD, or pneumonia, or for patients in whom intubation is not an option. Initial settings would be IPAP (inspiratory pressure) 12 cm; EPAP (expiratory pressure) 4 cm; Patient Assist Mode and backup rate, 12 breaths per minute. IPAP can then be titrated upward to increase the effective tidal volume. An experienced respiratory therapist is vital to the success of BiPAP. Starting at very low pressures and providing proper mask fit and a lot of reassurance are mandatory for success. Conventional ventilators can also be used to provide noninvasive ventilation via a face mask interface.

C. **CPAP or BiPAP** requires intensive respiratory therapy support for titration of O_2 and pressure as well as adjustments of the mask, since leaks are common. Necrosis of the bridge of the nose may occur.

    D. **Contraindications.** Rapidly progressive respiratory failure, coma (inability to protect the airway), vomiting, pneumothorax, and gastric distention are important contraindications. Partial ventilatory support should be initiated ideally in an ICU or stepdown unit.

III. Tracheal Intubation.
See Section III, Chapter 7, Endotracheal Intubation, p 434. Endotracheal intubation is actually the most difficult and complication-ridden part of ventilator initiation. Skill and experience are required for correct placement. Aspiration, esophageal intubation, and right mainstem bronchus intubation are common complications. Bilateral breath sounds always need to be confirmed by chest auscultation in each axilla. An immediate postintubation portable chest x-ray should be obtained. An inline CO_2 sensor can be used for rapid confirmation of tracheal intubation. Intubation can be accomplished by three routes:

    A. **Nasotracheal intubation.** This can be accomplished blindly and in an awake patient. Intubation requires experience and adequate local anesthesia. Complications include intubation of the esophagus, nosebleeds, kinking of the endotracheal tube (ETT), and postobstructive sinusitis. A smaller ETT is usually required for nasotracheal versus orotracheal intubation; this leads to a higher work of breathing because of increased resistance, difficulties with adequate suctioning, and higher ventilation pressures. Nasotracheal ETTs are more comfortable than orotracheal ETTs; they are less damaging to the larynx because they are better stabilized in the airway. This type of intubation should be avoided in the presence of facial trauma or in the anticoagulated patient.

    B. **Orotracheal intubation.** Placement of orotracheal tubes requires normal neck mobility to allow hyperextension of the neck for direct visualization of the vocal cords. Larger ETTs can be placed via this route. Adequate local anesthesia or sedation is necessary for safe placement without aspiration.

    C. **Tracheostomy.** Tracheostomy is recommended for patients who require more than 14–21 days of ventilatory support. It can be done percutaneously or surgically. Tracheostomy tubes facilitate the weaning process by decreasing tube resistance, since the tube is shorter and has a wider radius. Patients can eat with a tracheostomy and find the tubes more comfortable than those used for tracheal intubation.

IV. Ventilator Setup

    A. **The ventilator.** Contemporary ventilators are volume-cycled, pressure-targeted, or time-cycled. Elaborate alarm systems are present to alert personnel to inadequate minute ventilation or tidal volume, high peak pressure, disconnection of the ETT, and so forth.

        Effective ventilation is measured by changes in $paCO_2$. Minute ventilation ($\dot{V}_e$) can be calculated by tidal volume × breath rate. Thus, ventilation may be adjusted by changing the breath rate, tidal volume, or both. Tidal volumes > 10 mL/kg may cause overdistention of alveoli and increase the risk of pneumothorax. Recent ARDS research suggests that a tidal volume of 5–6 mL/kg ideal body weight (IBW) is optimal. (It is thought that excessive stretch may lead to increased inflammatory response and alveolar leak.) Most initial tidal volumes are therefore set at 5–8 mL/kg IBW.

Oxygenation is adjusted by changing FiO_2. Prolonged FiO_2 > 60% may cause pulmonary fibrosis. Thus, down-adjustment to "safe levels" sufficient to maintain O_2 saturation > 90% should be attempted as indicated by ABGs. If an O_2 saturation > 90% cannot be maintained when decreasing the FiO_2 < 60%, other means to increase oxygenation such as PEEP should be used.

The mode of ventilation should be specified:

1. **Assist control (AC) mode** allows the patient to trigger machine breaths once a threshold of inspiratory flow or effort is made. Each breath is a full machine breath. AC mode also supplies a backup rate in cases of apnea or paralysis. It is typically used in pulmonary edema states (both cardiogenic and noncardiogenic) as well as after cardiopulmonary resuscitation.

2. **Intermittent mandatory ventilation (IMV)** provides a set number of machine breaths per minute and allows the patient to make spontaneous breaths as well. Synchronized intermittent mandatory ventilation (SIMV) allows synchronization of the IMV breaths with patient efforts. As the rate is turned down, the patient assumes more and more of the work of breathing. Typically, SIMV is used in patients with obstructive airways disease (COPD or asthma).

3. **CPAP** allows completely spontaneous respirations while the patient is still connected to the ventilator. A set amount of continuous pressure may be applied as well (0–30 cm H_2O). It is almost always used in conjunction with pressure support.

4. **Pressure support.** Pressure support is an inspiratory boost given to augment spontaneous respiratory efforts. Thus, in CPAP mode or in SIMV, pressure support can be used to overcome the work of breathing imposed by the ventilatory system (endotracheal tube, tubing, demand valves) when a patient takes a spontaneous breath. Typically, an 8- to 10-cm pressure boost is used. Pressure support can also be used at higher levels during ventilator weaning (see Section VI, Chapter 4, Weaning, p 486).

5. **Pressure control.** Recent-model ventilators may be set to operate in a pressure-limited mode rather than volume-targeted. A set pressure boost is maintained for a measured time period in this mode. The primary goal is an improvement in oxygenation—often at the expense of ventilation (clearance of CO_2). Patients treated with PC (pressure control) or with APRV (airway pressure release ventilation) may have a respiratory acidosis. Another goal is the

limitation of peak airway pressures below 40 cm H_2O and thus minimization of barotrauma or overstretching of the lung. Pressure control is primarily used in ARDS. Often inverse ratio ventilation (increasing inspiratory time) is done simultaneously. Because this simulates a breath-holding maneuver, it feels unnatural to patients, and they usually require deep sedation and/or paralysis in this mode. Caution: Pressure control should be used only under supervision of ICU-trained faculty or fellows.

6. **Airway pressure release ventilation (APRV)** is very similar to pressure control. However, the patient is able to breathe throughout the machine cycles. Thus, deep sedation and paralysis can be avoided. Typical settings might be:
   - P—high 30
   - T (time)—high 3 seconds
   - P—low 8
   - T—low 0.5 seconds

   APRV is used primarily in patients with ARDS.

7. **Initial ventilator settings** should be dictated by the underlying condition as well as by previous blood gas results. An example of the initial settings for a 70-kg patient after respiratory arrest would be:
   - FiO_2 1.0 (100%)
   - Assist control mode
   - Rate 18
   - Tidal volume 560 mL

   An attempt should be made to supply the patient with at least as much minute ventilation as was required before intubation. Thus, a patient with pulmonary edema, ARDS, or neuromuscular disease may require a minute ventilation of 14–22 L/min. The AC mode is generally more comfortable and alleviates the work of breathing to a large extent. Sample settings might be:
   - FiO_2 1.0
   - Assist control mode
   - Rate 22
   - Tidal volume 550 mL

   The patient with COPD, on the other hand, should not be overventilated initially. Such patients may have a chronically high bicarbonate because of renal compensation, and overventilation may cause a severe alkalosis. (A pH > 7.55 is felt to be severely arrhythmogenic as well as moving the oxyhemoglobin curve to the right, which impedes oxygen release to the tissues.) Sample settings might be:
   - FiO_2 0.5 (50%)
   - SIMV mode
   - Pressure support 10 cm
   - Rate 12
   - Tidal volume 600 mL

B. Additional setup requirements
1. **Restrain the patient's hands,** because one's natural reaction to the ETT on awakening is to pull it out.
2. **Place a nasogastric tube** to decompress the stomach or to continue essential oral medications.
3. **Obtain a stat portable chest x-ray** to confirm ETT placement and to reassess any underlying pulmonary disease. The tip of the ETT should be 3–4 cm above the carina.
4. **Treat any underlying pulmonary disease** (maximize bronchodilators in status asthmaticus or vasodilators and diuretics in pulmonary edema).
5. **Consider prophylactic measures.** Heparin 5000 U SC Q 12 hr may reduce the incidence of pulmonary embolism while the patient is on bed rest. Stress ulceration bleeding can be prevented by the use of any of the following: proton pump inhibitors such as omeprazole, antacids, H_2 antagonists (cimetidine, ranitidine), sucralfate (Carafate), or tube feedings (enteral nutrition).
6. **Order other medications as needed,** such as morphine for pain and lorazepam (Ativan) for agitation. Often ventilator patients require continuous sedation with agents such as a versed (midazolam) drip or a propofol drip. Caution: All these agents cause hypotension in higher doses!

2. ROUTINE MODIFICATION OF SETTINGS

Arterial blood gases (ABGs) should be monitored and adjusted to a normal pH (7.37–7.44) and a paO_2 > 60 Torr on less than 60% O_2. Tachypnea should be investigated for adequacy of ventilation or for any other cause (eg, fever) before sedating the patient.

I. Adjusting paO_2

A. To decrease: Inspired fraction of oxygen (FiO_2) should be decreased in increments of 10–20% every 30 minutes. The "rule of sevens" states that there will be a 7-Torr fall in PaO_2 for each 1% decrease in FiO_2.

B. To increase
1. **Ventilation** has some effect on paO_2 (as shown by the alveolar air equation); therefore, correction of the respiratory acidosis will improve oxygenation.
2. **Positive end-expiratory pressure (PEEP)** can be added in increments of 2–4 cm H_2O. PEEP recruits previously collapsed alveoli, holds them open, and restores functional residual capacity (to a better physiologic level). It counteracts pulmonary shunts and raises paO_2. PEEP increases intrathoracic pressure and may thus impede venous return and decrease cardiac output. This is particularly true in the presence of volume depletion and shock. Consult

your ICU staff or fellow if high PEEP is needed or if the blood pressure drops with PEEP adjustment.

II. Adjusting $paCO_2$

A. To decrease
1. Increase the rate or tidal volume.
2. Check for leaks in the system.
3. Decrease CO_2 production by treating fever, minimizing shivering, and controlling agitation.

B. To increase
1. Decrease the rate.
2. You may have to switch from AC mode to SIMV mode to eliminate patient-driven central hyperventilation. Remember, every breath is a full machine breath in Assist Control mode!

3. TROUBLESHOOTING

3A. AGITATION

I. **Problem.** The ventilator patient becomes agitated, struggles constantly, tries to pull out all tubes, and actively fights the respirator.

II. **Immediate Questions**

A. **Is the patient still properly connected?** Hypoxemia or hypercarbia resulting from disconnection of the respirator may result in agitation. A patient who can speak is no longer intubated!

B. **Review the ventilator flow and pressure waveforms.** Look for auto-PEEP. Failure of the expiratory flow to flatten at zero indicates airtrapping or auto-PEEP. This may cause increased work of breathing and agitation (an experienced respiratory therapist will be able to measure it for you and then apply external positive end-expiratory pressure [PEEP] to counterbalance it). A double dip on the inspiratory flow curve usually indicates the patient has air hunger and wants a higher peak flow.

C. **What were the most recent arterial blood gas (ABG) values?** Again, hypoxemia or hypercarbia can cause agitation. Adjusting the settings can correct either problem.

D. **What does the chest x-ray show?** Atelectasis from mucous plugging or pneumothorax can occur spontaneously in asthma or as a result of barotrauma and can result in hypoxemia or hypercarbia. The endotracheal tube (ETT) touching the carina or the larynx almost always causes coughing and/or agitation.

E. **What is the underlying diagnosis? What are the current medications and IV fluids?** Agitation may be related to the underlying diagnosis or to a medication and may be unrelated to the patient's respiratory status. Cimetidine (Tagamet) and narcotics can cause confusion, especially in the elderly. Multiple metabolic disturbances (eg, hyponatremia and hypernatremia) can lead to confusion and possibly agitation. See Section I, Chapter 13, Coma, Acute Mental Status Changes, p 76.

F. What are the ventilator settings? The ventilator setting may have been set incorrectly, resulting in hypoxemia or hypercarbia. A high sensitivity setting may make it impossible for the fatigued patient to trigger a breath. Barotrauma resulting in pneumothorax is associated with high PEEP settings, high tidal volumes, and peak inspiratory pressures > 45 cm.

III. Differential Diagnosis

A. Causes of respiratory decompensation
1. **Worsening of underlying pulmonary disease**
2. **Pneumothorax**
3. **ETT displacement.** The tube may be outside the trachea, high in the glottis, or down the right mainstem bronchus.
4. **Mucous plugs.** May result in atelectasis and hypoxemia.
5. **Ventilator malfunction**
6. **Pulmonary embolism (PE).** Immobilization is a major risk for PE.
7. **Aspiration**
8. **Inadequate oxygenation or respiratory muscle fatigue**

B. Sepsis

C. ICU psychosis

D. Medications. Multiple medications such as digoxin (Lanoxin), lidocaine, theophylline, imipenem-cilastatin (Primaxin), diazepam (Valium) and other benzodiazepines, meperidine and other narcotics, and cimetidine may cause a toxic delirium, especially in high doses or with decreased clearance states.

E. Electrolyte imbalance. Hyponatremia, hypernatremia, hypercalcemia, hypocalcemia, and hypophosphatemia can cause confusion, which can lead to agitation.

IV. Database

A. Physical examination key points
1. **ETT.** Carefully check the patency, position, and function of the ETT.
2. **Vital signs.** Tachypnea may suggest hypoxemia. Tachycardia and hypertension can result from agitation or may be associated with respiratory failure or an underlying problem such as myocardial infarction (MI). Hypotension may be due to auto-PEEP, volume depletion, sepsis, cardiogenic shock, tension pneumothorax, or massive PE. An elevated temperature suggests sepsis, ventilator-associated nosocomial pneumonia, or pulmonary emboli. Tachycardia, tachypnea, and fever may be associated with PE or

MI. A pulsus paradoxus > 16 mm Hg implies severe respiratory distress or pericardial tamponade.

3. **HEENT.** Check for distended neck veins suggesting pericardial tamponade or congestive heart failure (CHF). Tracheal deviation may be caused by a tension pneumothorax.

4. **Chest.** Auscultate for bilateral breath sounds. Absent breath sounds on one side suggest pneumothorax or an improperly placed ETT. Bilaterally absent breath sounds can be secondary to either bilateral pneumothoraces or severe respiratory failure.

5. **Extremities.** Check for cyanosis.

6. **Skin.** Palpate for subcutaneous emphysema, which can result from a very high PEEP or may be seen in patients with asthma. Subcutaneous emphysema may portend more serious barotrauma such as a life-threatening tension pneumothorax.

B. Laboratory data

1. **ABGs.** To rule out hypoxemia and hypercarbia as well as severe acidosis or alkalosis.

2. **Electrolyte panel.** Including calcium and phosphorus.

C. Radiologic and other studies.
A chest x-ray to rule out atelectasis and pneumothorax and to evaluate underlying pulmonary pathology.

V. Plan

A. Emergency management

1. **Examine the patient** as outlined earlier. Carefully check the ETT function, ventilator connections, and chart.

2. **Suction the patient vigorously.** This confirms tube patency and clears out any mucous plugs.

3. **Bag the patient manually** to check for ease of ventilation. Marked difficulty can be seen with tension pneumothorax or mucous plugging. If auto-PEEP is suspected, use a slower rate and decrease the tidal volume. This allows trapped gas time to escape and thus allows decreased intrathoracic pressure and increased venous return to the heart.

4. **Obtain ABGs, electrolyte panel, and stat chest x-ray.**

5. **If the patient appears cyanotic** or "air hungry," turn the inspired fraction of oxygen (FiO_2) to 1.0 and the ventilator mode to "Assist Control" (AC).

6. **If hypotension and unilaterally absent breath sounds** are found concomitantly, consider chest tube insertion for tension pneumothorax. Patients on ventilators can rapidly die of tension pneumothoraces.

7. **If you suspect ICU psychosis,** reassure the patient. Have a family member help reorient the patient. Often a familiar voice works wonders! Ask the nurses to move the patient to a room with a window; this environmental feature has been shown to reduce ICU psychosis.

8. **Check the ventilator settings.** Perhaps too much effort is required to open the valves or to initiate a breath. Ask the respiratory therapist to lower the triggering sensitivity to 0.5 or 1.0 cm H_2O. Experiment with adding a little more pressure support for patient comfort.

9. **If everything else is stable** and the patient is endangering him- or herself, sedate the patient. Haloperidol (Haldol) 0.5–2.0 mg IM or IV and lorazepam (Ativan) 0.5–2.0 mg IV are the currently recommended agents.

3B. HYPOXEMIA

I. **Problem.** The respirator patient requires > 60% FiO_2 to maintain a paO_2 > 60 Torr.

II. **Immediate Questions**

A. **What is the sequence of ABGs?** In other words, is this an acute or a slowly developing change? A rapid deterioration implies an immediate life-threatening process such as a tension pneumothorax or a massive PE.

B. **What is the underlying diagnosis?** A patient with long-bone fractures may develop fat embolus syndrome, a patient with sepsis may develop acute respiratory distress syndrome (ARDS), and a patient with head injury may develop neurogenic pulmonary edema.

C. **What are the ventilator settings? Has a change been made recently?** An error may have been made with the ventilator settings, or recent changes may have been made too aggressively in an attempt to wean the patient from the ventilator. Some patients are very sensitive to PEEP changes.

III. **Differential Diagnosis**

A. **Shunts secondary to alveolar filling or by obstructed bronchi with consequent collapse**
   1. **Pneumonia**
   2. **Pulmonary contusion**
   3. **Atelectasis.** The ETT may be placed too far in the right mainstem bronchus, or there may be mucous plugs.
   4. **ARDS or cardiogenic pulmonary edema**

B. **Cardiac level shunt.** An acute ventricular septal defect, especially in the setting of an acute myocardial MI, may develop. Sudden pulmonary hypertension may occasionally lead to a patent foramen ovale and physiologic shunt at the atrial level. A tip-off to this is a worsening shunt and paO_2 as positive end-expiratory pressure (PEEP) is increased.

C. **Shunts secondary to pneumothorax**

D. **Ventilation/perfusion ($\dot{V}/\dot{Q}$) mismatch**

  1. **Bronchospasm**
  2. **Pulmonary embolism**
  3. **Aspiration.** Still possible, even when an ETT is in place.
  E. **Inadequate ventilation**
  1. **Ventilator disconnection or malfunction**
  2. **Incorrect settings.** Has the patient recently been changed to intermittent mandatory ventilation, which has resulted in hypoventilation?
  3. **Sedatives.** These can result in hypoxemia secondary to hypoventilation. Sedatives should be used cautiously, especially during weaning. Patients on ventilators may develop atelectasis due to failure to sigh or cough when sedated.
  4. **Neuromuscular disease.** Hypophosphatemia or aminoglycosides can cause neuromuscular weakness, which can cause hypoxemia secondary to hypoventilation and lack of sighing.

IV. **Database**
  A. **Physical examination key points**
  1. **ETT.** Confirm proper ETT position and listen for any leaks.
  2. **Vital signs.** Tachypnea implies worsening of the respiratory status. Tachycardia can be associated with a variety of conditions including PE, sepsis, MI, and worsening of underlying pulmonary pathology. Fever can be seen with PE, MI, or an infection.
  3. **Neck.** Stridor suggests upper airway obstruction.
  4. **Chest.** Check for bilateral breath sounds, signs of consolidation, or new onset of wheezing. Unilateral breath sounds suggest a pneumothorax or possibly displacement of the ETT in one of the mainstem bronchi. Palpate the chest for new subcutaneous emphysema, which can occur in asthmatics or as a result of high PEEP.
  5. **Heart.** New murmurs or a new S_3 or S_4 may be seen with an MI. A new systolic murmur may suggest a ventricular septal defect (VSD) or mitral regurgitation secondary to papillary muscle rupture.
  6. **Extremities.** Check the patient's nailbeds for cyanosis from worsening pulmonary status. Also, check legs for unilateral edema or other signs of phlebitis that point to PE.
  7. **Skin.** Check for new rashes, which may suggest a drug or anaphylactic reaction.
  B. **Laboratory data**
  1. **Repeat ABGs or check oximetry** to assess accuracy of initial ABGs and progression of deterioration.
  2. **Sputum appearance and Gram's stain** may direct antibiotic therapy if pneumonia is present.
  C. **Radiologic and other studies**
  1. **Stat chest x-ray.** To rule out atelectasis and pneumothorax, and to evaluate underlying pulmonary disease.

2. **Electrocardiogram.** An evolving MI may be evident. New right-axis deviation, right bundle branch block, P pulmonale, or an S wave in lead I, a Q wave in lead III, and a T wave in lead III ($S_1Q_3T_3$) suggest PE; however, these characteristic findings are often absent. Sinus tachycardia is the most common electrocardiographic finding with PE.

3. **V̇/Q̇ scan.** If clinical suspicion is high for PE. In some institutions, a fast-track CT chest scan may be done to look rapidly for central PE.

4. **Swan-Ganz catheter.** To measure pulmonary capillary wedge pressure (PCWP) and to exclude a cardiac shunt as well as to measure cardiac output and maximum O_2 consumption. A bedside echocardiogram may also provide similar information with the benefit of being noninvasive.

V. Plan

A. **Suction.** Vigorously suction the patient to prove patency of the ETT and dislodge mucous plugs.

B. **Treat underlying disorders**
   1. **Insert chest tube** for pneumothorax.
   2. **Reassess choice of antibiotic agents.** A pneumonia secondary to Legionella requires erythromycin (1 g IV Q 6 hr) or another macrolide.
   3. **Consider more vigorous chest physical therapy** or even bronchoscopy for recalcitrant mucous plugging or atelectasis.
   4. **Maximize bronchodilators** if bronchospasm is the problem. Corticosteroids such as hydrocortisone 125 mg or methylprednisolone 60 mg should be added and given IV Q 6 hr. Aerosolized albuterol should be given at least Q 4 hr.
   5. **Cardiogenic pulmonary edema** should be vigorously treated with afterload reduction and diuresis.

C. **Optimize ventilator settings**
   1. **Correct any hypoventilation.** This may mean giving up on weaning, and using the AC mode with the patient essentially controlled on a high minute ventilation.
   2. **Increase FiO_2 to 100%.** Your first priority is to prevent anoxic brain or cardiac damage. You may then reduce the FiO_2 as other maneuvers further improve the paO_2.
   3. **PEEP recruits unused, collapsed, or partially collapsed alveoli to overcome pulmonary shunts.** It should be added in 2–4 cm of H_2O increments while cardiac output and blood pressure are monitored.
   4. **Oxygen consumption ($\dot{V}O_2$)** can be markedly reduced by administering a neuromuscular blocking agent as a last resort. Remember to provide adequate analgesia and sedation as well. Nerve stimulation studies should be done routinely to monitor the neuro-

muscular blockade; otherwise, these agents should be used for < 24 hours.

D. Optimize hemodynamics

1. **Consider Swan-Ganz placement** when high levels of PEEP are in use, when shock of unclear cause is present, when a cardiac shunt is suspected, or when volume status is unclear.

2. **Correct any volume excess** because it will obviously worsen CHF and ARDS.

3. **Volume depletion** likewise alters both cardiac output and $\dot{V}/\dot{Q}$ ratios and may adversely affect oxygen delivery. A drop in blood pressure with the addition of PEEP almost always results from volume depletion.

4. **Correct anemia** to maximize O_2 delivery. Oxygen delivery to tissue depends on the hemoglobin as well as the cardiac output and SaO_2.

5. **Correct low cardiac output** to maximize O_2 delivery. Inotropic agents (eg, dobutamine) and agents for afterload reduction (eg, IV nitroglycerin or nitroprusside) can be used.

E. Prone positioning. If the primary lung disorder is ARDS or acute lung injury, consider prone positioning of the patient. Up to 70% of patients have a dramatic response. However, the nursing and respiratory therapy staff need experience in this technique since ETT dislodgement and unusual pressure sores may occur. Patients are left prone for 6–12 hours, flipped back supine for 1–2 hours, and then the cycle is repeated.

3C. HYPERCARBIA

I. Problem. The patient's $paCO_2$ remains > 40 Torr. $paCO_2$ is a direct reflection of both CO_2 production and alveolar ventilation. $PaCO_2$ increases when ventilation/perfusion ($\dot{V}/\dot{Q}$) mismatch worsens or dead space increases.

II. Immediate Questions

A. What is the sequence of ABGs? In other words, is this an acute or a slowly developing change? Rapid deterioration implies an immediate life-threatening process such as a tension pneumothorax or a massive pulmonary embolism.

B. What is the underlying diagnosis? Worsening of underlying pulmonary disease (pneumonia, atelectasis, or bronchospasm) can cause hypoventilation. CHF can cause $\dot{V}/\dot{Q}$ mismatch and CO_2 retention.

III. Differential Diagnosis

A. Inadequate minute ventilation ($\dot{V}_e$)

1. Too low a rate, inadequate tidal volume, or both

  2. **Patient tiring during synchronized intermittent mandatory ventilation or weaning**
  3. **ETT leak**
  4. **Worsening bronchospasm**
  5. **PE.** Keep in mind that immobilization is a major risk factor.

B. **Increased CO_2 production**
  1. **High-carbohydrate feedings**
  2. **Increased metabolism.** Causes include hyperthyroidism, fever, sepsis, and high work of breathing as well as rewarming after surgical procedures (a common but frequently overlooked cause of CO_2 production).

C. **Oversedation.** Decreases central ventilatory drive.

IV. Database

A. **Physical examination key points**
  1. **ETT.** Check ETT position and look for a leak.
  2. **Vital signs.** Tachycardia can be associated with fever, sepsis, worsening bronchospasm, PE, and hyperthyroidism. Tachypnea can be seen with PE, worsening bronchospasm, or sepsis. Fever suggests infection but can also be seen with hyperthyroidism and PE.
  3. **Chest.** Auscultate for new wheezes and look for inequality of breath sounds.
  4. **Heart.** Listen for a new loud P_2, which suggests a PE.
  5. **Extremities.** Check patient's legs for unilateral edema or other signs of thrombophlebitis.
  6. **Musculoskeletal exam.** Check for signs of respiratory fatigue such as abdominal paradox or accessory muscle use.

B. **Laboratory data**
  1. **ABGs.** Repeat ABGs or check oximetry to assess accuracy of initial ABGs and progression of deterioration.
  2. **Complete blood cell count with differential.** An increased white blood cell count with an increase in banded neutrophils suggests an infection or sepsis.

C. **Radiologic and other studies.** With a chest x-ray, proper ETT position can be ensured and new pulmonary infiltrates can be ruled out.

V. Plan

A. **Check position and functioning of ETT.** If there is a persistent leak, replace the tube.

B. **Verify proper ventilator function.** Check with particular care for leaky connections.

C. **Drugs.** Verify that the ordered sedatives are the drugs that were actually given and note time of last dose. If the patient is oversedated, you can either increase the minute ventilation ($\dot{V}_e$); or reverse sedation with naloxone (Narcan) 0.4 mg IV for narcotics or flumazenil (Romazicon) 1.0 mg IV over 5 minutes for benzodiazepines.

D. Look for a source of sepsis. Adjust antibiotics as indicated. Lower $\dot{V}O_2$ by treating fever with acetaminophen (Tylenol) or a cooling blanket.

E. Review ventilator settings. If the tidal volume is too low, dead space ventilation will be present. Correct this condition by increasing the tidal volume. If the patient is tiring on a low synchronized intermittent mandatory ventilation rate, switch to either a higher rate or change to AC mode.

F. Review the patient's nutrition regimen. If the patient is critically ill with bronchospasm or ARDS, you may be forced to reduce CO_2 production by decreasing the percentage of carbohydrates in tube feedings or IV hyperalimentation fluid.

3D. HIGH PEAK PRESSURES

I. Problem. The ventilator peak pressures remain consistently above 50 cm H_2O.

II. Immediate Questions

A. Is this a new problem or has it developed progressively? The answer to this question will be readily available on the respiratory therapy bedside flow sheet.

B. What is the underlying diagnosis? Severe status asthmaticus or ARDS can cause high ventilatory peak pressures.

C. What are the most recent ABGs? A decrease in the pO_2 or an increase in the pCO_2 may point to a worsening of the underlying pulmonary disease.

D. Has ETT function or position changed? Is it possible to suction the patient? The tube could be kinked or plugged by secretions.

III. Differential Diagnosis

A. ETT
1. **Too small or obstructed** by secretions.
2. **Kinked,** especially if placed nasotracheally.
3. **Migration** down the right mainstem so that the entire tidal volume flows into one lung. This condition also increases coughing and anxiety.

B. Incorrect ventilator settings
1. **High tidal volume.** Tidal volumes > 10 mL/kg may increase distention pressure tremendously.
2. **High PEEP.** PEEP should always be used at the lowest possible level.

3. **High minute ventilation.** A high minute ventilation may lead to the phenomenon of auto-PEEP, in which the patient has inadequate time to exhale, leading to "stacked breaths." Auto-PEEP may cause hypotension because of high intrathoracic pressure decreasing venous return.

C. **Worsening lung disease.** Lung compliance decreases in all of the following:
   1. **Severe status asthmaticus**
   2. **ARDS**
   3. **Cardiogenic pulmonary edema**
   4. **Interstitial lung disease**

D. **Uncooperative or agitated patient**
   1. **Biting the ETT**
   2. **Fighting the ventilator**
   3. **Coughing**

E. **Abdominal distention.** The recently described abdominal compartment syndrome can lead to both inability to ventilate and hypotension. It is diagnosed by measuring intravesicular (bladder) pressure and may result from severe ascites or intra-abdominal hemorrhage causing increased abdominal cavity pressure.

F. **Tension pneumothorax.** It is always imperative to exclude this as a cause of new onset of high peak pressures because death can occur quickly.

IV. Database

A. **Physical examination key points**
   1. **ETT.** Check position to rule out migration down the right mainstem bronchus; check patency of the ETT.
   2. **Vital signs.** Tachycardia and tachypnea can occur with worsening of the underlying pulmonary disease and with agitation. Hypotension and tachycardia are seen with tension pneumothorax, severe auto-PEEP, and the abdominal compartment syndrome.
   3. **HEENT.** An increase in jugular venous distention (JVD) implies CHF. Tracheal deviation can be seen with tension pneumothorax.
   4. **Chest.** Absent breath sounds, especially with hypotension, and unilateral hyperresonance to percussion point to tension pneumothorax. Rales suggest CHF.
   5. **Heart.** An S_3 over the apex implies left ventricular dysfunction/CHF.
   6. **Abdomen.** Examine for tenderness and distention.
   7. **Extremities.** New cyanosis is consistent with worsening of underlying pulmonary disease. Edema will be seen with biventricular or right-sided heart failure.
   8. **Skin.** Check for subcutaneous emphysema, which can be associated with barotrauma or with severe asthma.

B. Laboratory data
1. **ABGs.** Repeat ABGs or check oximetry to assess accuracy of initial ABGs and progression of deterioration.
2. **Complete blood count with differential.** An increased white blood count with an increase in banded neutrophils suggests an infection or sepsis.

C. Radiologic and other studies. Use a stat portable chest x-ray to check ETT position, rule out kinking, rule out pneumothorax, and assess any change in underlying pulmonary disease.

D. Ventilator. Ask the respiratory therapist to measure auto-PEEP or check for it via the waveforms. **View the peak airway pressure pattern.** A rapid rise and fall suggests a kinked or obstructed ETT. Check the patient's mouth to be sure the patient is not biting the tube. Suction the ETT to make sure it is not occluded and leading to artificially high pressures.

V. Plan

A. Try to suction the patient. If the patient is biting down, insert an oral airway or sedate the patient. If the patient is not biting down on the ETT but the suction tube will not go down the ETT, the ETT is kinked or blocked, possibly by a mucous plug, and must be replaced.

B. Ambu bag the patient and confirm equal breath sounds. Unequal breath sounds may result from a tension pneumothorax or from improper positioning of the ETT. Reposition the ETT if necessary. On an average-sized person, an oral ETT should not be in farther than 24 cm at the lip; however, there is considerable variability among patients, and the chest x-ray should always be reviewed. If there is considerable resistance to bagging, a tension pneumothorax, auto-PEEP, or a mucous plug may be present.

C. Place a chest tube if a pneumothorax is present.

D. Adjust the ventilator. Try to reduce the PEEP to the minimum needed for adequate oxygenation. Try reducing high tidal volumes to 5–6 mL/kg body weight. Increase FiO_2 as needed to ensure adequate oxygenation.

E. Sedation may have to be increased.

F. Consider switching to airway pressure release ventilation or pressure control modes. These modes exquisitely control high peak pressures while often improving oxygenation as well.

4. WEANING

I. Requirements. Once the underlying cause of respiratory failure has been corrected, it is time for the most arduous task of all: weaning the patient from the respirator.

A. Stabilization. The underlying disease is under optimum control.

B. Initiation of weaning. The process is begun in the early morning. Patients prefer to rest at night rather than work at breathing. Desirable conditions are:

1. **PaO_2 > 60 Torr on no positive end-expiratory pressure (PEEP); and $FiO_2 \leq 0.5$**
2. **Minute ventilation < 10 L/min**
3. **Negative inspiratory force more negative than – 20 cm H_2O**
4. **Vital capacity > 800 mL**
5. **Tidal volume > 300 mL**
6. **Rapid shallow breathing index < 90 (60-second breath rate/tidal volume in liters).** This is the most predictive indicator of success.

II. Weaning Techniques

A. T-piece (or T-tube bypass). The patient is taken off the respirator for a limited period of time, and the endotracheal tube (ETT) is connected to a constant flow of O_2 (usually 40%). If the patient tolerates breathing independently for 2 hours, he or she is extubated immediately. In research studies, this technique has been the most rapid.

This technique, however, has important drawbacks. No alarms are available because the patient is totally disconnected from the ventilator. The technique is time-consuming for the respiratory therapists and nurses. Perhaps most important, it is much more work for the patient than breathing spontaneously without an ETT. This is due to the relatively small diameter of the tube. (Remember that resistance increases by the fourth power of the radius of a tube.) T-tube trials are thus usually limited to 2-hour trials or less.

B. Synchronized intermittent mandatory ventilation (SIMV). In this method, fewer and fewer machine breaths are given as the patient begins taking spontaneous breaths in the intervals. For example, a patient breathing at a rate of 14 in AC mode is switched to SIMV mode, rate 14. The rate is then decreased to 10, to 6, to 4, and then to 0. Most physicians either place the patient on continuous positive airway pressure (CPAP) mode at this juncture or observe the patient briefly on a T piece.

This method has several theoretical advantages over T-piece weaning. Backup alarms, including automatic rates in case of apnea, are in place. A graded assumption of work is done, allowing respiratory muscle "retraining"; however, this method has never proved to be clearly superior to T-piece weaning. Moreover, there is still a high work of breathing because of the ETT resistance as well as the inherent resistance of the SIMV circuit valves.

One way to decrease the work of breathing with the SIMV weaning technique is to add pressure support (PS) to the system. Pressure support is a positive pressure boost that is initiated when a certain liter flow rate during inspiration is sensed by the respirator. It then supplies a set amount of positive pressure (and by Boyle's law, it also supplies some tidal volume). A PS level of 8–12 cm will overcome the increased work caused by the ETT resistance.

C. **CPAP and PS.** In this method, the patient is switched to the spontaneous breathing mode, which in some ventilators is the CPAP mode. In current usage, CPAP is equivalent to PEEP, except that it is used exclusively in spontaneously breathing mode. Anywhere from 0 to 30 cm pressure may be used, but generally the lowest level possible (usually 0–5 cm) is preferred. Pressure support may be used concomitantly to augment the patient's spontaneous breaths. It can then be progressively decreased as the patient increases tidal volumes. For example, PS levels of 25, then 20, then 15, and finally 10 can be used while monitoring the patient's breath rate, tidal volumes, and ABGs.

This method requires an alert, cooperative patient who is breathing spontaneously; if those conditions do not pertain, why wean anyway? Machine backup functions remain in place in case of apnea or other inadequate parameters.

D. **Extubation to BIPAP (bi-level positive airway pressure).** Patients with advanced lung disease may never reach standard weaning criteria. Extubation to partial ventilatory support is often successful. It decreases risk of ventilator-associated pneumonia and saves the patient from having a tracheostomy tube. This should also be considered in patients with poor left ventricular cardiac function. Rapidly going off positive pressure may induce pulmonary edema in these fragile patients.

III. **Timing.** Deciding when to extubate the patient is part of the art of medicine. Still, the fulfillment of certain criteria ensures success. The following weaning parameters (as discussed earlier) are acceptable:

A. Respiratory rate is < 30/min.

B. ABGs show a pH > 7.35 and adequate oxygenation on ≤ 5 FiO_2.

C. The patient is awake and alert.

D. A normal gag reflex is present.

E. The stomach is not distended.

IV. **Postextubation care.** After extubation, it is important to encourage the patient to cough frequently and forcefully. Respiratory therapy treatments should be continued. Incentive spirometry should be used several times an hour while the patient is awake to encourage deep breathing. The patient must be carefully observed for stridor, respiratory muscle fatigue, or other signs of failure. Oxygen should be given at the same level or at a level slightly higher than was given via the respirator before intubation. The ABGs should be checked 2–4 hours after extubation to confirm adequate ventilation and oxygenation.

REFERENCES

Albert RK: Prone ventilation (ARDS). Clin Chest Med 2000;21:511.

Glauser FL, Polatty C, Sessler CN: Worsening oxygenation in the mechanically ventilated patient: Causes, mechanisms and early detection. Am Rev Respir Dis 1988;138:458.

Luce JM et al: Intermittent mandatory ventilation. Chest 1981;79:678.

MacIntyre NR: Weaning from mechanical ventilatory support: Volume-assisting intermittent breaths versus pressure-assisting every breath. Respir Care 1988;33:121.

Marcy TW, Marini JJ: Respiratory distress in the ventilated patient. Clin Chest Med 1994;15:55.

Raoof S, Khan FA: Mechanical Ventilation Manual. American College of Physicians Press;1998.

Slutsky AS: ACCP consensus conference: Mechanical ventilation. Chest 1993;104:1833.

Tobin MJ: Mechanical ventilation. N Engl J Med 1994;330:1056.

VII. THERAPEUTICS

The Therapeutics Section is designed to serve as a quick reference to commonly used medications. You should be familiar with all of the indications, contraindications, side effects, and drug interactions of any medications that you prescribe. Such detailed information is beyond the scope of this manual and can be found in the package insert, Physicians' Desk Reference (PDR), or the *American Hospital Formulary Service (AHFS) Drug Information.*

MEDICATION KEY

Medications are listed by prescribing class, and the individual medications are then listed in alphabetical order by generic name. Some of the more commonly recognized trade names are listed for each medication (in parentheses after the generic name).

CONTROLLED SUBSTANCE CLASSIFICATION

Medications under the control of the US Drug Enforcement Agency (Schedule I–V controlled substances) are indicated by the symbol [C]. Most medications are "uncontrolled" and do not require a DEA prescriber number on the prescription. The following is a general description for the schedules of DEA controlled substances:

Schedule (CI) I: All nonresearch use forbidden (e.g., heroin, LSD, mescaline, etc.).

Schedule (CII) II: High addictive potential; medical use accepted. No telephone call-in prescriptions; no refills. Some states require special prescription form (e.g., cocaine, morphine, methadone).

Schedule (CIII) III: Low to moderate risk of physical dependence, high risk of psychologic dependence; prescription must be rewritten after 6 months or five refills (e.g., acetaminophen plus codeine).

Schedule (CIV) IV: Limited potential for dependence; prescription rules same as for schedule III (e.g., benzodiazepines, propoxyphene)

Schedule (CV) V: Very limited abuse potential; prescribing regulations often same as for uncontrolled medications; some states have additional restrictions.

FDA FETAL RISK CATEGORIES

Category A: Adequate studies in pregnant women have not demonstrated a risk to the fetus in the first trimester of pregnancy; there is no evidence of risk in the last two trimesters.

Category B: Animal studies have not demonstrated a risk to the fetus, but no adequate studies have been done in pregnant women.

or

Animal studies have shown an adverse effect, but adequate studies in pregnant women have not demonstrated a risk to the fetus during the first trimester of pregnancy and there is no evidence of risk in the last two trimesters.

Category C: Animal studies have shown an adverse effect on the fetus, but no adequate studies have been done in humans. The potential risks of using the drug during pregnancy may be acceptable given the benefits of using the drug.

or

No animal reproduction studies and no adequate studies in humans have been done.

Category D: There is evidence of human fetal risk, but the potential risks from the use of the drug in pregnant women may outweigh any benefits.

Category X: Studies in animals or humans or adverse reaction reports, or both, have demonstrated fetal abnormalities. The risk of use in pregnant women clearly outweighs any possible benefit.

Category ?:   No data available (not a formal FDA classification; included to provide complete data set).

BREASTFEEDING

No formally recognized classification exists for drugs and breastfeeding. This shorthand was developed for the *Clinician's Pocket Drug Reference*.

+   Compatible with breastfeeding
M   Monitor patient or use with caution
+/–   Excreted, or likely excreted, with unknown effects or at unknown concentrations
?/–   Unknown excretion, but effects likely to be of concern
–   Contraindicated in breastfeeding
?   No data available

Generic Drug Name (Selected Common Brand Names [Controlled Substance]) **WARNING:** Summary of the "Black Box" precautions that are deemed necessary by the FDA. These are significant precautions and contraindications concerning the individual medication. **Uses:** This includes both FDA-labeled indications (in **bold** type) and other off-label uses of the medication. Because the uses of many medications are based on the medical literature and are not listed in package inserts, we list common uses of the medication rather than the official labeled indications (FDA-approved) based on input from our editorial board. **Action:** How the drug works. This information is helpful in comparing classes of drugs and understanding side effects and contraindications. **Dose: Caution:** [pregnancy/fetal risk categories, breastfeeding] Fetal risk categories and breastfeeding concerns (see above for classifications) and other cautions. **Contra:** Other common contraindications or cautions **Supplied:** Common dosing forms. **SE:** Common or significant side effects. **Notes:** Lists other key information about the drug.

1. CLASSES OF GENERIC DRUGS, MINERALS, NATURAL PRODUCTS, AND VITAMINS

Analgesic/Anti-Inflammatory/Antipyretic Agents

Acetaminophen
Acetaminophen with butalbital and caffeine
Acetaminophen with codeine
Aspirin
Aspirin with butalbital and caffeine
Aspirin with butalbital, caffeine, and codeine
Aspirin with codeine
Buprenorphine
Butorphanol
Capsaicin
Celecoxib
Cocaine
Codeine
Dezocine
Diclofenac sodium
Diflunisal
Etodolac
Fenoprofen
Fentanyl
Fentanyl transdermal system
Fentanyl, transmucosal
Flurbiprofen
Hydrocodone and acetaminophen
Hydrocodone and aspirin
Hydrocodone and ibuprofen
Hydromorphone
Ibuprofen
Indomethacin
Ketoprofen
Ketorolac
Meloxicam
Meperidine
Methadone
Morphine sulfate
Nabumetone
Nalbuphine
Naproxen
Oxaprozin
Oxycodone
Oxycodone and acetaminophen
Oxycodone and aspirin
Oxymorphone
Pentazocine
Piroxicam
Propoxyphene
Sulindac
Tolmetin
Tramadol

Antacids/Antigas

Aluminum carbonate
Aluminum hydroxide
Aluminum hydroxide with magnesium carbonate
Aluminum hydroxide with magnesium hydroxide
Aluminum hydroxide with magnesium hydroxide and simethicone
Aluminum hydroxide with magnesium trisilicate
Calcium carbonate
Magaldrate
Simethicone

Antianxiety Agents

Alprazolam
Amoxapine
Buspirone
Chlordiazepoxide
Clorazepate
Diazepam
Doxepin
Hydroxyzine
Lorazepam
Meprobamate
Oxazepam

Antiarrhythmics

Adenosine
Amiodarone
Digoxin
Diltiazem
Disopyramide
Dofetilide

Esmolol
Flecainide
Ibutilide
Lidocaine
Mexiletine
Procainamide

Propafenone
Quinidine
Sotalol
Tocainide
Verapamil

Antibiotics

Amikacin
Amoxicillin
Amoxicillin/potassium clavu-
   lanate
Ampicillin
Ampicillin/sulbactam
Atovaquone
Atovaquone/proguanil
Azithromycin
Aztreonam
Cefaclor
Cefadroxil
Cefazolin
Cefdinir
Cefepime
Cefditoren
Cefixime
Cefoperazone
Cefotaxime
Cefotetan
Cefoxitin
Cefpodoxime
Cefprozil
Ceftazidime
Ceftibuten
Ceftizoxime
Ceftriaxone
Cefuroxime
Cephalexin
Cephapirin
Cephradine

Ciprofloxacin
Clarithromycin
Clindamycin
Clofazimine
Cloxacillin
Cortisporin, otic
Dalfopristin/quinupristin
Dapsone
Demeclocycline
Dicloxacillin
Dirithromycin
Doxycycline
Ertapenem
Erythromycin
Ethambutol
Fosfomycin
Gatifloxacin
Gentamicin
Imipenem/cilastatin
Isoniazid
Levofloxacin
Linezolid
Lomefloxacin
Loracarbef
Meropenem
Metronidazole
Mezlocillin
Moxifloxacin
Mupirocin
Nafcillin
Nalidixic acid

Neomycin sulfate
Nitrofurantoin
Norfloxacin
Ofloxacin
Oxacillin
Penicillin G aqueous
Penicillin G benzathine
Penicillin G procaine
Penicillin V
Pentamidine
Piperacillin
Piperacillin/tazobactam
Pyrazinamide
Quinupristin/dalfopristin
Rifabutin
Rifampin
Rifapentine
Silver sulfadiazine
Sparfloxacin
Streptomycin
Tetracycline
Ticarcillin
Ticarcillin/potassium clavu-
   lanate
Tobramycin
Trimethoprim
Trimethoprim/sulfamethoxa-
   zole
Trimetrexate
Trovafloxacin
Vancomycin

Anticoagulant/Thrombolytic and Related Agents

Abciximab
Alteplase, recombinant
   (TPA)
Aminocaproic acid
Anistreplase
Antihemophilic Factor VIII
Aprotinin
Ardeparin
Argatroban
Bivalirudin
Cilostazol

Clopidogrel
Dalteparin
Danaparoid
Desmopressin (DDAVP)
Dipyridamole
Dipyridamole and aspirin
Enoxaparin
Fondaparinux
Heparin
Lepirudin
Pentoxifylline

Protamine sulfate
Reteplase
Streptokinase
Tenecteplase
Ticlopidine
Tinzaparin
Tirofiban
Urokinase
Warfarin

Anticonvulsants

Carbamazepine
Clonazepam

Diazepam
Ethosuximide

Fosphenytoin
Gabapentin

Lamotrigine
Levetiracetam
Lorazepam
Oxcarbazepine

Pentobarbital
Phenobarbital
Phenytoin
Tiagabine

Topiramate
Valproic acid
Zonisamide

Antidepressants

Amitriptyline
Bupropion
Citalopram
Desipramine
Doxepin
Escitalopram

Fluoxetine
Imipramine
Lithium carbonate
Maprotiline
Mirtazapine
Nefazodone

Nortriptyline
Paroxetine
Phenelzine
Sertraline
Trazodone
Venlafaxine

Antidiabetic Agents

Acarbose
Acetohexamide
Becaplermin
Chlorpropamide
Glimepiride
Glipizide

Glyburide
Glyburide/metformin
Glyburide micronized
Insulin
Metformin
Miglitol

Pioglitazone
Repaglinide
Rosiglitazone
Tolazamide
Tolbutamide

Antidiarrheal Agents

Bismuth subsalicylate
Diphenoxylate with atropine

Kaolin/pectin
Lactobacillus

Loperamide
Octreotide

Antidotes

Acetylcysteine
Charcoal
Dexrazoxane
Digoxin immune Fab

Flumazenil
Fomepizole
Ipecac syrup
Mesna

Naloxone
Sodium polystyrene sul-
    fonate
Succimer

Antiemetics

Aprepitant
Buclizine
Chlorpromazine
Dimenhydrinate
Dolasetron
Dronabinol

Droperidol
Granisetron
Meclizine
Metoclopramide
Ondansetron
Palonosetron

Prochlorperazine
Promethazine
Scopolamine
Thiethylperazine
Trimethobenzamide

Antifungal Agents

Amphotericin B
Amphotericin B cholesteryl
Amphotericin B lipid com-
    plex
Amphotericin B liposomal
Caspofungin
Ciclopirox
Clotrimazole
Econazole

Fluconazole
Flucytosine
Halciprogin
Itraconazole
Ketoconazole
Miconazole
Naftifine
Nystatin
Nystatin and triamcinolone

Oxiconazole
Terbinafine
Terconazole
Tioconazole
Triamcinolone and nystatin
Tolnaftate
Voriconazole

Antigout Agents

Allopurinol
Colchicine

Probenecid

Sulfinpyrazone

Antihistamines

Azelastine
Cetirizine
Chlorpheniramine
Clemastine fumarate

Cyproheptadine
Desloratadine
Diphenhydramine
Fexofenadine

Hydroxyzine
Loratadine

Antihyperlipidemics

Atorvastatin
Cholestyramine
Colesevelam
Colestipol
Ezetimibe/simvastatin
Ezetimibe/Simvastatin
Fenofibrate
Fluvastatin
Gemfibrozil
Lovastatin
Niacin
Pravastatin
Rosuvastatin
Simvastatin

Antihypertensives

Acebutolol
Amlodipine
Atenolol
Benazepril
Betaxolol
Bisoprolol
Candesartan
Captopril
Carteolol
Carvedilol
Clonidine
Diazoxide
Diltiazem
Doxazosin
Enalapril
Eplerenone
Eprosartan
Felodipine
Fenoldopam
Fosinopril
Guanabenz
Guanadrel
Guanethidine
Guanfacine
Hydralazine
Irbesartan
Isradipine
Labetalol
Lisinopril
Losartan
Methyldopa
Metoprolol
Minoxidil
Moexipril
Nadolol
Nicardipine
Nifedipine
Nisoldipine
Nitroglycerin
Nitroprusside
Penbutolol
Perindopril
Pindolol
Prazosin
Propranolol
Quinapril
Ramipril
Telmisartan
Terazosin
Timolol
Trandolapril
Valsartan
Verapamil

Antineoplastic Agents and Related Medications

Aldesleukin (IL-2)
Altretamine
Amifostine
Aminoglutethimide
Anastrozole
Asparaginase
Bacillus Calmette-Guérin
Bexarotene
Bicalutamide
Bleomycin
Bortezomib
Busulfan
Capecitabine
Carboplatin
Carmustine
Chlorambucil
Cisplatin
Cladribine
Cyclophosphamide
Cytarabine
Cytarabine liposome
Dacarbazine
Dactinomycin
Daunorubicin
Docetaxel
Doxorubicin
Epirubicin
Estramustine
Etoposide
Exemestane
Floxuridine
Fludarabine phosphate
Fluorouracil
Fluorouracil, topical
Fluoxymesterone
Flutamide
Fulvestrant
Gefitinib
Gemcitabine
Gemtuzumab ozagamicin
Goserelin
Hydroxyurea
Idarubicin
Ifosfamide
Imatinib
Irinotecan
Letrozole
Leuprolide
Levamisole
Lomustine
Mechlorethamine
Megestrol acetate
Melphalan
Mercaptopurine
Methotrexate
Mitomycin
Mitotane
Mitoxantrone
Nilutamide
Paclitaxel
Procarbazine
Streptozocin
Tamoxifen citrate
Teniposide
6-Thioguanine
Thiotepa (See Triethylene-triphosphamide)
Topotecan
Trastuzumab
Triethylene-triphosphamide
Valrubicin
Vinblastine
Vincristine
Vinorelbine

Antiparkinsonism Agents

Amantadine
Benztropine
Bromocriptine
Carbidopa/levodopa
Entacapone
Pergolide
Pramipexole
Selegiline
Trihexyphenidyl

Antipsychotic Agents

Aripiprazole
Chlorpromazine
Clozapine
Fluphenazine
Haloperidol
Lithium carbonate
Mesoridazine
Molindone
Olanzapine
Perphenazine
Prochlorperazine
Quetiapine
Risperidone
Thioridazine
Thiothixine
Trifluoperazine

Antitussive, Decongestant, Expectorant, and Mucolytic Agents

Acetylcysteine
Benzonatate
Codeine
Dextromethorphan
Guaifenesin
Guaifenesin and codeine
Guaifenesin and dextromethorphan
Pseudoephedrine
Hydrocodone and guaifenesin
Hydrocodone and homatropine
Hydrocodone and pseudoephedrine
Hydrocodone, chlorpheniramine, phenylephrine, acetaminophen and caffeine
Phenylephrine

Antiviral Agents

Abacavir
Acyclovir
Adefovir
Amantadine
Amprenavir
Atazanavir
Cidofovir
Delavirdine
Didanosine
Efavirenz
Emtricitabine
Enfuvirtide
Famciclovir
Foscarnet
Ganciclovir
Imiquimod cream
Indinavir
Lamivudine
Lamivudine and zidovudine
Lopinavir and ritonavir
Nelfinavir
Nevirapine
Oseltamivir
Penciclovir
Ribavirin
Rimantadine
Ritonavir
Ritonavir and lopinavir
Saquinavir
Stavudine
Trifluridine
Valacyclovir
Zalcitabine
Zanamivir
Zidovudine
Zidovudine and lamivudine

Bronchodilators (Also see Respiratory and Nasal Inhalants)

Albuterol
Albuterol and ipratropium
Aminophylline
Bitolterol
Levalbuterol
Metaproterenol
Pirbuterol
Salmeterol
Terbutaline
Theophylline

Cardiovascular Agents

Acebutolol
Atenolol
Atropine
Candesartan
Cilostazol
Clopidogrel
Digoxin
Diltiazem
Dobutamine
Dopamine
Eplerenone
Epoprostenol
Eprosartan
Eptifibatide
Ephedrine
Epinephrine
Esmolol
Hydralazine
Inamrinone
Irbesartan
Isoproterenol
Isosorbide dinitrate
Isosorbide mononitrate
Labetalol
Losartan
Metoprolol
Milrinone
Nadolol
Nicardipine
Nifedipine
Nimodipine
Nitroglycerin
Nitroprusside
Norepinephrine
Perindopril
Pindolol
Propranolol
Sodium polystyrene sulfonate
Telmisartan
Timolol
Tolazoline
Trandolapril
Treprostinil
Valsartan
Verapamil

Cathartics/Laxatives

Bisacodyl
Docusate calcium
Docusate potassium
Docusate sodium
Glycerin suppositories
Lactulose

Magnesium citrate
Magnesium hydroxide
Mineral oil

Polyethylene glycol-electrolyte solution

Psyllium
Sorbitol

Dermatologic Agents

Acitretin
Alefacept
Anthralin
Bacitracin
Bacitracin and polymyxin B
Bacitracin, neomycin, and polymyxin B
Bacitracin, neomycin, polymyxin B, and hydrocortisone
Bacitracin, neomycin, polymyxin B,

and lidocaine
Calcipotriene
Clotrimazole
Clotrimazole and betamethasone
Dibucaine
Doxepin
Haloprogin
Isotretinoin
Lactic acid and ammonium hydroxide
Neomycin and polymyxin B

Neomycin, bacitracin, and polymyxin B
Selenium sulfide
Silver nitrate
Triamcinolone and nystatin
Tazarotene
Tretinoin

Diuretics

Acetazolamide
Amiloride
Bumetanide
Chlorothiazide
Chlorthalidone
Furosemide
Hydrochlorothiazide

Hydrochlorothiazide and amiloride
Hydrochlorothiazide and spironolactone
Hydrochlorothiazide and triamterene

Indapamide
Mannitol
Metolazone
Spironolactone
Torsemide
Triamterene

Estrogens

Esterified estrogens
Esterified estrogens with methyltestosterone
Estradiolcypionate/medroxyprogesterone
Estradiol topical
Estradiol transdermal
Estrogen, conjugated
Estrogen, conjugated with methylprogesterone

Estrogen, conjugated methyltestosterone
Ethinyl estradiol
Ethinyl estradiol/levonorgestrel
Ethinyl estradiol/norelgestromin
Etonogestrel cypionate/medroxyprogesterone
Norethindrone

Norgestrel
Oral contraceptives
Raloxifene

Gastrointestinal Agents

Alosetron
Balsalazide
Cimetidine
Cisapride
Dexpanthenol
Dicyclomine
Esomeprazole
Famotidine
Hyoscyamine
Hyoscyamine, atropine, scopolamine, and phenobarbital

Infliximab
Lactulose
Lansoprazole
Loperamide
Mesalamine enema
Metoclopramide
Misoprostol
Neomycin sulfate
Nizatidine
Octreotide
Olsalazine
Omeprazole

Pancreatin/pancrelipase
Pantoprazole
Paregoric
Propantheline
Rabeprazole
Sodium phosphate
Ranitidine
Sulfasalazine
Sucralfate
Tegaserod
Vasopressin

Hormones/Synthetic Substitutes (Also see Estrogens and Thyroid/Antithyroid)

Alpha-protease inhibitor
Aminoglutethimide
Betamethasone
Calcitonin

Cortisone
Darbepoetin alfa
Desmopressin
Dexamethasone

Drotecogin
Epoetin alfa (Erythropoietin)
Filgrastim (G-CSF)
Fludrocortisone acetate

Glucagon
Gonadorelin
Hydrocortisone
Insulin
Interferon alfa
Interferon alfa-2B
Interferon alfacon-1
Interferon beta-1b
Interferon gamma-1b
Levonorgestrel Implants

Medroxyprogesterone
Methylprednisolone
Metyrapone
Nicotine gum
Nicotine nasal spray
Nicotine, transdermal
Oxytocin
Pancreatin/pancrelipase
Peg interferon alfa 2a
Peg interferon alfa 2b

Prednisolone
Prednisone
Sargramostim (GM-CSF)
Steroids
Teriparatide
Triptorelin
Vasopressin
Zoledronic acid

Immunosuppressive Agents

Adalimumab
Anakinra
Antithymocyte globulin
  (ATG)
Azathioprine
Basiliximab

Cyclosporine
Daclizumab
Etanercept
Leflunomide
Methotrexate
Muromonab-CD3 (OKT-3)

Mycophenolate mofetil
Omalizumab
Sirolimus
Tacrolimus (FK-506)
Thalidomide

Local Anesthetic Agents

Bupivacaine
Dibucaine

Lidocaine
Lidocaine and prilocaine

Pramoxine and hydrocorti-
  sone

Muscle Relaxants

Atracurium
Baclofen
Carisoprodol
Chlorzoxazone
Cyclobenzaprine

Dantrolene
Diazepam
Metaxalone
Methocarbamol
Orphenadrine

Pancuronium
Rocuronium
Succinylcholine
Vecuronium

Neurologic Drugs (Also see Antiparkinsonism Agents, Anticonvulsants)

Almotriptan
Atomoxetine
Demeclocycline
Disulfiram
Edrophonium
Eletriptan

Frovatriptan
Galantamine
Modafinil
Naltrexone
Naratriptan
Physostigmine

Rivastigmine
Rizatriptan
Sodium oxybate
Sumatriptan
Tacrine
Zolmitriptan

Ophthalmic Agents

Apraclonidine
Artificial tears
Betaxolol
Brimonidine
Brinzolamide
Carbachol
Chloramphenicol
Ciprofloxacin
Cortisporin
Demecarium
Dexamethasone
Dipivefrin
Dorzolamide
Dorzolamide and timolol
Echothiophate iodide

Emedastine
Erythromycin
Gentamicin
Gentamicin and pred-
  nisolone
Ketotifen
Latanoprost
Levobetaxolol
Levobunolol
Lodoxamide
Metipranolol
Naphazoline and antazoline
Naphazoline and pheni-
  ramine acetate
Neomycin

Neomycin and dexametha-
  sone
Pemirolast
Pilocarpine
Prednisolone
Rimexolone
Sulfacetamide
Sulfacetamide and pred-
  nisolone
Timolol
Tobramycin
Tobramycin and dexam-
  ethasone

Otic Agents

Acetic acid/aluminum ac-
  etate
Benzocaine and antipyrine

Ciprofloxacin
Cortisporin

Neomycin, colistin, and hydrocortisone

Neomycin, colistin, hydrocortisone, and thonzo-
nium

Neomycin, polymyxin, and
hydrocortisone
Polymyxin B and hydrocortisone

Ofloxacin
Triethanolamine

Plasma Volume Expanders
Albumin
Dextran 40

Hetastarch

Plasma protein fraction

Respiratory and Nasal Inhalants (Also see Bronchodilators)
Alpha-protease inhibitor
Beclomethasone
Budesonide
Cromolyn sodium
Dexamethasone
Dornase alfa
Flunisolide
Fluticasone

Fluticasone/salmeterol
Formoterol
Ipratropium
Montelukast
Nedocromil
Omalizumab
Potassium iodide (see
SSKI)

Salmeterol
Salmeterol/fluticasone
SSKI (see potassium iodide)
Triamcinolone
Zafirlukast
Zileuton

Sedatives/Hypnotics
Diphenhydramine
Estazolam
Flurazepam
Hydroxyzine

Midazolam
Quazepam
Secobarbital
Temazepam

Triazolam
Zaleplon
Zolpidem

Supplements (Also see Minerals, Natural Products, and Vitamins)
Calcitrol
Calcium acetate
Calcium salts
Cholecalciferol
Cyanocobalamin (B$_{12}$)
Ferric gluconate
Ferric gluconate complex
Ferrous sulfate
Folic acid

Iron dextran
Iron sucrose
Leucovorin
Magnesium oxide
Magnesium sulfate
Oprelvekin
Oral contraceptives
Phytonadione (vitamin K)
Potassium supplements

Pyridoxine (B$_6$)
Sodium bicarbonate
Thiamine (B$_1$)
Vitamin B$_1$ (thiamine)
Vitamin B$_6$ (pyridoxine)
Vitamin B$_{12}$ (cyanocobal-
amin)
Vitamin K (phytonadione)

Thyroid/Antithyroid
Levothyroxine
Liothyronine
Methimazole

Potassium iodide (see
SSKI)
Propylthiouracil

SSKI (see Potassium io-
dide)

Toxoids/Vaccines/Serums
Bacillus Calmette-Guérin
Cytomegalovirus immune
globulin
Haemophilus B conjugate
vaccine
Hepatitis A vaccine
Hepatitis A/hepatitis B vac-
cine

Hepatitis B immune globulin
Hepatitis B vaccine
Immune globulin, intra-
venous
Influenza vaccine
Influenza vaccine, intranasal
Lyme disease vaccine

Pneumococcal vaccine,
polyvalent
Smallpox vaccine
Tetanus immune globulin
Tetanus toxoid
Varicella vaccine

Urinary (and Genitourinary) Tract Agents
Alfuzosin
Alprostadil
Amino-cerv pH 5.5 cream
Ammonium aluminum sul-
fate
Belladonna and opium sup-
positories

Bethanechol
Dimethyl sulfoxide
Dutasteride
Finasteride
Flavoxate
Hyoscyamine

Hyoscyamine, atropine,
scopolamine, and pheno-
barbital
Mesna
Methenamine
Oxybutynin
Oxybutynin transdermal

Pentosan polysulfate sodium	Sildenafil	Terazosin
Phenazopyridine	Sodium citrate	Tolterodine
	Tamsulosin	Vardenafil

Miscellaneous

Alendronate	Lindane (γ-benzene hexa-chloride)	Physostigmine
Cevimeline HCl		Propofol
Demeclocycline	Methylergonovine	Risedronate
Diazoxide	Naltrexone	Sevelamer
Disulfiram	Orlistat	Sibutramine
Etidronate	Pamidronate	Silver nitrate
Gallium nitrate	Permethrin	

Minerals (Also see under specific generic drugs)

Calcium	Iron	Selenium
Chromium	Magnesium	Zinc
Copper		

Natural Products

Black cohosh	Garlic	Melatonin
Chamomile	Ginger	Milk thistle
Cranberry	Ginkgo biloba	Saw palmetto
Dong quai	Ginseng	St. John's wort
Echinacea	Glucosamine/chondroitin sulfate	Valerian
Ephedra/Ma huang		Yohimbine
Feverfew	Kava kava	

Unsafe Herbs

Aconite	Coltsfoot	Licorice
Aristocholic acid	Comfrey	Life root
Calamus	Ephedra/Ma huang	Pokeweed
Chaparral	Juniper	Sassafrass
Chinese herbal mixtures	Kava kava	Usnic acid

Vitamins (Also see under specific generic drugs)

Vitamin A	Vitamin B_6	Vitamin D
Folate	Vitamin B_{12}	Vitamin E
Thiamine	Vitamin C	Vitamin K

2. GENERIC DRUGS: INDICATIONS, ACTIONS, DOSE, CAUTION, CONTRAINDICATIONS, SUPPLIED, SIDE EFFECTS, & NOTES

Abacavir (Ziagen) **WARNING:** Hypersensitivity manifested as fever, rash, fatigue, GI, and respiratory reported; stop drug immediately and do not rechallenge; lactic acidosis and hepatomegaly/steatosis reported **Uses: HIV infection Action:** Nucleoside reverse transcriptase inhibitor **Dose: *Adults.*** 300 mg PO bid **Caution:** [C, −] CDC recommends HIV-infected mothers not breastfeed because of risk of infant HIV transmission **Supplied:** Tabs 300 mg; soln 20 mg/mL **SE:** See warning, increased LFTs, fat redistribution **Notes:** Numerous drug interactions

Abciximab (ReoPro) **Uses: Prevent acute ischemic complications in PTCA Action:** Inhibits platelet aggregation (glycoprotein IIb/IIIa inhibitor) **Dose:** 0.25 mg/kg bolus 10–60 min before PTCA, then 0.125 mcg/kg/min (max = 10 mcg/min) cont inf for 12 h **Caution:** [C, ?/−] **Contra:** Active or recent (within 6 wk) internal hemorrhage, CVA within 2 y or CVA with significant neurologic deficit, bleeding diathesis or administration of oral anticoagulants within 7 d (unless PT ≤ 1.2 × control), thrombocytopenia (< 100,000 cells/μL), recent trauma or major surgery (within 6 wk), CNS tumor, AVM, aneurysm, severe uncontrolled HTN, vasculitis, use of dextran prior to or during PTCA, hypersensitivity to murine proteins **Sup-**

plied: Inj 2 mg/mL **SE:** Allergic reactions, bleeding, thrombocytopenia possible **Notes:** Use with heparin

Acarbose (Precose) **Uses:** Type 2 DM **Action:** α-Glucosidase inhibitor; delays digestion of carbohydrates, thus reduces glucose levels **Dose:** 25–100 mg PO tid (with 1st bite of each meal) **Caution:** [B, ?] Avoid if CrCl < 25 mL/min **Contra:** IBD, cirrhosis **Supplied:** Tabs 25, 50, 100 mg **SE:** Abdominal pain, diarrhea, flatulence, increased LFTs **Notes:** May take with sulfonylureas; can affect digoxin levels; check LFTs q3mo for 1st year of therapy

Acebutolol (Sectral) [See Table VII–7, p 617]

Acetaminophen [APAP, N-acetyl-p-aminophenol] (Tylenol) [OTC]
Uses: Mild to moderate pain, HA, and fever **Action:** Nonnarcotic analgesic; inhibits synthesis of prostaglandins in the CNS; inhibits hypothalamic heat-regulating center **Dose:** 650 mg PO or PR q4–6h or 1000 mg PO q6h; max 4 g/24 h **Caution:** [B, +] Hepatotoxicity reported in elderly and with alcohol use at doses > 4 g/day; alcoholic liver disease **Contra:** G6PD deficiency **Supplied:** Tabs 160, 325, 500, 650 mg; chew tabs 80, 160 mg; liq 100 mg/mL, 120 mg/2.5 mL, 120 mg/5 mL, 160 mg/5 mL, 167 mg/5 mL, 325 mg/5 mL, 500 mg/15 mL; drops 48 mg/mL, 60 mg/0.6 mL; supp 80, 120, 125, 300, 325, 650 mg **SE:** Overdose causes hepatotoxicity, which is treated with N-acetylcysteine **Notes:** No anti-inflammatory or platelet-inhibiting action; avoid alcohol intake

Acetaminophen + Butalbital ± Caffeine (Fioricet, Medigesic, Repan, Sedapap-10, Two-Dyne, Triapin, Axocet, Phrenilin Forte) [C-III] **Uses: Mild pain; HA, especially associated with stress** **Action:** Nonnarcotic analgesic with barbiturate **Dose:** 1–2 tabs or caps PO q4/6h PRN; 4 g/24 h APAP max **Caution:** [D, +] Alcoholic liver disease **Contra:** G6PD deficiency **Supplied:** Caps *Medigesic, Repan, Two-Dyne:* Butalbital 50 mg, caffeine 40 mg + APAP 325 mg. Caps *Axocet, Phrenilin Forte:* Butalbital 50 mg + APAP 650 mg; *Triapin:* Butalbital 50 mg + APAP 325 mg. Tabs *Medigesic, Fioricet, Repan:* Butalbital 50 mg, caffeine 40 mg, + APAP 325 mg; *Phrenilin:* Butalbital 50 mg + APAP 325 mg; *Sedapap-10:* Butalbital 50 mg + APAP 650 mg **SE:** drowsiness, dizziness, "hangover" effect **Notes:** Butalbital is habit-forming; avoid alcohol intake

Acetaminophen + Codeine (Tylenol No. 1, No. 2, No. 3, No. 4) [C-III, C-V]
Uses: No. 1, No. 2, and No. 3 for mild–moderate pain; No. 4 for moderate–severe pain **Action:** Combined effects of APAP and a narcotic analgesic **Dose:** 1–2 tabs q3–4h PRN (max dose APAP = 4 g/d); adjust in renal/hepatic impairment **Caution:** [C, +] Alcoholic liver disease **Contra:** G6PD deficiency **Supplied:** Tabs 300 mg of APAP + codeine; caps 325 mg of APAP + codeine; helix, susp (C-V) APAP 120 mg + codeine 12 mg/5 mL **SE:** Drowsiness, dizziness, N/V **Notes:** Codeine in No. 1 = 7.5 mg, No. 2 = 15 mg, No. 3 = 30 mg, No. 4 = 60 mg

Acetazolamide (Diamox) **Uses: Diuresis, glaucoma, prevent and treat high-altitude sickness, refractory epilepsy** **Action:** Carbonic anhydrase inhibitor; decreases renal excretion of hydrogen and ↑ renal excretion of sodium, potassium, bicarbonate, and water **Dose:** *Diuretic:* 250–375 mg IV or PO q24h *Glaucoma:* 250–1000 mg PO q24h in ÷ doses *Epilepsy:* 8–30 mg/kg/d PO in ÷ doses *Altitude sickness (treatment):* 250 mg PO Q 8–12 h or SR 500 mg PO Q 12–24 h *Altitude sickness (prevention):* 250 mg PO Q 8–12 h or SR 500 mg PO Q12–24h starting 24–48 h before ascent and 48 h after highest ascent. Adjust in renal impairment; avoid if CrCl < 10 mL/min **Caution:** [C, +] **Contra:** Renal/hepatic failure, sulfa hypersensitivity **Supplied:** Tabs 125, 250 mg; SR caps 500 mg; inj 500 mg/vial **SE:** Malaise, metallic taste, drowsiness, photosensitivity, hyperglycemia **Notes:** Follow Na^+ and K^+; watch for metabolic acidosis; SR dosage forms not recommended for use in epilepsy

Acetic Acid and Aluminum Acetate (Otic Domeboro) **Uses: Otitis externa** **Action:** Anti-infective **Dose:** 4–6 drops in ear(s) q2–3h **Caution:** [C,?] **Contra:** Perforated tympanic membranes **Supplied:** 2% otic soln

Acetohexamide (Dymelor) [See Table VII–13, p 626]

Acetylcysteine (Mucomyst)   **Uses:** Mucolytic agent as adjuvant Rx for chronic bronchopulmonary diseases and CF; **antidote to APAP hepatotoxicity**, best results used within 24 h   **Action:** Splits disulfide linkages between mucoprotein molecular complexes; protects liver by restoring glutathione levels in APAP overdose   **Dose:** *Nebulizer:* 3–5 mL of 20% soln diluted with equal vol of water or NS tid–qid *Antidote:* PO or NG: 140 mg/kg loading dose, then 70 mg/kg q4h for 17 doses. (Dilute 1:3 in carbonated beverage or orange juice)   **Caution:** [C, ?]   **Supplied:** Soln 10%, 20%   **SE:** Bronchospasm when used by inhalation in asthmatics; N/V, drowsiness   **Notes:** Activated charcoal adsorbs acetylcysteine when given PO for acute APAP ingestion

Acitretin (Soriatane)   WARNING: Must not be used by women who are pregnant or intend to become pregnant during therapy or for up to 3 y after discontinuation of therapy; ethanol must not be ingested during therapy or for 2 months after cessation of therapy; do not donate blood during or up to 3 y after cessation of therapy   **Uses: Severe psoriasis** and other keratinization disorders (lichen planus, etc)   **Action:** Retinoid-like activity   **Dose:** 25–50 mg/d PO, with main meal; can ↑ if no response by 4 wk to 75 mg/d   **Caution:** [X, −] Caution in renal/hepatic impairment; caution in women of reproductive potential   **Contra:** See Warning   **Supplied:** Caps 10, 25 mg   **SE:** Cheilitis, skin peeling, alopecia, pruritus, rash, arthralgia, GI upset, photosensitivity, thrombocytosis, hypertriglyceridemia   **Notes:** Follow LFTs; response often takes 2–3 mo; must sign a patient agreement/informed consent prior to use

Acyclovir (Zovirax)   **Uses: Herpes simplex and herpes zoster viral infections** **Action:** Interferes with viral DNA synthesis   **Dose:** *Oral: Initial genital herpes:* 200 mg PO q4h while awake, total of 5 caps/d for 10 d or 400 mg PO tid for 7–10 d *Chronic suppression:* 400 mg PO bid *Intermittent Rx:* As for initial treatment, except treat for 5 d, or 800 mg PO bid, initiate at earliest prodrome *Herpes zoster:* 800 mg PO 5 ×/d for 7–10 d *IV:* 5–10 mg/kg/dose IV q8h *Topical initial herpes genitalis:* Apply q3h (6 ×/d) for 7 d; ↓ for CrCl < 50 mL/min   **Caution:** [C, +]   **Supplied:** Caps 200 mg; tabs 400, 800 mg; susp 200 mg/5 mL; inj 500 mg/vial; oint 5%   **SE:** Dizziness, lethargy, confusion, rash, inflammation at IV injection site   **Notes:** PO better than topical for herpes genitalis .

Adalimumab (Humira)   WARNING: Cases of TB have been observed, check tuberculin skin test prior to use   **Uses: Treatment of moderate to severe rheumatoid arthritis in patients with an inadequate response to one or more DMARDs**   **Action:** Tumor necrosis factor alpha inhibitor   **Dose:** 40 mg subcutaneously every other wk; may increase to 40 mg every wk if not on methotrexate   **Caution:** [B, ?/−] Serious infections and sepsis have been reported   **Supplied:** Pre-filled 1-mL (40 mg) syringe   **SE:** Injection site reactions, serious infections, neurologic events, malignancies   **Notes:** Refrigerate pre-filled syringe, rotate injection sites; may be used with other DMARDs

Adefovir (Hepsera)   WARNING: Acute exacerbations of hepatitis may occur upon discontinuation of therapy (monitor hepatic function); chronic administration may lead to nephrotoxicity, especially in patients with underlying renal dysfunction (monitor renal function); HIV resistance may emerge; lactic acidosis and severe hepatomegaly with steatosis have been reported when used alone or in combination with other antiretrovirals   **Uses: Chronic active hepatitis B virus**   **Action:** Nucleotide analogue   **Dose:** CrCl ≥ 50 mL/min: 10 mg PO daily; CrCl 20–49 mL/min: 10 mg PO q48h; CrCl 10–19 mL/min: 10 mg PO q72h; Hemodialysis: 10 mg PO q7d postdialysis; adjust dose when CrCl < 50 mL/min   **Caution:** [C,−]   **Supplied:** Tabs 10 mg   **SE:** Asthenia, headache, abdominal pain, see Warning

Adenosine (Adenocard)   **Uses: PSVT,** including associated with WPW   **Action:** Class IV antiarrhythmic; slows AV node conduction   **Dose:** 6 mg IV bolus; may repeat in 1–2 min; max 12 mg IV   **Caution:** [C, ?]   **Contra:** 2nd- or 3rd-degree AV block or SSS (without pacemaker); recent MI or cerebral hemorrhage   **Supplied:** Inj 6 mg/2 mL   **SE:** Facial flushing, HA, dyspnea, chest pressure, hypotension   **Notes:** Doses > 12 mg not recommended; can cause momentary asystole when administered; caffeine and theophylline antagonize effects of adenosine

Albumin (Albuminar, Buminate, Albutein) Uses: **Plasma volume expansion for shock** (burns, surgery, hemorrhage, or other trauma) **Action:** Maintenance of plasma colloid oncotic pressure **Dose:** Initially, 25 g IV; subsequent dose based on response. 250 g/48 h max **Caution:** [C, ?] Severe anemia; caution with cardiac, renal, or hepatic insufficiency due to added protein load and possible hypervolemia **Contra:** Cardiac failure **Supplied:** Soln 5%, 25% **SE:** Chills, fever, CHF, tachycardia, hypotension, hypervolemia **Notes:** Contains 130–160 mEq Na$^+$/L. May precipitate pulmonary edema

Albuterol (Proventil, Ventolin, Volmax) Uses: **Asthma; prevent exercise-induced bronchospasm** **Action:** β-Adrenergic sympathomimetic bronchodilator; relaxes bronchial smooth muscle **Dose:** *Inhaler:* 2 inhal q4–6h PRN; 1 Rotacap inhaled q4–6h *Oral:* 2–4 mg PO tid–qid; *Neb:* 1.25–5 mg (0.25–1 mL of 0.5% soln in 2–3 mL of NS) tid–qid **Caution:** [C, +] **Supplied:** Tabs 2, 4 mg; ER tabs 4, 8 mg; syrup 2 mg/5 mL; 90 mcg/dose metdose inhaler; Rotacaps 200 mcg; soln for neb 0.083, 0.5% **SE:** Palpitations, tachycardia, nervousness, GI upset

Albuterol and Ipratropium (Combivent) Uses: **COPD** **Action:** Combination of β-adrenergic bronchodilator and quaternary anticholinergic compound **Dose:** 2 inhal qid **Caution:** [C, +] **Contra:** Allergy to peanut/soybean **Supplied:** Met-dose inhaler, 18 mcg ipratropium/103 mcg albuterol/puff **SE:** Palpitations, tachycardia, nervousness, GI upset, dizziness, blurred vision

Aldesleukin [IL-2] (Proleukin) WARNING: Use restricted to patients with normal pulmonary and cardiac function Uses: **Renal cell carcinoma (RCC), melanoma** **Action:** Acts via IL-2 receptor; numerous immunomodulatory effects **Dose:** 600,000 IU/kg q8h × 14 doses (FDA-approved dose/schedule for RCC). Multiple cont inf and alternate schedules (including "high dose" using 24 × 10^6 IU/m^2 IV q8h on days 1–5 and 12–16) **Caution:** [C, ?/–] **Contra:** Organ allografts **Supplied:** Inj 1.1 mg/mL (22 × 10^6 IU) **SE:** Flu-like syndrome (malaise, fever, chills), N/V/D, ↑ bilirubin; capillary leak syndrome with ↓ BP, pulmonary edema, fluid retention, and weight gain; renal toxicity and mild hematologic toxicity (anemia, thrombocytopenia, leukopenia) and secondary eosinophilia; cardiac toxicity (myocardial ischemia, atrial arrhythmias); neurologic toxicity (CNS depression, somnolence, rarely coma, delirium). Pruritic rashes, urticaria, and erythroderma common **Notes:** Cont inf schedules less likely to cause severe hypotension and fluid retention

Alefacept (Amevive) WARNING: Must monitor CD4 before each dose; withhold if < 250; discontinue if < 250 × 1 month Uses: **Treatment of adults with moderate to severe chronic plaque psoriasis** **Action:** Fusion protein inhibitor **Dose:** 7.5 mg IV OR 15 mg IM once weekly × 12 wk **Caution:** [B, ?/–] Pregnancy registry; associated with serious infections **Contra:** Lymphopenia **Supplied:** 7.5, 15 mg vials **SE:** Chills, pharyngitis, myalgia, injection site reaction, malignancy **Notes:** Different formulations for IV or IM administration; may repeat course 12 wk later if CD4 acceptable

Alendronate (Fosamax) Uses: **Treatment and prevention of osteoporosis, treatment of steroid-induced osteoporosis and Paget's disease** **Action:** Reduce normal and abnormal bone resorption **Dose:** *Osteoporosis: Treatment:* 10 mg/d PO or 70 mg q wk *Steroid-induced osteoporosis: Treatment:* 5 mg/d PO *Prevention:* 5 mg/d PO or 35 mg q wk *Paget's disease:* 40 mg/d PO **Caution:** [C, ?] Not recommended if CrCl < 35 mL/min; NSAID use **Contra:** Abnormalities of the esophagus, inability to sit or stand upright for 30 min, hypocalcemia **Supplied:** Tabs 5, 10, 35, 40, 70 mg **SE:** GI disturbances, HA, pain **Notes:** Take 1st thing in AM with water (8 oz) at least 30 min before 1st food or beverage of the day. Do not lie down for 30 min after taking. Adequate calcium and vitamin D supplements are necessary

Alfuzosin (Uroxatral) WARNING: May prolong QTc interval Uses: **Benign prostatic hypertrophy** **Action:** Alpha blocker **Dose:** 10 mg PO daily immediately after the same meal each day **Caution:** [B, –] **Contra:** Concomitant CYP3A4 inhibitors; moderate/severe hepatic impairment **Supplied:** Tabs 10 mg **SE:** Postural hypotension, dizziness, HA, fatigue **Notes:** Extended-release tablet—do not halve or crush; fewest reports of ejaculatory disorders compared with other drugs in class

Allopurinol (Zyloprim, Lopurin, Aloprim) **Uses:** Gout, hyperuricemia of malignancy, and uric acid urolithiasis **Action:** Xanthine oxidase inhibitor; decreases uric acid production **Dose:** *PO:* Initially, 100 mg/d; usual 300 mg/d; max 800 mg/d *IV:* 200–400 mg/m^2/d (max 600 mg/24 h); adjust for renal impairment; take after meal with plenty of fluid **Caution:** [C, M] **Supplied:** Tabs 100, 300 mg; inj 500 mg/30 mL (Aloprim) **SE:** Skin rash, N/V, renal impairment, angioedema **Notes:** Aggravates acute gout; begin after acute attack resolves; administer after meals; IV dose of 6 mg/mL final conc as single daily infusion or ÷ 6-, 8-, or 12-h intervals

Almotriptan (Axert) [See Table VII–16, p 629]

α_1-Protease Inhibitor (Prolastin) **Uses:** α_1-antitrypsin deficiency; panacinar emphysema **Action:** Replacement of human α_1-protease inhibitor **Dose:** 60 mg/kg IV once/wk **Caution:** [C, ?] **Contra:** Selective IgA deficiencies with known antibodies to IgA **Supplied:** Inj 500 mg/20 mL, 1000 mg/40 mL **SE:** Fever, dizziness, flu-like symptoms, allergic reactions

Alosetron (Lotronex) **WARNING:** Serious GI side effects, some fatal, including ischemic colitis, have been reported. May be prescribed only through participation in the Prescribing Program for Lotronex **Uses:** Treatment of severe diarrhea-predominant IBS in women who have failed conventional therapy **Action:** Selective 5-HT$_3$ receptor antagonist **Dose:** Adults: 1 mg PO qd × 4 wk; titrate to max of 1 mg bid; discontinue after 4 wk at max dose if IBS symptoms not controlled **Caution:** [B, ?/–] **Contra:** History of chronic or severe constipation, intestinal obstruction, strictures, toxic megacolon, GI perforation, adhesions, ischemic colitis, Crohn's disease, ulcerative colitis, diverticulitis, thrombophlebitis, or hypercoagulable state **Supplied:** Tabs 1 mg **SE:** Constipation, abdominal pain, nausea **Notes:** Discontinue immediately if constipation or symptoms of ischemic colitis develop; must sign a patient agreement/informed consent before use

Alprazolam (Xanax) [C-IV] **Uses:** Anxiety and panic disorders + anxiety with depression **Action:** Benzodiazepine; antianxiety agent **Dose:** *Anxiety:* Initially, 0.25–0.5 mg tid; ↑ to a max of 4 mg/d in ÷ doses *Panic:* Initially, 0.5 mg tid; may gradually ↑ to desired response; ↓ dose in elderly, debilitated, and hepatic impairment **Caution:** [D, –] **Contra:** Narrow angle glaucoma, concomitant itra-/ketoconazole **Supplied:** Tabs 0.25, 0.5, 1, 2 mg, soln 1 mg/mL **SE:** Drowsiness, fatigue, irritability, memory impairment, sexual dysfunction **Notes:** Avoid abrupt discontinuation after prolonged use

Alprostadil, Intracavernosal (Caverject, Edex) **Uses:** Erectile dysfunction **Action:** Relaxes smooth muscles, dilates cavernosal arteries, increases lacunar spaces and entrapment of blood by compressing venules against tunica albuginea **Dose:** 2.5–60 mcg intracavernosal; adjusted to individual needs **Caution:** [X, –] **Contra:** Conditions predisposing to priapism; anatomic deformities of the penis; penile implants; men in whom sexual activity is inadvisable **Supplied:** *Caverject:* 6–10 or 6–20 mcg vials ± diluent syringes *Caverject Impulse:* self-contained syringe (29-gauge) 10 and 20 mcg *Edex:* 5-, 10-, 20-, 40-mcg vials + syringes **SE:** Penile pain common; pain with injection **Notes:** Counsel patients about possible priapism, penile fibrosis, and hematoma; titrate dose at physician's office

Alprostadil, Urethral Suppository (Muse) **Uses:** Erectile dysfunction **Action:** Alprostadil (PGE$_1$) absorbed through urethral mucosa; vasodilator and smooth muscle relaxant of corpus cavernosa **Dose:** 125–1000 mcg system 5–10 min before sexual activity **Caution:** [X, –] **Contra:** Conditions predisposing to priapism; anatomic deformities of the penis; penile implants; men in whom sexual activity is inadvisable **Supplied:** 125, 250, 500, 1000 mcg with a transurethral delivery system **SE:** Hypotension, dizziness, syncope, penile pain, testicular pain, urethral burning/bleeding, and priapism **Notes:** Dose titration under physician's supervision

Alteplase, Recombinant [tPA] (Activase) **Uses:** Acute MI, PE, acute ischemic stroke and CV cath occlusion **Action:** Thrombolytic; initiates local fibrinolysis by binding to fibrin in the thrombus **Dose:** *AMI and PE:* 100 mg IV over 3 h (10 mg over 2 min, then 50 mg over 1 h, then 40 mg over 2 h) *Stroke:* 0.9 mg/kg (max 90 mg) infused over 60 min; *Cath occlusion:* 10–29 kg: 1 mg/mL; ≥ 30 kg: 2 mg/mL **Caution:** [C, ?] **Contra:** Active internal bleeding; uncontrolled HTN (systolic BP = 185 mm Hg/diastolic = 110 mm Hg); recent (within 3 mo) CVA, GI bleed, trauma, surgery, prolonged external cardiac massage; intracranial neoplasm, suspected aortic dissection, AV malformation or aneurysm, bleeding diathesis, hemostatic defects, seizure at the time of stroke, suspicion of subarachnoid hemorrhage **Supplied:** Powder for inj 50, 100 mg **SE:** Bleeding, bruising (especially from venipuncture sites), hypotension **Notes:** Give heparin to prevent reocclusion; in AMI doses of > 150 mg associated with intracranial bleeding

Altretamine (Hexalen) **Uses: Epithelial ovarian CA** **Action:** Unknown; cytotoxic agent, possibly alkylating agent; inhibits nucleotide incorporation into DNA and RNA **Dose:** 260 mg/m²/d in 4 ÷ doses for 14–21 d of a 28-d treatment cycle; dose ↑ to 150 mg/m²/d for 14 d in multiagent regimens (refer to specific protocols) **Caution:** [D, ?/–] **Contra:** Preexisting severe bone marrow depression or neurologic toxicity **Supplied:** Caps 50, 100 mg **SE:** Vomiting, diarrhea, and cramps; neurologic toxicity (peripheral neuropathy, CNS depression); minimally myelosuppressive

Aluminum Hydroxide (Amphojel, AlternaGEL) [OTC] **Uses: Relief of heartburn, upset or sour stomach, or acid indigestion**; supplement to Rx of hyperphosphatemia **Action:** Neutralizes gastric acid; binds phosphate **Dose:** 10–30 mL or 2 tabs PO q4–6h **Caution:** [C, ?] **Supplied:** Tabs 300, 600 mg; chew tabs 500 mg; susp 320, 600 mg/5 mL **SE:** Constipation **Notes:** Can use in renal failure

Aluminum Hydroxide + Magnesium Carbonate (Gaviscon) [OTC] **Uses: Relief of heartburn, upset or sour stomach, or acid indigestion** **Action:** Neutralizes gastric acid **Dose:** 15–30 mL PO pc and hs; avoid in renal impairment **Caution:** [C, ?] **Supplied:** Liq containing aluminum hydroxide 95 mg + magnesium carbonate 358 mg/15 mL **SE:** May cause ↑ Mg²⁺ (with renal insufficiency), constipation, diarrhea **Notes:** Doses are best given pc and hs; may affect absorption of some drugs

Aluminum Hydroxide + Magnesium Hydroxide (Maalox) [OTC] **Uses: Hyperacidity** (peptic ulcer, hiatal hernia, etc) **Action:** Neutralizes gastric acid **Dose:** 10–60 mL or 2–4 tabs PO qid or PRN **Caution:** [C, ?] **Supplied:** Tabs, susp **SE:** May cause ↑ Mg²⁺ in renal insufficiency, constipation, diarrhea **Notes:** Doses qid best given pc and hs

Aluminum Hydroxide + Magnesium Hydroxide and Simethicone (Mylanta, Mylanta II, Maalox Plus) [OTC] **Uses: Hyperacidity with bloating** **Action:** Neutralizes gastric acid and defoaming **Dose:** 10–60 mL or 2–4 tabs PO qid or PRN; avoid in renal impairment **Caution:** [C, ?] **Supplied:** Tabs, susp **SE:** Hypermagnesemia in renal insufficiency, diarrhea, constipation **Notes:** Mylanta II contains twice the aluminum and magnesium hydroxide of Mylanta; may affect absorption of some drugs

Aluminum Hydroxide + Magnesium Trisilicate (Gaviscon, Gaviscon-2) [OTC] **Uses: Relief of heartburn, upset or sour stomach, or acid indigestion** **Action:** Neutralizes gastric acid **Dose:** Chew 2–4 tabs qid; avoid in renal impairment **Caution:** [C, ?] **Supplied:** *Gaviscon:* Aluminum hydroxide 80 mg and magnesium trisilicate 20 mg; *Gaviscon-2:* Aluminum hydroxide 160 mg and magnesium trisilicate 40 mg **SE:** Hypermagnesemia in renal insufficiency, constipation, diarrhea **Notes:** Concomitant administration may affect absorption of some drugs

Amantadine (Symmetrel) **Uses: Treatment or prophylaxis of influenza A viral infections, parkinsonism, and drug-induced EPS** **Action:** Prevents release of infectious viral nucleic acid into the host cell; releases dopamine from intact dopaminergic terminals **Dose:** *Influenza A:* 200 mg/d PO or 100 mg PO bid *Parkinsonism:* 100 mg PO qd–bid; reduce dose in renal impairment **Caution:** [C, M] **Supplied:** Caps 100 mg; tabs 100 mg; soln 50 mg/5 mL **SE:** Orthostatic hypotension, edema, insomnia, depression, irritability, hallucinations, dream abnormalities

Amifostine (Ethyol) Uses: **Xerostomia prophylaxis during radiation therapy (head and neck, ovarian, or non–small cell lung CA). Reduces renal toxicity associated with repeated administration of cisplatin** Action: Prodrug, dephosphorylated by alkaline phosphatase to the pharmacologically active thiol metabolite Dose: 910 mg/m^2/d as a 15-min IV inf 30 min prior to chemotherapy Caution: [C, ±] Supplied: 500-mg vials of lyophilized drug with 500 mg of mannitol, reconstituted in sterile NS SE: Transient hypotension in > 60%, N/V, flushing with hot or cold chills, dizziness, hypocalcemia, somnolence, and sneezing Notes: Does not reduce the effectiveness of cyclophosphamide plus cisplatin chemotherapy

Amikacin (Amikin) Uses: **Serious infections caused by gram(–) bacteria and mycobacteria** Action: Aminoglycoside antibiotic; inhibits protein synthesis Spectrum: Good gram(–) bacterial coverage including *Pseudomonas* sp; *Mycobacterim* sp Dose: 5–7.5 mg/kg/dose ÷ q8–24h based on renal function Caution: [C, +/–] Supplied: Inj 100, 500 mg/2 mL SE: Nephrotoxicity, ototoxicity, neurotoxicity; avoid use with potent diuretics Notes: May be effective against gram(–) bacteria resistant to gentamicin and tobramycin; monitor renal function carefully for dosage adjustments; monitor serum levels (see Table VII–18, p 000)

Amiloride (Midamor) Uses: **HTN, CHF, and thiazide-induced hypokalemia** Action: K$^+$-sparing diuretic; interferes with K$^+$/Na$^+$ exchange in the distal tubules Dose: 5–10 mg PO daily; reduce dose in renal impairment Caution: [B, ?] Contra: Hyperkalemia, SCr > 1.5, BUN > 30 Supplied: Tabs 5 mg SE: Hyperkalemia possible; monitor serum K$^+$ levels; HA, dizziness, dehydration, impotence

Aminocaproic Acid (Amicar) Uses: **Excessive bleeding resulting from systemic hyperfibrinolysis and urinary fibrinolysis** Action: Inhibits fibrinolysis via inhibition of TPA substances Dose: 5 g IV or PO (1st h) followed by 1–1.25 g/h IV or PO; max dose 18 g/m^2/d; reduce dose in renal failure Caution: [C, ?] Hematuria of upper urinary tract Contra: DIC Supplied: Tabs 500 mg; syrup 250 mg/mL; inj 250 mg/mL SE: ↓ BP, bradycardia, dizziness, HA, fatigue, rash, GI disturbance, ↓ platelet function Notes: Administer for 8 h or until bleeding is controlled; not for upper urinary tract bleeding

Amino-Cerv pH 5.5 Cream Uses: **Mild cervicitis,** postpartum cervicitis/cervical tears, postcauterization, postcryosurgery, and postconization Action: Hydrating agent; removes excess keratin in hyperkeratotic conditions Dose: 1 Applicatorful intravaginally hs for 2–4 wk Caution: [C, ?] Use in viral skin infection Supplied: Vaginal cream SE: Transient stinging, local irritation Notes: Also called carbamide or urea; contains 8.34% urea, 0.5% sodium propionate, 0.83% methionine, 0.35% cystine, 0.83% inositol, and benzalkonium chloride

Aminoglutethimide (Cytadren) Uses: **Adrenocortical carcinoma, Cushing's syndrome,** breast and prostate CA Action: Inhibits adrenal steroidogenesis and adrenal conversion of androgens to estrogens Dose: 750–1500 mg/d in ÷ doses plus hydrocortisone 20–40 mg/d; reduce in renal insufficiency Caution: [D, ?] Supplied: Tabs 250 mg SE: Adrenal insufficiency ("medical adrenalectomy"), hypothyroidism, masculinization, hypotension, vomiting, rare hepatotoxicity, rash, myalgia, fever

Aminophylline Uses: **Asthma, COPD, and bronchospasm** Action: Relaxes smooth muscle of the bronchi, pulmonary blood vessels; stimulates diaphragm Dose: *Acute asthma:* Load 6 mg/kg IV, then 0.4–0.9 mg/kg/h IV cont inf *Chronic asthma:* 24 mg/kg/24 h PO or PR ÷ q6h; reduce in hepatic insufficiency and with certain drugs (macrolide and quinolone antibiotics, cimetidine, and propranolol) Caution: [C, +] Uncontrolled arrhythmias, hyperthyroidism, peptic ulcers, uncontrolled seizure disorder Supplied: Tabs 100, 200 mg; soln 105 mg/5 mL; supp 250, 500 mg; inj 25 mg/mL SE: N/V, irritability, tachycardia, ventricular arrhythmias, and seizures Notes: Individualize dosage; follow serum levels carefully (see Table VII–16, p 000); aminophylline is about 85% theophylline; erratic absorption with rectal doses

Amiodarone (Cordarone, Pacerone)
Uses: **Recurrent VF or hemodynamically unstable VT**, supraventricular arrhythmias, AF **Action:** Class III antiarrhythmic **Dose:** *Ventricular arrhythmias:* *Intravenous:* 15 mg/min for 10 min, followed by 1 mg/min for 6 h, then a maintenance dose of 0.5 mg/min continuous infusion OR *Oral loading dose:* 800–1600 mg/d PO for 1–3 wk *Maintenance:* 600–800 mg/d PO for 1 month, then 200–400 mg/d *Supraventricular arrhythmias:* *Intravenous:* 300 mg IV over 1 h, then 20 mg/kg for 24 h, then 600 mg PO q day for 1 wk; then a maintenance dose of 100–400 mg q day OR *Oral Loading dose:* 600–800 mg/d PO for 1–4 wk *Maintenance:* Gradually reduce dose to 100–400 mg q day; reduce in severe liver insufficiency **Caution:** [D, –] **Contra:** Sinus node dysfunction, 2nd- or 3rd-degree AV block, sinus bradycardia (without pacemaker) **Supplied:** Tabs 200 mg; inj 50 mg/mL **SE:** Pulmonary fibrosis, exacerbation of arrhythmias, prolongs QT interval; CHF, arrhythmias, hypo-/hyperthyroidism, increased LFTs, liver failure, corneal microdeposits, optic neuropathy/neuritis, peripheral neuropathy, photosensitivity **Notes:** Half-life is 53 d; IV conc of > 0.2 mg/mL administer via a central catheter; alters digoxin and warfarin levels, may require reduced digoxin and warfarin dose. A Medication Guide must be provided with each prescription

Amitriptyline (Elavil)
WARNING: *Pediatric:* Antidepressants may increase risk of suicidality; consider risks and benefits of use. Patients should be closely monitored for clinical worsening, suicidality, or unusual changes in behavior **Uses:** **Depression**, peripheral neuropathy, chronic pain, and tension and migraine headaches **Action:** Tricyclic antidepressant (TCA); inhibits reuptake of serotonin and norepinephrine by the presynaptic neurons **Dose:** Initially, 30–50 mg PO hs; may ↑ to 300 mg hs; caution in hepatic impairment; taper when discontinuing **Caution:** [D, +/–] Narrow-angle glaucoma **Contra:** With MAOIs, during acute recovery following MI **Supplied:** Tabs 10, 25, 50, 75, 100, 150 mg; inj 10 mg/mL **SE:** Strong anticholinergic side effects; overdose may be fatal; may cause urine retention and sedation; ECG changes; photosensitivity

Amlodipine (Norvasc)
Uses: **HTN and stable or unstable angina** **Action:** Ca channel blocker; relaxation of coronary vascular smooth muscle **Dose:** 2.5–10 mg/d PO **Caution:** [C, ?] **Supplied:** Tabs 2.5, 5, 10 mg **SE:** Peripheral edema, HA, palpitations, flushing **Notes:** May be taken without regard to meals

Ammonium Aluminum Sulfate (Alum) [OTC]
Uses: Hemorrhagic cystitis when bladder irrigation fails **Action:** Astringent **Dose:** 1–2% soln used with constant bladder irrigation with NS **Caution:** [+/–] **Supplied:** Powder for reconstitution **SE:** Encephalopathy possible; obtain aluminum levels, especially in renal insufficiency; can precipitate and occlude catheters **Notes:** Safe to use without anesthesia and with vesicoureteral reflux

Amoxicillin (Amoxil, Polymox)
Uses: **Ear, nose, and throat, lower respiratory, skin, urinary tract infections resulting from susceptible gram(+) and gram(–) bacteria**, endocarditis prophylaxis **Action:** β-Lactam antibiotic; inhibits cell wall synthesis *Spectrum:* Gram(+) coverage including *Streptococcus* sp, *Enterococcus* sp; some gram(–) coverage including *H influenzae*, *E coli*, *P mirabilis*, *N gonorrhoeae*, and *H pylori* **Dose:** 250–500 mg PO tid or 500–875 mg bid; reduce in renal impairment **Caution:** [B, +] **Supplied:** Caps 250, 500 mg; chew tabs 125, 200, 250, 400 mg; susp 50 mg/mL, 125, 200, 250, 400 mg/5 mL; tabs 500, 875 mg **SE:** Diarrhea; skin rash common **Notes:** Cross-hypersensitivity with penicillin; many hospital strains of *E coli* are resistant

Amoxicillin and Clavulanic Acid (Augmentin, Augmentin 600 ES, Augmentin XR)
Uses: **Ear, lower respiratory, sinus, urinary tract, skin infections caused by β-lactamase-producing *H influenzae*, *S aureus*, and *E coli*** **Action:** Combination of a β-lactam antibiotic and a β-lactamase inhibitor *Spectrum:* Gram(+) coverage same as amox alone, though β-lactamase sp with amox alone, β-lactamase producing *H influenzae*, *Klebsiella* sp, *M catarrhalis* **Dose:** 250–500 mg PO q8h or 875 mg q12h; XR 2000 mg PO q12h; adjust in renal impairment; take with food **Caution:** [B, ?] **Supplied** (expressed as amoxicillin/clavulanic acid): Tabs 250/125, 500/125, 875/125 mg; chew tabs 125/31.25, 200/28.5, 250/62.5, 400/57 mg; susp 125/31.25, 250/62.5, 200/28.5, 400/57 mg/5 mL;600-ES 600/42.9 mg tab; XR tab 1000/62.5 mg **SE:** Abdominal discomfort, N/V/D, allergic reaction,

vaginitis **Notes:** Do not substitute two 250-mg tabs for one 500-mg tab or an overdose of clavulanic acid will occur

Amphotericin B (Fungizone)   Uses: Severe, systemic fungal infections; oral and cutaneous candidiasis   **Action:** Binds ergosterol in the fungal membrane, altering membrane permeability   **Dose:** *Intravenous:* Test dose of 1 mg in adults, then 0.25–1.5 mg/kg/24 h IV over 2–6 h (range 25–50 mg/d or qod). Total dose varies with indication *Oral:* 1 mL qid *Topical:* Apply bid–qid for 1–4 wk depending on infection; adjust dose in renal impairment   **Caution:** [B, ?]   **Supplied:** Powder for inj 50 mg/vial, oral susp 100 mg/mL, cream, lotion, oint 3%   **SE:** Reduced K⁺ and Mg²⁺ from renal wasting; anaphylaxis reported, HA, fever, chills, nephrotoxicity, hypotension, anemia   **Notes:** Monitor renal function/LFTs; pretreatment with APAP and antihistamines (Benadryl) helps minimize adverse effects with IV infusion (e.g., fever, chills)

Amphotericin B Cholesteryl (Amphotec)   Uses: Aspergillosis in persons intolerant or refractory to conventional amphotericin B, systemic candidiasis   **Action:** Binds to sterols in the cell membrane, alters membrane permeability   **Dose:** Test dose 1.6–8.3 mg, over 15–20 min, followed by a dose of 3–4 mg/kg/d; infuse at rate of 1 mg/kg/h; reduce in renal insufficiency   **Caution:** [B, ?]   **Supplied:** Powder for inj 50 mg/vial (final conc 0.6 mg/mL)   **SE:** Anaphylaxis reported; fever, chills, HA, ↓ K⁺, ↓ Mg⁺, nephrotoxicity, hypotension, anemia   **Notes:** Do not use in-line filter; monitor LFTs and electrolytes

Amphotericin B Lipid Complex (Abelcet)   Uses: Refractory invasive fungal infection in persons intolerant to conventional amphotericin B   **Action:** Binds to sterols in the cell membrane, alters membrane permeability   **Dose:** 5 mg/kg/d IV as a single daily dose; infuse at rate of 2.5 mg/kg/h   **Supplied:** Inj 5 mg/mL   **Caution:** [B, ?]   **SE:** Anaphylaxis reported; fever, chills, HA, ↓ K⁺,↓ Mg⁺, nephrotoxicity, hypotension, anemia   **Notes:** Filter soln with a 5-mm filter needle; do not mix in electrolyte-containing solns. If inf > 2 h, manually mix bag

Amphotericin B Liposomal (Ambisome)   Uses: Refractory invasive fungal infection in persons intolerant to conventional amphotericin B, cryptococcal meningitis in HIV, empiric treatment for febrile neutropenia, visceral leishmaniasis   **Action:** Binds to sterols in the cell membrane, resulting in changes in membrane permeability   **Caution:** [B, ?]   **Supplied:** Powder for inj 50 mg   **Dose:** 3–5 mg/kg/d, infused over 60–120 min; reduce in renal insufficiency   **Caution:** [B, ?]   **Supplied:** Powder for inj 50 mg   **SE:** Anaphylaxis reported; fever, chills, HA, ↓ K⁺, ↓ Mg²⁺, nephrotoxicity, hypotension, anemia   **Notes:** Filter with no less than 1 μm filter

Ampicillin (Amcill, Omnipen)   Uses: Respiratory tract, GU tract, GI tract infections and meningitis due to susceptible bacteria, endocarditis prophylaxis   **Action:** β-Lactam antibiotic; inhibits cell wall synthesis *Spectrum:* Gram(+) coverage, including Streptococcus sp, *Staphylococcus* sp, *Listeria,* gram(−) coverage, including *Klebsiella* sp, *E coli, H influenzae, P mirabilis, Shigella* sp, *Salmonella* sp   **Dose:** 500 mg–2 g IM or IV q6h or 250–500 mg PO q6h; reduce in renal impairment. Take on an empty stomach   **Caution:** [B, M] Cross-hypersensitivity with penicillin   **Supplied:** Caps 250, 500 mg; susp 100 mg/mL (reconstituted as drops), 125 mg/5 mL, 250 mg/5 mL, 500 mg/5 mL; powder for inj 125 mg, 250 mg, 500 mg, 1 g, 2 g, 10 g/vial   **SE:** Diarrhea, skin rash, allergic reaction   **Notes:** Many hospital strains of *E coli* now resistant

Ampicillin-Sulbactam (Unasyn)   Uses: Gynecologic, intra-abdominal, skin infections caused by β-lactamase-producing strains of *S aureus, Enterococcus, H influenzae, P mirabilis,* and *Bacteroides* sp   **Action:** Combination of a β-lactam antibiotic and a β-lactamase inhibitor *Spectrum:* Gram(+) coverage as amp alone, gram- coverage as amp alone also *Enterobacter, Acinetobacter, Bacteroides* **Dose:** 1.5–3 g IM or IV q6h; reduce in renal impairment   **Caution:** [B, M]   **Supplied:** Powder for inj 1.5, 3 g/vial   **SE:** Hypersensitivity reactions, rash, diarrhea, pain at injection site   **Notes:** A 2:1 ratio of ampicillin:sulbactam

Amprenavir (Agenerase)   **WARNING:** Oral solution contraindicated in children < 4 y due to potential toxicity from large volume of excipient polypropylene glycol in the formulation

Uses: HIV infection **Action:** Protease inhibitor; prevents the maturation of the virion to mature viral particle **Dose:** 1200 mg bid **Caution:** [C, ?] CDC recommends HIV-infected mothers not breastfeed because of risk of transmission of HIV to infant; previous allergic reaction to sulfonamides **Contra:** CYP450 3A4 substrates (ergot derivatives, midazolam, triazolam, etc); soln < 4 years, pregnancy, hepatic or renal failure, disulfiram or metronidazole **Supplied:** Caps 50, 150 mg; soln 15 mg/mL **SE:** Life-threatening rash, hyperglycemia, hypertriglyceridemia, fat redistribution, N/V/D, depression **Notes:** Caps and soln contain vitamin E exceeding RDA intake amounts; avoid high-fat meals with administration; many drug interactions

Anakinra (Kineret) WARNING: Associated with an increased incidence of serious infections; DC with serious infection **Uses: Reduce signs and symptoms of moderately to severely active RA, failed one or more disease-modifying antirheumatic drugs** **Action:** Human IL-1–receptor antagonist **Dose:** 100 mg SC qd **Caution:** [B, ?] **Contra:** Hypersensitivity to *E coli*–derived proteins, active infection, < 18 y **Supplied:** 100 mg prefilled syringes **SE:** Neutropenia especially when used with TNF blocking agents, injection site reactions, infections

Anastrozole (Arimidex) **Uses: Breast CA: postmenopausal women with metastatic breast CA, adjuvant treatment of postmenopausal women with early hormone receptor–positive breast CA** **Action:** Selective nonsteroidal aromatase inhibitor, ↓ circulating estradiol **Dose:** 1 mg/d **Caution:** [C, ?] **Contra:** Pregnancy **Supplied:** Tabs 1 mg **SE:** May ↑ cholesterol levels; diarrhea, hypertension, flushing, increased bone and tumor pain, HA, somnolence **Notes:** No detectable effect on adrenal corticosteroids or aldosterone

Anistreplase (Eminase) **Uses: Acute MI** **Action:** Thrombolytic agent; activates the conversion of plasminogen to plasmin, promoting thrombolysis **Dose:** 30 units IV over 2–5 min **Caution:** [C, ?] **Contra:** Active internal bleeding, history of CVA, recent (< 2 mo) intracranial or intraspinal surgery or trauma, intracranial neoplasm, AV malformation, aneurysm, bleeding diathesis, severe uncontrolled hypertension **Supplied:** Vials containing 30 units **SE:** Bleeding, hypotension, hematoma **Notes:** May not be effective if re-administered > 5 d after the previous dose of anistreplase or streptokinase, or streptococcal infection, because of the production of antistreptokinase antibody

Anthralin (Anthra-Derm) **Uses: Psoriasis** **Action:** Keratolytic **Dose:** Apply daily **Caution:** [C, ?] **Contra:** Acutely inflamed psoriatic eruptions, erythroderma **Supplied:** Cream, oint 0.1, 0.2, 0.25, 0.4, 0.5, 1% **SE:** Irritation; discoloration of hair, fingernails, skin

Antihemophilic Factor [Factor VIII] [AHF] (Monoclate) **Uses: Classic hemophilia A, von Willebrand disease** **Action:** Provides factor VIII needed to convert prothrombin to thrombin **Dose:** 1 AHF unit/kg ↑ factor VIII level ~2%. Units required = (kg) (desired factor VIII ↑ as % normal) × (0.5). Prophylaxis of spontaneous hemorrhage = 5% normal. Hemostasis after trauma/surgery = 30% normal. Head injuries, major surgery, or bleeding = 80–100% normal. Determine patient's % of normal factor VIII before dosing **Caution:** [C, ?] **Supplied:** Check each vial for units contained **SE:** Rash, fever, HA, chills, N/V

Antithymocyte Globulin (ATG) (ATGAM) **Uses: Management of allograft rejection in transplant patients** **Action:** Reduces the number of circulating, thymus-dependent lymphocytes **Dose:** 10–15 mg/kg/d **Caution:** [C, ?/–] **Contra:** Do not administer to a patient with a history of severe systemic reaction to any other equine gamma-globulin preparation **Supplied:** Inj 50 mg/mL **SE:** Thrombocytopenia, leukopenia **Notes:** Discontinue treatment if severe, unremitting thrombocytopenia or leukopenia occurs

Apraclonidine (Iopidine) [See Table VII–12, p 623]

Aprepitant (Emend) **Uses: Prevention of nausea and vomiting associated with highly emetogenic cancer chemotherapy, including cisplatin (used in combination with other antiemetic agents)** **Action:** Substance P/neurokinin 1(NK$_1$) receptor antagonist **Dose:** 125 mg PO on day 1, 1 h before chemotherapy, then 80 mg PO q AM on days 2 and 3 **Caution:** [B, ?/–] Substrate and moderate inhibitor of CYP3A4; inducer of CYP2C9 **Contra:**

Use with pimozide   **Supplied:** Caps 80, 125 mg   **SE:** Fatigue, asthenia, hiccups   **Notes:** Decreases effectiveness of oral contraceptives; decreases anticoagulant effect of warfarin

Aprotinin (Trasylol)   **Uses: Reduce/prevent blood loss in patients undergoing CABG**   **Action:** Protease inhibitor, antifibrinolytic   **Dose:** 1-mL IV test dose to assess for allergic reaction *High dose:* 2 million KIU load, 2 million KIU to prime pump, then 500,000 KIU/h until surgery ends *Low dose:* 1 million KIU load, 1 million KIU to prime pump, then 250,000 KIU/h until surgery ends. 7 million KIU max total   **Caution:** [B, ?] Thromboembolic disease requiring anticoagulants or blood factor administration   **Supplied:** Inj 1.4 mg/mL (10,000 KIU/mL)   **SE:** AF, MI, heart failure, dyspnea, postoperative renal dysfunction   **Notes:** 1000/KIU = 0.14 mg of aprotinin

Ardeparin (Normiflo)   **Uses: Prevent DVT/PE after knee replacement**   **Action:** LMW heparin   **Dose:** 35–50 units/kg SC q12h. Begin day of surgery, continue up to 14 d; caution in ↓ renal function   **Caution:** [C, ?]   **Contra:** Active hemorrhage; hypersensitivity to pork products   **Supplied:** Inj 5000, 10,000 units/0.5 mL   **SE:** Bleeding, bruising, thrombocytopenia, pain at injection site, increased serum transaminases   **Notes:** Laboratory monitoring usually not necessary

Argatroban (Acova)   **Uses: Prophylaxis or treatment of thrombosis in HIT, PCI in patients with risk of HIT**   **Action:** Anticoagulant, direct thrombin inhibitor   **Dose:** 2 mcg/kg/min IV; adjust until aPTT 1.5–3 × baseline value not to exceed 100 s; 10 mcg/kg/min max; reduce dose in hepatic impairment   **Caution:** [B, ?] Avoid oral anticoagulants, ↑ risk of bleeding; avoid concomitant use of thrombolytics   **Contra:** Overt major bleeding   **Supplied:** Inj 100 mg/mL   **SE:** Atrial fibrillation, cardiac arrest, cerebrovascular disorder, hypotension, ventricular tachycardia, N/V/D, sepsis, cough, renal toxicity, decrease in Hgb   **Notes:** Steady state typically achieved 1–3 h after initiation of therapy

Aripiprazole (Abilify)   **Uses: Schizophrenia**   **Action:** Dopamine and serotonin antagonist   **Dose:** *Adults:* 10–15 mg PO daily; ↓ when used in combination with potent CYP3A4 or CYP2D6 inhibitors; ↑ when used in combination with inducer of CYP3A4   **Caution:** [C, –]   **Supplied:** Tabs 10, 15, 20, 30 mg   **SE:** Neuroleptic malignant syndrome, tardive dyskinesia, orthostatic hypotension, cognitive and motor impairment, hyperglycemia

Artificial Tears (Tears Naturale) [OTC]   **Uses:** Dry eyes   **Action:** Ocular lubricant   **Dose:** 1–2 drops tid–qid   **Supplied:** OTC soln

L-Asparaginase (Elspar, Oncaspar)   **Uses: ALL** (in combination with other agents)   **Action:** Protein synthesis inhibitor   **Dose:** 500–20,000 IU/m^2 /d for 1–14 d (refer to specific protocols)   **Caution:** [C, ?]   **Contra:** Active/history of pancreatitis   **Supplied:** Inj 10,000 IU   **SE:** Hypersensitivity reactions in 20–35% (spectrum of urticaria to anaphylaxis), test dose recommended; rare GI toxicity (mild nausea/anorexia, pancreatitis)

Aspirin (Bayer, Ecotrin, St. Joseph) [OTC]   **Uses: Angina, CABG, PTCA, carotid endarterectomy, ischemic stroke, TIA, MI, arthritis, pain, HA, fever, inflammation, Kawasaki disease**   **Action:** Prostaglandin inhibitor   **Dose:** *Pain, fever:* 325–650 mg q4–6h PO or PR *RA:* 3–6 g/d PO in ÷ doses *Platelet inhibitory action:* 81–325 mg PO daily *Prevention of MI:* 81–325 mg PO daily; avoid use with CrCl < 10 mL/min and in severe liver disease   **Caution:** [C, M] Use linked to Reye's syndrome; avoid use with viral illness in children   **Contra:** Allergy to ASA, chickenpox or flu symptoms, syndrome of nasal polyps, asthma, rhinitis   **Supplied:** Tabs 325, 500 mg; chew tabs 81 mg; EC tabs 165, 325, 500, 650, 975 mg; SR tabs 650, 800 mg; effervescent tabs 325, 500 mg; supp 120, 200, 300, 600 mg   **SE:** GI upset and erosion   **Notes:** Discontinue use 1 wk before surgery to avoid postoperative bleeding complications; avoid or limit alcohol intake. See drug levels for salicylates (Table VII–16, p 000)

Aspirin and Butalbital Compound (Fiorinal, Others) [C-III]   **Uses: Tension HA, pain**   **Action:** Combination barbiturate and analgesic   **Dose:** 1–2 PO q4h PRN, max 6 tabs/d; avoid use with CrCl < 10 mL/min and in severe liver disease   **Caution:** [C (D if used for prolonged periods or high doses at term), ?]   **Contra:** Allergy to ASA, GI ulceration, bleeding disorder, porphyria, syndrome of nasal polyps, angioedema and bronchospasm to NSAIDs   **Supplied:** Caps Fiorgen PF, Fiorinal. Tabs Fiorinal, Lanorinal: ASA 325 mg/butalbital 50 mg/caffeine 40 mg **SE:** Drowsiness, dizziness, GI upset, ulceration, bleeding **Notes:** Butalbital habit-forming; avoid or limit alcohol intake

Aspirin + Butalbital, Caffeine, and Codeine (Fiorinal + Codeine) [C-III]
Uses: Mild pain; HA, especially when associated with stress **Action:** Sedative analgesic, narcotic analgesic **Dose:** 1–2 tabs (caps) PO q4–6h PRN **Caution:** [D, ?] **Contra:** Allergy to ASA **Supplied:** Each cap or tab contains 325 mg ASA, 40 mg caffeine, 50 mg of butalbital, codeine: No. 3 = 30 mg **SE:** Drowsiness, dizziness, GI upset, ulceration, bleeding

Aspirin + Codeine (Empirin No. 2, No. 3, No. 4) [C-III]
Uses: Mild to moderate pain **Action:** Combined effects of ASA and codeine **Dose:** 1–2 tabs PO q4–6h PRN **Caution:** [C, M] **Contra:** Allergy to ASA/codeine, PUD, bleeding, anticoagulant therapy, children with chickenpox or flu symptoms **Supplied:** Tabs 325 mg of ASA and codeine as in Notes **SE:** Drowsiness, dizziness, GI upset, ulceration, bleeding **Notes:** Codeine in No. 2 = 15 mg, No. 3 = 30 mg, No. 4 = 60 mg

Atazanavir (Reyataz)
WARNING: Hyperbilirubinemia may require drug discontinuation **Uses: HIV-1 infection** **Action:** Protease inhibitor **Dose:** 400 mg PO daily with food; when given with efavirenz 600 mg, administer atazanavir 300 mg + ritonavir 100 mg once daily; separate doses from buffered didanosine administration; reduce dose in hepatic impairment **Caution:** [B, –] Increases levels of statins, sildenafil, antiarrhythmics, warfarin, cyclosporine, TCAs; atazanavir concentrations reduced by St. John's wort **Contra:** Concomitant use of midazolam, triazolam, ergots, cisapride, pimozide **Supplied:** 100-, 150-, 200-mg capsules **SE:** Headache, nausea, vomiting, diarrhea, rash, abdominal pain, diabetes mellitus, photosensitivity, PR-interval prolongation **Notes:** May have lesser effects on cholesterol profile

Atenolol (Tenormin) [See Table VII–7, p 617]

Atomoxetine (Strattera)
WARNING: Severe liver injury may occur in rare cases. Discontinue in patients with jaundice or laboratory evidence of liver injury **Uses: ADHD** **Action:** Selective norepinephrine reuptake inhibitor **Dose:** Adults and children > 70 kg: 40 mg × 3 days, then titrate up to 80–100 mg divided daily–bid **Caution:** [C, ?/–] **Contra:** Narrow angle glaucoma, use with or within 2 wk of discontinuing an MAOI **Supplied:** Caps 10, 18, 25, 40, 60 mg **SE:** Hypertension, tachycardia, weight loss, sexual dysfunction **Notes:** ↓ dose with hepatic insufficiency, ↓ dose when used in combination with inhibitors of CYP2D6

Atorvastatin (Lipitor) [See Table VII–15, p 628]

Atovaquone (Mepron)
Uses: Treatment and prevention of PCP **Action:** Inhibits nucleic acid and ATP synthesis **Dose:** *Treatment:* 750 mg PO bid for 21 d *Prevention:* 1500 mg PO once/d. Take with meals **Caution:** [C, ?] **Supplied:** Suspension 750 mg/5 mL **SE:** Fever, HA, anxiety, insomnia, rash, N/V

Atovaquone/Proguanil (Malarone)
Uses: Prevention or treatment of *P falciparum* malaria **Action:** Antimalarial **Dose:** *Prevention:* 1 tab PO 2 d before, during, and 7 d after leaving endemic region; *Treatment:* 4 tabs PO as single dose qd × 3 d **Caution:** [C, ?] **Contra:** CrCl < 30 mL/min **Supplied:** Tab atovaquone 250 mg/proguanil 100 mg; pediatric 62.5/25 mg **SE:** HA, fever, myalgia

Atracurium (Tracrium)
Uses: Adjunct to anesthesia to facilitate ET intubation **Action:** Nondepolarizing neuromuscular blocker **Dose:** 0.4–0.5 mg/kg IV bolus, then 0.08–0.1 mg/kg q20–45 min PRN **Caution:** [C, ?] **Supplied:** Inj 10 mg/mL **SE:** Flushing **Notes:** Patient must be intubated and on controlled ventilation. Use adequate amounts of sedation and analgesia

Atropine
Uses: Preanesthetic; symptomatic bradycardia and asystole **Action:** Antimuscarinic agent; blocks acetylcholine at parasympathetic sites **Dose:** *Emergency cardiac care, bradycardia:* 0.5 mg –1 mg IV q3–5min up to 2 mg total; asystole 1 mg IV, repeat in 5 min *Preanesthetic:* 0.3–0.6 mg IM **Caution:** [C, +] **Contra:** Glaucoma **Supplied:** Tabs 0.3, 0.4, 0.6 mg; inj 0.05, 0.1, 0.3, 0.4, 0.5, 0.8, 1 mg/mL; ophthalmic 0.5, 1, 2% **SE:** Blurred vision, urinary retention, constipation, dried mucous membranes

Azathioprine (Imuran)   Uses: **Adjunct for the prevention of rejection following kidney transplantation; RA; SLE**   Action: Immunosuppressive agent; antagonizes purine metabolism   Dose: 1–3 mg/kg/d IV or PO (reduce in renal failure)   Caution: [D, ?]   Contra: Pregnancy   Supplied: Tabs 50 mg; inj 100 mg/20 mL   SE: GI intolerance, fever, chills, leukopenia, thrombocytopenia; chronic use may ↑ neoplasia   Notes: Inj should be handled with cytotoxic precautions; interaction with allopurinol; do not administer live vaccines to a patient taking azathioprine

Azelastine (Astelin, Optivar)   Uses: **Allergic rhinitis (rhinorrhea, sneezing, nasal pruritus); allergic conjunctivitis**   Action: Histamine H$_1$-receptor antagonist   Dose: *Nasal spray:* 2 sprays/nostril bid; *Ophthalmic solution:* 1 drop into each affected eye bid   Caution: [C, ?/–]   Supplied: Nasal spray 137 mcg/spray; ophthalmic solution 0.05%   SE: Somnolence, bitter taste

Azithromycin (Zithromax)   Uses: **Community-acquired pneumonia, pharyngitis, otitis media, skin infections, nongonococcal urethritis, and PID; treatment and prevention of MAC in HIV**   Action: Macrolide antibiotic; inhibits protein synthesis *Spectrum: Chlamydia, H ducreyi, H influenzae, Legionella, M catarrhalis, M pneumoniae, M hominis, N gonorrhoeae, S aureus, S agalactiae, S pneumoniae, S pyogenes* Dose: *Oral: Respiratory tract infections:* 500 mg day 1, then 250 mg/d PO × 4 d or 500 mg/d PO × 3 d *Nongonococcal urethritis:* 1 g PO single dose *Prevention of MAC:* 1200 mg PO once/wk *IV:* 500 mg × 2 d, then 500 mg PO × 7–10 d; take susp on empty stomach; tabs may be taken with or without food   Caution: [B, +]   Supplied: Tabs 250, 600 mg; Z-Pack (5-day regimen); Tri-Pak (500 mg tabs × 3); susp 1-g single-dose packet; susp 100, 200 mg/5 mL; inj 500 mg   SE: GI upset

Aztreonam (Azactam)   Uses: **Aerobic gram(–) bacterial UTIs, lower respiratory tract, intra-abdominal, skin, gynecologic infections, and septicemia**   Action: Monobactam antibiotic; inhibits cell wall synthesis *Spectrum:* Gram(–) coverage including *Pseudomonas, E coli, Klebsiella, H influenzae, Serratia, Proteus, Enterobacter, Citrobacter* Dose: 1–2 g IV/IM q6–12h; reduce dose in renal impairment   Caution: [B, +]   Supplied: Inj 500 mg, 1 g, 2 g   SE: N/V/D, rash, pain at injection site   Notes: No gram(+) or anaerobic activity; may be given to penicillin-allergic patients

Bacillus Calmette-Guerin (TheraCys, Tice BCG, Pacis)   Uses: **Bladder carcinoma, TB prophylaxis**   Action: Immunomodulator   Dose: Bladder CA, contents of 1 vial prepared and instilled in bladder for 2 h. Repeat once weekly for 6 wk; repeat 1 treatment at 3, 6, 12, 18, and 24 mo after initial therapy   Caution: [C, ?] Asthma   Contra: Immunosuppression, UTI steroid use, acute illness, fever of unknown origin   Supplied: Inj 81 mg (10.5 + 8.7 × 10^8 CFU)/vial (TheraCys), 1 to 8 × 10^8 CFU/vial (Tice BCG)   SE: *Intravesical:* Hematuria, urinary frequency, dysuria, bacterial UTI, rare BCG sepsis   Notes: Routine US adult BCG immunization not recommended; occasionally used in high-risk children who are PPD(–) and cannot take INH

Bacitracin, Topical (Baciguent); Bacitracin and Polymyxin B, Topical (Polysporin); Bacitracin, Neomycin, and Polymyxin B, Topical (Neosporin Ointment); Bacitracin, Neomycin, Polymyxin B, and Hydrocortisone, Topical (Cortisporin); Bacitracin, Neomycin, Polymyxin B, and Lidocaine, Topical (Clomycin)   Uses: **Prevention and treatment of minor skin infections**   Action: Topical antibiotic with added effects based on components (anti-inflammatory and analgesic)   Dose: Apply sparingly bid–qid   Caution: [C, ?]   Supplied: Bacitracin 500 units/g oint. Bacitracin 500 units/polymyxin B sulfate 10,000 units/g oint and powder. Bacitracin 400 units/neomycin 3.5 mg/polymyxin B 5000 units/g oint (for Neosporin Cream, see p 000). Bacitracin 400 units/neomycin 3.5 mg/polymyxin B/10,000 units/hydrocortisone 10 mg/g oint. Bacitracin 500 units/neomycin 3.5 g/ polymyxin B 5000 units/lidocaine 40 mg/g oint   Notes: Systemic and irrigation forms of bacitracin available but not generally used because of potential toxicity

Bacitracin, Ophthalmic (AK-Tracin Ophthalmic); Bacitracin and Polymyxin B, Ophthalmic (AK Poly Bac Ophthalmic, Polysporin Oph-

thalmic); **Bacitracin, Neomycin, and Polymixin B, Ophthalmic (AK Spore Ophthalmic, Neosporin Ophthalmic); Bacitracin, Neomycin, Polymyxin B, and Hydrocortisone, Ophthalmic (AK Spore HC Ophthalmic, Cortisporin Ophthalmic)** Uses: Blepharitis, conjunctivitis, prophylactic treatment of corneal abrasions **Action:** Topical antibiotic with added effects based on components (anti-inflammatory) **Dose:** Apply q3–4h into conjunctival sac **Caution:** [C, ?] **Contra:** Viral, mycobacterial, or fungal eye infection **Supplied:** See Topical equivalents this page

Baclofen (Lioresal) Uses: **Spasticity secondary to severe chronic disorders such as MS, ALS, or spinal cord lesions, trigeminal neuralgia** **Action:** Centrally acting skeletal muscle relaxant; inhibits transmission of both monosynaptic and polysynaptic reflexes at the spinal cord **Dose:** Initially, 5 mg PO tid; ↑ q3d to max effect; max 80 mg/d *Intrathecal:* Through implantable pump; adjust in renal impairment; avoid abrupt withdrawal; take with food or milk **Caution:** [C, +] Use caution in epilepsy and neuropsychiatric disturbances; withdrawal may occur with abrupt discontinuation **Supplied:** Tabs 10, 20 mg; IT inj 10 mg/20 mL, 10 mg/5 mL **SE:** Dizziness, drowsiness, insomnia, ataxia, weakness, hypotension

Balsalazide (Colazal) Uses: **Ulcerative colitis** **Action:** 5-Aminosalicylic acid derivative, anti-inflammatory; reduces leukotriene synthesis **Dose:** 2.25 g (3 caps) tid × 8–12 wk **Caution:** [B, ?] Severe renal/hepatic failure **Contra:** Hypersensitivity to mesalamine or salicylates **Supplied:** Caps 750 mg **SE:** Dizziness, HA, nausea, agranulocytosis, pancytopenia, renal impairment, allergic reactions **Notes:** Each daily dose of 6.75 g is equivalent to 2.4 g of mesalamine

Basiliximab (Simulect) Uses: **Prevention of acute organ transplant rejections** **Action:** IL-2 receptor antagonist **Dose:** 20 mg IV 2 h before transplantation, then 20 mg IV 4 d after transplantation **Caution:** [B, ?/–] **Contra:** Known hypersensitivity to murine proteins **Supplied:** Inj 20 mg **SE:** Edema, HTN, HA, dizziness, fever, pain, infection, GI effects, electrolyte disturbances **Notes:** Murine/human monoclonal antibody

Becaplermin (Regranex Gel) Uses: **Adjunct to local wound care in diabetic foot ulcers** **Action:** Recombinant human platelet derived growth factor (PDGF), enhanced formation of granulation tissue **Dose:** Based on size of lesion; 1½-in. ribbon from 2-g tube, ⅔ in. ribbon from 7.5- or 15-g tube/square inch of ulcer; apply and cover with moist gauze; rinse after 12 h; do not reapply; repeat process 12 h later **Caution:** [C, ?] **Contra:** Neoplasm or active infection at site **Supplied:** 0.01% gel in 2-, 7.5-, 15-g tubes **SE:** Erythema, local pain **Notes:** Use along with good wound care; wound must be vascularized

Beclomethasone (Beconase, Vancenase Nasal Inhaler) Uses: Allergic **rhinitis** refractory to conventional therapy with antihistamines and decongestants; **nasal polyps** **Action:** Inhaled steroid **Dose:** 1 spray intranasally bid–qid; *aqueous inhal:* 1–2 sprays/nostril qd–bid **Caution:** [C, ?] **Supplied:** Nasal met-dose inhaler **SE:** Local irritation, burning, epistaxis **Notes:** Nasal spray delivers 42 mcg/dose and 84 mcg/dose

Beclomethasone (QVAR) Uses: **Chronic asthma** **Action:** Inhaled corticosteroid **Dose:** 1–4 inhal BID (Rinse mouth/throat after use) **Caution:** [C, ?] **Contra:** Acute asthma exacerbation **Supplied:** Oral met-dose inhaler; 40, 80 mcg/inhal **SE:** HA, cough, hoarseness, oral candidiasis **Notes:** Not effective for acute asthmatic attacks

Belladonna and Opium Suppositories (B & O Supprettes) [C-II] Uses: **Bladder spasms; moderate/severe pain** **Action:** Antispasmodic **Dose:** Insert 1 supp PR q6h PRN. 15A = 30 mg powdered opium/16.2 mg belladonna extract. 16A = 60 mg powdered opium/16.2 mg belladonna extract **Caution:** [C, ?] **Supplied:** Supp 15A, 16A **SE:** Anticholinergic side effects (sedation, urinary retention, and constipation)

Benazepril (Lotensin) [See Table VII–3, p 614]

Benzocaine and Antipyrine (Auralgan) Uses: **Analgesia in severe otitis media** **Action:** Anesthetic and local decongestant **Dose:** Fill the ear and insert a moist cotton plug; repeat 1–2 h PRN **Caution:** [C, ?] **Contra:** Do not use with perforated eardrum **Supplied:** Soln **SE:** Local irritation

Benzonatate (Tessalon Perles) **Uses:** Symptomatic relief of cough **Action:** Anesthetizes the stretch receptors in the respiratory passages **Dose:** 100 mg PO tid **Caution:** [C, ?] **Supplied:** Caps 100 mg **SE:** Sedation, dizziness, GI upset **Notes:** Do not chew or puncture the caps

Benztropine (Cogentin) **Uses: Parkinsonism and drug-induced extrapyramidal disorders** **Action:** Partially blocks striatal cholinergic receptors **Dose:** 0.5–6 mg PO, IM, or IV in ÷ doses/d **Caution:** [C, ?] **Contra:** < 3 y **Supplied:** Tabs 0.5, 1, 2 mg; inj 1 mg/mL **SE:** Anticholinergic side effects **Notes:** Physostigmine 1–2 mg SC/IV can reverse severe symptoms

Betamethasone (Celestone) [See Table VII–2, p 613]

Betaxolol (Kerlone) [See Table VII–7, pp 617–18]

Betaxolol, Ophthalmic (Betoptic) [See Table VII–12, pp 624–25]

Bethanechol (Urecholine, Duvoid, others) **Uses: Neurogenic bladder atony with retention, acute postoperative and postpartum functional (nonobstructive) urinary retention** **Action:** Stimulates cholinergic smooth muscle receptors in bladder and GI tract **Dose:** 10–50 mg PO tid–qid or 2.5–5 mg SC tid–qid and PRN (take on empty stomach) **Caution:** [C, ?/–] **Contra:** Bladder outlet obstruction, PUD, epilepsy, hyperthyroidism, bradycardia, COPD, AV conduction defects, parkinsonism, hypotension, vasomotor instability **Supplied:** Tabs 5, 10, 25, 50 mg; inj 5 mg/mL **SE:** Abdominal cramps, diarrhea, salivation, hypotension **Notes:** Do not administer IM or IV

Bicalutamide (Casodex) **Uses: Advanced prostate CA (in combination with GnRH agonists such as leuprolide or goserelin)** **Action:** Nonsteroidal antiandrogen **Dose:** 50 mg/d **Caution:** [X, ?] **Contra:** Women **Supplied:** Caps 50 mg **SE:** Hot flashes, loss of libido, impotence, diarrhea, N/V, gynecomastia, and LFT elevation

Bisacodyl (Dulcolax) [OTC] **Uses: Constipation; preoperative bowel preparation** **Action:** Stimulates peristalsis **Dose:** 5–15 mg PO or 10 mg PR PRN; (Do not chew tabs; do not give within 1 h of antacids or milk) **Caution:** [B, ?] **Contra:** Acute abdomen or bowel obstruction, appendicitis, gastroenteritis **Supplied:** EC tabs 5 mg; supp 10 mg **SE:** Abdominal cramps, proctitis, and inflammation with suppositories

Bismuth Subsalicylate (Pepto-Bismol) [OTC] **Uses: Indigestion, nausea, and diarrhea; combination for treatment of H pylori infection** **Action:** Antisecretory and antiinflammatory effects **Dose:** 2 tabs or 30 mL PO PRN (max 8 doses/24 h); avoid in patients with renal failure **Caution:** [C, D (3rd trimester), –] **Contra:** Influenza or chickenpox (↑ risk of Reye's syndrome), ASA allergy **Supplied:** Chew tabs 262 mg; liq 262, 524 mg/15 mL **SE:** May turn tongue and stools black

Bisoprolol (Zebeta) [See Table VII–7, pp 617–18]

Bitolterol (Tornalate) **Uses: Prophylaxis and Rx of asthma and reversible bronchospasm** **Action:** Sympathomimetic bronchodilator; stimulates β_2-adrenergic receptors in the lungs **Dose:** 2 inhal q8h **Caution:** [C, ?] **Supplied:** Aerosol 0.8% **SE:** Dizziness, nervousness, trembling, HTN, palpitations

Bivalirudin (Angiomax) **Uses: Anticoagulant used with ASA in unstable angina undergoing PTCA** **Action:** Anticoagulant, direct thrombin inhibitor **Dose:** 1 mg/kg IV bolus, then 2.5 mg/kg/h over 4 h; if needed, use 0.2 mg/kg/h for up to 20 h. Give with aspirin 300–325 mg/day; start pre-PTCA; adjust dose in renal impairment **Caution:** [B, ?] **Contra:** Major bleeding **Supplied:** Powder for inj **SE:** Bleeding, back pain, nausea, HA

Bleomycin Sulfate (Blenoxane) **Uses: Testicular carcinomas; Hodgkin's lymphoma and NHL; cutaneous lymphomas; and squamous cell carcinomas of the head and neck, larynx, cervix, skin, penis; sclerosing agent for malignant pleural effusion** **Action:** Induces breakage (scission) of single- and double-stranded DNA **Dose:** 10–20 units/m^2 1–2/wk (refer to specific protocols); adjust in renal impairment   **Supplied:** Inj 15 units/vial   **Caution:** [D, ?] Severe pulmonary disease   **SE:** Hyperpigmentation (skin staining) and hypersensitivity (rash to anaphylaxis); fever in 50%; lung toxicity (idiosyncratic and dose related); pneumonitis may progress to fibrosis; Raynaud's phenomenon, N/V   **Notes:** Test dose of 1 unit recommended, especially in lymphoma patients; lung toxicity likely when the total dose > 400 units

Bortezomib (Velcade)   WARNING: May worsen pre-existing neuropathy   Uses: Progression of multiple myeloma despite two previous treatments   Action: Proteasome inhibitor   Dose: 1.3 mg/m^2 bolus IV twice weekly for 2 wk, with 10-day rest period (= 1 cycle); adjust for hematologic toxicity, neuropathy   Caution: [D, ?/–]   Supplied: 3.5 mg vial   SE: Asthenia, GI upset, anorexia, dyspnea, headache, orthostatic hypotension, edema, insomnia, dizziness, rash, pyrexia, arthralgia, neuropathy   Notes: May interact with drugs metabolized via CYP450 system

Brimonidine (Alphagan) [See Table VII–12, p 623–25]

Brinzolamide (Azopt) [See Table VII–12, pp 623–25]

Bromocriptine (Parlodel)   Uses: Parkinson's syndrome, hyperprolactinemia, acromegaly, pituitary tumors   Action: Direct-acting on the striatal dopamine receptors; inhibits prolactin secretion   Dose: Initially, 1.25 mg PO bid; titrate to effect   Caution: [C, ?]   Contra: Severe ischemic heart disease or peripheral vascular disease   Supplied: Tabs 2.5 mg; caps 5 mg   SE: Hypotension, Raynaud's phenomenon, dizziness, nausea, hallucinations

Budesonide (Rhinocort, Pulmicort)   Uses: Allergic and nonallergic rhinitis, asthma   Action: Steroid   Dose: *Intranasal:* 2 sprays/nostril bid or 4 sprays/nostril/d *Aqueous:* 1 spray/nostril/d *Oral inhaled:* 1–4 inhal bid; (Rinse mouth after oral use)   Caution: [C, ?/–]   Supplied: Met-dose inhal, Turbuhaler, nasal inhaler, and aqueous spray   SE: HA, cough, hoarseness, *Candida* infection, epistaxis

Bumetanide (Bumex)   Uses: Edema from CHF, hepatic cirrhosis, and renal disease   Action: Loop diuretic; inhibits reabsorption of sodium and chloride in the ascending loop of Henle and the distal renal tubule   Dose: 0.5–2 mg/d PO; 0.5–1 mg IV q8–24h (max 10 mg/d)   Caution: [D, ?]   Contra: Anuria, hepatic coma, severe electrolye depletion   Supplied: Tabs 0.5, 1, 2 mg; inj 0.25 mg/mL   SE: Hypokalemia, hyperuricemia, hypochloremia, hyponatremia, dizziness, increased serum creatinine, ototoxicity   Notes: Monitor fluid and electrolyte status during treatment

Bupivacaine (Marcaine)   Uses: Local, regional, and spinal anesthesia, local and regional analgesia   Action: Local anesthetic   Dose: Dose-dependent on procedure, tissue vascularity, depth of anesthesia, and degree of muscle relaxation required   Caution: [C, ?]   Contra: Severe bleeding, severe hypotension, shock and arrhythmias, local infections at anesthesia site, septicemia   Supplied: Inj 0.25, 0.5, 0.75%   SE: Hypotension, bradycardia, dizziness, anxiety

Buprenorphine (Buprenex) [C-V]   Uses: Moderate/severe pain   Action: Opiate agonist-antagonist   Dose: 0.3–0.6 mg IM or slow IV push q6h PRN   Caution: [C, ?/–]   Supplied: Inj 0.324 mg/mL (= 0.3 mg of buprenorphine)   SE: Sedation, hypotension, respiratory depression   Notes: May induce withdrawal syndrome in opioid-dependent patients

Bupropion (Wellbutrin, Wellbutrin SR, Wellbutrin XL, Zyban) WARNING: *Pediatric:* Antidepressants may increase risk of suicidality; consider risks and benefits of use. Patients should be closely monitored for clinical worsening, suicidality, or unusual changes in behavior   Uses: Depression, adjunct to smoking cessation   Action: Weak inhibitor of neuronal uptake of serotonin and norepinephrine; inhibits the neuronal reuptake of dopamine   Dose: *Depression:* 100–450 mg/d ÷ bid–tid; SR 100-200 mg bid; XL 150–300 mg daily; *Smoking cessation:* 150 mg/d × 3 d, then 150 mg bid × 8–12 wk; ↓ in renal/hepatic impairment   Caution: [B, ?/–]   Contra: Seizure disorder, prior diagnosis of anorexia nervosa or bulimia, MAOI, abrupt discontinuation of alcohol or sedatives   Supplied: Tabs 75, 100 mg; SR tabs

100, 150, 200 mg; XL tabs 150, 300 mg   **SE:** Associated with seizures; agitation, insomnia, HA, tachycardia   **Notes:** Avoid use of alcohol and other CNS depressants

Buspirone (BuSpar)   **Uses: Short-term relief of anxiety**   **Action:** Antianxiety agent; selectively antagonizes CNS serotonin receptors   **Dose:** 5–10 mg PO tid; ↑ to desired response; usual dose 20–30 mg/d; max 60 mg/d; reduce dose in severe hepatic/renal insufficiency   **Caution:** [B, ?/–]   **Supplied:** Tabs 5, 10, 15, 30 mg dividose   **SE:** Drowsiness, dizziness; HA, nausea   **Notes:** No abuse potential or physical or psychologic dependence

Busulfan (Myleran, Busulfex)   **Uses: CML, preparative regimens for allogeneic and autologous BMT in high doses**   **Action:** Alkylating agent   **Dose:** Refer to specific protocols   **Caution:** [D, ?]   **Supplied:** Tabs 2 mg, inj 60 mg/10 mL   **SE:** Myelosuppression, pulmonary fibrosis, nausea (high-dose therapy), gynecomastia, adrenal insufficiency, and skin hyperpigmentation

Butorphanol (Stadol) [C-IV]   **Uses: Anesthesia adjunct, pain, and migraine headaches**   **Action:** Opiate agonist-antagonist with central analgesic actions   **Dose:** *Pain:* 1–4 mg IM or IV q3–4h PRN *Headaches:* 1 spray in 1 nostrll, may repeat × 1 if pain not relieved in 60–90 min; reduce dose in renal impairment   **Caution:** [C (D if used in high doses or for prolonged periods at term), +]   **Supplied:** Inj 1, 2 mg/mL; nasal spray 10 mg/ mL   **SE:** Drowsiness, dizziness, nasal congestion   **Notes:** May induce withdrawal in opioid-dependent patients

Calcipotriene (Dovonex)   **Uses: Plaque psoriasis**   **Action:** Keratolytic   **Dose:** Apply bid   **Caution:** [C, ?]   **Contra:** Hypercalcemia; vitamin D toxicity; do not apply to face   **Supplied:** Cream; oint; soln 0.005%   **SE:** Skin irritation, dermatitis

Calcitonin (Cibacalcin, Miacalcin)   **Uses: Paget's disease of bone; hypercalcemia; osteogenesis imperfecta, postmenopausal osteoporosis**   **Action:** Polypeptide hormone   **Dose:** *Paget's (salmon form):* 100 units/d IM/SC initially, 50 units/d or 50–100 units q 1–3d maintenance *Paget's (human form):* 0.5 mg/d initially; maintenance 0.5 mg 2–3 times/wk or 0.25 mg/d, max 0.5 mg bid *Hypercalcemia (salmon calcitonin):* 4 units/kg IM/SC q12h; ↑ to 8 units/kg q12h, max q6h *Osteoporosis (salmon calcitonin):* 100 units/d IM/SC; intranasal 200 units = 1 nasal spray/d   **Caution:** [C, ?]   **Supplied:** Spray, nasal 200 units/activation; inj, human (Cibacalcin) 0.5 mg/ vial, salmon 200 units/mL (2 mL)   **SE:** Facial flushing, nausea, edema at injection site, nasal irritation, polyuria   **Notes:** Human (Cibacalcin) and salmon forms; human only approved for Paget's bone disease

Calcitriol (Rocaltrol)   **Uses: Reduction of elevated parathyroid hormone levels, hypocalcemia associated with dialysis**   **Action:** 1,25-Dihydroxycholecalciferol, a vitamin D analogue   **Dose:** *Renal failure:* 0.25 mcg/d PO, ↑0.25 mcg/d q4–6wk PRN; 0.5 mcg 3×/wk IV, ↑ PRN *Hyperparathyroidism:* 0.5–2 mcg/d   **Caution:** [C, ?]   **Contra:** Hypercalcemia; vitamin D toxicity   **Supplied:** Inj 1, 2 mcg/mL (in 1-mL volume); caps 0.25, 0.5 mcg   **SE:** Hypercalcemia possible   **Notes:** Monitor dosing to keep Ca$^+$ WNL

Calcium Acetate (Calphron, Phos-Ex, PhosLo)   **Uses: ESRD-associated hyperphosphatemia**   **Action:** Ca supplement to treat ESRD hyperphosphatemia without aluminum   **Dose:** 2–4 tabs PO with meals   **Caution:** [C, ?]   **Contra:** Hypercalcemia   **Supplied:** Caps Phos-Ex 500 mg (125 mg Ca); tabs Calphron and PhosLo 667 mg (169 mg Ca)   **SE:** Can cause ↑ Ca^{2+}, hypophosphatemia, constipation   **Notes:** Monitor Ca^{2+} levels

Calcium Carbonate (Tums, Alka-Mints) [OTC]   **Uses: Hyperacidity associated with peptic ulcer disease, hiatal hernia,** etc   **Action:** Neutralizes gastric acid   **Dose:** 500 mg–2 g PO PRN; adjust in renal impairment   **Caution:** [C, ?]   **Supplied:** Chew tabs 350, 420, 500, 550, 750, 850 mg; susp   **SE:** Hypercalcemia, hypophosphatemia, constipation

Calcium Salts (Chloride, Gluconate, Gluceptate)   **Uses: Ca replacement, VF, Ca blocker toxicity, Mg^{2+} intoxication, tetany, hyperphosphatemia in ESRD**   **Action:** Calcium supplement/replacement, increased myocardial contractility, binding phosphate   **Dose:** *Replacement:* 1–2 g/d PO *Cardiac emergencies:* CaCl 0.5–1 g IV q 10 min or Ca gluconate 1–2 g IV q 10 min *Hyperphosphatemia in end-stage renal disease*: 2 tabs with each meal **Caution:** [C, ?] **Contra:** Hypercalcemia **Supplied:** CaCl inj 10% = 100 mg/mL = Ca 27.2 mg/mL = 10-mL ampule. Ca gluconate inj 10% = 100 mg/mL = Ca 9 mg/mL; tabs 500 mg = 45 mg Ca, 650 mg = 58.5 mg Ca, 975 mg = 87.75 mg Ca, 1 g = 90 mg Ca. Ca glucep-tate inj 220 mg/mL = 18 mg/mL Ca **SE:** Bradycardia, cardiac arrhythmias, hypercalcemia **Notes:** CaCl contains 270 mg (13.6 mEq) elemental Ca/g, and calcium gluconate contains 90 mg (4.5 mEq) Ca/g. RDA for Ca: Adults = 800 mg/d

Candesartan (Atacand) [See Table VII–4, p 615]

Capecitabine (Xeloda) WARNING: Clinically significant increases in INR have been observed with concomitant use of Xeloda and Warfarin—frequent monitoring of INR is neces-sary: **Uses: Metastatic breast cancer and colorectal cancer Action:** Enzymatically converted to 5-fluorouracil; inhibitor of thymidylate synthetase **Dose:** Refer to specific proto-cols; adjust in renal impairment **Caution:** [D, –] **Contra:** Known dihydropyrimidine dehy-drogenase (DPD) deficiency; severe renal impairment **Supplied:** Tabs 150, 500 mg **SE:** N/V/D, stomatitis, hand-and-foot syndrome, neutropenia, fever

Capsaicin (Capsin, Zostrix, others) [OTC] **Uses: Pain due to postherpetic neuralgia, chronic neuralgia, arthritis, diabetic neuropathy, postoperative pain, psoria-sis, intractable pruritus Action:** Topical analgesic **Dose:** Apply tid–qid **Caution:** [?, ?] **Supplied:** OTC creams; gel; lotions; roll-ons **SE:** Local irritation, neurotoxicity, cough

Captopril (Capoten) [See Table VII–3, p 614]

Carbachol (Isopto Carbachol) [See Table VII–12, pp 623–25]

Carbamazepine (Tegretol) WARNING: Aplastic anemia and agranulosytosis have been reported with carbamazepine **Uses: Epilepsy, trigeminal neuralgia, alcohol with-drawal Action:** Anticonvulsant **Dose:** Initially, 200 mg PO bid; ↑ by 200 mg/d; usual 800–1200 mg/d in ÷ doses; reduce dose in renal impairment; take with food **Caution:** [D, +] **Contra:** MAOI use, history of bone marrow depression **Supplied:** Tabs 200 mg; chew tabs 100 mg; XR tabs 100, 200, 400 mg; susp 100 mg/5 mL **SE:** Drowsiness, dizziness, blurred vision, N/V, rash, hyponatremia, leukopenia, agranulocytosis **Notes:** Monitor CBC and serum levels (see Table VII–17, p 000); generic products not interchangeable

Carbidopa/Levodopa (Sinemet) **Uses: Parkinson's disease Action:** ↑ CNS levels of dopamine **Dose:** 25/100 mg bid–qid; ↑ as needed (max 200/2000 mg/d) **Cau-tion:** [C, ?] **Contra:** Narrow-angle glaucoma, suspicious skin lesion (may activate melanoma), melanoma, MAOI use **Supplied:** Tabs (mg carbidopa/mg levodopa) 10/100, 25/100, 25/250; tabs SR (mg carbidopa/mg levodopa) 25/100, 50/200 **SE:** Psychiatric distur-bances, orthostatic hypotension, dyskinesias, and cardiac arrhythmias

Carboplatin (Paraplatin) **Uses: Ovarian, lung, head and neck, testicular, urothe-lial and brain CAs, NHL and allogeneic and autologous BMT in high doses Action:** DNA cross-linker; forms DNA-platinum adducts **Dose:** Refer to specific protocols **Cau-tion:** [D, ?] **Contra:** Severe bone marrow suppression, excessive bleeding **Supplied:** Inj 50, 150, 450 mg **SE:** Myelosuppression, N/V/D, nephrotoxicity, hematuria, neurotoxicity, ↑ LFTs **Notes:** Physiologic dosing based on either Culvert's or Egorin's formula allows for larger doses with reduced toxicity

Carisoprodol (Soma) **Uses: Adjunct to sleep and physical therapy for the relief of painful musculoskeletal conditions Action:** Centrally acting muscle relaxant **Dose:** 350 mg PO tid–qid **Caution:** [C, M] tolerance may result; caution in renal/hepatic impair-ment **Contra:** Hypersensitivity to meprobamate; acute intermittent porphyria **Supplied:** Tabs 350 mg **SE:** CNS depression; drowsiness; dizziness, tachycardia **Notes:** Avoid alco-hol and other CNS depressants; available in combination with ASA or codeine

Carmustine [BCNU] (BiCNU; Gliadel) **Uses: Primary brain tumors, melanoma, Hodgkin's and non-Hodgkin's lymphomas, multiple myeloma, and induction for allogeneic and autologous BMT in high doses; adjunct to surgery in patients with recurrent glioblastoma multiforme Action:** Alkylating agent; nitrosourea forms DNA

cross-links; inhibitor of DNA synthesis   **Dose:** Refer to specific protocols; dosage adjustment may be necessary in hepatic impairment   **Caution:** [D, ?] Administer with caution in patients with depressed platelet, leukocyte, or erythrocyte counts, renal or hepatic impairment   **Contra:** Myelosuppression; pregnancy   **Supplied:** Inj 100 mg/vial; wafer: 7.7 mg   **SE:** Hypotension, N/V, myelosuppression (especially leukocytes and platelets), phlebitis, facial flushing, hepatic and renal dysfunction, pulmonary fibrosis, and optic neuroretinitis. Hematologic toxicity may persist up to 4–6 wk after dose   **Notes:** Do not give courses more frequently than every 6 wk because toxicity is cumulative. Baseline pulmonary function tests are recommended

Carteolol (Cartrol) [See Table VII–7, pp 617–18]

Carteolol (Ocupress) [See Table VII–12, pp 623–25]

Carvedilol (Coreg) [See Table VII–7, pp 617–18]

Caspofungin (Cancidas)   Uses: **Invasive aspergillosis refractory/intolerant to standard therapy, esophageal candidiasis**   **Action:** An echinocandin; inhibits fungal cell wall synthesis; highest activity in regions of active cell growth   **Dose:** 70 mg IV load day 1, 50 mg/d IV; slow infusion; adjust dose in hepatic impairment   **Caution:** [C, ?/–] Do not use with cyclosporine; has not been studied as initial therapy   **Contra:** Hypersensitivity to any component   **Supplied:** IV infusion   **SE:** Fever, HA, N/V, thrombophlebitis at injection site, altered LFTs   **Notes:** Monitor during infusion; limited experience beyond 2 wk of therapy

Cefaclor (Ceclor) [See Table VII–9, p 619]

Cefadroxil (Duricef, Ultracef) [See Table VII–8, p 619]

Cefazolin (Ancef, Kefzol) [See Table VII–8, p 619]

Cefdinir (Omnicef) [See Table VII–10, p 620]

Cefditoren (Spectracef) [See Table VII–10, p 620]

Cefepime (Maxipime) [See Table VII–10, p 620]

Cefixime (Suprax) [See Table VII–10, p 620]

Cefoperazone (Cefobid) [See Table VII–10, p 620]

Cefotaxime (Claforan) [See Table VII–10, p 620]

Cefotetan (Cefotan) [See Table VII–9, p 619]

Cefoxitin (Mefoxin) [See Table VII–9, p 619]

Cefpodoxime (Vantin) [See Table VII–10, p 620]

Cefprozil (Cefzil) [See Table VII–9, p 619]

Ceftazidime (Fortaz, Ceptaz, Tazidime, Tazicef) [See Table VII–10, p 620]

Ceftibuten (Cedax) [See Table VII–10, p 620]

Ceftizoxime (Cefizox) [See Table VII–10, p 620]

Ceftriaxone (Rocephin) [See Table VII–10, p 620]

Cefuroxime (Ceftin [oral], Zinacef [parenteral]) [See Table VII–9, p 619]

Celecoxib (Celebrex) [See Table VII–11, pp 621–22]

Cephalexin (Keflex, Keftab) [See Table VII–8, p 619]

Cephradine (Velosef) [See Table VII–8, p 619]

Cetirizine (Zyrtec) Uses: **Allergic rhinitis and other allergic symptoms including urticaria**   **Action:** Nonsedating antihistamine   **Dose:** 5–10 mg/d; ↓ dosage in renal/hepatic

impairment **Caution:** [B, ?/–] Use with caution in elderly and nursing mothers; doses > 10 mg/day may cause drowsiness **Contra:** Hypersensitivity to cetirizine, hydroxyzine **Supplied:** Tabs 5, 10 mg; syrup 5 mg/5 mL **SE:** HA, drowsiness, dry mouth **Notes:** Can cause sedation

Cevimeline HCL (Evoxac) **Uses:** Treatment of symptoms of dry mouth in patients with Sjögren's syndrome **Action:** A cholinergic agent **Dose:** 30 mg tid **Caution:** [C, ?/–] history of nephrolithiasis or cholelithiasis **Contra:** Uncontrolled asthma, narrow angle glaucoma **Supplied:** Caps 30 mg **SE:** Excessive sweating, salivation, rhinitis, nausea, visual disturbances, alteration in cardiac conduction and/or heart rate

Charcoal, Activated (Superchar, Actidose, Liqui-Char) **Uses:** Emergency treatment in poisoning by most drugs and chemicals **Action:** Adsorbent detoxicant **Dose:** *Acute intoxication:* 30–100 g/dose *GI dialysis:* 20–50 g q6h for 1–2 days; also give 70% sorbitol solution (2 mL/kg body weight). Repeated use of sorbitol not recommended **Caution:** [C, ?] If ipecac used, induce vomiting with ipecac before administering charcoal; may cause vomiting, which is hazardous in petroleum distillate and caustic ingestions; do not mix with milk, ice cream, or sherbet **Contra:** Not effective for cyanide, mineral acids, caustic alkalis, organic solvents, iron, ethanol, methanol lithium poisoning. Do not use sorbitol in patients with fructose intolerance **Supplied:** Powder, liq, caps **SE:** Some liq dosage forms in sorbitol base (a cathartic); vomiting, diarrhea, black stools, constipation **Notes:** Charcoal with sorbitol not recommended in children < 1yr; monitor for hypokalemia and hypomagnesemia; protect the airway in lethargic or comatose patients

Chlorambucil (Leukeran) **Uses:** CLL, Hodgkin's disease, Waldenström's macroglobulinemia **Action:** Alkylating agent **Dose:** Refer to specific protocol **Caution:** [D, ?] Use with caution in patients with seizure disorder and bone marrow suppression; affects human fertility **Contra:** Previous resistance; hypersensitivity to alkylating agents **Supplied:** Tabs 2 mg **SE:** Myelosuppression, CNS stimulation, N/V, drug fever, skin rash, chromosomal damage that can result in secondary leukemias, alveolar dysplasia, pulmonary fibrosis, hepatotoxicity **Notes:** Monitor LFTs, CBC, leukocyte counts, platelets, serum uric acid; reduce initial dosage if patient has received radiation therapy

Chloramphenicol, Ophthalmic (Chloromycetin Ophthalmic) [See Table VII–12, pp 623–25]

Chlordiazepoxide (Librium) [C-IV] **Uses:** Anxiety, tension, alcohol withdrawal, and preoperative apprehension **Action:** Benzodiazepine; antianxiety agent **Dose:** *Mild anxiety:* 5–10 mg PO tid–qid or PRN *Severe anxiety:* 25–50 mg IM, IV, or PO q6–8h or PRN *Alcohol withdrawal:* 50–100 mg IM or IV; repeat in 2–4 h if needed up to 300 mg in 24 h; gradually taper the daily dosage; adjust dose in renal impairment **Caution:**[D, ?] **Contra:** Pre-existing CNS depression **Supplied:** Caps 5, 10, 25 mg; tabs 10, 25 mg; inj 100 mg **SE:** Drowsiness, CP, rash, fatigue, memory impairment, xerostomia, weight gain **Notes:** Erratic IM absorption; reduce dose in the elderly; avoid in hepatic impairment

Chlorothiazide (Diuril) **Uses:** HTN, edema **Action:** Thiazide diuretic **Dose:** 500 mg–1 g PO or IV daily–bid **Caution:** [D, +] Do not administer inj IM or SQ **Contra:** Cross-sensitivity to thiazides/sulfonamides, anuria **Supplied:** Tabs 250, 500 mg; susp 250 mg/5 mL; inj 500 mg/vial **SE:** Hypokalemia, hyponatremia, dizziness, hyperglycemia, hyperuricemia, hyperlipidemia, photosensitivity **Notes:** May be taken with food/milk; take early in the day to avoid nocturia; use sunblock; monitor serum electrolytes

Chlorpheniramine (Chlor-Trimeton, Others) [OTC] **Uses:** Allergic reactions; common cold **Action:** Antihistamine **Dose:** 4 mg PO q4–6h or 8–12 mg PO bid of SR **Caution:** [C, ?/–] bladder obstruction; narrow-angle glaucoma; hepatic insufficiency **Contra:** Hypersensitivity **Supplied:** Tabs 4 mg; chew tabs 2 mg; SR tabs 8, 12 mg; syrup 2 mg/5 mL; inj 10, 100 mg/mL **SE:** Anticholinergic SE and sedation common, postural hypotension, QT changes, extrapyramidal reactions, photosensitivity

Chlorpromazine (Thorazine) **Uses:** Psychotic disorders, N/V, apprehension, intractable hiccups **Action:** Phenothiazine antipsychotic; antiemetic **Dose:** *Acute anxiety, agitation:* 10–25 mg PO or PR bid–tid (usual 30–800 mg/d in ÷ doses) *Severe symptoms:* 25 mg IM, may repeat in 1 h; then 25–50 mg PO or PR tid *Hiccups:* 25–50 mg PO bid–tid **Caution:** [C, ?/–] Avoid in hepatic impairment; caution in those with seizures; bone marrow suppression **Contra:** Cross-sensitivity with other phenothiazines may exist; avoid use in patients with narrow-angle glaucoma **Supplied:** Tabs 10, 25, 50, 100, 200 mg; SR caps 30, 75, 150 mg; syrup 10 mg/5 mL; conc 30, 100 mg/mL; supp 25, 100 mg; inj 25 mg/mL **SE:** Extrapyramidal SE and sedation; α-adrenergic blocking properties; hypotension; prolongs QT interval **Notes:** Do not stop abruptly; oral concentrate must be diluted in 2–4 oz of liquid

Chlorpropamide (Diabinese) [See Table VII–13, p 626]

Chlorthalidone (Hygroton, Others) **Uses:** HTN, edema associated with CHF **Action:** Thiazide diuretic **Dose:** 50–100 mg PO q day; reduce dose in renal impairment **Caution:** [D, +] **Contra:** Cross-sensitivity with other thiazides or sulfonamides; anuria **Supplied:** Tabs 15, 25, 50, 100 mg **SE:** Hypokalemia, dizziness, photosensitivity, hyperglycemia, hyperuricemia, sexual dysfunction **Notes:** May take with food/milk

Chlorzoxazone (Paraflex, Parafon Forte DSC, Others) **Uses:** Adjunct to rest and physical therapy for the relief of discomfort associated with acute, painful musculoskeletal conditions **Action:** Centrally acting skeletal muscle relaxant **Dose:** 250–500 mg PO tid–qid **Caution:** [C, ?] Avoid alcohol and CNS depressants **Contra:** Severe liver disease **Supplied:** Tabs 250; caps 250, 500 mg **SE:** Drowsiness, tachycardia, dizziness, hepatotoxicity, angioedema

Cholecalciferol [Vitamin D3] (Delta D) **Uses:** Dietary supplement for treatment of vitamin D deficiency **Action:** Enhances intestinal calcium absorption **Dose:** 400–1000 IU/d PO **Caution:** [A (D doses above the RDA), +] **Contra:** Hypercalcemia; hypervitaminosis; hypersensitivity **Supplied:** Tabs 400, 1000 IU **SE:** Vitamin D toxicity (renal failure, HTN, psychosis) **Notes:** 1 mg of cholecalciferol = 40,000 IU of vitamin D activity

Cholestyramine (Questran) **Uses:** Hypercholesterolemia; treatment of pruritus associated with partial biliary obstruction; diarrhea associated with excess fecal bile acids **Action:** Binds intestinal bile acids to form insoluble complexes **Dose:** Individualize: 4 g/d–bid (↑ to max 24 g/d and 6 doses/d) **Caution:** [C, ?] Caution in patients with constipation and phenylketonuria **Contra:** Avoid in complete biliary obstruction; hypolipoproteinemia types III, IV, V **Supplied:** 4 g of cholestyramine resin/9 g of powder; with aspartame: 4 g resin/5 g of powder **SE:** Constipation, abdominal pain, bloating, HA, rash **Notes:** Overdose may result in GI obstruction; mix 4 g of cholestyramine in 2–6 oz of noncarbonated beverage; take other meds 1–2 h before or 6 h after cholestyramine

Ciclopirox (Loprox) **Uses:** Tinea pedis, tinea cruris, tinea corporis, cutaneous candidiasis, tinea versicolor **Action:** Antifungal antibiotic **Dose:** *Adults & Peds > 10:* Massage into affected area bid **Caution:** [B, ?] **Supplied:** Cream; lotion 1% **SE:** Pruritus, local irritation, burning **Notes:** Discontinue if irritation occurs; avoid occlusive wrappings or dressings

Cidofovir (Vistide) **WARNING:** Renal impairment is the major toxicity. Follow administration instructions **Uses: CMV retinitis in patients with HIV** **Action:** Selective inhibition of viral DNA synthesis **Dose:** *Treatment:* 5 mg/kg IV over 1 h once/wk for 2 wk; administered with probenecid; *Maintenance:* 5 mg/kg IV once/2 wk; administered with probenecid *Probenecid:* 2 g PO 3 h prior to cidofovir, and then 1 g PO at 2 h and 8 h after cidofovir; decrease dose in renal impairment **Caution:** [C, –] SCr > 1.5 mg/dL or CrCl = 55 mL/min or urine protein > 100 mg/dL; other nephrotoxic drugs **Contra:** Hypersensitivity to probenecid or sulfa **Supplied:** Inj 75 mg/mL **SE:** Renal toxicity, chills, fever, HA, N/V/D, thrombocytopenia, neutropenia **Notes:** Hydrate with NS prior to each infusion

Cilostazol (Pletal) **Uses: Reduce symptoms of intermittent claudication** **Action:** Phosphodiesterase III inhibitor. Increases cAMP in platelets and blood vessels, leading to inhibition of platelet aggregation and vasodilation **Dose:** 100 mg PO bid, taken 30 min before or

2 h after breakfast and dinner   **Caution:** [C, +/–] Dosage adjustments may be necessary when used in conjunction with other drugs known to inhibit CYP3A4 and CYP2C19   **Contra:** Use in patients with CHF of any severity   **Supplied:** Tabs 50, 100 mg   **SE:** HA, palpitation, diarrhea

Cimetidine (Tagamet, Tagamet HB [OTC])   **Uses:** Duodenal ulcer; ulcer prophylaxis in hypersecretory states, e.g., trauma, burns, surgery; and GERD   **Action:** H_2-receptor antagonist   **Dose:** *Active ulcer:* 2400 mg/d IV cont inf or 300 mg IV q6h; 400 mg PO bid or 800 mg hs *Maintenance:* 400 mg PO hs *GERD:* 800 mg PO bid; maintenance 800 mg PO hs; ↑ dosing interval with renal insufficiency; ↓ dose in the elderly   **Caution:** [B, +] Many drug interactions (p-450 system)   **Supplied:** Tabs 200, 300, 400, 800 mg; liq 300 mg/5 mL; inj 300 mg/2 mL   **SE:** Dizziness, HA, agitation, thrombocytopenia, gynecomastia   **Notes:** Take 1 h before or 2 h after antacids; avoid excessive alcohol

Ciprofloxacin (Cipro)   **Uses:** Treatment of lower respiratory tract, sinuses, skin and skin structure, bone/joints, and urinary tract including prostatitis **Spectrum:** Effective against susceptible strains of *Pseudomonas*, complicated gram(–) infections due to *E coli*, *P mirabilis*, *K pneumoniae*, *Campylobacter jejuni* or *Shigella*   **Action:** Quinolone antibiotic; inhibits DNA gyrase   **Dose:** 250–750 mg PO q12h; XR 500-1000 mg PO q24h; or 200–400 mg IV q12h; adjust in renal impairment   **Caution:** [C, ?/–] Children < 18 y   **Supplied:** Tabs 100, 250, 500, 750 mg; Tabs XR 500, 1000 mg; susp 5 g/100 mL, 10 g/100 mL; inj 200, 400 mg   **SE:** Restlessness, N/V/D, rash, ruptured tendons, ↑ LFTs   **Notes:** Avoid antacids; reduce/restrict caffeine intake; little activity against streptococci; interactions with theophylline, caffeine, sucralfate, warfarin, antacids

Ciprofloxacin, Ophthalmic (Ciloxan) [See Table VII–12, pp 623–25]

Ciprofloxacin, Otic (Cipro HC Otic)   **Uses:** Otitis externa   **Action:** Quinolone antibiotic; inhibits DNA gyrase   **Dose:** 1–2 drops in ear(s) bid for 7 d   **Caution:** [C, ?/–]   **Contra:** Perforated tympanic membrane, viral infections of the external canal   **Supplied:** Susp ciprofloxacin 0.2% and hydrocortisone 1%   **SE:** HA, pruritus

Cisplatin (Platinol, Platinol AQ)   **Uses:** Testicular, small-cell and non-small-cell lung, bladder, ovarian, breast, head and neck, and penile CAs; osteosarcoma; pediatric brain tumors   **Action:** DNA-binding; denatures double helix; intrastrand cross-linking; formation of DNA adducts   **Dose:** Refer to specific protocols; adjust dose in renal impairment   **Caution:** [D, –] Cumulative renal toxicity may be severe; serum magnesium, as well as other electrolytes, should be monitored both before and within 48 h after cisplatin therapy   **Contra:** Preexisting renal insufficiency, myelosuppression, hearing impairment   **Supplied:** Inj 1 mg/mL   **SE:** Allergic reactions, N/V, nephrotoxicity (exacerbated by concurrent administration of other nephrotoxic drugs and minimized by NS infusion and mannitol diuresis), high-frequency hearing loss in 30%, peripheral "stocking glove"-type neuropathy, cardiotoxicity (ST-, T-wave changes), hypomagnesemia, mild myelosuppression, hepatotoxicity; renal impairment is dose-related and cumulative   **Notes:** Taxane derivatives should be administered before platinum derivatives

Citalopram (Celexa)   **WARNING:** *Pediatric:* Aantidepressants may increase risk of suicidality; consider risks and benefits of use. Patients should be closely monitored for clinical worsening, suicidality, or unusual changes in behavior   **Uses:** Depression   **Action:** SSRI   **Dose:** Initial 20 mg/d, may be ↑ to 40 mg/d; adjust dose in elderly and hepatic insufficiency; renal insufficiency   **Caution:** [C, +/–] History of mania; history of seizures and patients at risk for suicide   **Contra:** Use with MAOI or within 14 d of MAOI administration   **Supplied:** Tabs 10, 20, 40 mg; soln 10 mg/5mL   **SE:** Somnolence, insomnia, anxiety, xerostomia, diaphoresis, sexual dysfunction   **Notes:** May cause hyponatremia/SIADH

Cladribine (Leustatin)   **Uses:** Hairy cell leukemia (HCL), CLL, non-Hodgkin's lymphoma, progressive multiple sclerosis   **Action:** Induces DNA strand breakage; interferes with DNA repair/synthesis; purine nucleoside analogue   **Dose:** Refer to specific protocols   **Caution:** [D, ?/–] observe for signs of neutropenia and infection   **Supplied:** Inj 1 mg/mL   **SE:** Myelosuppression; T-lymphocyte suppression may be prolonged (26–34 wk); fever in

46% (possibly tumor lysis); infections (especially lung and IV sites); rash (50%), HA; fatigue **Notes:** Consider prophylactic allopurinol; monitor CBC

Clarithromycin (Biaxin, Biaxin XL)   **Uses: Upper and lower respiratory tract infections, skin and skin structure infections, H pylori infections, infections caused by non-tuberculosis (atypical) Mycobacterium, prevention of MAC infections in HIV-infected persons** **Action:** Macrolide antibiotic; inhibits protein synthesis **Spectrum:** Effective against susceptible strains of *H influenzae, M catarrhalis, S pneumoniae, Mycoplasma pneumoniae, H pylori* **Dose:** 250–500 mg PO bid or 1000 mg (2 × 500 mg ER tab)/d *Mycobacterium:* 500–1000 mg PO bid; ↓ in renal/hepatic impairment   **Caution:** [C, ?] Antibiotic-associated colitis; rare QT prolongation and ventricular arrhythmias, including torsades de pointes **Supplied:** Tabs 250, 500 mg; susp 125, 250 mg/ 5 mL; 500 mg ER tab **SE:** Prolongs QT interval, multiple drug interactions; causes metallic taste, diarrhea, nausea, abdominal pain, HA, rash **Notes:** Increases theophylline and carbamazepine levels; do not refrigerate oral suspension

Clemastine Fumarate (Tavist; Tavist-1) [OTC]   **Uses: Allergic rhinitis and symptoms of urticaria** **Action:** Antihistamine **Dose:** 1.34 mg bid–2.68 mg tid; max 8.04 mg/d   **Caution:** [C, M] bladder neck obstruction, asthma, symptomatic prostate hypertrophy **Contra:** Narrow-angle glaucoma **Supplied:** Tabs 1.34, 2.68 mg; syrup 0.67 mg/5 mL **SE:** Drowsiness; dyscoordination; epigastric distress **Notes:** Avoid alcohol

Clindamycin (Cleocin, Cleocin-T)   **Uses: For treatment of susceptible aerobic and anaerobic bacteria; topical for severe acne and vaginal infections** **Action:** Bacteriostatic; interferes with protein synthesis **Spectrum:** Susceptible strains of streptococci, pneumococci, staphylococci, and gram(+) and gram(–) anaerobes; no activity against gram(–) aerobes and bacterial vaginosis **Dose:** *Oral:* 150–450 mg PO qid *Intravenous:* 300–600 mg IV q6h or 900 mg IV q8h *Vaginal:* 1 applicatorful qhs for 7 d *Topical:* Apply 1% gel, lotion, or soln bid; adjust dose in hepatic impairment   **Caution:** [B, +] Can cause fatal colitis   **Contra:** Previous pseudomembranous colitis **Supplied:** Caps 75, 150, 300 mg; susp 75 mg/5 mL; inj 300 mg/2 mL; vaginal cream 2% **SE:** Diarrhea may be pseudomembranous colitis caused by *C difficile*, rash, ↑ LFTs **Notes:** Discontinue drug if significant diarrhea

Clofazimine (Lamprene)   **Uses: Leprosy and combination therapy for MAC in AIDS** **Action:** Bactericidal; inhibits DNA synthesis **Spectrum:** Effective against multibacillary dapsone-sensitive leprosy; erythema nodosum leprosum; *Mycobacterium avium-intracellulare* **Dose:** 100–300 mg PO daily   **Caution:** [C, +/–] Use with caution in patients with GI problems; dosages > 100 mg/d should be used for as short a duration as possible   **Supplied:** Caps 50, 100 mg **SE:** Pink to brownish-black discoloration of the skin and conjunctiva, dry skin, GI intolerance **Notes:** Orphan drug for the treatment of dapsone-resistant leprosy; take with meals; monitor for GI complaints

Clonazepam (Klonopin) [C-IV]   **Uses: Lennox-Gastaut syndrome, akinetic and myoclonic seizures, absence seizures, panic attacks, restless legs syndrome, neuralgia, parkinsonian dysarthria, bipolar disorder** **Action:** Benzodiazepine; anticonvulsant **Dose:** 1.5 mg/d PO in 3 ÷ doses; ↑ by 0.5–1 mg/d q3d PRN up to 20 mg/d; avoid abrupt withdrawal   **Caution:** [D, M] Elderly patients, respiratory disease, CNS depression, severe hepatic impairment, narrow-angle glaucoma **Supplied:** Tabs 0.5, 1, 2 mg **SE:** CNS side effects, including drowsiness, dizziness, ataxia, memory impairment **Notes:** Can cause retrograde amnesia; CYP3A4 substrate

Clonidine, Oral (Catapres)   **Uses: HTN; opioid, alcohol, and tobacco withdrawal** **Action:** Centrally acting α-adrenergic stimulant **Dose:** 0.1 mg PO bid, adjust daily by 0.1- to 0.2-mg increments (max 2.4 mg/d); adjust dose in renal impairment   **Caution:** [C, +/–] Avoid with β-blocker; withdrawl slowly **Supplied:** Tabs 0.1, 0.2, 0.3 mg **SE:** Rebound HTN with abrupt cessation of doses > 0.2 mg bid; drowsiness, orthostatic hypotension, dry mouth, constipation, bradycardia, dizziness **Notes:** More effective for HTN if combined with diuretics

Clonidine, Transdermal (Catapres TTS)   **Uses: HTN** **Action:** Centrally acting α-adrenergic stimulant **Dose:** Apply 1 patch q7d to hairless area (upper arm/torso); titrate to effect; ↓ in severe renal impairment, do not discontinue abruptly (rebound HTN)   **Caution:**

[C, +/–] Avoid with β-blocker; withdraw slowly **Supplied:** TTS-1, TTS-2, TTS-3 (delivers 0.1, 0.2, 0.3 mg, respectively, of clonidine/d for 1 wk) **SE:** Drowsiness, orthostatic hypotension, dry mouth, constipation, bradycardia **Notes:** Doses > 2 TTS-3 usually not associated with ↑ efficacy; steady state in 2–3 days

Clopidogrel (Plavix) **Uses: Reduction of atherosclerotic events** **Action:** Inhibits platelet aggregation **Dose:** 75 mg/d **Caution:** [B, ?] Active bleeding; TTP; liver disease **Contra:** Active pathologic bleeding; intracranial bleeding **Supplied:** Tabs 75 mg **SE:** Prolongs bleeding time, GI intolerance, HA, dizziness, rash, thrombocytopenia, leukopenia **Notes:** Use with caution in persons at risk of bleeding from trauma and other causes; platelet aggregation returns to baseline ~ 5 d after discontinuing; platelet transfusion reverses effects acutely; 300 mg PO × 1 dose can be used to load patients

Clorazepate (Tranxene) [C-IV] **Uses: Acute anxiety disorders, acute alcohol withdrawal symptoms, adjunctive therapy in partial seizures** **Action:** Benzodiazepine; antianxiety agent **Dose:** 15–60 mg/d PO single or ÷ doses *Elderly and debilitated patients:* Start at 7.5–15 mg/d in ÷ doses *Alcohol withdrawal:* Day 1: Initially, 30 mg; then 30–60 mg in ÷ doses. Day 2: 45–90 mg in ÷ doses. Day 3: 22.5–45 mg in ÷ doses. Day 4: 15–30 mg in ÷ doses **Caution:** [D, ?/–] **Contra:** Narrow-angle glaucoma **Supplied:** Tabs 3.75, 7.5, 15 mg; Tabs-SD (once-daily) 11.25, 22.5 mg **SE:** CNS depressant effects (drowsiness, dizziness, ataxia, memory impairment), hypotension **Notes:** Monitor patients with renal/hepatic impairment (drug may accumulate); avoid abrupt withdrawal; may cause dependence

Clotrimazole (Lotrimin, Mycelex) [OTC] **Uses: Candidiasis and tinea infections** **Action:** Antifungal agent; alters cell wall permeability **Spectrum:** Oropharyngeal candidiasis, dermatophytoses, superficial mycoses, and cutaneous vulvovaginal candidiasis **Dose:** *Oral:* One troche dissolved in mouth 5 ×/d for 14 d *Vaginal 1% Cream:* 1 applicatorful hs for 7 d; *2% Cream:* 1 applicatorful hs for 3 days *Tabs:* 100 mg vaginally hs for 7 d or 200 mg (2 tabs) vaginally hs for 3 d or 500-mg tabs vaginally hs once *Topical:* Apply bid for 10–14 d **Caution:** [B,(C if oral)/?] Do not use for treatment of systemic fungal infection **Supplied:** 1% cream; soln; lotion; troche 10 mg; vaginal tabs 100, 500 mg; vaginal cream 1%, 2% **SE:** *Topical:* Local irritation; *Oral:* N/V, elevated LFTs **Notes:** Oral prophylaxis common in immunosuppressed patients

Clotrimazole and Betamethasone (Lotrisone) **Uses: Fungal skin infections** **Action:** Imidazole antifungal and anti-inflammatory **Spectrum:** Tinea pedis, cruris, and corporis in patients ≥ 17 y **Dose:** Apply and massage into area bid for 2–4 wk **Caution:** [C, ?] Varicella infection **Contra:** Do not use in children < 12 y **Supplied:** Cream 15, 45 g, lotion 30 mL **SE:** Local irritation, rash **Notes:** Do not use for diaper dermatitis or under occlusive dressings

Cloxacillin (Cloxapen, Tegopen) [See Table VII–5, p 616]

Clozapine (Clozaril) **WARNING:** Myocarditis, agranulocytosis, seizures, and orthostatic hypotension have been associated with clozapine **Uses: Refractory severe schizophrenia** **Action:** Tricyclic "atypical" antipsychotic **Dose:** Initially, 25 mg daily–bid; ↑ to 300–450 mg/d over 2 wk. Maintain at the lowest dose possible; do not discontinue abruptly **Caution:** [B, +/–] Monitor patients for psychosis and cholinergic rebound **Contra:** Uncontrolled epilepsy; comatose state; WBC count = 3500 cells/mm^3 before treatment or < 3000 cells/mm^3 during treatment **Supplied:** Tabs 25, 100 mg **SE:** Tachycardia, drowsiness, weight gain, constipation, urinary incontinence, rash, seizures, CNS stimulation, hyperglycemia **Notes:** Benign, self-limiting temperature elevations may occur during the 1st 3 wk of treatment, weekly CBC mandatory for 1st 6 mo, then every other wk

Cocaine [C-II] **Uses: Topical anesthetic for mucous membranes** **Action:** Narcotic analgesic, local vasoconstrictor **Dose:** Apply lowest amount of topical soln that provides relief; 1 mg/kg max **Caution:** [C, ?] **Contra:** Ophthalmologic anesthesia **Supplied:** Topical soln and viscous preparations 4%, 10%; powder, soluble tabs (135 mg) for soln **SE:** CNS stimulation, nervousness, loss of taste/smell, chronic rhinitis **Notes:** Use only on mucous membranes of the oral, laryngeal, and nasal cavities, do not use on extensive areas of broken skin

Codeine [C-II]   **Uses: Mild/moderate pain; symptomatic relief of cough**   **Action:** Narcotic analgesic; depresses cough reflex   **Dose:** *Analgesic:* 15–60 mg PO or IM qid PRN *Antitussive:* 10–20 mg PO q4h PRN; max 120 mg/d; ↓ in renal/hepatic impairment   **Caution:** [C (D if prolonged use or high doses at term), +]   **Supplied:** Tabs 15, 30, 60 mg; soln 15 mg/5 mL; inj 30, 60 mg/mL   **SE:** Drowsiness, constipation   **Notes:** Usually combined with APAP for pain or with agents (e.g., terpin hydrate) as an antitussive; 120 mg IM = 10 mg IM morphine

Colchicine   **Uses: Acute gouty arthritis attacks and prevention of recurrences; management of familial Mediterranean fever; primary biliary cirrhosis**   **Action:** Inhibits migration of leukocytes; reduces production of lactic acid by leukocytes   **Dose:** *Initially:* 0.5–1.2 mg PO, then 0.5–0.6 mg q1–2h until relief or GI side effects develop (max 8 mg/d); do not repeat for 3 d *IV:* 1–3 mg, then 0.5 mg q6h until relief (max 4 mg/d); do not repeat for 7 d *Prophylaxis:* PO: 0.5–0.6 mg/d or 3–4 d/wk; ↓ dose with renal impairment; caution in elderly   **Caution:** [D, +]   **Contra:** Serious renal, GI, hepatic, or cardiac disorders; blood dyscrasias   **Supplied:** Tabs 0.5, 0.6 mg; inj 1 mg/2 mL   **SE:** N/V/D, abdominal pain, bone marrow suppression, hepatotoxicity   **Notes:** Colchicine 1–2 mg IV within 24–48 h of an acute attack diagnostic/therapeutic in monoarticular arthritis

Colesevelam (Welchol)   **Uses: Reduction of LDL and total cholesterol when used alone or in combination with an HMG-CoA reductase inhibitor**   **Action:** Bile acid sequestrant   **Dose:** 3 tabs PO bid with meals   **Caution:** [B, ?] Severe GI motility disorders   **Contra:** Bowel obstruction   **Supplied:** Tabs 625 mg   **SE:** Constipation, dyspepsia, myalgia, weakness   **Notes:** May decrease absorption of fat-soluble vitamins

Colestipol (Colestid)   **Uses: Adjunct to ↓ serum cholesterol in primary hypercholesterolemia**   **Action:** Binds intestinal bile acids to form an insoluble complex   **Dose:** Granules: 5–30 g/d ÷ into 2–4 doses; tabs: 2–16 g/d daily–bid   **Caution:** [C, ?] Avoid in patients with high triglycerides, GI dysfunction   **Contra:** Bowel obstruction   **Supplied:** Tabs 1 g; granules 5 g   **SE:** Constipation, abdominal pain, bloating, HA   **Notes:** Do not use dry powder; mix with beverages, soups, cereals, etc; may decrease absorption of other medications; may decrease absorption of fat-soluble vitamins

Cortisone (Cortone) [See Table VII–2, p 613]

Cortisporin Ophthalmic [See Table VII–12, pp 623–25]

Cortisporin Otic   **Uses: Treatment of superficial bacterial infections of the external auditory canal by organisms sensitive to neomycin and polymyxin; suspension used in the treatment of infections of the mastoid and fenestrated cavities**   **Actions:** Topical antibiotic combination   **Dose:** 4 drops instilled into external auditory canal 3–4 times daily   **Caution:** [C, ?]   **Supplied:** Otic solution and suspension   **Notes:** Use suspension in cases of ruptured eardrum

Cromolyn Sodium (Intal, NasalCrom, Opticrom)   **Uses: Adjunct to the treatment of asthma; prevent exercise-induced asthma; allergic rhinitis; ophth allergic manifestations**   **Action:** Antiasthmatic; mast cell stabilizer   **Dose:** *Inhal:* 20 mg (as powder in caps) inhaled qid or met-dose inhaler 2 puffs qid *Oral:* 200 mg qid 15–20 min ac, up to 400 mg qid *Nasal instillation:* Spray once in each nostril 2–6×/d *Ophth:* 1–2 drops in each eye 4–6×/d   **Caution:** [B, ?]   **Contra:** Acute asthmatic attacks   **Supplied:** Oral conc 100 mg/5 mL; soln for neb 20 mg/2 mL; met-dose inhaler; nasal soln 40 mg/mL; ophth soln 4%   **SE:** Unpleasant taste, hoarseness, coughing   **Notes:** No benefit in acute treatment; 2–4 wk for maximal effect in perennial allergic disorders

Cyanocobalamin [Vitamin B$_{12}$]   **Uses: Pernicious anemia and other vitamin B$_{12}$ deficiency states**   **Action:** Dietary supplement of vitamin B$_{12}$ **Dose:** 100 mcg IM or SC qd for 7 d, then 100 mcg IM 2×/wk for 1 mo, then 100 mcg weekly for 1 month, then 1000 mcg IM monthly   **Caution:** [A (C if dose exceeds RDA), +]   **Supplied:** Tabs 50, 100, 250, 500, 1000 mcg; inj 100, 1000 mcg/mL; gel 500 mcg/0.1 mL **SE:** Itching, diarrhea, HA, anxiety **Notes:** Oral absorption erratic, altered by many drugs and not recommended; for use with hyperalimentation

Cyclobenzaprine (Flexeril) Uses: Relief of muscle spasm Action: Centrally acting skeletal muscle relaxant; reduces tonic somatic motor activity Dose: 10 mg PO 2–4×/d (2–3 wk max) Caution: [B, ?] Shares the toxic potential of the TCAs; urinary hesitancy or angle-closure glaucoma Contra: Do not use concomitantly or within 14 days of MAOIs; hyperthyroidism; heart failure; arrhythmias Supplied: Tabs 10 mg SE: Sedation, anticholinergic side effects Notes: May inhibit mental alertness or physical coordination

Cyclophosphamide (Cytoxan, Neosar) Uses: Hodgkin's and non-Hodgkin's lymphomas, multiple myeloma, small cell lung, breast, and ovarian CAs, mycosis fungoides, neuroblastoma, retinoblastoma, acute leukemias, and allogeneic and autologous BMT in high doses; severe rheumatoid disorders Action: Converted to acrolein and phosphoramide mustard, the active alkylating moieties Dose: Refer to specific protocols; adjust in renal/hepatic impairment Caution: [D, ?] Patients with bone marrow suppression Supplied: Tabs 25, 50 mg; inj 100 mg SE: Myelosuppression (leukopenia and thrombocytopenia); hemorrhagic cystitis, SIADH, alopecia, anorexia; N/V; hepatotoxicity and rarely interstitial pneumonitis; irreversible testicular atrophy possible; cardiotoxicity rare; 2nd malignancies (bladder CA and acute leukemias); cumulative risk 3.5% at 8 y, 10.7% at 12 y Notes: Hemorrhagic cystitis prophylaxis: continuous bladder irrigation and mesna uroprotection; encourage adequate hydration

Cyclosporine (Sandimmune, Neoral) Uses: Organ rejection in kidney, liver, heart, and bone marrow transplants with steroids; RA; psoriasis Action: Immunosuppressant; reversible inhibition of immunocompetent lymphocytes Dose: Oral: 15 mg/kg/d 12 h pretransplantation; after 2 wk, taper by 5 mg/wk to 5–10 mg/kg/d IV: If NPO, give ⅓ oral dose IV; ↓ in renal/hepatic impairment Caution: [C, ?] Dose-related risk of nephrotoxicity/hepatotoxicity; live, attenuated vaccines may be less effective Contra: Abnormal renal function; uncontrolled HTN Supplied: Caps 25, 50, 100 mg; oral soln 100 mg/mL; inj 50 mg/mL SE: May ↑ BUN and creatinine and mimic transplant rejection; HTN; HA; hirsutism Notes: Administer in glass containers; many drug interactions; Neoral and Sandimmune not interchangeable; interaction with St. John's wort

Cyproheptadine (Periactin) Uses: Allergic reactions; itching Action: Phenothiazine antihistamine; serotonin antagonist Dose: 4–20 mg PO ÷ q8h; max 0.5 mg/kg/d; reduce dose in hepatic impairment Caution: [B, ?] Symptomatic prostate hypertrophy Contra: Narrow-angle glaucoma; bladder neck obstruction; acute asthma attack; GI obstruction Supplied: Tabs 4 mg; syrup 2 mg/5 mL SE: Anticholinergic, drowsiness Notes: May stimulate appetite

Cytarabine [ARA-C] (Cytosar-U) Uses: Acute leukemias, CML, NHL; intrathecal (IT) administration for leukemic meningitis or prophylaxis Action: Antimetabolite; interferes with DNA synthesis Dose: Refer to specific protocols; ↓ in renal/hepatic impairment Caution: [D, ?] Marked bone marrow suppression necessitates dosage reduction by a decrease in the number of days of administration Supplied: Inj 100, 500 mg, 1, 2 g SE: Myelosuppression, N/V/D, stomatitis, flu-like syndrome, rash on palms/soles, hepatic dysfunction, cerebellar dysfunction, noncardiogenic pulmonary edema, neuropathy Notes: Of little use in solid tumors; toxicity of high-dose regimens (conjunctivitis) ameliorated by corticosteroid ophth soln

Cytarabine Liposome (DepoCyt) Uses: Lymphomatous meningitis Action: Antimetabolite; interferes with DNA synthesis Dose: 50 mg IT q14d for 5 doses, then 50 mg IT q28d for 4 doses; use dexamethasone prophylaxis Caution: [D, ?] May cause neurotoxicity; blockage to CSF flow may increase the risk of neurotoxicity Contra: Active meningeal infection Supplied: IT inj 50 mg/5 mL SE: Neck pain/rigidity, HA, confusion, somnolence, fever, back pain, N/V, edema, neutropenia, thrombocytopenia, anemia Notes: Cytarabine li-

posomes are similar in appearance to WBCs, care must be taken in interpreting CSF examinations in patients

Cytomegalovirus Immmune Globulin [CMV-IG IV] (CytoGam)   Uses: **Attenuation of primary CMV disease associated with transplantation**   Action: Exogenous IgG antibodies to CMV   Dose: Administered for 16 weeks post-transplantation; see product information for dosing schedule   Caution: [C, ?] Monitor for anaphylactic reactions; use with caution in renal dysfunction   Contra: Hypersensitivity to immunoglobulins; immunoglobulin A deficiency   Supplied: Inj 50–10 mg/mL   SE: Flushing, N/V, muscle cramps, wheezing, HA, fever   Notes: IV use only; administer by separate line; do not shake

Dacarbazine (DTIC)   Uses: **Melanoma, Hodgkin's disease, sarcoma**   Action: Alkylating agent; antimetabolite activity as a purine precursor; inhibits synthesis of protein, RNA, and especially DNA   Dose: Refer to specific protocols; adjust in renal impairment   Caution: [C, ?] Use with caution in patients with bone marrow suppression; renal/hepatic impairment; avoid extravasation   Supplied: Inj 100, 200, 500 mg   SE: Myelosuppression, severe N/V, hepatotoxicity, flu-like syndrome, hypotension, photosensitivity, alopecia, facial flushing, facial paresthesias, urticaria, phlebitis at injection site

Daclizumab (Zenapax)   Uses: **Prevent acute organ rejection**   Action: IL-2 receptor antagonist   Dose: 1 mg/kg IV/dose; 1st dose pretransplantation, then 4 doses 14 d apart post-transplantation   Caution: [C, ?]   Supplied: Inj 5 mg/mL   SE: Hyperglycemia, edema, hypertension, hypotension, constipation, HA, dizziness, anxiety, nephrotoxicity, pulmonary edema, pain   Notes: Administer within 4 h of preparation

Dactinomycin (Cosmegen)   Uses: **Choriocarcinoma, Wilms' tumor, Kaposi's sarcoma, Ewing's sarcoma, rhabdomyosarcoma, testicular CA**   Action: DNA intercalating agent   Dose: Refer to specific protocols; ↓ in renal impairment   Caution: [C, ?]   Contra: Patients with concurrent or recent chickenpox or herpes zoster   Supplied: Inj 0.5 mg   SE: Myelosuppression, immunosuppression, severe N/V, alopecia, acne, hyperpigmentation, radiation recall phenomenon, tissue damage with extravasation, hepatotoxicity

Dalteparin (Fragmin)   Uses: **Unstable angina, non–Q-wave MI, prevention of ischemic complications due to clot formation in patients on concurrent ASA, prevention and treatment of DVT after surgery**   Action: LMW heparin   Dose: *Angina/MI:* 120 IU/kg (max 10,000 IU) SC q12h with ASA *DVT prophylaxis:* 2500–5000 IU SC 1–2 h preop, then qd for 5–10 d *Systemic anticoagulation:* 200 IU/kg/d SC or 100 IU/kg bid SC; use with caution in renal/hepatic impairment   Caution: [B, ?] Active hemorrhage, cerebrovascular disease, cerebral aneurysm, severe uncontrolled HTN   Contra: HIT; hypersensitivity to pork products; not for IM or IV use   Supplied: Inj 2500 IU (16 mg/0.2 mL), 5000 IU (32 mg/0.2 mL), 10,000 IU (64 mg/mL)   SE: Bleeding, pain at injection site, thrombocytopenia   Notes: Predictable antithrombotic effects eliminate need for laboratory monitoring

Danaparoid (Orgaron)   Uses: **Prophylaxis of DVT which may lead to PE, in patients undergoing hip replacement surgery**   Action: Antithrombotic agent that acts by inhibition of factors Xa and IIa   Dose: 750 anti-Xa units bid administered by SC injection beginning 1–4 h preoperatively and starting no sooner than 2 h after surgery; reduce dose with severe renal impairment   Caution: [B, ?/–]   Contra: Active major bleeding, hemophilia, ITP, type II thrombocytopenia with a positive antiplatelet antibody test   Supplied: Ampoules and prefilled syringes 0.6 mL (750 anti-Xa units)   SE: Bleeding, fever, injection site pain, increased risk of epidural and spinal hematoma in patients receiving epidural/spinal anesthesia   Notes: aPTT monitoring is not necessary

Dantrolene (Dantrium)   Uses: **Clinical spasticity due to upper motor neuron disorders, e.g., spinal cord injuries, strokes, CP, MS; treatment of malignant hyperthermia**   Action: Skeletal muscle relaxant   Dose: *Spasticity:* Initially, 25 mg PO qd; ↑ to effect by 25 mg to a max dose of 100 mg PO qid PRN *Malignant hyperthermia: Treatment:* Continuous rapid IV push beginning at 1 mg/kg until symptoms subside or 10 mg/kg is reached *Postcrisis follow-up:* 4–8 mg/kg/d in 3–4 ÷ doses for 1–3 d to prevent recurrence   Caution: [C, ?] Impaired cardiac function or pulmonary function; potential for hepatotoxicity   Contra: Active he-

patic disease; should not be used where spasticity is used to maintain posture or balance **Supplied:** Caps 25, 50, 100 mg; powder for inj 20 mg/vial **SE:** Elevated LFTs, drowsiness, dizziness, rash, muscle weakness, pleural effusion with pericarditis, diarrhea, blurred vision, hepatitis **Notes:** Monitor transaminases

Dapsone (Avlosulfon) **Uses: Treatment and prevention of PCP; toxoplasmosis prophylaxis; leprosy** **Action:** Unknown; bactericidal **Dose:** Prophylaxis of PCP 50–100 mg/d PO; treatment of PCP 100 mg/d PO with TMP 15–20 mg/kg/d for 21 d **Caution:** [C, +] Caution in G6PD deficiency; severe anemia **Supplied:** Tabs 25, 100 mg **SE:** Hemolysis, methemoglobinemia, agranulocytosis, rash, cholestatic jaundice **Notes:** Absorption ↑ by an acidic environment; with leprosy, combine with rifampin and other agents

Darbepoetin Alfa (Aranesp) **Uses: Anemia associated with CRF** **Action:** Stimulates erythropoiesis, recombinant variant of erythropoietin **Dose:** 0.45 mcg/kg single IV or SC qwk; titrate dose, do not exceed target Hgb of 12 g/dL; see insert for converting from Epogen **Caution:** [C, ?] May increase risk of cardiovascular and/or neurologic SE in renal failure; HTN; history of seizures **Contra:** Uncontrolled hypertension, allergy to components **Supplied:** 25, 40, 60, 100 mcg/mL, in polysorbate or albumin excipient **SE:** May ↑ risk of cardiac events, chest pain, hypo-/hypertension, N/V/D, myalgia, arthralgia, dizziness, edema, fatigue, fever, ↑ risk infection **Notes:** Longer half-life than Epogen; follow weekly CBC until stable

Daunorubicin (Daunomycin, Cerubidine) WARNING: Cardiac function should be monitored because of potential risk for cardiac toxicity and CHF **Uses: Acute leukemias** **Action:** DNA intercalating agent; inhibits topoisomerase II; generates oxygen free radicals **Dose:** Refer to specific protocols; adjust dose in renal/hepatic impairment **Caution:** [D, ?] **Supplied:** Inj 20 mg **SE:** Myelosuppression, mucositis, N/V, alopecia, radiation recall phenomenon, hepatotoxicity (hyperbilirubinemia), tissue necrosis on extravascular extravasation, and cardiotoxicity (1–2% CHF risk with 550 mg/m^2 cumulative dose) **Notes:** Prevent cardiotoxicity with dexrazoxane

Delavirdine (Rescriptor) **Uses: HIV infection** **Action:** Nonnucleoside reverse transcriptase inhibitor **Dose:** 400 mg PO tid **Caution:** [C, ?] CDC recommends HIV-infected mothers not breastfeed because of risk of HIV transmission to infant; use caution in renal/hepatic impairment **Contra:** Concomitant use with drugs highly dependent on CYP 3A for clearance (i.e., alprazolam, ergot alkaloids, midazolam, pimozide, triazolam) **Supplied:** Tabs 100 mg **SE:** HA, fatigue, rash, ↑ serum transaminases, N/V/D **Notes:** Avoid antacids; inhibits cytochrome P-450 enzymes; numerous drug interactions; monitor LFTs

Demecarium (Humorsol) [See Table VII–12, pp 623–25]

Demeclocycline (Declomycin) **Uses:** SIADH **Action:** Antibiotic, antagonizes action of ADH on renal tubules **Dose:** 300–600 mg PO q12h on an empty stomach; ↓ in renal failure; avoid antacids **Caution:** [D, +] Avoid use in hepatic/renal dysfunction **Contra:** Hypersensitivity to tetracyclines **Supplied:** Tabs 150, 300 mg **SE:** Diarrhea, abdominal cramps, photosensitivity, diabetes insipidus **Notes:** Avoid prolonged exposue to sunlight

Desipramine (Norpramin) WARNING: *Pediatric:* Antidepressants may increase risk of suicidality; consider risks and benefits of use. Patients should be closely monitored for clinical worsening, suicidality, or unusual changes in behavior **Uses: Endogenous depression, chronic pain, and peripheral neuropathy** **Action:** TCA; increases synaptic concentration of serotonin or norepinephrine in CNS **Dose:** 25–200 mg/d single or ÷ doses; usually a single hs dose (max 300 mg/d) **Caution:** [C, ?/–] Caution in cardiovascular disease, seizure disorder, hypothyroidism **Contra:** Use of MAO inhibitors within 14 days; pt in recovery phase of MI **Supplied:** Tabs 10, 25, 50, 75, 100, 150 mg; caps 25, 50 mg **SE:** Anticholinergic (blurred vision, urinary retention, dry mouth); orthostatic hypotension; prolongs QT interval, arrythmias **Notes:** Numerous drug interactions

Desloratadine (Clarinex) **Uses: Symptoms of seasonal and perennial allergic rhinitis; chronic idiopathic urticaria** **Action:** The active metabolite of loratadine, H$_1$-antihistamine, blocks inflammatory mediators **Dose:** 5 mg PO qd; hepatic/renal impairment: 5 mg

PO qod **Caution:** [C, ?/–] RediTabs contain phenylalanine **Supplied:** Tabs and Reditabs 5 mg **SE:** Hypersensitivity reactions, anaphylaxis, somnolence, HA, dizziness, fatigue, pharyngitis, dry mouth, nausea, dyspepsia, myalgia **Notes:** May be taken with or without food

Desmopressin (DDAVP, Stimate)
Uses: Diabetes insipidus (intranasal and parenteral); bleeding due to uremia, hemophilia A, and type I von Willebrand's disease (parenteral), nocturnal enuresis **Action:** Synthetic analogue of vasopressin, a naturally occurring human ADH; ↑ factor VIII **Dose:** *DI: Intranasal:* 0.1–0.4 mL (10–40 mcg)/d in 1–4 ÷ doses *Parenteral:* 0.5–1 mL (2–4 mcg)/d in 2 ÷ doses. If converting from nasal to parenteral, use ¹⁄₁₀ nasal dose *Oral:* 0.05 mg bid; ↑ to max of 1.2 mg *Hemophilia A and von Willebrand's disease (type I):* 0.3 mcg/kg in 50 mL NS, infuse over 15–30 min **Caution:** [B, M] Avoid overhydration **Contra:** Hemophilia B; severe classic von Willebrand's disease; patients with factor VIII antibodies **Supplied:** Tabs 0.1, 0.2 mg; inj 4 mcg/mL; nasal soln 0.1, 1.5 mg/mL **SE:** Facial flushing, HA, dizziness, vulval pain, nasal congestion, pain at injection site, hyponatremia, water intoxication **Notes:** In very young and old patients, ↓ fluid intake to avoid water intoxication and hyponatremia

Dexamethasone (Decadron) [See Table VII–2, p 613]

Dexamethasone, Nasal (Dexacort Phosphate Turbinaire)
Uses: Chronic nasal inflammation or allergic rhinitis **Action:** Antiinflammatory corticosteroid **Dose:** 2 sprays/nostril bid–tid, max 12 sprays/d **Caution:** [C, ?] **Supplied:** Aerosol, 84 mcg/activation **SE:** Local irritation

Dexamethasone, Ophthalmic (AK-Dex Ophthalmic, Decadron Ophthalmic) [See Table VII–12, pp 623–25]

Dexpanthenol (Ilopan-Choline Oral, Ilopan)
Uses: Minimize paralytic ileus, treatment of postop distention **Action:** Cholinergic agent **Dose:** *Relief of gas:* 2–3 tabs PO tid *Prevent postop ileus:* 250–500 mg IM stat, repeat in 2 h, then q6h PRN *Ileus:* 500 mg IM stat, repeat in 2 h, followed by doses q6h, if needed **Caution:** [C, ?] **Contra:** Hemophilia, mechanical obstruction **Supplied:** Inj; tabs 50 mg; cream **SE:** GI cramps

Dexrazoxane (Zinecard)
Uses: Prevent anthracycline-induced cardiomyopathy **Action:** Chelates heavy metals; binds intracellular iron and prevents anthracycline-induced free radicals **Dose:** 10:1 ratio dexrazoxane:doxorubicin 30 min prior to each dose **Caution:** [C, ?] **Supplied:** Inj 10 mg/mL **SE:** Myelosuppression (especially leukopenia), fever, infection, stomatitis, alopecia, N/V/D; mild ↑ transaminase, pain at injection site

Dextran 40 (Rheomacrodex)
Uses: Shock, prophylaxis of DVT and thromboembolism, adjunct in peripheral vascular surgery **Action:** Expands plasma volume; ↓ blood viscosity **Dose:** *Shock:* 10 mL/kg infused rapidly; 20 mL/kg max in the 1st 24 h; beyond 24 h 10 mL/kg max; discontinue after 5 d *Prophylaxis of DVT and thromboembolism:* 10 mL/kg IV day of surgery, then 500 mL/d IV for 2–3 d, then 500 mL IV q2–3d based on risk for up to 2 wk **Caution:** [C, ?] Infusion reactions; patients receiving corticosteroids **Contra:** Marked hemostatic defects of all types; marked cardiac decompensation; renal disease with severe oliguria/anuria **Supplied:** 10% dextran 40 in 0.9% NaCl or 5% dextrose **SE:** Hypersensitivity/anaphylactoid reaction (observe patient closely during 1st minute of infusion), arthralgia, cutaneous reactions, hypotension, fever; monitor renal function and electrolytes **Notes:** Observe patients for anaphylactic reactions; patients should be well hydrated

Dextromethorphan (Mediquell, Benylin DM, PediaCare 1, Others) [OTC]
Uses: Controlling nonproductive cough **Action:** Depresses the cough center in the medulla **Dose:** 10–30 mg PO q4–8h PRN (max 120 mg/24 h) **Caution:** [C,?/–] Should not be used for persistent or chronic cough **Supplied:** Caps 30 mg; lozenges 2.5, 5, 7.5, 15 mg; syrup 15 mg/15 mL, 10 mg/5 mL; liq 10 mg/15 mL, 3.5, 7.5, 15 mg/5 mL; sustained-action liq 30 mg/5 mL **SE:** GI disturbances **Notes:** May be found in combination products with guaifenesin

Dezocine (Dalgan)
Uses: Moderate to severe pain **Action:** Narcotic agonist-antagonist **Dose:** 5–20 mg IM or 2.5–10 mg IV q2–4h PRN; ↓ in renal impairment **Caution:**

[C, ?] **Contra:** Not recommended for patients < 18 y **Supplied:** Inj 5, 10, 15 mg/mL **SE:** Sedation, dizziness, vertigo, N/V, injection site reaction **Notes:** Withdrawal possible in patients dependent on narcotics

Diazepam (Valium) [C-IV]
Uses: **Anxiety, alcohol withdrawal, muscle spasm, status epilepticus, panic disorders, amnesia, preoperative sedation** **Action:** Benzodiazepine **Dose:** *Status epilepticus:* 5–10 mg q10–20 min to 30 mg max in 8-h period *Anxiety, muscle spasm:* 2–10 mg PO bid–qid or IM/IV q3–4h PRN *Preop:* 5–10 mg PO or IM 20–30 min or IV just before procedure *Alcohol withdrawal:* Initial 2–5 mg IV, then 5–10 mg q5–10 min, 100 mg in 1 h max. May require up to 1000 mg in 24-h period for severe withdrawal. Titrate to agitation; avoid excessive sedation; may lead to aspiration or respiratory arrest; ↓ in hepatic impairment; avoid abrupt withdrawal **Caution:** [D, ?/–] **Supplied:** Tabs 2, 5, 10 mg; soln 1, 5 mg/mL; inj 5 mg/mL; rectal gel 5 mg/mL **SE:** Sedation, amnesia, bradycardia, hypotension, rash, decreased respiratory rate **Notes:** Do not exceed 5 mg/min IV in adults because respiratory arrest possible; IM absorption erratic

Diazoxide (Hyperstat, Proglycem)
Uses: **Hypoglycemia due to hyperinsulinism (Proglycem); hypertensive crisis (Hyperstat)** **Action:** Inhibits pancreatic insulin release; antihypertensive **Dose:** *Hypertensive crisis:* IV: 1–3 mg/kg (maximum: 150 mg in a single injection); repeat dose in 5–15 min until BP controlled; repeat every 4–24 h; monitor BP closely *Hypoglycemia:* 3–8 mg/kg/24 h PO ÷ q8–12h **Caution:** [C, ?] ↓ effect w/ phenytoin; ↑ effect w/ diuretics, warfarin **Contra:** Hypersensitivity to thiazides or other sulfonamide-containing products; HTN associated with aortic coarctation, arteriovenous shunt, or pheochromocytoma **Supplied:** Inj 15 mg/mL; caps 50 mg; oral susp 50 mg/mL **SE:** Hyperglycemia, hypotension, dizziness, sodium and water retention, N/V, weakness **Notes:** Can give false-negative insulin response to glucagons; treat extravasation w/ warm compress

Dibucaine (Nupercainal)
Uses: **Hemorrhoids and minor skin conditions** **Action:** Topical anesthetic **Dose:** Insert PR with applicator bid and after each bowel movement; apply sparingly to skin **Caution:** [C, ?] **Supplied:** 1% oint with rectal applicator; 0.5% cream **SE:** Local irritation, rash

Diclofenac (Cataflam, Voltaren) [See Table VII–11, pp 621–22, and Table VII–12, pp 623–25]

Dicloxacillin (Dynapen, Dycill) [See Table VII–5, p 616]

Dicyclomine (Bentyl)
Uses: **Functional irritable bowel syndromes** **Action:** Smooth muscle relaxant **Dose:** 20 mg PO qid; ↑ to a max dose of 160 mg/d or 20 mg IM q6h **Caution:** [B, –] **Contra:** Narrow-angle glaucoma, myasthenia gravis, severe ulcerative colitis, obstructive uropathy, nursing mothers **Supplied:** Caps 10, 20 mg; tabs 20 mg; syrup 10 mg/5 mL; inj 10 mg/mL **SE:** Anticholinergic side effects may limit dose **Notes:** Take 30–60 min before meal; avoid alcohol

Didanosine [ddI] (Videx)
WARNING: Hypersensitivity manifested as fever, rash, fatigue, GI/respiratory symptoms reported; stop drug immediately and do not rechallenge; lactic acidosis and hepatomegaly/steatosis reported **Uses:** **HIV infection in zidovudine-intolerant patients** **Action:** Nucleoside antiretroviral agent **Dose:** > 60 kg: 400 mg/d PO or 200 mg PO bid < 60 kg: 250 mg/d PO or 125 mg PO bid; adults should take 2 tabs/administration; adjust dose in renal impairment, thoroughly chew tablets, do not mix with fruit juice or other acidic beverages; reconstitute powder with water **Caution:** [B, –] CDC recommends HIV-infected mothers not breastfeed because of risk of transmission of HIV to the infant **Supplied:** Chew tabs 25, 50, 100, 150, 200 mg; powder packets 100, 167, 250, 375 mg; powder for soln 2, 4 g **SE:** Pancreatitis, peripheral neuropathy, diarrhea, HA **Notes:** Do not take with meals

Diflunisal (Dolobid) [See Table VII–11, pp 621–22]

Digoxin (Lanoxin, Lanoxicaps)
Uses: **CHF, AF and flutter, and paroxysmal atrial tachycardia** **Action:** Positive inotrope; ↑ AV node refractory period **Dose:** *PO digitalization:* 0.50–0.75 mg PO, then 0.25 mg PO q6–8h to total 1–1.5 mg or until therapeutic ef-

fect at lower dose *IV digitalization:* 0.25–0.5 mg IV, then 0.25 mg q4–6h to total ~ 1 mg *Daily maintenance:* 0.125–0.5 mg/d PO or IV (average daily dose 0.125–0.25 mg); ↓ in renal impairment, follow serum levels **Caution:** [C, +] **Contra:** AV block; idiopathic hypertrophic subaortic stenosis; constrictive pericarditis **Supplied:** Caps 0.05, 0.1, 0.2 mg; tabs 0.125, 0.25, 0.5 mg; elixir 0.05 mg/mL; inj 0.1, 0.25 mg/mL **SE:** Can cause heart block; ↓ K⁺ potentiates toxicity; N/V, HA, fatigue, visual disturbances (yellow-green halos around lights), cardiac arrhythmias **Notes:** Multiple drug interactions; IM inj painful, has erratic absorption, and should not be used; therapeutic levels 0.5–2 ng/mL (See Table VII–17, p 630)

Digoxin Immune Fab (Digibind) Uses: Life-threatening digoxin intoxication
Action: Antigen-binding fragments bind and inactivate digoxin **Dose:** Based on serum level and patient's weight; see charts provided with the drug **Caution:** [C, ?] **Contra:** Hypersensitivity to sheep products **Supplied:** Inj 38 mg/vial **SE:** Worsening of cardiac output or CHF, hypokalemia, facial swelling, and redness **Notes:** Each vial binds ~ 0.6 mg of digoxin; in renal failure may require redosing in several days because of breakdown of the immune complex

Diltiazem (Cardizem, Cardizem CD, Cardizem SR, Cartia XT, Dilacor XR, Diltia XT, Tiamate, Tiazac) Uses: Angina, prevention of reinfarction, HTN, AF or flutter, and paroxysmal atrial tachycardia Action: Ca channel blocker Dose: *Oral:* Initially, 30 mg PO qid; ↑ to 180–360 mg/d in 3–4 ÷ doses PRN *SR:* 60–120 mg PO bid; ↑ to 360 mg/d max *CD or XR:* 120–360 mg/d (max 480 mg/d) *IV:* 0.25 mg/kg IV bolus over 2 min; may repeat in 15 min at 0.35 mg/kg; may begin inf of 5–15 mg/h **Caution:** [C, +] **Contra:** Sick sinus syndrome, AV block, hypotension, acute MI, pulmonary congestion **Supplied:** Cardizem CD: Caps 120, 180, 240, 300, 360 mg; Cardizem SR: caps 60, 90, 120 mg; Cardizem: Tabs 30, 60, 90, 120mg; Cartia XT: Caps 120, 180, 240, 300 mg; Dilacor XR: Caps 180, 240 mg; Diltia XT: Caps 120, 180, 240 mg; Tiazac: Caps 120, 180, 240, 300, 360, 420 mg; Tiamate (ext rel): Tabs 120, 180, 240 mg; inj: 5 mg/mL **SE:** Gingival hyperplasia, bradycardia, AV block, ECG abnormalities, peripheral edema, dizziness, HA **Notes:** Cardizem CD, Dilacor XR, and Tiazac not interchangeable

Dimenhydrinate (Dramamine, others) Uses: Prevention and treatment of nausea, vomiting, dizziness, or vertigo of motion sickness Action: Antiemetic Dose:
50–100 mg PO q4–6h, max 400 mg/d; 50 mg IM/IV PRN **Caution:** [B, ?] **Supplied:** Tabs 50 mg; chew tabs 50 mg; liq 12.5 mg/4 mL, 12.5 mg/5 mL, 15.62 mg/5 mL; inj 50 mg/mL **SE:** Anticholinergic side effects

Dimethyl Sulfoxide [DMSO] (Rimso 50) Uses: Interstitial cystitis Action:
Unknown **Dose:** Intravesical, 50 mL, retain for 15 min; repeat q2wk until relief **Caution:** [C, ?] **Supplied:** 50% soln in 50 mL **SE:** Cystitis, eosinophilia, GI, and taste disturbance

Diphenhydramine (Benadryl) Uses: Treat and prevent allergic reactions, motion sickness, potentiate narcotics, sedation, cough suppression, and treatment of extrapyramidal reactions Action: Antihistamine, antiemetic Dose: 25–50 mg PO, IV, or IM bid–tid; ↑ dosing interval in moderate/severe renal failure **Caution:** [B, –] **Contra:** Do not use in acute asthma attack **Supplied:** Tabs and caps 25, 50 mg; chew tabs 12.5 mg; elixir 12.5 mg/5 mL; syrup 12.5 mg/5 mL; liq 6.25 mg/5 mL, 12.5 mg/5 mL; inj 50 mg/mL **SE:** Anticholinergic side effects (dry mouth, urinary retention, sedation)

Diphenoxylate + Atropine (Lomotil) [C-V] Uses: Diarrhea Action: Constipating meperidine congener, reduces GI motility Dose: Initially, 5 mg PO tid–qid until under control, then 2.5–5.0 mg PO bid **Caution:** [C, +] **Contra:** Obstructive jaundice, diarrhea due to bacterial infection **Supplied:** Tabs 2.5 mg of diphenoxylate/0.025 mg of atropine; liq 2.5 mg diphenoxylate/0.025 mg atropine/5 mL **SE:** Drowsiness, dizziness, dry mouth, blurred vision, urinary retention, constipation

Dipivefrin (Propine) [See Table VII–12, pp 623–25]

Dipyridamole (Persantine) Uses: Prevent postoperative thromboembolic disorders, often in combination with ASA or warfarin (e.g., CABG, vascular graft; with warfarin after artificial heart valve; chronic angina; with ASA to prevent coronary artery

thrombosis); dipyridamole IV used in place of exercise stress test for CAD **Action:** Antiplatelet activity; coronary vasodilator **Dose:** 75–100 mg PO tid–qid; stress test 0.14 mg/kg/min (max 60 mg over 4 min) **Caution:** [B, ?/–] Caution with other drugs that affect coagulation **Supplied:** Tabs 25, 50, 75 mg; inj 5 mg/mL **SE:** HA, hypotension, nausea, abdominal distress, flushing rash, dyspnea **Notes:** IV can worsen angina

Dipyridamole and Aspirin (Aggrenox)
Uses: ↓ risk of stroke; reduce rate of reinfarction after MI; prevent occlusion after CABG; **Action:** ↓ platelet aggregation (both agents) **Dose:** 1 cap PO bid **Caution:** [C, ?] **Contra:** Contra in ulcers, bleeding diathesis **Supplied:** Caps Dipyridamole extended-release 200 mg/aspirin 25 mg **SE:** ASA component: allergic reactions, skin reactions, ulcers/GI bleed, bronchospasm; dipyridamole component: dizziness, HA, rash **Notes:** Swallow capsule whole

Dirithromycin (Dynabac)
Uses: Bronchitis, community-acquired pneumonia, and skin and skin structure infections **Action:** Macrolide antibiotic **Spectrum:** *M catarrhalis, S pneumoniae, Legionella, H influenzae, S pyogenes, S aureus* **Dose:** 500 mg/d PO; take with food **Caution:** [C, M] **Supplied:** Tabs 250 mg **SE:** Abdominal discomfort, HA, rash, hyperkalemia **Notes:** Swallow whole

Disopyramide (Norpace)
Uses: Suppression and prevention of ventricular arrhythmias **Action:** Class 1A antiarrhythmic **Dose:** 400–800 mg/d ÷ q6h for regular-release and q12h for SR; ↓ in renal/hepatic impairment **Caution:** [C, +] **Contra:** AV block, cardiogenic shock **Supplied:** Caps 100, 150 mg; SR caps 100, 150 mg **SE:** Anticholinergic side effects; negative inotropic properties may induce CHF

Disulfiram (Antabuse)
Uses: Alcohol consumption deterrent **Action:** Blocks oxidation of alcohol to produce unpleasant reaction when alcohol is consumed **Dose:** 500 mg PO daily for 1–2 weeks, then 250 mg PO daily **Caution:** [C, ?] **Contra:** alcohol use, metronidazole use, severe CAD **Supplied:** Tabs 250, 500 mg **Notes:** Instruct patients to avoid hidden forms of alcohol (cough syrup, mouthwashes, sauces, etc); CBC and LFTs should be checked periodically

Dobutamine (Dobutrex)
Uses: Short-term use in cardiac decompensation secondary to depressed contractility **Action:** Positive inotropic agent **Dose:** Cont IV inf of 2.5–15 mcg/kg/min; rarely, 40 mcg/kg/min may be required; titrate according to response **Caution:** [C, ?] **Supplied:** Inj 250 mg/20 mL **SE:** Chest pain, hypertension, dyspnea **Notes:** Monitor PWP and cardiac output if possible, check ECG for ↑ heart rate, ectopic activity, follow BP

Docetaxel (Taxotere)
Uses: Breast (anthracycline resistant), lung, ovarian, and prostate CAs **Action:** Antimitotic agent; promotes microtubular aggregation; semisynthetic taxoid **Dose:** Refer to specific protocols; Start dexamethasone 8 mg bid prior to docetaxel and continue for 3–4 d; ↓ dose with ↑ bilirubin levels **Caution:** [D, –] **Supplied:** Inj 20, 40, 80 mg/mL **SE:** Myelosuppression, neuropathy, N/V, alopecia, fluid retention syndrome with cumulative doses of 300–400 mg/m^2 without steroid prep and post-treatment and 600–800 mg/m^2 with steroid prep; hypersensitivity reactions possible, but rare with steroid prep

Docusate Calcium (Surfak, Others) (See Docusate Sodium)

Docusate Potassium (Dialose) (See Docusate Sodium)

Docusate Sodium (DOSS, Colace, Others)
Uses: Constipation; adjunct to painful anorectal conditions (hemorrhoids) **Action:** Stool softener **Dose:** 50–500 mg PO ÷ daily–qid **Caution:** [C, ?] **Contra:** Concomitant use of mineral oil; intestinal obstruction, acute abdominal pain, N/V **Supplied:** *Ca:* Caps 50, 240 mg. *K:* Caps 100, 240 mg. *Na:* Caps 50, 100, 250 mg; syrup 50, 60 mg/15 mL; liq 150 mg/15 mL; soln 50 mg/mL **SE:** No significant side effects, rare abdominal cramping, diarrhea; no laxative action

Dofetilide (Tikosyn)
WARNING: To minimize the risk of induced arrhythmia, patients initiated or reinitiated on tikosyn should be placed for a minimum of 3 d in a facility that can provide calculations of creatinine clearance, continuous ECG monitoring, and cardiac resuscitation **Uses:** Maintain NSR in AF/A flutter after conversion **Action:** Class III antiar-

rhythmic   **Dose:** The dosage is individualized based on calculated creatinine clearance and QTc.

- $Cl_{cr} > 60$ mL/min: 500 mcg PO bid
- $Cl_{cr} = 40$–60 mL/min: 250 mcg PO bid
- $Cl_{cr} = 20$–<40 mL/min: 125 mcg PO bid

Determine QTc 2–3 h after first dose. If increase in QTc is = 15%, continue current dose. If QTc increase is > 15% or > 500 msec (550 msec in patients with ventricular conduction abnormalities), adjust dose as follows:

Starting Dose	Adjusted Dose
500 mcg PO bid	250 mcg PO bid
250 mcg PO bid	125 mcg PO bid
125 mcg PO bid	125 mcg PO qd

Continue to check QTc 2–3 h after each subsequent dose for a minimum of 3 d. If at any time QTc increases to > 500 msec (550 msec in patients with ventricular conduction abnormalities), discontinue dofetilide   **Caution:** [C, –]   **Contra:** Baseline QTc is > 440 msec (500 msec in patients with ventricular conduction abnormalities) or Clcr < 20 mL/min; concomitant use of verapamil, cimetidine, trimethoprim, or ketoconazole   **Supplied:** Caps 125, 250, 500 mcg   **SE:** Serious ventricular arrhythmias, HA, chest pain, dizziness   **Notes:** Avoid use with other drugs that prolong the QT interval. Class I or III antiarrhythmic agents should be withheld for at least 3 half-lives before dosing with dofetilide. Amiodarone level should be < 0.3 mg/L prior to dosing with dofetilide

Dolasetron (Anzemet)   **Uses: Prevent chemotherapy-associated N/V**   **Action:** 5-HT3-receptor antagonist   **Dose:** *IV:* 1.8 mg/kg IV as single dose 30 min prior to chemotherapy. *Oral:* 100 mg PO as a single dose 1 h prior to chemotherapy.   **Caution:** [B, ?]   **Supplied:** Tabs 50, 100 mg; inj 20 mg/mL   **SE:** Prolongs QT interval, HTN, HA, abdominal pain, urinary retention, transient ↑ LFTs

Dopamine (Intropin)   **Uses: Short-term use in cardiac decompensation secondary to decreased contractility; increases organ perfusion (at low dose)**   **Action:** Positive inotropic agent with dose-related response; 2–10 mcg/kg/min β-effects (increases cardiac output and renal perfusion); 10–20 mcg/kg/min β-effects (peripheral vasoconstriction, pressor); > 20 mcg/kg/min peripheral and renal vasoconstriction   **Dose:** 5 mcg/kg/min by cont inf, ↑ increments of 5 mcg/kg/min to 50 mcg/kg/min max based on effect   **Caution:** [C, ?]   **Supplied:** Inj 40, 80, 160 mg/mL   **SE:** Tachycardia, vasoconstriction, hypotension, HA, N/V, dyspnea   **Notes:** Dosage > 10 mcg/kg/min may ↓ renal perfusion; monitor urinary output; monitor ECG for ↑ in heart rate, BP, and ectopic activity; monitor PCWP and cardiac output if possible

Dornase Alfa (Pulmozyme)   **Uses: ↓ Frequency of respiratory infections in patients with CF**   **Action:** Enzyme that selectively cleaves DNA   **Dose:** Inhal 2.5 mg/d   **Caution:** [B, ?]   **Supplied:** Soln for inhalation 1 mg/mL   **SE:** Pharyngitis, voice alteration, chest pain, rash   **Notes:** Use with recommended nebulizer

Dorzolamide (Trusopt) [See Table VII–12, pp 623–25]

Dorzolamide and Timolol (Cosopt) [See Table VII–12, pp 623–25]

Doxazosin (Cardura)   **Uses: HTN and symptomatic BPH**   **Action:** α_1-Adrenergic blocker; relaxes bladder neck smooth muscle   **Dose:** *HTN:* Initially 1 mg/d PO; may increase to 16 mg/d PO *BPH:* Initially 1 mg/d PO, may increase to 8 mg/d PO   **Caution:** [B, ?]   **Supplied:** Tabs 1, 2, 4, 8 mg   **SE:** Dizziness, HA, drowsiness, sexual dysfunction, doses > 4 mg ↑ likelihood of postural hypotension   **Notes:** Take first dose at bedtime

Doxepin (Sinequan, Adapin)   **WARNING:** *Pediatric:* Antidepressants may increase risk of suicidality; consider risks and benefits of use. Patients should be closely monitored for clinical worsening, suicidality, or unusual changes in behavior   **Uses: Depression, anxiety,**

chronic pain **Action:** TCA; increases the synaptic CNS concentrations of serotonin or norepinephrine **Dose:** 25–150 mg/d PO, usually hs but can be in $\div$ doses; $\downarrow$ dose in hepatic impairment **Caution:** [C, ?/–] **Supplied:** Caps 10, 25, 50, 75, 100, 150 mg; oral conc 10 mg/mL **SE:** Anticholinergic side effects, hypotension, tachycardia, drowsiness, photosensitivity

Doxepin, Topical (Zonalon)
Uses: Short-term treatment of pruritus (atopic dermatitis or lichen simplex chronicus) **Action:** Antipruritic; H_1- and H_2-receptor antagonism **Dose:** Apply thin coating qid for max 8 d **Caution:** [C, ?/–] **Supplied:** 5% cream **SE:** Limit application area to avoid systemic toxicity (hypotension, tachycardia, drowsiness, photosensitivity)

Doxorubicin (Adriamycin, Rubex)
Uses: Acute leukemias; Hodgkin's and non-Hodgkin's lymphomas; breast CA; soft tissue and osteosarcomas; Ewing's sarcoma; Wilms' tumor; neuroblastoma; bladder, ovarian, gastric, thyroid, and lung CAs **Action:** Intercalates DNA; inhibits DNA topoisomerases I and II **Dose:** Refer to specific protocols **Caution:** [D, ?] **Contra:** Severe CHF, cardiomyopathy, pre-existing myelosuppression, impaired cardiac function, patients who received previous treatment with complete cumulative doses of doxorubicin, idarubicin, daunorubicin **Supplied:** Inj 10, 20, 50, 75, 200 mg **SE:** Myelosuppression, venous streaking and phlebitis, N/V, diarrhea, mucositis, radiation recall phenomenon, cardiomyopathy rare but dose related; limit of 550 mg/m^2 cumulative dose (400 mg/m^2 if prior mediastinal irradiation) **Notes:** Dexrazoxane may limit cardiac toxicity; extravasation leads to tissue damage; discolors urine red/orange

Doxycycline (Vibramycin)
Uses: Broad-spectrum antibiotic **Action:** Tetracycline; interferes with protein synthesis **Spectrum:** Activity against *Rickettsia* spp, *Chlamydia,* and *M pneumoniae* **Dose:** 100 mg PO q12h on 1st day, then 100 mg PO daily–bid or 100 mg IV q12h **Supplied:** Tabs 50, 100 mg; caps 20, 50, 100 mg; syrup 50 mg/5 mL; susp 25 mg/5 mL; inj 100, 200 mg/vial **Caution:** [D, +] **Contra:** Children < 8yo, severe hepatic dysfunction **SE:** Diarrhea, GI disturbance, photosensitivity **Notes:** Useful for chronic bronchitis; $\downarrow$ effect w/ antacids containing aluminum, calcium, magnesium; tetracycline of choice in renal impairment

Dronabinol (Marinol) [C-II]
Uses: N/V associated with cancer chemotherapy; appetite stimulation **Action:** Antiemetic; inhibits the vomiting center in the medulla **Dose:** *Antiemetic:* 5–15 mg/m^2/dose q4–6h PRN *Appetite stimulant:* 2.5 mg PO before lunch and dinner **Caution:** [C, ?] **Contra:** Should not be used in patients with history of schizophrenia **Supplied:** Caps 2.5, 5, 10 mg **SE:** Drowsiness, dizziness, anxiety, mood change, hallucinations, depersonalization, orthostatic hypotension, tachycardia **Notes:** Principal psychoactive substance present in marijuana

Droperidol (Inapsine)
Uses: N/V; anesthetic premedication **Action:** Tranquilization, sedation, and antiemetic **Dose:** *Nausea:* 2.5–5 mg IV or IM q3–4h PRN *Premed:* 2.5–10 mg IV, 30–60 min preop **Caution:** [C, ?] **Supplied:** Inj 2.5 mg/mL **SE:** Drowsiness, moderate hypotension, occasional tachycardia and extrapyramidal reactions, QT interval prolongation, arrhythmias **Notes:** Give IVP slowly over 2–5 min

Drotrecogin Alfa (Xigris)
Uses: Reduce mortality in adults with severe sepsis (associated with acute organ dysfunction) who have a high risk of death (e.g., as determined by APACHE II) **Action:** Recombinant form of human activated protein C; exact mechanism unknown **Dose:** 24 mcg/kg/h for a total of 96 h **Caution:** [C, ?] **Contra:** Active bleeding, recent stroke or CNS surgery, head trauma, epidural catheter, CNS lesion at risk for herniation **Supplied:** 5-, 20-mg vials for reconstitution **SE:** Bleeding most common SE **Notes:** For percutaneous procedures stop infusion 2 h before the procedure and resume 1 h after; for major surgery stop infusion 2 h before surgery and resume 12 h after surgery in absence of bleeding

Dutasteride (Avodart)
Uses: Symptomatic BPH **Action:** 5α-reductase inhibitor **Dose:** 0.5 mg PO daily **Caution:** [X, –] Caution in hepatic impairment; pregnant women should avoid handling pills **Contra:** Women and children **Supplied:** Caps 0.5 mg **SE:** $\downarrow$

PSA levels, impotence, ↓ libido, gynecomastia   **Notes:** Do not donate blood until 6 months after discontinuation of this drug

Echothiophate Iodide (Phospholine Iodide) [See Table VII–12, pp 623–25]

Econazole (Spectazole)   **Uses:** Most tinea, cutaneous *Candida,* and tinea versicolor infections   **Action:** Topical antifungal   **Dose:** Apply to areas bid (daily for tinea versicolor) for 2–4 wk   **Caution:** [C, ?]   **Supplied:** Topical cream 1%   **SE:** Local irritation, pruritus, erythema   **Notes:** Symptom/clinical improvement seen early in treatment must carry out course of therapy to avoid recurrence

Edrophonium (Tensilon)   **Uses: Diagnosis of myasthenia gravis (MyG); acute myasthenic crisis; curare antagonist**   **Action:** Anticholinesterase   **Dose:** *Test for MyG:* 2 mg IV in 1 min; if tolerated, give 8 mg IV; positive test is a brief increase in strength; ↓ in renal impairment   **Caution:** [C, ?]   **Contra:** GI or GU obstruction; hypersensitivity to sulfite   **Supplied:** Inj 10 mg/mL   **SE:** N/V/D, excessive salivation, stomach cramps   **Notes:** ↑ aminotransferases; can cause severe cholinergic effects; keep atropine available

Efavirenz (Sustiva)   **Uses:** HIV infections   **Action:** Antiretroviral; non-nucleoside reverse transcriptase inhibitor   **Dose:** 600 mg/d PO, take qhs; avoid high-fat meals   **Caution:** [C, ?] CDC recommends HIV-infected mothers not breastfeed because of risk of transmission of HIV to infant   **Supplied:** Caps 50, 100, 200 mg   **SE:** Somnolence, vivid dreams, dizziness, rash, N/V/D   **Notes:** monitor transaminases, cholesterol

Eletriptan (Relpax)[See Table VII–16, p 629]

Emedastine (Emadine)   **Uses: Allergic conjunctivitis**   **Action:** Antihistamine; selective H_1-antagonist   **Dose:** 1 drop in eye/s up to qid   **Caution:** [B, ?]   **Contra:** Hypersensitivity to ingredients (preservatives benzalkonium, tromethamine)   **Supplied:** 0.05% soln   **SE:** HA, blurred vision, burning/stinging, corneal infiltrates/staining, dry eyes, foreign body sensation, hyperemia, keratitis, tearing, pruritus, rhinitis, sinusitis, asthenia, bad taste, dermatitis, discomfort   **Notes:** Do not use contact lenses if eyes are red; take care to prevent contaminating dropper tip

Emtricitabine (Emtriva)   **WARNING:** Class warning for lipodystrophy, lactic acidosis, and severe hepatomegaly   **Uses: HIV-1 infection**   **Action:** Nucleoside reverse transcriptase inhibitor (NRTI)   **Dose:** 200 mg PO daily; adjust dose for renal dysfunction   **Caution:** [B, –]   **Supplied:** 200 mg capsules   **SE:** Headache, diarrhea, nausea, rash;   **Notes:** Rarely causes hyperpigmentation of feet and hands; post-treatment exacerbation of hepatitis; first NRTI with once-daily dosing

Enalapril (Vasotec) [See Table VII–3, p 614]

Enfuvirtide (Fuzeon)   **WARNING:** Rarely causes hypersensitivity, never rechallenge patient   **Uses: Combination with antiretroviral agents for treatment of HIV-1 infection in treatment-experienced patients with evidence of viral replication despite ongoing antiretroviral therapy**   **Action:** Fusion inhibitor   **Dose:** 90 mg (1 mL) sq twice daily in upper arm, anterior thigh or abdomen   **Caution:** [B, –]   **Contra:** Previous hypersensitivity to drug   **Supplied:** 90 mg/mL upon reconstitution; dispensed as patient convenience kit with monthly supplies   **SE:** Injection site reactions (in nearly all patients); pneumonia, diarrhea, nausea, fatigue, insomnia, peripheral neuropathy   **Notes:** Rotate injection site; available only via restricted drug distribution system; must be immediately administered upon reconstitution or refrigerated for up to 24 hours before use

Enoxaparin (Lovenox)   **WARNING:** Recent or anticipated epidural/spinal anesthesia increase risk of spinal/epidural hematoma with subsequent paralysis   **Uses: Prevention and treatment of DVT; treatment of PE; unstable angina and non–Q-wave MI**   **Action:** LMW heparin   **Dose:** *DVT Prevention:* 30 mg SC bid or 40 mg SC q24h *DVT/PE treatment:* 1 mg/kg SC q12h or 1.5 mg/kg SC q24h *Angina:* 1 mg/kg SC q12h; ↓ dosage adjustment necessary with severe renal impairment (Crcl < 30 ml/min)   **Caution** [B, ?] Not recommended for thromboprophylaxis for prosthetic heart valves   **Contra:** Active bleeding, HIT antibody positive   **Supplied:** Inj 10 mg/0.1 mL (30-, 40-, 60-, 80-, 100-, 120-, 150-mg syringes)   **SE:** Bleeding,

hemorrhage, bruising, thrombocytopenia, pain/hematoma at injection site, ↑ AST/ALT **Notes:** Does not significantly affect bleeding time, platelet function, PT, or APTT; monitor platelets, bleeding; may monitor anti-factor Xa

Entacapone (Comtan)
Uses: Parkinson's disease **Action:** Selective and reversible catechol-*o*-methyltransferase (COMT) inhibitor **Dose:** 200 mg concurrently with each levodopa/carbidopa dose to a max 1600 mg/d; reduce levodopa/carbidopa dose by 25% if levodopa dose > 800 mg **Caution:** [C, ?] Hepatic impairment **Contra:** Concurrent use with nonselective MAOI **Supplied:** Tabs 200 mg **SE:** Dyskinesia, hyperkinesia, nausea, dizziness, hallucinations, orthostatic hypotension, brown-orange urine, diarrhea **Notes:** Monitor LFT; do not withdraw therapy abruptly

Ephedrine
Uses: Acute bronchospasm, bronchial asthma, nasal congestion, hypotension, narcolepsy, enuresis, and myasthenia gravis **Action:** Sympathomimetic; stimulates α- and β-receptors **Dose:** 25–50 mg IM or IV q 10 min to a max of 150 mg/d; 25–50 mg PO q3–4h PRN; 2–3 sprays each nostril q4h **Caution:** [C, ?/—] **Contra:** Cardiac arrhythmias; angle-closure glaucoma **Supplied:** Inj 50 mg/mL; caps 25, 50 mg; nasal spray 0.25% **SE:** CNS stimulation (nervousness, anxiety, trembling), tachycardia, arrhythmia, HTN, xerostomia, painful urination

Epinephrine (Adrenalin, Sus-Phrine, Others)
Uses: Cardiac arrest, anaphylactic reaction, bronchospasm, manage open-angle glaucoma **Action:** β-adrenergic agonist with some α-effects **Dose:** *Emergency cardiac care:* 0.5–1 mg (5–10 mL of 1:10,000) IV q5min to response *Anaphylaxis:* 0.3–0.5 SC of 1:1000 dilution, may repeat q5–15 min to a max of 1 mg/dose and 5 mg/d *Asthma:* 0.1–0.5 SC of 1:1000 dilution, repeated at 20-min to 4-h intervals or 1 inhal (met-dose) repeat in 1–2 min or susp 0.1–0.3 mL SC for extended effect **Caution:** [C, ?] ↓ Bronchodilation with β-blockers; **Contra:** Cardiac arrhythmias, angle-closure glaucoma **Supplied:** Inj 1:1000, 1:2000, 1:10,000, 1:100,000; susp for inj 1:200; aerosol 220 mcg/spray; soln for inhal 1% **SE:** CV (tachycardia, HTN, vasoconstriction), CNS stimulation (nervousness, anxiety, trembling), ↓ renal blood flow **Notes:** Can give via ET tube if no central line (2–2.5 × IV dose)

Epirubicin (Ellence)
Uses: Adjuvant therapy in patients with evidence of axillary node tumor involvement following resection of primary breast cancer **Actions:** An anthracycline cytotoxic agent **Dose:** Refer to specific protocols; reduce dose with hepatic impairment **Caution:** [D, –] **Contra:** Baseline neutrophil count < 1500 cells/mm^3, severe myocardial insufficiency, recent MI, severe arrhythmias, severe hepatic dysfunction, previous treatment with anthracyclines up to max cumulative dose **Supplied:** Inj 50 mg/25 mL, 200 mg/100 mL **SE:** Mucositis, N/V/D, alopecia, myelosuppression, cardiotoxicity, secondary acute myelogenous leukemia, severe tissue necrosis if extravasation occurs

Eplerenone (Inspra)
Uses: HTN **Action:** Selective aldosterone antagonist **Dose:** *Adults:* 50 mg PO daily to bid, doses > 100 mg/d no benefit with ↑ hyperkalemia; ↓ dose to 25 mg PO qd if giving with weak CYP3A4 inhibitors **Caution:** [B, +/–] Use of CYP3A4 inhibitors (ketoconazole, itraconazole, erythromycin, fluconazole, verapamil, saquinavir); monitor potassium with ACEI, ARB, NSAIDs, potassium-sparing diuretics; grapefruit juice, St. John's wort **Contra:** Potassium > 5.5 mEq/L; NIDDM with microalbuminuria; SCr > 2 mg/dL (males), > 1.8 mg/dL (females); CrCl < 50 mL/min; concurrent use of potassium supplements/potassium-sparing diuretics **Supplied:** Tabs 25, 50, 100 mg **SE:** Hypertriglyceridemia, hyperkalemia, headache, dizziness, gynecomastia, hypercholesterolemia, diarrhea, orthostatic hypotension **Notes:** May take 4 wk to see full effect

Epoetin Alfa [Erythropoietin, EPO] (Epogen, Procrit)
Uses: Anemia associated with CRF, zidovudine treatment in HIV-infected patients, CA chemotherapy; reduction in transfusions associated with surgery **Action:** Erythropoietin supplementation **Dose:** 50–150 units/kg IV/SC 3×/wk; adjust the dose q4–6wk as needed *Surgery:* 300 units/kg/d × 10 d before surgery to 4 d after. Decrease dose if Hct approaches 36% or Hgb ↑ > 4 points in 2-wk period **Caution:** [C, +] **Contra:** Uncontrolled HTN **Supplied:** Inj 2000,

3000, 4000, 10,000, 20,000, 40,000 units/mL **SE:** HTN, HA, tachycardia, fatigue, fever, N/V **Notes:** Store in refrigerator; monitor baseline and post-treatment Hct/Hgb, BP, ferritin

Epoprostenol (Flolan) **Uses:** Pulmonary HTN **Action:** Dilates the pulmonary and systemic arterial vascular beds; inhibits platelet aggregation **Dose:** Initial 2 ng/kg/min, ↑ by 2 ng/kg/min q15 min until dose-limiting SE (chest pain, dizziness, N/V, HA, hypotension, flushing). IV cont infusion 4 ng/kg/min **less than** maximum-tolerated rate; adjustments based on response and package insert guidelines **Caution:** [B, ?] ↑ Toxicity with diuretics, vasodilators, acetate in dialysis fluids, anticoagulants **Contra:** Chronic use in CHF 2nd-degree severe LVSD **Supplied:** Inj 0.5, 1.5 mg **SE:** Flushing, tachycardia, CHF, fever, chills, nervousness, HA, N/V/D, jaw pain, flu-like symptoms **Notes:** Abrupt discontinuation/interruptions can cause rebound pulmonary HTN. Monitor bleeding if using other antiplatelet/anticoagulants; watch hypotensive effects with other vasodilators/diuretics

Eprosartan (Teveten) [See Table VII–4, p 615]

Eptifibatide (Integrilin) **Uses: Acute coronary syndrome, PCI** **Action:** Glycoprotein IIb/IIIa inhibitor **Dose:** 180-mcg/kg IV bolus, then 2-mcg/kg/min continuous inf; ↓ dose in renal impairment (SCr > 2 mg/dL, < 4 mg/dL: 135-mcg/kg bolus and 0.5-mcg/kg/min infusion) **Caution:** [B, ?] Monitor bleeding with other anticoagulants **Contra:** Other GPIIb/IIIa inhibitors, h/o abnormal bleeding or hemorrhagic stroke (within 30 d), severe HTN, major surgery (within 6 wk), platelet count < 100,000 cells/mm^3, renal dialysis **Supplied:** Inj 0.75, 2 mg/mL **SE:** Bleeding, hypotension, injection site reaction, thrombocytopenia **Notes:** Monitor bleeding, coags, platelets, SCr, ACT with PCI (maintain ACT b/w 200–300 sec)

Ertapenem (Invanz) **Uses: Complicated intra-abdominal, acute pelvic and skin infections, pyelonephritis, community-acquired pneumonia** **Action:** A carbapenem; β-lactam antibiotic, inhibits cell wall synthesis *Spectrum*: Good gram(+)/(–) and anaerobic coverage, but not *Pseudomonas,* PCN-resistant pneumococci, MRSA, *Enterococcus,* β-lactamase(+) *H influenzae, Mycoplasma, Chlamydia* **Dose:** 1 g IM/IV once daily; 500 mg/d in CrCl < 30 mL/min **Caution:** [C, ?/–] Probenecid ↓ renal clearance of ertapenem **Contra:** < 18 yo, caution in PCN allergy **Supplied:** Inj 1 g/vial **SE:** HA, N/V/D, injection site reactions, thrombocytosis, ↑ LFTs **Notes:** Can give IM × 7 d, IV × 14 d; 137 mg sodium (~6 mEq)/g ertapenem

Erythromycin (E-Mycin, E.E.S., Ery-Tab, Others) **Uses:** Bacterial infections; bowel decontamination; GI motility; acne vulgaris **Action:** Bacteriostatic; interferes with protein synthesis *Spectrum:* Group A streptococci (*S pyogenes*), *S pneumoniae, N meningitides, N gonorrhoeae* (in penicillin-allergic patients), *Legionella, M pneumoniae* **Dose:** 250–500 mg PO q6–12h or 500 mg–1 g IV q6h *Prokinetic:* 250 mg PO tid 30 min before meals **Caution:** [B, +] ↑ Toxicity of carbamazepine, cyclosporine, digoxin, methylprednisolone, theophylline, felodipine, warfarin, simvastatin/lovastatin **Contra:** Hepatic impairment, pre-existing liver disease (estolate), concomitant use with pimozide **Supplied:** *Powder for inj as lactobionate:* 500 mg, 1 g *Base:* Tabs 250, 333, 500 mg; caps 250 mg *Estolate:* Caps 125, 250 mg; susp 125, 250 mg/5 mL *Stearate:* Tabs 250, 500 mg *Ethylsuccinate:* Chew tabs 200 mg; tabs 400 mg; susp 200, 400 mg/5 mL **SE:** HA, abdominal pain, N/V/D, [QT prolongation, torsades de pointes, ventricular arrhythmias/tachycardias (rare)]; cholestatic jaundice (estolate) **Notes:** 400 mg ethylsuccinate = 250 mg base/state/estolate; take with food to minimize GI upset

Erythromycin, Ophthalmic (Ilotycin) [See Table VII–12, pp 623–25]

Escitalopram (Lexapro) **WARNING:** *Pediatric:* Antidepressants may increase risk of suicidality; consider risks and benefits of use. Patients should be closely monitored for clinical worsening, suicidality, or unusual changes in behavior **Uses: Antidepressant, anxiety** **Action:** SSRI **Dose:** 10–20 mg PO daily; 10 mg/d in elderly and hepatic impairment **Caution:** [C, +/–] ↑ Risk of serotonin syndrome with other SSRI, tramadol, linezolid, sumatriptan **Contra:** Use with or within 14 d of discontinuing a MAOI **Supplied:** Tabs 5, 10, 20 mg; soln 1 mg/mL **SE:** N/V/D, sweating, insomnia, dizziness, dry mouth, sexual dysfunction **Notes:** Full effects may take 3 wk

Esmolol (Brevibloc)   Uses: **Supraventricular tachycardia and noncompensatory sinus tachycardia**   Action: β_1 Adrenergic blocker; class II antiarrhythmic   Dose: Initiate treatment with 500 mcg/kg load over 1 min, then 50 mcg/kg/min × 4 min; if inadequate response, repeat the loading dose and follow with maintenance infusion of 100 mcg/kg/min × 4 min; titrate by repeating loading, then incremental ↑ in the maintenance dose of 50 mcg/kg/min for 4 min until desired heart rate reached or BP decreases; average dose 100 mcg/kg/min   Caution: [C (1st trimester); D 2nd or 3rd trimester), ?]   Contra: Sinus bradycardia, heart block, uncompensated CHF, cardiogenic shock, hypotension   Supplied: Inj 10, 250 mg/mL; premix infusion 10 mg/mL   SE: Hypotension (↓ or discontinuing infusion reverses hypotension in ~30 min); bradycardia, diaphoresis, dizziness, pain on injection   Notes: Hemodynamic effects back to baseline within 20–30 min after discontinuing infusion

Esomeprazole (Nexium) [See Table VII–14, p 627]

Estazolam (ProSom) [C-IV]   Uses: **Short-term management of insomnia**   Action: Benzodiazepine   Dose: 1–2 mg PO qhs PRN; ↓ in hepatic impairment/elderly/debilitated; avoid abrupt withdrawal   Caution: [X, –] ↑ Effects with CNS depressants; cross-sensitivity with other benzodiazepines may occur   Supplied: Tabs 1, 2 mg   SE: Somnolence, weakness, palpitations   Notes: May cause psychological/physical dependence; avoid abrupt discontinuation after prolonged use

Esterified Estrogens (Estratab, Menest)   WARNING: Do not use in the prevention of cardiovascular disease   Uses: **Vasomotor symptoms or vulvar/vaginal atrophy associated with menopause; female hypogonadism**   Action: Estrogen supplement   Dose: *Menopause:* 0.3–1.25 mg/d, cyclically 3 wk on, 1 wk off *Hypogonadism:* 2.5–7.5 mg/d PO × 20 d, off × 10 d; not recommended in severe hepatic impairment   Caution: [X, –]   Contra: Genital bleeding of unknown etiology, breast CA, estrogen-dependent tumors, thromboembolic disorders, thrombophlebitis, recent MI, pregnancy   Supplied: Tabs 0.3, 0.625, 1.25, 2.5 mg   SE: Nausea, HA, bloating, breast enlargement/tenderness, edema, venous thromboembolism, ↑ triglycerides   Notes: Use at lowest dose for shortest period of time; refer to Womens Health Initiatives (WHI) data

Esterified Estrogens + Methyltestosterone (Estratest, Estratest HS)   Uses: **Vasomotor symptoms; postpartum breast engorgement**   Action: Estrogen and androgen supplement   Dose: 1 tab/d for 3 wk, then 1 wk off   Caution: [X, –]   Contra: Genital bleeding of unknown etiology, breast CA, estrogen-dependent tumors, thromboembolic disorders, thrombophlebitis, recent MI, pregnancy   Supplied: Tabs (estrogen/methyltestosterone) (HS) 0.625 mg/1.25 mg, 1.25 mg/2.5 mg   SE: Nausea, HA, bloating, breast enlargement/tenderness, edema, ↑ triglycerides, venous thromboembolism, gallbladder disease   Notes: Use at lowest dose for shortest period of time

Estradiol (Estrace)   Uses: **Atrophic vaginitis, vasomotor symptoms associated with menopause, osteoporosis**   Action: Estrogen supplement   Dose: *Oral:* 1–2 mg/d, adjust PRN to control symptoms *Vaginal cream:* 2–4 g/d × 2 wk, then 1 g 1–3 ×/wk   Caution: [X,–]   Contra: Genital bleeding of unknown etiology, breast CA, estrogen-dependent tumors, thromboembolic disorders, thrombophlebitis; recent MI; not recommended in severe hepatic impairment   Supplied: Tabs 0.5, 1, 2 mg; vaginal cream 0.1 mg/g   SE: Nausea, HA, bloating, breast enlargement/tenderness, edema, ↑ triglycerides, venous thromboembolism, gallbladder disease

Estradiol, Transdermal (Estraderm, Climara, Vivelle)   Uses: **Severe menopausal vasomotor symptoms; female hypogonadism**   Action: Estrogen supplementation   Dose: 0.1 mg/d patch 1–2 ×/wk depending on product; adjust PRN to control symptoms   Caution: [X, –] (See estradiol above)   Contra: Pregnancy, undiagnosed genital bleeding, carcinoma of breast, estrogen-dependent tumors, history of thrombophlebitis, thrombosis, thromboembolic disorders associated with estrogen use   Supplied: TD patches (delivers _____ mg/24 h) 0.025, 0.0375, 0.05, 0.075, 0.1   SE: Nausea, bloating, breast enlargement/tenderness, edema, HA, hypertriglyceridemia, gallbladder disease   Notes: Do not apply to breasts, place on trunk of body and rotate sites

Estradiol cypionate and medroxyprogesterone acetate (Lunelle)
WARNING: Cigarette smoking ↑ risk of serious cardiovascular side effects from contraceptives containing estrogen. This risk increases with age and with heavy smoking (> 15 cigarettes/d) and is quite marked in women > 35 y. Women who use LUNELLE should be strongly advised not to smoke **Uses:** Contraceptive **Action:** Estrogen and progestin **Dose:** 0.5 mL IM (deltoid, ant thigh, buttock) monthly, do not exceed 33 d **Caution:** [X, M] HTN, gallbladder disease, ↑ lipids, migraines, sudden HA, valvular heart disease with complications **Contra:** Pregnancy, heavy smokers > 35 y, DVT, PE, cerebro/cardiovascular disease, estrogen-dependent neoplasm, undiagnosed abnormal uterine bleeding, hepatic tumors, cholestatic jaundice **Supplied:** Estradiol cypionate (5 mg), medroxyprogesterone acetate (25 mg) single-dose vial or prefilled syringe (0.5 mL) **SE:** Arterial thromboembolism, hypertension, cerebral hemorrhage, myocardial infarction, amenorrhea, acne, breast tenderness **Notes:** Start within 5 d of menstruation

Estramustine Phosphate (Estracyt, Emcyt) **Uses:** Advanced prostate CA
Action: Anti-microtubule agent; weak estrogenic and antiandrogenic activity **Dose:** 14 mg/kg/d in 3–4 ÷ doses; preferable to take on empty stomach, do not take with milk or milk products **Caution:** [NA, not used in females] **Contra:** Active thrombophlebitis or thromboembolic disorders **Supplied:** Caps 140 mg **SE:** N/V, exacerbation of preexisting CHF, thrombophlebitis, MI, PE; gynecomastia in 20–100%

Estrogen, Conjugated (Premarin) **WARNING:** Should not be used for the prevention of cardiovascular disease. The WHI reported increased risk of MI, stroke, breast CA, PE, and DVT when combined with methoxyprogesterone over 5 years of treatment; increased risk of endometrial CA **Uses:** Moderate to severe menopausal vasomotor symptoms; atrophic vaginitis; palliative therapy of advanced prostatic carcinoma; prevention and treatment of estrogen deficiency-induced osteoporosis **Action:** Hormonal replacement **Dose:** 0.3–1.25 mg/d PO cyclically; prostatic carcinoma requires 1.25–2.5 mg PO tid; **Caution:** [X, –] **Contra:** Not recommended in severe hepatic impairment, genital bleeding of unknown etiology, breast CA, estrogen-dependent tumors, thromboembolic disorders, thrombosis, thrombophlebitis, recent MI **Supplied:** Tabs 0.3, 0.625, 0.9, 1.25, 2.5 mg; inj 25 mg/mL **SE:** ↑ risk of endometrial carcinoma, gallbladder disease, thromboembolism, HA, and possibly breast CA; generic products not equivalent

Estrogen, Conjugated—Synthetic (Cenestin) **Uses:** Treatment of moderate to severe vasomotor symptoms associated with menopause **Action:** Hormonal replacement **Dose:** 0.625–1.25 mg PO qd **Caution:** [X,–] **Contra:** See estrogen, conjugated **Supplied:** Tabs 0.625, 0.9, 1.25 mg **SE:** Associated with an increased risk of endometrial CA, gallbladder disease, thromboembolism, and possibly breast CA

Estrogen, Conjugated + Medroxyprogesterone (Prempro, Premphase)
WARNING: Should not be used for the prevention of cardiovascular disease; the WHI study reported increased risk of MI, stroke, breast CA, PE, and DVT over 5 years of treatment **Uses:** Moderate to severe menopausal vasomotor symptoms; atrophic vaginits; prevention of postmenopausal osteoporosis **Action:** Hormonal replacement **Dose:** Prempro 1 tab PO qd; Premphase 1 tab PO qd **Caution:** [X,–] **Contra:** Not recommended in severe hepatic impairment, genital bleeding of unknown etiology, breast CA, estrogen-dependent tumors, thromboembolic disorders, thrombosis, thrombophlebitis **Supplied:** (Expressed as estrogen/medroxyprogesterone) *Prempro:* Tabs 0.625/2.5, 0.625/5 mg *Premphase:* Tabs 0.625/0 (days 1–14) and 0.625/5 mg (days 15–28) **SE:** Gallbladder disease, thromboembolism, HA, breast tenderness

Estrogen, Conjugated + Methylprogesterone (Premarin + Methylprogesterone) **Uses:** Menopausal vasomotor symptoms; osteoporosis **Action:** Estrogen and androgen combination **Dose:** 1 tab/d **Caution:** [X, –] **Contra:** Genital bleeding of unknown etiology, breast CA, estrogen-dependent tumors, thromboembolic disorders, thrombosis, thrombophlebitis **Supplied:** Tabs 0.625 mg of estrogen, conjugated, and 2.5 or 5 mg of methylprogesterone **SE:** Nausea, bloating, breast enlargement/tenderness, edema,

HA, hypertriglyceridemia, gallbladder disease **Notes:** Not recommended in severe hepatic impairment

Estrogen, Conjugated + Methyltestosterone (Premarin + Methyltestosterone)
Uses: Moderate to severe menopausal vasomotor symptoms; postpartum breast engorgement **Action:** Estrogen and androgen combination **Dose:** 1 tab/d × 3 wk, then 1 wk off **Caution:** [X, –] **Contra:** Not recommended in severe hepatic impairment, genital bleeding of unknown etiology, breast CA, estrogen-dependent tumors, thromboembolic disorders, thrombosis, thrombophlebitis **Supplied:** Tabs (estrogen/methyltestosterone) 0.625 mg/5 mg, 1.25 mg/10 mg **SE:** Nausea, bloating, breast enlargement/tenderness, edema, HA, hypertriglyceridemia, gallbladder disease

Etanercept (Enbrel)
Uses: Reduce signs and symptoms of RA in patients who have failed other DMARDs (disease-modifying antirheumatic drugs), Crohn's **Action:** Binds TNF **Dose:** 25 mg SC 2 × wk (separated by at least 72–96 h); **Caution:** [B, ?] **Contra:** Active infection; caution in conditions that predispose to infection (i.e., DM) **Supplied:** Inj 25 mg/vial **SE:** HA, rhinitis, inj site reaction **Notes:** Rotate injection sites

Ethambutol (Myambutol)
Uses: Pulmonary TB and other mycobacterial infections **Action:** Inhibits RNA synthesis **Dose:** 15–25 mg/kg/d PO as a single dose; adjust in renal impairment, take with food **Caution:** [B, +] **Contra:** Optic neuritis **Supplied:** Tabs 100, 400 mg **SE:** HA, hyperuricemia, acute gout, abdominal pain, ↑ LFTs, optic neuritis, GI upset **Notes:** Avoid antacids

Ethinyl Estradiol (Estinyl, Feminone)
Uses: Menopausal vasomotor symptoms; female hypogonadism **Action:** Estrogen supplement **Dose:** 0.02–1.5 mg/d ÷ daily–tid; **Caution:** [X, –] **Contra:** Not recommended in severe hepatic impairment; genital bleeding of unknown etiology, breast CA, estrogen-dependent tumors, thromboembolic disorders, thrombosis, thrombophlebitis **Supplied:** Tabs 0.02, 0.05, 0.5 mg **SE:** Nausea, bloating, breast enlargement/tenderness, edema, HA, hypertriglyceridemia, gallbladder disease

Ethinyl estradiol and Levonorgestrel (Preven)
Uses: Emergency contraceptive ("morning-after pill"); prevent pregnancy after contraceptive failure or unprotected intercourse **Actions:** Estrogen and progestin; interferes with implantation **Dose:** 4 tabs, take 2 tabs q12h × 2 (within 72 h of intercourse) **Supplied:** Kit ethinyl estradiol (0.05), levonogestrel (0.25) blister pack with 4 pills and urine pregnancy test **Caution:** [X, M] **Contra:** Known/suspected pregnancy, abnormal uterine bleeding **SE:** Peripheral edema, N/V/D, bloating, abdominal pain, fatigue, HA, and menstrual changes **Notes:** Will not induce abortion; may increase risk of ectopic pregnancy

Ethinyl estradiol and Norelgestromin (Ortho Evra)
Uses: Contraceptive patch **Action:** Estrogen and progestin **Dose:** Apply patch to abdomen, buttocks, upper torso (not breasts), or upper outer arm at the beginning of the menstrual cycle; new patch is applied weekly for 3 weeks; week 4 is patch-free **Caution:** [X, M] **Contra:** Thrombophlebitis, undiagnosed vaginal bleeding, pregnancy, carcinoma of breast, estrogen-dependent tumor **Supplied:** 20-cm^2 patch (6 mg norelgestromin [active metabolite norgestrate] and 0.75 mg of ethinyl estradiol) **SE:** Breast discomfort, HA, application site reactions, nausea, menstrual cramps; thrombosis risks similar to OCP **Notes:** Less effective in women > 90 kg

Ethosuximide (Zarontin)
Uses: Absence (petit mal) seizures **Action:** Anticonvulsant; increases the seizure threshold **Dose:** Initial dose 500 mg PO divided bid; ↑ by 250 mg/d q4–7d PRN (max 1500 mg/d) **Caution:** [C, +] Renal/hepatic impairment **Supplied:** Caps 250 mg; syrup 250 mg/5 mL **SE:** Blood dyscrasias, GI upset, drowsiness, dizziness, irritability **Notes:** Monitor serum levels (see Table VII–17, p 630)

Etidronate Disodium (Didronel)
Uses: Hypercalcemia of malignancy, Paget's disease, and heterotopic ossification **Action:** Inhibition of normal and abnormal bone resorption **Dose:** *Paget's:* 5–10 mg/kg/d PO in divided doses (duration 3–6 mo) *Hypercalcemia:* 7.5 mg/kg/d IV infusion over 2 h × 3 d **Caution:** [B oral (C parenteral), ?] **Contra:** SCr > 5 mg/dL **Supplied:** Tabs 200, 400 mg; inj 50 mg/mL **SE:** GI intolerance (↓ by divid-

ing daily doses); hypophosphatemia, hypomagnesemia, bone pain, abnormal taste, fever, convulsions, nephrotoxicity **Notes:** Take oral on empty stomach 2 h before any meal

Etodolac (Lodine) [See Table VII–11, pp 621–22]

Etonogestrel/Ethinyl Estradiol (NuvaRing)   **Uses:** Contraceptive **Action:** Estrogen and progestin combination **Dose:** Rule out pregnancy first; insert ring vaginally for 3 wk, remove for 1 wk; insert new ring 7 d after last removed (even if still bleeding) at same time of day ring removed. First day of menses is day 1, insert before day 5 even if still bleeding. Use other contraception for first 7 days of starting therapy. See insert if converting from other forms of contraception. After delivery or 2nd-trimester abortion, insert ring 4 wk postpartum (if not breastfeeding) **Caution:** [X, ?/–] HTN, gallbladder disease, ↑ lipids, migraines, sudden HA **Contra:** Pregnancy, heavy smokers > 35 yrs, DVT, PE, cerebro/cardiovascular disease, estrogen-dependent neoplasm, undiagnosed abnormal genital bleeding, hepatic tumors, cholestatic jaundice **Supplied:** Intravaginal ring: ethinyl estradiol 0.015 mg/d and etonogestrel 0.12 mg/d **Notes:** If ring accidentally removed, rinse with cool/lukewarm water (not hot) and reinsert ASAP; if not reinserted within 3 h, effectiveness decreased. Do not use with diaphragm

Etoposide [VP-16] (VePesid, Toposar)   **Uses:** Testicular CA, non–small cell lung CA, Hodgkin's and non-Hodgkin's lymphomas, pediatric ALL, and allogeneic/autologous BMT in high doses **Action:** Topoisomerase II inhibitor **Dose:** Refer to specific protocols; ↓ in renal/hepatic impairment **Caution:** [D, –] Intrathecal administration **Supplied:** Caps 50 mg; inj 20 mg/mL **SE:** Myelosuppression, N/V, alopecia, hypotension if infused too rapidly, anorexia, anemia, leukopenia **Notes:** Emetic potential moderately low (10–30%)

Exemestane (Aromasin)   **Uses:** Treatment of advanced breast cancer in postmenopausal women whose disease has progressed following tamoxifen therapy **Action:** An irreversible, steroidal aromatase inhibitor, which lowers circulating estrogen concentrations **Dose:** 25 mg PO daily after a meal **Caution:** [D, ?/–] **Supplied:** Tabs 25 mg **SE:** Hot flashes, nausea, fatigue

Ezetimibe (Zetia)   **Uses:** Primary hypercholesterolemia alone or in combination with an HMG-CoA reductase inhibitor **Action:** Inhibits intestinal absorption of cholesterol and phytosterols **Dose:** 10 mg/d PO **Caution:** [C, +/–] Bile acid sequestrants ↓ bioavailability **Contra:** Hepatic impairment **Supplied:** Tabs 10 mg **SE:** HA, diarrhea, abdominal pain, ↑ transaminases used in combination with an HMG-CoA reductase inhibitor

Ezetimibe/simvastatin (Vytorin) [See Table VII–15, p 628]

Famciclovir (Famvir)   **Uses:** Acute herpes zoster (shingles) and genital herpes **Action:** Inhibits viral DNA synthesis **Dose:** *Zoster:* 500 mg PO q8h × 7 d *Simplex:* 125–250 mg PO bid; ↓ in renal impairment **Caution:** [B, –] **Supplied:** Tabs 125, 250, 500 mg **SE:** Fatigue, dizziness, HA, pruritus, nausea, diarrhea **Notes:** Most effective if given within 72 h of initial lesion

Famotidine (Pepcid)   **Uses:** Short-term treatment of active duodenal ulcer and benign gastric ulcer; maintenance treatment for duodenal ulcer, hypersecretory conditions, GERD, and heartburn **Action:** H₁-antagonist; inhibits gastric acid secretion **Dose:** *Ulcer:* 20–40 mg PO qhs or 20 mg IV q12h × 4–8 wk *Hypersecretion:* 20–160 mg PO q6h *GERD:* 20 mg PO bid × 6 wk; maintenance 20 mg PO hs *Heartburn:* 10 mg PO prn q12h; ↓ dose in severe renal insufficiency **Caution:** [B, M] **Supplied:** Tabs 10, 20, 40 mg; chew tabs 10 mg; susp 40 mg/5 mL; inj 10 mg/2 mL **SE:** Dizziness, HA, constipation, diarrhea, thrombocytopenia **Notes:** Chewable tablets contain phenylalanine

Felodipine (Plendil)   **Uses:** HTN and CHF **Action:** Ca channel blocker **Dose:** 2.5–10 mg PO daily; ↓ in hepatic impairment **Caution:** [C, ?] ↑ Effect with azole antifungals, erythromycin; bioavailability ↑ with grapefruit juice **Supplied:** ER tabs 2.5, 5, 10 mg **SE:** Peripheral edema, flushing, tachycardia, HA, gingival hyperplasia **Notes:** Follow BP in elderly and in impaired hepatic function, do not use doses > 10 mg in these patients; swallow whole

Fenofibrate (TriCor) **Uses: Hypertriglyceridemia** **Action:** Inhibits triglyceride synthesis **Dose:** 54–160 mg QD; take with meals; ↓ in renal impairment **Caution:** [C, ?] **Contra:** Hepatic/severe renal dysfunction, 1st-degree biliary cirrhosis, unexplained persistent LFT abnormalities, pre-existing gallbladder disease **Supplied:** Tabs 48, 145 mg **SE:** GI disturbances, cholecystitis, arthralgia, myalgia, dizziness **Notes:** Monitor LFTs

Fenoldopam (Corlopam) **Uses: Hypertensive emergency** **Action:** Rapid vasodilator **Dose:** Initial dose 0.03–0.1 mcg/kg/min IV cont infusion; titrate to effect q15min with 0.05–0.1 mcg/kg/min increments **Caution:** [B, ?] ↑ Levels with APAP; hypotension with BB **Contra:** Hypersensitivity to sulfites **Supplied:** Inj 10 mg/mL **SE:** Hypotension, edema, facial flushing, N/V/D, atrial flutter/fibrillation, ↑ intraocular pressure **Notes:** Avoid concurrent use with β-blockers

Fenoprofen (Nalfon) [Table VII–11, pp 621–22]

Fentanyl (Sublimaze) [C-II] **Uses: Short-acting analgesic used in conjunction with anesthesia** **Action:** Narcotic analgesic **Dose:** *Adults:* 25–100 mcg/kg/dose IV/IM prn; ↓ in renal impairment **Caution:** [B, +] **Contra:** Increased ICP, respiratory depression, severe renal/hepatic impairment **Supplied:** Inj 0.05 mg/mL **SE:** Sedation, hypotension, bradycardia, constipation, nausea, respiratory depression, miosis **Notes:** 0.1 mg of fentanyl = 10 mg of morphine IM

Fentanyl, Transdermal (Duragesic) [C-II] **Uses: Chronic pain** **Action:** Narcotic **Dose:** Apply patch to upper torso q72h; dose calculated from narcotic requirements in previous 24 h; ↓ in renal impairment **Caution:** [B, +] **Contra:** ↑ ICP, respiratory depression, severe renal/hepatic impairment **Supplied:** TD patches 25, 50, 75, 100 mcg/h **SE:** Sedation, ↓ BP, bradycardia, constipation, nausea, respiratory depression, miosis **Notes:** 0.1 mg of fentanyl = 10 mg of morphine IM

Fentanyl, Transmucosal System (Actiq) [C-II] **Uses: Induction of anesthesia; breakthrough CA pain** **Action:** Narcotic **Dose:** Anesthesia: 5–15 mcg/kg *Pain:* 200 mcg over 15 min, titrate to effect; ↓ in renal impairment **Caution:** [B, +] **Contra:** ↑ ICP, respiratory depression, severe renal/hepatic impairment **Supplied:** Lozenges on stick 200, 400, 600, 800, 1200, 1600 mcg **SE:** Sedation, ↓ BP, bradycardia, constipation, nausea, respiratory depression, miosis **Notes:** 0.1 mg of fentanyl = 10 mg of morphine IM

Ferrous Gluconate (Fergon, Others) **Uses: Iron deficiency anemia** and iron supplementation **Action:** Dietary supplementation **Dose:** 100–200 mg of elemental Fe/d in ÷ doses; take on empty stomach (take with meals if GI upset occurs) **Caution:** [A, ?] Avoid antacids **Contra:** Hemochromatosis, hemolytic anemia **Supplied:** Tabs 300 (34 mg Fe), 325 mg (36 mg Fe) **SE:** GI upset, constipation, dark stools, discoloration of urine, stain teeth **Notes:** 12% elemental Fe

Ferrous Gluconate Complex (Ferrlecit) **Uses: Iron deficiency anemia or supplement to erythropoietin therapy** **Action:** Supplemental iron **Dose:** Test Dose: 2 mL (25 mg Fe) infused over 1 h. If no reaction, 125 mg (10 mL) IV over 1 h. Usual cumulative dose 1 g Fe administered over 8 sessions (until favorable hematocrit achieved) **Caution:** [B, ?] **Contra:** Use in any anemia not caused by iron deficiency; heart failure; iron overload **Supplied:** Inj 12.5 mg/mL Fe **SE:** Hypotension, serious hypersensitivity reactions, GI disturbance, injection site reaction **Notes:** Dosage expressed as mg Fe; may be infused during dialysis

Ferrous Sulfate **Uses: Iron deficiency anemia and iron supplementation** **Action:** Dietary supplementation **Dose:** *Adults:* 100–200 mg of elemental Fe/d in ÷ doses; take on empty stomach (take with meals if GI upset occurs); avoid antacids **Caution:** [A, ?] ↑ Absorption with vitamin C; ↓ absorption with tetracycline, fluoroquinolones, antacids, H_2 blockers, proton pump inhibitors **Contra:** Hemochromatosis, hemolytic anemia **Supplied:** Tabs 187 (60 mg Fe), 200 (65 mg Fe), 324 (65 mg Fe), 325 mg (65 mg Fe); SR caplets and tabs 160 mg (50 mg Fe), 200 mg (65 mg Fe); drops 75 mg/0.6 mL (15 mg Fe/0.6 mL); elixir 220 mg/5 mL (44 mg Fe/5 mL); syrup 90 mg/5 mL (18 mg Fe/5 mL) **SE:** GI upset, constipation, dark stools, discolored urine

Fexofenadine (Allegra)   Uses: **Allergic rhinitis**   Action: Antihistamine   Dose: 60 mg PO bid or 180 mg/d; adjust in renal impairment   Caution: [C, ?]   Supplied: Caps 60 mg, tabs 30, 60, 180 mg; Allegra-D (60 mg fexofenadine/120 mg pseudoephedrine)   SE: Drowsiness (uncommon)

Filgrastim [G-CSF] (Neupogen)   Uses: **Decrease incidence of infection in febrile neutropenic patients; treatment of chronic neutropenia**   Action: Recombinant G-CSF   Dose: 5 mcg/kg/d SC or IV single daily dose; discontinue therapy when ANC > 10,000   Caution: [C, ?] Drug interaction with drugs that potentiate release of neutrophils (e.g., lithium)   Contra: Hypersensitivity to *E coli*-derived proteins or G-CSF   Supplied: Inj 300 mcg/mL   SE: Fever, alopecia, N/V/D, splenomegaly, bone pain, HA, rash   Notes: Monitor blood cell count and platelets; monitor for cardiac events; no clinical benefit with ANC > 10,000/mm³

Finasteride (Proscar, Propecia)   Uses: **BPH and androgenetic alopecia**   Action: Inhibits 5α-reductase   Dose: *BPH:* 5 mg/d PO *Alopecia:* 1 mg/d PO; food may delay rate/reduce extent of oral absorption   Caution: [X, −] Caution in hepatic impairment   Contra: Pregnant women should avoid handling pills   Supplied: Tabs 1 mg (Propecia), 5 mg (Proscar)   SE: ↓ PSA levels; ↓ libido, impotence (rare)   Notes: Reestablish PSA baseline at 6 mo; 3–6 mo for effect on urinary symptoms; must continue therapy to maintain new hair

Flavoxate (Urispas)   Uses: **Symptomatic relief of dysuria, urgency, nocturia, suprapubic pain, urinary frequency, and incontinence**   Action: Antispasmotic   Dose: 100–200 mg PO tid–qid   Caution: [B, ?]   Contra: Pyloric or duodenal obstruction, GI hemorrhage, GI obstruction, ileus, achalasia, BPH   Supplied: Tabs 100 mg   SE: Drowsiness, blurred vision, dry mouth

Flecainide (Tambocor)   Uses: **Prevent AF/flutter and PSVT, prevent/suppress life-threatening ventricular arrhythmias**   Action: Class 1C antiarrhythmic   Dose: 100 mg PO q12h; ↑ by 50 mg q12h q4d to max 400 mg/d; ↓ in renal impairment, monitor closely in hepatic impairment   Caution: [C, +] ↑ Conc with amiodarone, digoxin, quinidine, ritonavir/amprenavir, BB, verapamil,   Contra: 2nd-/3rd-degree AV block, RBBB with bifascicular or trifascicular block, cardiogenic shock, CAD, ritonavir/amprenavir; alkalinizing agents   Supplied: Tabs 50, 100, 150 mg   SE: Dizziness, visual disturbances, dyspnea, palpitations, edema, tachycardia, CHF, HA, fatigue, rash, nausea   Notes: May cause new/worsened arrhythmias; initiate medication in hospital; may dose q8h if patient is intolerant/condition is uncontrolled at 12-h intervals

Floxuridine (FUDR)   Uses: **Gastrointestinal adenoma, liver, renal cell carcinoma; colon and pancreatic CAs;**   Action: Inhibitor of thymidylate synthase; interferes with DNA synthesis (S-phase specific)   Dose: Refer to specific protocols   Caution: [D, −] Drug interaction with live and rotavirus vaccine   Contra: Bone marrow suppression, poor nutritional status, potentially serious infection   Supplied: Inj 500 mg   SE: Myelosuppression, anorexia, abdominal cramps, N/V/D, mucositis, alopecia, skin rash, and hyperpigmentation; rare neurotoxicity (blurred vision, depression, nystagmus, vertigo, and lethargy); intra-arterial catheter-related problems (ischemia, thrombosis, bleeding, and infection)   Notes: Need effective birth control; palliative treatment for inoperable/incurable patients

Fluconazole (Diflucan)   Uses: **Candidiasis (esophageal, oropharyngeal, urinary tract, vaginal, prophylaxis); cryptococcal meningitis**   Action: Antifungal; inhibits fungal cytochrome P-450 sterol demethylation   Dose: 100–400 mg/d PO or IV *Vaginitis:* 150 mg PO as a single dose *Cryptococcus:* 400 mg day 1, then 200 mg × 10–12 wk after CSF (−); ↓ in renal impairment   Caution: [C, −]   Supplied: Tabs 50, 100, 150, 200 mg; susp 10, 40 mg/mL; inj 2 mg/mL   SE: HA, rash, GI upset, hypokalemia, ↑ LFTs   Notes: PO use produces the same blood levels as IV, PO preferred when possible

Flucytosine (Ancobon)   Uses: **Serious infections caused by susceptible strains of *Candida* or *Cryptococcus***   Action: Antifungal   Dose: 50–150 mg/kg/d divided q6h; reduce dose with impaired renal function   Caution: [C, −]   Supplied: Caps 250, 500 mg   SE: Myelosuppression, N/V/D, chest pain, dyspnea, rash   Notes: Instruct patient to take caps a few at a time over 15 min

Fludarabine Phosphate (Flamp, Fludara) Uses: **Autoimmune hemolytic anemia, CLL, cold agglutinin hemolysis, low-grade lymphoma, mycosis fungoides** Action: Inhibits ribonucleotide reductase; blocks DNA polymerase-induced DNA repair Dose: Refer to specific protocols Caution: [D, –] Cytarabine given before fludarabine ↓ its metabolism Contra: Pregnancy Supplied: Inj 50 mg SE: Myelosuppression, N/V/D, LFT elevations; edema, CHF, fever, chills, fatigue, dyspnea, nonproductive cough, pneumonitis; severe CNS toxicity rare in leukemia Notes: Not recommended in CrCl < 30 mL/min

Fludrocortisone Acetate (Florinef) Uses: **Adrenocortical insufficiency, Addison's, salt-wasting syndrome** Action: Mineralocorticoid replacement Dose: 0.1–0.2 mg/d PO Caution: [C, ?] Contra: Systemic fungal infections; known hypersensitivity Supplied: Tabs 0.1 mg SE: HTN, edema, CHF, HA, dizziness, convulsions, acne, rash, bruising, hyperglycemia, HPA suppression, cataracts Notes: For adrenal insufficiency, must use with glucocorticoid supplement; dosage changes based on plasma renin activity

Flumazenil (Romazicon) Uses: **Reversal of the sedative effects of benzodiazepines and general anesthesia** Action: Benzodiazepine receptor antagonist Dose: 0.2 mg IV over 15 sec; repeat dose if desired level of consciousness not obtained, to 1 mg max (3 mg max benzodiazepine overdose); ↓ in hepatic impairment Caution: [C, ?] Contra: Patients showing signs of serious cyclic-antidepressant overdose, patients given benzodiazepine for control of life-threatening conditions (ICP/status epi) Supplied: Inj 0.1 mg/mL SE: N/V, palpitations, HA, anxiety, nervousness, hot flashes, tremor, blurred vision, dyspnea, hyperventilation, withdrawal syndrome Notes: Does not reverse narcotic symptoms (amnesia)

Flunisolide (AeroBid, Nasalide) Uses: **Control of bronchial asthma in patients requiring chronic steroid therapy; relief of seasonal/perennial allergic rhinitis** Action: Topical steroid Dose: *MDI:* 2 inhal bid (max 8/d) *Nasal:* 2 sprays/nostril bid (max 8/d) Caution: [C, ?] Contra: Status asthmaticus Supplied: Aerosol 250 mcg/actuation; nasal spray 0.025% SE: Tachycardia, bitter taste, local effects, oral candidiasis Notes: Not for acute asthma attack

Fluorometholone (FML, Flarex) [See Table VII–12, pp 623–25]

Fluorouracil [5-FU] (Adrucil) Uses: **Colorectal, gastric, pancreatic, breast, basal cell, head, neck, bladder CAs** Action: Inhibitor of thymidylate synthetase (interferes with DNA synthesis, S-phase specific) Dose: Refer to specific protocol Caution: [D, ?] ↑ Toxicity with allopurinol; do not give MTX before 5-FU Contra: Poor nutritional status, depressed bone marrow function, thrombocytopenia, major surgery within past month, DPD enzyme deficiency, pregnancy, serious infection, daily doses > 800 mg, bilirubin > 5 mg/dL Supplied: Inj 50 mg/mL SE: Stomatitis, esophagopharyngitis, N/V/D, anorexia; myelosuppression (leukocytopenia, thrombocytopenia, and anemia); rash/dry skin/photosensitivity; tingling in hands/feet with pain (palmar-plantar erythrodysesthesia); phlebitis, discoloration at inj sites Notes: ↑ Thiamine intake; sun sensitivity; contraception recommended

Fluorouracil, Topical [5-FU] (Efudex) Uses: **Basal cell carcinoma; actinic/solar keratosis** Action: Inhibitor of thymidylate synthetase (interferes with DNA synthesis, S-phase specific) Dose: Apply 5% cream bid × 3–6 wk Caution: [D, ?] Irritant chemotherapy Supplied: Cream 1, 5%; soln 1, 2, 5% SE: Rash, dry skin, photosensitivity Notes: Complete healing may not be evident for 1–2 months; wash hands thoroughly; avoid occlusive dressings; do not overuse

Fluoxetine (Prozac, Sarafem) WARNING: *Pediatric:* Antidepressants may increase risk of suicidality; consider risks and benefits of use. Patients should be closely monitored for clinical worsening, suicidality, or unusual changes in behavior Uses: **Depression, OCD, panic disorder, bulimia, PMDD (Sarafem)** Action: SSRI Dose: *Depression:* 20 mg/d PO (max 80 mg/d divided); weekly regimen 90 mg/wk after 1–2 wk of standard dose *Bulimia:* 60 mg daily q AM *Panic disorder:* 20 mg/d *OCD:* 20–80 mg/d *PMDD:* 20 mg or 20 mg intermittently starting 14 d before menses, repeat with each cycle; adjust dose in hepatic failure Caution: [B, ?/–] Risk of serotonin syndrome with MAOI, SSRI, serotonin agonists, linezolid; risk of QT prolongation with phenothiazines **Contra:** MAOI/thioridazine (use within 5 wk) **Supplied:** *Prozac:* Caps 10, 20, 40 mg; scored tabs 10 mg; SR cap 90 mg; soln 20 mg/5 mL *Sarafem:* 10, 20 mg caps **SE:** Nausea, nervousness, weight loss, HA, insomnia

Fluoxymesterone (Halotestin) **Uses: Androgen-responsive metastatic breast CA, hypogonadism** **Action:** Inhibition of secretion of LH and FSH by feedback inhibition **Dose:** Refer to specific protocol **Caution:** [X, ?/–] ↑ Effect with anticoagulants, cyclosporine, insulin, lithium, narcotics **Contra:** Serious cardiac, liver, or kidney disease; pregnancy **Supplied:** Tabs 2, 5, 10 mg **SE:** Virilization, amenorrhea and menstrual irregularities, hirsutism, alopecia and acne, nausea, and cholestasis *Hematologic toxicity:* Suppression of clotting factors II, V, VII, and X and polycythemia; ↑ libido, HA, and anxiety **Notes:** ↓ Total T$_4$ levels

Fluphenazine (Prolixin, Permitil) **Uses: Schizophrenia** **Action:** Phenothiazine antipsychotic; blocks postsynaptic mesolimbic dopaminergic receptors in the brain **Dose:** 0.5–10 mg/d in ÷ doses PO q6–8h, average maintenance 5 mg/d; or 1.25 mg IM initially, then 2.5–10 mg/d in ÷ doses q6–8h PRN; ↓ dose in elderly **Caution:** [C, ?/–] **Contra:** Severe CNS depression, coma, subcortical brain damage, blood dyscrasias, hepatic disease **Supplied:** Tabs 1, 2.5, 5, 10 mg; conc 5 mg/mL; elixir 2.5 mg/5 mL; inj 2.5 mg/mL; depot inj 25 mg/mL **SE:** May cause drowsiness; do not administer conc with caffeine, tannic acid, or pectin-containing products; extrapyramidal effects **Notes:** Monitor LFT; less sedative/hypotensive effects than chlorpromazine

Flurazepam (Dalmane) [C-IV] **Uses: Insomnia** **Action:** Benzodiazepine **Dose:** 15–30 mg PO q hs PRN; ↓ in elderly **Caution:** [X, ?/–] Caution in elderly, low albumin, hepatic dysfunction; ↑ levels with CNS depressants, ethanol, azole antifungals, kava, St. John's wort, warfarin **Contra:** Narrow-angle glaucoma; pregnancy **Supplied:** Caps 15, 30 mg **SE:** Hangover due to accumulation of metabolites, apnea

Flurbiprofen (Ansaid, Ocufen) [See Table VII–11, pp 621–22 or Table VII–12, pp 623–25]

Flutamide (Eulexin) **WARNING:** Liver failure and death have been reported. Measure LFT before, monthly × 4 months, and periodically after; discontinue immediately if ALT is 2 × upper limits of normal or jaundice develops **Uses: Advanced prostate CA (in combination with GnRH agonists, e.g., leuprolide or goserelin); with radiation and GnRH for localized prostate CA** **Action:** Nonsteroidal antiandrogen **Dose:** 250 mg PO tid (750 mg total) **Caution:** [D, ?] **Contra:** Severe hepatic impairment; pregnancy **Supplied:** Caps 125 mg **SE:** Hot flashes, loss of libido, impotence, diarrhea, N/V, gynecomastia **Notes:** Follow LFTs; can mix with applesauce (not with beverage)

Fluticasone, Nasal (Flonase) **Uses: Seasonal allergic rhinitis** **Action:** Topical steroid **Dose:** 1–2 sprays/nostril/d **Caution:** [C, M] **Contra:** Primary treatment of status asthmaticus **Supplied:** Nasal spray 50 mcg/actuation **SE:** HA, dysphonia, oral candidiasis

Fluticasone, Oral (Flovent, Flovent Rotadisk) **Uses: Chronic treatment of asthma** **Action:** Topical steroid **Dose:** 2–4 puffs bid **Caution:** [C, M] **Contra:** Primary treatment of status asthmaticus **Supplied:** MDI 44, 110, 220 mcg/activation; Rotadisk dry powder 50, 100, 250 mcg/activation **SE:** HA, dysphonia, oral candidiasis **Notes:** Risk of thrush; instruct patients to rinse mouth after use; counsel patients carefully on use of device

Fluticasone propionate and Salmeterol xinafoate (Advair Diskus) **Uses: Maintainence therapy for asthma** **Action:** Corticosteroid/long-acting bronchodilator **Dose:** 1 inhal bid q12h **Caution:** [C, M] **Contra:** Not for acute attack or in conversion from oral steroids; status asthmaticus **Supplied:** MDI powder (fluticasone/salmeterol in mcg)100/50, 250/50, 500/50 **SE:** Upper respiratory infection, pharyngitis, HA **Notes:** Combination of Flovent and Serevent; do not use with spacer, do not wash mouthpiece, do not exhale into device

Fluvastatin (Lescol) [See Table VII–15, p 628]

Fluvoxamine (Luvox) **WARNING:** *Pediatric:* Antidepressants may increase risk of suicidality; consider risks and benefits of use. Patients should be closely monitored for clinical worsening, suicidality, or unusual changes in behavior **Uses: OCD** **Action:** SSRI **Dose:** Initial 50 mg as single q hs dose, ↑ to 300 mg/d in ÷ doses; ↓ dose in elderly/hepatic dysfunction, titrate slowly **Caution:** [C, ?/–] Numerous drug interactions (MAOIs, phenothiazines, SSRI, serotonin agonists) **Contra:** Concurrent use with astemizole/thioridazine/cisapride; MAOI within 14 d **Supplied:** Tabs 25, 50, 100 mg **SE:** HA, GI upset, somnolence, insomnia **Notes:** Divide doses > 100 mg

Folic Acid **Uses: Megaloblastic anemia; folate deficiency** **Action: Dietary supplementation** **Dose:** *Supplement:* 0.4 mg/d PO *Pregnancy:* 0.8 mg/d PO *Folate deficiency:* 1 mg PO daily–tid **Caution:** [A, +] **Contra:** Pernicious, aplastic, normocytic anemias **Supplied:** Tabs 0.4, 0.8, 1 mg; inj 5 mg/mL **SE:** Well tolerated **Notes:** Recommended for all women of childbearing age; ↓ incidence of fetal neural tube defects by 50%; no effect on normocytic anemias

Fomepizole (Antizol) **Uses: Antidote for ethylene glycol and methanol toxicity** **Action:** Complexes and inactivates alcohol dehydrogenase **Dose:** 15 mg/kg IV load, followed by 10 mg/kg q12h for 4 doses, then 15 mg/kg q12h until ethylene glycol levels < 20 mg/dL **Caution:** [C, ?/–] **Supplied:** 1 g/mL (1.5-mL vials) **SE:** HA, nausea, dizziness, drowsiness, bad taste/metallic taste **Notes:** Dosage adjustment for hemodialysis

Fondaparinux (Arixtra) **WARNING:** When epidural/spinal anesthesia or spinal puncture is used, patients anticoagulated or scheduled to be anticoagulated with LMW heparins, heparinoids, or fondaparinux for prevention of thromboembolic complications are at risk for epidural or spinal hematoma, which can result in long-term or permanent paralysis **Uses: DVT prophylaxis in hip fracture or replacement or knee replacement surgery** **Action:** Synthetic and specific inhibitor of activated factor X; a LMW heparin **Dose:** 2.5 mg SC qd, up to 5–9 d; start at least 6 h postop **Caution:** [B, ?] ↑ Bleeding risk with anticoagulants, antiplatelets, drotrecogin alfa, NSAIDs **Contra:** Wt < 50 kg, CrCl < 30 mL/ min, active major bleeding, bacterial endocarditis, thrombocytopenia associated with antiplatelet antibody **Supplied:** Prefilled syringes 2.5 mg/0.5mL **SE:** Thrombocytopenia, anemia, fever, nausea **Notes:** Discontinue if platelets < 100,000 mm^3; only give SC; may monitor anti–factor Xa levels

Formoterol (Foradil Aerolizer) **Uses: Maintenance treatment of asthma and prevention of bronchospasm with reversible obstructive airways disease; exercise-induced bronchospasm; COPD** **Action:** Long-acting β_2-adrenergic receptor agonist, bronchodilator **Dose:** *Asthma:* Inhalation of one 12 mcg capsule q12h using the aerolizer inhaler, 24 mcg/d max *Exercise-induced bronchospasm:* One inhalation 12 mcg capsule 15 min before exercise **Caution:** [C, ?] **Contra:** Need for acute bronchodilation; use within 2 wk of MAOI **Supplied:** 12 mcg blister pack for use in aerolizer **SE:** Paradoxical bronchospasm, can be life-threatening; URI, pharyngitis, back pain **Notes:** Do not swallow capsule—for use only with inhaler; do not start with significantly worsening or acutely deteriorating asthma which may be life-threatening

Foscarnet (Foscavir) **Uses: CMV retinitis; acyclovir-resistant herpes infections** **Action:** Inhibits viral DNA polymerase and reverse transcriptase **Dose:** *CMV retinitis:Induction:* 60 mg/kg IV q8h or 100 mg/kg q12h × 14–21 d *Maintenance:* 90–120 mg/kg/d IV (Monday–Friday) *Acyclovir-resistant HSV induction:* 40 mg/kg IV q8–12h × 14–21 d; adjust dose with ↓ renal function **Caution:** [C, –] ↑ Seizure potential with flouroquinolones; avoid nephrotoxic medication (cyclosporine, aminoglycosides, ampho B, protease inhibitors) **Contra:** Significant renal impairment (CrCl < 0.4mL/min/kg during treatment) **Supplied:** Inj 24 mg/mL **SE:** Nephrotoxicity; causes electrolyte abnormalities **Notes:** Sodium loading with 500 mL 0.9% NaCl before and after helps minimize nephrotoxicity; monitor ionized calcium closely; administer through central line

Fosfomycin (Monurol) **Uses: Uncomplicated UTI** **Action:** Inhibits bacterial cell wall synthesis *Spectrum:* Gram(+) *S saprophiticus*, pneumococci, enterococcus; gram(–) (*E*

coli, Salmonella, Shigella, H influenzae, Neisseria, indole-negative *Proteus, Providencia*); *B fragilis* and anaerobic gram(–) cocci are resistant **Dose:** 3 g PO dissolved in 90–120 mL water as single dose; ↓ in renal impairment **Caution:** [B, ?] ↓ Absorption with antacids/calcium salts **Supplied:** Granule packets 3 g **SE:** HA, GI upset **Notes:** May take 2–3 d for symptoms to improve

Fosinopril (Monopril) [See Table VII–3, p 614]

Fosphenytoin (Cerebyx) Uses: **Status epilepticus** Action: Inhibits seizure spread in motor cortex **Dose:** Dosed as phenytoin equivalents (PE), *Loading:* 15–20 mg PE/kg, *Maintenance:* 4–6 mg PE/kg/d; dosage adjustment/plasma monitoring necessary in hepatic impairment **Caution:** [D, +] May ↑ phenobarbital concn **Contra:** Sinus bradycardia, sino-atrial block, second/third degree A-V block, Adams-Stokes syndrome, rash development during treatment **Supplied:** Inj 75 mg/mL **SE:** Hypotension, dizziness, ataxia, pruritus, nystagmus **Notes:** Requires 15 min to convert fosphenytoin to phenytoin; administer at < 150 mg PE/min to prevent hypotension; administer with BP monitoring

Frovatriptan (Frova) [See Table VII–16, p 629]

Fulvestrant (Faslodex) Uses: **Hormone receptor-positive metastatic breast CA in postmenopausal women with disease progression following anti-estrogen therapy** Action: Estrogen receptor antagonist **Dose:** 250 mg IM monthly, either a single 5-mL injection or two concurrent 2.5-mL IM injections into buttocks **Caution:** [X, ?/–] ↑ Effects with CYP3A4 inhibitors (amiodarone, clarithromycin, fluoxetine, grapefruit juice, ketoconazole, ritonavir, etc.) **Contra:** Pregnancy **Supplied:** Prefilled syringes 50 mg/mL (single 5 mL, dual 2.5 mL) **SE:** N/V/D, constipation, abdominal pain, HA, back pain, hot flushes, pharyngitis, injection site reactions **Notes:** Only use IM; caution in hepatic impairment

Furosemide (Lasix) Uses: **CHF, HTN, edema, ascites** Action: Loop diuretic; inhibits Na and Cl reabsorption in ascending loop of Henle and distal tubule **Dose:** 20–80 mg PO or IV daily–bid **Caution:** [C, +] Hypokalemia may ↑ risk of digoxin toxicity; ↑ risk of ototoxicity with aminoglycosides, cisplatin (esp in renal dysfunction) **Contra:** Hypersensitivity to sulfonylureas; anuria; hepatic coma/severe electrolyte depletion **Supplied:** Tabs 20, 40, 80 mg; soln 10 mg/mL, 40 mg/5 mL; inj 10 mg/mL **SE:** Hypotension, hyperglycemia, hypokalemia **Notes:** Monitor for hypokalemia, I&O, electrolytes, renal function; high doses of the IV form may cause ototoxicity

Gabapentín (Neurontin) Uses: **Adjunctive therapy in the treatment of partial seizures; postherpetic neuralgia; chronic pain syndromes** Action: Anticonvulsant **Dose:** 300–1200 mg PO TID, (max 3600 mg/d); dosage adjustment in renal impairment **Caution:** [C, ?] **Supplied:** Caps 100, 300, 400 mg; soln 250 mg/5 mL; tab 600, 800 mg **SE:** Somnolence, dizziness, ataxia, fatigue **Notes:** Not necessary to monitor levels

Galantamine (Reminyl) Uses: **Alzheimer's disease** Action: Acetylcholinesterase inhibitor **Dose:** 4 mg PO bid, increasing to 8 mg bid after at least 4 wk; may increase to 12 mg in 4 wk **Caution:** [B, ?] ↑ Effect with succinylcholine, amiodarone, diltiazem, verapamil, NSAIDs, digoxin; ↓ effect with anticholinergics **Contra:** Severe renal or hepatic impairment **Supplied:** Tabs 4, 8, 12 mg; soln 4 mg/mL **SE:** GI disturbances, weight loss, sleep disturbances, dizziness, HA **Notes:** Caution with urinary outflow obstruction, Parkinson's, severe asthma/COPD, severe heart disease or hypotension

Gallium Nitrate (Ganite) Uses: **Hypercalcemia of malignancy; bladder CA** Action: Inhibits resorption of Ca^{2+} from the bones; antitumor activity **Dose:** Refer to specific protocol **Caution:** [C, ?] Do not give with live vaccines or rotavirus vaccine **Contra:** SCr > 2.5 mg/dL **Supplied:** Inj 25 mg/mL **SE:** Can cause renal insufficiency; hypocalcemia, hypophosphatemia, decreased bicarbonate; < 1% acute optic neuritis **Notes:** Bladder CA: use in combination with vinblastine and ifosfamide

Ganciclovir (Cytovene, Vitrasert) Uses: **Treatment and prevention of CMV retinitis, prevention of CMV disease in transplant recipients** Action: Inhibits viral DNA synthesis **Dose:** *IV:* 5 mg/kg IV q12h for 14–21 d, then maintenance of 5 mg/kg/d IV for 7 d/wk

or 6 mg/kg/d IV for 5 d/wk *PO:* Following induction, 1000 mg PO tid *Prevention:* 1000 mg PO tid; take with food *Ocular implant:* One implant q5–8mo; ↓ dose in renal impairment **Caution:** [C, –] ↑ Effect with immunosuppressives, imipenem/cilastatin, zidovudine, didanosine, other nephrotoxic medication **Contra:** Neutropenia (ANC < 500), thrombocytopenia (plt < 25,000), intravitreal implant **Supplied:** Caps 250, 500 mg; inj 500 mg; ocular implant 4.5 mg **SE:** Granulocytopenia and thrombocytopenia are major toxicities; fever, rash, GI upset **Notes:** Not a cure for CMV; injection should be handled with cytotoxic cautions; implant confers no systemic benefit

Gatifloxacin (Tequin)
Uses: Bronchitis, sinusitis, community-acquired pneumonia, UTI, uncomplicated skin/soft tissue infection **Action:** Quinolone antibiotic, inhibits DNA-gyrase *Spectrum:* Gram(+) (except MRSA, *Listeria*), gram(–) (except *Pseudomonas*), atypicals, some anaerobes (*Clostridium* – not *difficile*) **Dose:** 400 mg/d PO or IV; ↓ dose in renal impairment **Caution:** [C, M] **Contra:** Known prolongation of QT interval, uncorrected hypokalemia, concurrent administration with other medications that prolong QT interval (class Ia and III antiarrhythmics, erythromycin, antipsychotics, TCAs); do not use in children < 18 y or in pregnant or lactating women **Supplied:** Tabs 200, 400 mg; inj 10 mg/mL; premixed infuse D$_5$W 200 mg, 400 mg **SE:** Prolonged QT interval, HA, N/D, tendon rupture, photosensitivity **Notes:** Reliable activity against *S pneumoniae*; take 4 h after antacids containing Mg, Fe, Zn; drink plenty of fluids; avoid direct sunlight

Gefitinib (Iressa)
Uses: Treatment of locally advanced or metastatic non–small cell lung cancer after failure of both platinum-based and docetaxel chemotherapies **Action:** Inhibition of intracellular phosphorylation of numerous tyrosine kinases **Dose:** 250 mg PO daily **Caution:** [D, –] **Supplied:** Tabs 250 mg **SE:** Diarrhea, rash, acne, dry skin, nausea, vomiting, interstitial lung disease, increased liver transaminases **Notes:** Periodically check LFTs

Gemcitabine (Gemzar)
Uses: Pancreatic CA, brain mets, NSCLC, gastric CA **Action:** Antimetabolite; inhibits ribonucleotide reductase; produces false nucleotide base-inhibiting DNA synthesis **Dose:** Refer to specific protocol; dose modifications based on hematologic function **Caution:** [D, ?/–] **Supplied:** Inj 200 mg, 1 g **SE:** Myelosuppression, N/V/D, drug fever, and skin rash **Notes:** Reconstituted soln has concentration of 38 mg/mL; monitor hepatic and renal function before treatment and periodically

Gemfibrozil (Lopid)
Uses: Hypertriglyceridemia, reduction of CHD risk **Action:** Fibric acid **Dose:** 1200 mg/d PO ÷ bid, 30 min ac AM and PM **Caution:** [C, ?] May enhance the effect of warfarin, sulfonylureas; ↑ risk of rhabdomyopathy with HMG-CoA reductase inhibitors; ↓ effects with cyclosporine **Contra:** Renal/hepatic impairment (SCr > 2.0 mg/dL), gallbladder disease, primary biliary cirrhosis **Supplied:** Tabs 600 mg **SE:** Cholelithiasis may occur secondary to treatment; GI upset **Notes:** Avoid concurrent use with the HMG-CoA reductase inhibitors; monitor LFTs and serum lipids

Gemtuzumab Ozagamicin (Mylotarg)
WARNING: Can cause severe hypersensitivity reactions and other infusion-related reactions including severe pulmonary events; Hepatotoxicity, including severe hepatic veno-occlusive disease has been reported **Uses: Relapsed CD33+ acute myelogenous leukemia in patients > 60 y who are poor candidates for chemotherapy** **Action:** Monoclonal antibody linked to calicheamicin; selective for myeloid cells **Dose:** Refer to specific protocol **Caution:** [D,?/–] Should be used only as single-agent chemo and not in combination with other chemotherapeutic agents **Supplied:** 5 mg/20 mL vial **SE:** Myelosuppression, hypersensitivity reactions (including anaphylaxis), infusion reactions (chills, fever, N/V, HA), pulmonary events, hepatotoxicity **Notes:** Premedicate with diphenhydramine and acetaminophen

Gentamicin (Garamycin, G-Mycitin, Others)
Uses: Serious infections caused by Pseudomonas, Proteus, E coli, Klebsiella, Enterobacter, and Serratia and initial treatment of gram(–) sepsis **Action:** Bactericidal; inhibits protein synthesis *Spectrum:* Synergism with penicillins; gram(–) (not *Neisseria, Legionella, Acinetobacter*) **Dose:** See Aminoglycoside Dosing (see Tables VII–18, VII–19, VII–20, VII–21, pp 630–634); ↓ dose with

renal insufficiency   **Caution:** [C, +/–] Avoid other nephrotoxic medications; monitor CrCl and serum concentration for dosage adjustments (see Table VII–18, p 630)   **Supplied:** Premixed Infusion 40, 60, 70, 80, 90, 100, 120 mg; ADD-Vantage inj vials 10 mg/mL; inj 40 mg/mL; IT preservative-free 2 mg/mL   **SE:** Nephrotoxic/ototoxic/neurotoxic   **Notes:** Once daily dosing becoming popular; follow SCr; use IBW to dose (use adjusted if obese > 30% IBW)

Gentamicin, Ophthalmic (Garamycin, Genoptic, Gentacidin, Gentak, others) [See Table VII–12, pp 623–25]

Gentamicin, Topical (Garamycin, G-Mycitin)   Uses: **Skin infections caused by susceptible organisms**   Action: Bactericidal; inhibits protein synthesis   Dose: Apply 3–4 × d   **Caution:** [C, ?]   **Contra:** Pts with absent/perforated tympanic membranes   **Supplied:** Cream and oint 0.1%;   **SE:** Irritation

Gentamicin and Prednisolone, Ophthalmic (Pred-G Ophthalmic) [See Table VII–12, pp 623-25]

Glimepiride (Amaryl) [See Table VII–13, p 626]

Glipizide (Glucotrol, Glucotrol XL) [See Table VII–13, p 626]

Glucagon   Uses: **Severe hypoglycemic reactions in DM with sufficient liver glycogen stores or b-blocker overdose**   Action: Accelerates liver gluconeogenesis   Dose: *Usual:* 0.5–1 mg SC, IM, or IV; repeat after 20 min PRN β-*Blocker overdose:* 3–10 mg IV; repeat in 10 min PRN; may be given as cont inf   **Caution:** [B, M]   **Contra:** Known pheochromocytoma   **Supplied:** Inj 1 mg   **SE:** N/V, hypotension   **Notes:** Administration of glucose IV necessary; ineffective in states of starvation, adrenal insufficiency, or chronic hypoglycemia

Glyburide (DiaBeta, Micronase, Glynase) [See Table VII–13, p 626]

Glyburide/Metformin (Glucovance)   Uses: **Type 2 DM**   Action: Sulfonylurea: stimulates pancreatic insulin release; Metformin: ↑ peripheral insulin sensitivity, ↓ hepatic glucose output and production, ↓ intestinal absorption of glucose   Dose: 1st line (naive patients), 1.25/250 mg PO qd–bid; 2nd line, 2.5/500 mg or 5/500 mg bid (max 20/2000 mg); take with meals, ↑ dose gradually   **Caution:** [C, –]   **Contra:** SCr > 1.3 in females or > 1.4 in males; hypoxemic conditions (CHF, sepsis, recent MI); alcoholism; metabolic acidosis; liver disease; hold dose before and 48 h after ionic contrast media   **Supplied:** Tabs 1.25/250 mg, 2.5/500 mg, 5/500 mg   **SE:** HA, hypoglycemia, lactic acidosis, anorexia, N/V, rash   **Notes:** Avoid alcohol; hold dose if NPO; monitor folate levels for megaloblastic anemia

Glycerin Suppository   Uses: **Constipation**   Action: Hyperosmolar laxative   Dose: 1 adult supp PR PRN   **Caution:** [C, ?]   **Supplied:** Supp (adult, infant); liq 4 mL/applicatorful   **SE:** Can cause diarrhea

Gonadorelin (Lutrepulse)   Uses: **Primary hypothalamic amenorrhea**   Action: Stimulates the pituitary to release the gonadotropins LH and FSH   Dose: 5 mcg IV q90min × 21 d using Lutrepulse pump kit   **Caution:** [B, M] ↑ Levels with androgens, estrogens, progestins, glucocorticoids, spironolactone, levodopa; ↓ levels with OCP, digoxin, dopamine antagonists   **Contra:** Any condition exacerbated by pregnancy, ovarian cysts/causes of anovulation other than hypothalamic, conditions worsened by reproductive hormones, hormonally-dependent tumor   **Supplied:** Inj 100 mcg   **SE:** Risk of multiple pregnancies; injection site pain   **Notes:** Monitor LH, FSH

Goserelin (Zoladex)   Uses: **Advanced prostate CA and with radiation for localized prostate CA; endometriosis, breast CA**   Action: LHRH agonist, inhibits LH, resulting in ↓ testosterone   Dose: 3.6 mg SC (implant) q28d or 10.8 mg SC q3mo; usually into lower abdominal wall   **Caution:** [X,]   **Contra:** Pregnancy, breastfeeding, 10.8 mg implant not for women   **Supplied:** Subcutaneous implant 3.6 (1 month), 10.8 mg (3 month)   **SE:** Hot flashes, ↓ libido, gynecomastia, and transient exacerbation of CA-related bone pain ("flare reaction" 7–10 d after 1st dose)   **Notes:** Inject into SC fat in upper abdominal wall; do not aspirate; females must use contraception

Granisetron (Kytril) Uses: **Prevention of N/V** Action: Serotonin receptor antagonist Dose: 10 mcg/kg/dose IV 30 min before initiation of chemotherapy; OR 2 mg PO 1 h before chemotherapy, then 12 h later; *Postop N/V*: 1 mg IV before end of operative case Caution: [B, +/–] St. John's wort may ↓ levels Contra: Liver disease, pregnant/breastfeeding, children < 2 yo Supplied: Tabs 1 mg; inj 1 mg/mL; soln 2 mg/10 mL SE: HA, constipation

Guaifenesin (Robitussin, others) Uses: **Symptomatic relief of dry, nonproductive cough** Action: Expectorant Dose: 200–400 mg (10–20 mL) PO q4h (max 2.4 g/d) Caution: [C, ?] Supplied: Tabs 100, 200; SR tab 600, 1200 mg; caps 200 mg; SR caps 300 mg; liq 100 mg/5 mL SE: GI upset Notes: Give with large amount of water; some dosage forms contain alcohol

Guaifenesin and Codeine (Robitussin AC, Brontex, others) [C-V] Uses: **Symptomatic relief of dry, nonproductive cough** Action: Antitussive with expectorant Dose: 5–10 mL or 1 tab PO q6–8h (max 60 mL/24 h) Caution: [C, +] Supplied: Brontex tab 10 mg codeine/guaif 300 mg; liq 2.5 mg codeine/75 mg guaif/5 mL; others 10 mg codeine/100 mg guaif/5 mL SE: Somnolence

Guaifenesin and Dextromethorphan (many OTC brands) Uses: **Cough due to upper respiratory tract irritation** Action: Antitussive with expectorant Dose: 10 mL PO q6–8h (max 40 mL/24 h) Caution: [C, +] Contra: Administration with MAOI Supplied: Many OTC formulations SE: Somnolence Notes: Give with plenty of fluids

***Haemophilus* B Conjugate Vaccine (ActHIB, HibTITER, PedvaxHIB, Prohibit, Others)** Uses: **Routine immunization of children against H influenzae type B diseases** Action: Active immunization against *Haemophilus* B Dose: 0.5 mL (25 mcg) IM in deltoid or vastus lateralis Caution: [C, +] Contra: Febrile illness, immunosuppression, hypersensitivity to thimerosal Supplied: Inj 7.5, 10, 15, 25 mcg/0.5 mL SE: Observe for anaphylaxis; edema, ↑ risk of *Haemophilus* B infection in the week after vaccination Notes: Booster not required; report all serious adverse reaction to VAERS 1-800-822-7967

Haloperidol (Haldol) Uses: **Psychotic disorders, agitation, Tourette's disorders, and hyperactivity in children** Action: Antipsychotic, neuroleptic Dose: *Moderate symptoms:* 0.5–2 mg PO bid–tid *Severe symptoms/agitation:* 3–5 mg PO bid–tid or 1–5 mg IM q4h PRN (max 100 mg/d); ↓ dose in elderly Caution: [C, ?] ↑ Effects with SSRI, CNS depressants, TCA, indomethacin, metoclopramide; avoid levodopa (inhibits antiparkinsonian effects of levodopa) Contra: Narrow-angle glaucoma, severe CNS depression, Parkinson's, bone marrow suppression, severe cardiac/hepatic disease, coma Supplied: Tabs 0.5, 1, 2, 5, 10, 20 mg; conc liq 2 mg/mL; inj 5 mg/mL; decanoate inj 50, 100 mg/mL SE: Extrapyramidal symptoms, hypotension, anxiety, dystonias Notes: Do not administer decanoate IV; dilute oral concn liquid with water/juice; monitor for EPS

Haloprogin (Halotex) Uses: **Topical treatment of tinea pedis, tinea cruris, tinea corporis, tinea manus** Action: Topical antifungal Dose: Apply bid for up to 2 wk; intertriginous may require up to 4 wk Caution: [B, ?] Supplied: 1% Cream; soln SE: Local irritation Notes: Avoid contact with eyes; improvement should occur within 4 wk

Heparin Uses: **Treatment and prevention of DVT and PE, unstable angina, AF with emboli formation, and acute arterial occlusion** Action: Acts with antithrombin III to inactivate thrombin and inhibit thromboplastin formation Dose: *Prophylaxis:* 3000–5000 units SC q8–12h *Thrombosis treatment:* Loading dose 50–80 units/kg IV, then 10–20 units/kg IV qh (adjust based on PTT) Caution: [B, +] ↑ Risk of hemorrhage with anticoagulants, aspirin, antiplatelets, cephalosporins that contain MTT side chain Contra: Uncontrolled bleeding, severe thrombocytopenia, suspected ICH Supplied: Inj 10, 100, 1000, 2000, 2500, 5000, 7500, 10,000, 20,000, 40,000 units/mL SE: Bruising, bleeding, thrombocytopenia Notes: Follow PTT, thrombin time, or activated clotting time to assess effectiveness; little effect on the PT; therapeutic PTT is 1.5–2 for most conditions; monitor for thrombocytopenia (HIT); follow platelet counts

Hepatitis A Vaccine (Havrix, VAQTA) Uses: **Prevent hepatitis A in high-risk individuals (e.g., travelers, certain professions, or high-risk behaviors)** Action: Provides active immunity Dose: (Expressed as ELISA units [EL.U]) *Havrix:* 1440 EL.U. single IM dose *VAQTA:* 50 units single IM dose Caution: [C, +] Contra: Hypersensitivity to any component of formulation Supplied: Inj 720 EL.U./0.5 mL, 1440 EL.U./1 mL.; 50 units/mL SE: Fever, fatigue, pain at injection site, HA Notes: Booster recommended 6–12 mo after primary vaccination; report all serious adverse reactions to VAERS: 1-800-822-7967

Hepatitis A (inactivated) and Hepatitis B (recombinant) vaccine (Twinrix) Uses: **Active immunization against hepatitis A/B** Action: Provides active immunity Dose: I mL IM at 0, 1, and 6 mo Caution: [C, +] Supplied: Single-dose vials, syringes SE: Fever, fatigue, pain at injection site, HA Notes: Booster recommended 6–12 mo after primary vaccination; report all serious adverse reactions to VAERS: 1-800-822-7967

Hepatitis B Immune Globulin (HyperHep, H-BIG) Uses: **Exposure to HBsAg-positive materials, e.g., blood, plasma, or serum (accidental needle-stick, mucous membrane contact, or oral ingestion)** Action: Passive immunization Dose: 0.06 mL/kg IM to a max of 5 mL; within 24 h of needle-stick or percutaneous exposure; within 14 d of sexual contact; repeat 1 and 6 mo after exposure Caution: [C, ?] Contra: Allergies to gamma globulin or anti-immunoglobulin antibodies; allergies to thimerosal, IgA deficiency Supplied: Inj SE: Pain at site, dizziness Notes: Administered in gluteal or deltoid muscle (IM only); if exposure continues, patient should also receive the hepatitis B vaccine

Hepatitis B Vaccine (Engerix-B, Recombivax HB) Uses: **Prevention of hepatitis B** Action: Active immunization Dose: 3 IM doses of 1 mL each, the 1st 2 doses given 1 mo apart, the 3rd dose 6 mo after the 1st Caution: [C, +] ↓ Effect with immunosuppressives Contra: Yeast hypersensitivity Supplied: *Engerix-B:* Inj 20 mcg/mL *Recombivax HB:* Inj 10 and 40 mcg/mL SE: Fever, inj site soreness Notes: Administer IM injections in the deltoid; derived from recombinant DNA technology

Hetastarch (Hespan) Uses: **Plasma volume expansion as an adjunct in the treatment of shock and leukapheresis** Action: Synthetic colloid with actions similar to those of albumin Dose: *Volume expansion:* 500–1000 mL (do not exceed 1500 mL/d) IV at a rate not to exceed 20 mL/kg/h *Leukapheresis:* 250–700 mL; reduce dose in renal failure Caution: [C, +] Contra: Severe bleeding disorders, severe CHF, or renal failure with oliguria or anuria Supplied: Inj 6 g/100 mL SE: Bleeding side effect (prolongs PT, PTT, bleed time, etc) Notes: Not a substitute for blood or plasma

Hydralazine (Apresoline, Others) Uses: **Moderate to severe HTN; CHF (with Isordil)** Action: Peripheral vasodilator Dose: Begin at 10 mg PO qid, then ↑ to 25 mg qid to max of 300 mg/d; ↓ in renal impairment; check CBC and ANA before starting Caution: [C, +] Caution with impaired hepatic function and CAD; ↑ toxicity with MAOI, indomethacin, β-blockers Contra: Dissecting aortic aneurysm, mitral valve rheumatic heart disease Supplied: Tabs 10, 25, 50, 100 mg; inj 20 mg/mL SE: chronically high doses cause SLE-like syndrome; SVT following IM administration, peripheral neuropathy Notes: Compensatory sinus tachycardia eliminated with use of a β-blocker

Hydrochlorothiazide (HydroDIURIL, Esidrix, others) Uses: **Edema, HTN** Action: Thiazide diuretic; inhibits Na reabsorption in the distal tubule Dose: 25–100 mg/d PO in single or ÷ doses Caution: [D, +] Contra: Anuria; sulfonamide allergy, renal decompensation Supplied: Tabs 25, 50, 100 mg; caps 12.5 mg; oral soln 50 mg/5 mL SE: Hypokalemia frequent; hyperglycemia, hyperuricemia, hyponatremia Notes: May cause sun sensitivity

Hydrochlorothiazide and Amiloride (Moduretic) Uses: **HTN** Action: Combined effects of a thiazide diuretic and a potassium-sparing diuretic Dose: 1–2 tabs/d PO Caution: [D, ?] Contra: Do not give to patients with renal failure, sulfonamide allergy Supplied: Tabs (amiloride/hydrochlorothiazide) 5 mg/50 mg SE: Hypotension, photosensitivity, hyper-/hypokalemia, hyperglycemia, hyponatremia, hyperlipidemia, hyperuricemia

Hydrochlorothiazide and Spironolactone (Aldactazide) Uses: **Edema, HTN** Action: Combined effects of a thiazide diuretic and a K-sparing diuretic Dose:

25–200 mg each component/d in ÷ doses **Caution:** [D, +] **Contra:** Sulfonamide allergy **Supplied:** Tabs (hydrochlorothiazide/spironolactone) 25 mg/25 mg, 50 mg/50 mg **SE:** Photosensitivity, hypotension, hyper-/hypokalemia, hyperglycemia, hyponatremia, hyperlipidemia, hyperuricemia

Hydrochlorothiazide and Triamterene (Dyazide, Maxzide) Uses: Edema and HTN

Action: Combined effects of a thiazide diuretic and a K-sparing diuretic **Dose:** *Dyazide:* 1–2 caps PO daily–bid *Maxzide:* 1 tab/d PO **Caution:** [D, +/–] **Contra:** Sulfonamide allergy **Supplied:** (Triamterene/HCTZ) 37.5 mg/25 mg, 50 mg/25 mg, 75 mg/50 mg **SE:** Photosensitivity, hypotension, hyper-/hypokalemia, hyperglycemia, hyponatremia, hyperlipidemia, hyperuricemia **Notes:** HCTZ component in Maxzide more bioavailable than in Dyazide

Hydrocodone and Acetaminophen (Lorcet, Vicodin, others) [C-III]

Uses: Moderate to severe pain; hydrocodone has antitussive properties **Action:** Narcotic analgesic with nonnarcotic analgesic **Dose:** 1–2 caps or tabs PO q4–6h PRN **Caution:** [C, M] **Contra:** CNS depression, severe respiratory depression **Supplied:** Many different combinations; specify hydrocodone/APAP dose. Caps 5/500; tabs 2.5/500, 5/400, 5/500, 7.5/400, 10/400, 7.5/500, 7.5/650, 7.5/750, 10/325, 10/400, 10/500, 10/650; elixir and soln (fruit punch flavor) 2.5 mg hydrocodone/167 mg APAP/5 mL **SE:** GI upset, sedation, fatigue **Notes:** Do not exceed > 4 g acetaminophen/d

Hydrocodone and Aspirin (Lortab ASA, others) [C-III] Uses: Moderate to

severe pain **Action:** Narcotic analgesic with NSAID **Dose:** 1–2 PO q4–6h PRN **Caution:** [C, M] Caution in impaired renal function, gastritis/PUD; do not use in children for chicken pox (Reye's syndrome) **Supplied:** 5 mg hydrocodone/500 mg ASA/tab **SE:** GI upset, sedation, fatigue **Notes:** Give with food/milk; monitor for GI bleed

Hydrocodone and Guaifenesin (Hycotuss Expectorant, Others) [C-III]

Uses: Nonproductive cough associated with respiratory infection **Action:** Expectorant plus cough suppressant **Dose:** 5 mL q4h, pc and hs **Caution:** [C, M] **Supplied:** Hydrocodone 5 mg/guaifenesin 100 mg/5 mL **SE:** GI upset, sedation, fatigue

Hydrocodone and Homatropine (Hycodan, Hydromet, Others) [C-III]

Uses: Relief of cough **Action:** Combination antitussive **Dose:** (Dose based on hydrocodone) 5–10 mg q4–6h **Caution:** [C, M] **Contra:** Narrow-angle glaucoma; ↑ ICP; depressed ventilation **Supplied:** Syrup 5 mg hydrocodone/5 mL; tabs 5 mg hydrocodone **SE:** Sedation, fatigue, GI upset

Hydrocodone and Ibuprofen (Vicoprofen) [C-III] Uses: Moderate to severe

pain (< 10 d) **Action:** Narcotic with NSAID **Dose:** 1–2 tabs q4–6h PRN **Caution:** [C, M] Caution in renal insufficiency; ↓ effect with ACEI and diuretics; ↑ effect with CNS depressants, alcohol, MAOI, aspirin, TCA, anticoagulants **Supplied:** Tabs 7.5 mg hydrocodone/200 mg ibuprofen **SE:** Sedation, fatigue, GI upset

Hydrocodone and Pseudoephedrine (Detussin, Histussin-D, Others)

[C-III] **Uses: Cough and nasal congestion** **Action:** Narcotic cough suppressant with decongestant **Dose:** 5 mL qid, PRN **Caution:** [C, M] **Contra:** MAOIs **Supplied:** 5 mg hydrocodone/60 mg pseudoephedrine/5 mL **SE:** Increased blood pressure, GI upset, sedation, fatigue

Hydrocodone, Chlorpheniramine, Phenylephrine, Acetaminophen, and Caffeine (Hycomine Compound)[C-III] Uses: Cough and symptoms of upper

respiratory infections **Action:** Narcotic cough suppressant with decongestants and analgesic **Dose:** 1 tab PO q4h PRN **Caution:** [C, M] **Contra:** Narrow-angle glaucoma **Supplied:** Hydrocodone 5 mg/chlorpheniramine 2 mg/phenylephrine 10 mg/APAP 250 mg/caffeine 30 mg/tab **SE:** Increased blood pressure, GI upset, sedation, fatigue

Hydrocortisone [See Table VII–2, p 613]

Hydrocortisone, Rectal (Anusol-HC Suppository, Cortifoam Rectal, Proctocort, Others)

Uses: Painful anorectal conditions; radiation proctitis, management of ulcerative colitis   **Action:** Anti-inflammatory steroid   **Dose:** *Ulcerative colitis:* 10–100 mg rectally daily–bid for 2–3 wk   **Caution:** [B, ?/]   **Supplied:** *Hydrocortisone acetate;* Rectal aerosol 90 mg/applicator; supp 25 mg *Hydrocortisone base:* Rectal 1%; rectal susp 100 mg/60 mL   **SE:** Minimal systemic effect

Hydromorphone (Dilaudid) [C–II]   Uses: Moderate/severe pain   Action: Narcotic analgesic

Dose: 1–4 mg PO, IM, IV, or PR q4–6h PRN; 3 mg PR q6–8h PRN; ↓ with hepatic failure   **Caution:** [B (D if prolonged use or high doses near term), ?] ↑ effects with CNS depressants, phenothiazines, TCAs   **Supplied:** Tabs 1, 2, 3, 4, 8 mg; liq 5 mg/mL; inj 1, 2, 4, 10 mg/mL; supp 3 mg   **SE:** Sedation, dizziness, GI upset   **Notes:** Morphine 10 mg IM = hydromorphone 1.5 mg IM

Hydroxyurea (Hydrea, Droxia)   Uses: CML, head and neck, ovarian and colon CA, melanoma, acute leukemia, sickle cell anemia, polycythemia vera, HIV   Action:

Probable inhibitor of the ribonucleotide reductase system   **Dose:** (Refer to specific protocols) 50–75 mg/kg for WBC counts of > 100,000 cells/mL; 20–30 mg/kg in refractory CML *HIV:* 1000–1500 mg/d in single or ÷ doses; ↓ in renal insufficiency   **Caution:** [D, –] ↑ Effects with zidovudine, zalcitabine, didanosine, stavudine, fluorouracil   **Contra:** Severe anemia, severe bone marrow suppression; WBC < 2500 or platelet < 100,000; pregnancy   **Supplied:** Caps 200, 300, 400, 500 mg, tab 1000 mg   **SE:** Myelosuppression (primarily leukopenia), N/V, rashes, facial erythema, radiation recall reactions, and renal dysfunction   **Notes:** Capsules can be opened and emptied into water

Hydroxyzine (Atarax, Vistaril)   Uses: Anxiety, sedation, itching   Action: Antihistamine, anti-anxiety

Dose: *Anxiety or sedation:* 50–100 mg PO or IM qid or PRN (max 600 mg/d) *Itching:* 25–50 mg PO or IM tid–qid; ↓ in hepatic failure   **Caution:** [C, +/–] ↑ Effects with CNS depressants, anticholinergics, alcohol   **Supplied:** Tabs 10, 25, 50, 100 mg; caps 25, 50, 100 mg; syrup 10 mg/5 mL; susp 25 mg/5 mL; inj 25, 50 mg/mL   **SE:** Drowsiness and anticholinergic effects   **Notes:** Useful in potentiating effects of narcotics; not for IV/SC use due to thrombosis and digital gangrene

Hyoscyamine (Anaspaz, Cystospaz, Levsin, others)   Uses: Spasm associated with GI and bladder disorders   Action: Anticholinergic

Dose: 0.125–0.25 mg (1–2 tabs) SL/PO 3–4 times/d, ac and hs; 1 SR caps q12h   **Caution:** [C, +] ↑ Effects with amantadine, antihistamines, antimuscarinics, haloperidol, phenothiazines, TCAs, MAOI   **Contra:** Obstructive uropathy, GI obstruction; glaucoma, myasthenia gravis, paralytic ileus, severe ulcerative colitis, MI   **Supplied:** (Cystospaz-M, Levsinex): Cap timed release 0.375 mg; elixir (alcohol), soln 0.125 mg/5 mL; inj 0.5 mg/mL; tab 0.125 mg; tab (Cystospaz) 0.15 mg; ext rel tab (Levbid): 0.375 mg; SL (Levsin SL) 0.125 mg   **SE:** Dry skin, xerostomia, constipation, anticholinergic SE   **Notes:** Administer tabs before meals/food; heat prostration may occur in hot weather

Hyoscyamine, Atropine, Scopolamine, and Phenobarbital (Donnatal, Others)   Uses: Irritable bowel, spastic colitis, peptic ulcer, spastic bladder

Dose: 0.125–0.25 mg (1–2 tabs) 3–4×/d, 1 cap q12h (SR), 5–10 mL elixir 3–4×/d or q8h   **Caution:** [D, M]   **Contra:** Narrow-angle glaucoma   **Supplied:** Many combinations/manufacturers available *Cap (Donnatal, others):* Hyoscyamine 0.1037 mg/atropine 0.0194 mg/scopolamine 0.0065 mg/phenobarbital 16.2 mg *Tabs (Donnatal, others):* Hyoscyamine 0.1037 mg/atropine 0.0194 mg/scopolamine 0.0065 mg/phenobarbital 16.2 mg *Long-acting (Donnatal):* Hyoscyamine 0.311 mg/atropine 0.0582 mg/scopolamine 0.0195 mg/phenobarbital 48.6 mg *Elixirs (Donnatal, others):* Hyoscyamine 0.1037 mg/atropine 0.0194 mg/scopolamine 0.0065 mg/phenobarbital 16.2 mg/5 mL   **SE:** Sedation, xerostomia, constipation

Ibuprofen (Motrin, Rufen, Advil, Others) [See Table VII–11, pp 621–22]

Ibutilide (Corvert)   Uses: Rapid conversion of AF or flutter   Action: Class III antiarrhythmic agent

Dose: 0.01 mg/kg (max 1 mg) IV inf over 10 min; may be repeated once   **Caution:** [C, –] Do not administer class I or III antiarrhythmics concurrently or within 4 h of ibutilide infusion   **Contra:** QTc > 440 msec   **Supplied:** Inj 0.1 mg/mL   **SE:** Arrhythmias, HA   **Notes:** Observe patient with continuous ECG monitoring

Idarubicin (Idamycin) **Uses:** Acute leukemias (AML, ALL, ANLL), **CML in blast crisis, breast CA** **Action:** DNA intercalating agent; inhibits DNA topoisomerases I and II **Dose:** Refer to specific protocol; ↓ in renal/hepatic dysfunction **Caution:** [D, –] **Contra:** bilirubin > 5 mg/dL, pregnancy **Supplied:** Inj 1 mg/mL (5-, 10-, 20-mg vials) **SE:** Myelosuppression, cardiotoxicity, N/V, mucositis, alopecia, and irritation at sites of IV administration; rare changes in renal/hepatic function **Notes:** Avoid extravasation—potent vesicant; only given IV

Ifosfamide (Ifex, Holoxan) **Uses:** Lung, breast, pancreatic and gastric CA, HL/NHL, soft tissue sarcoma **Action:** Alkylating agent **Dose:** Refer to specific protocol; ↓ in renal, hepatic impairment **Caution:** [D, M] ↑ Effect with phenobarbital, carbamazepine, phenytoin; St. John's wort may ↓ levels **Contra:** Severely depressed bone marrow function, pregnancy **Supplied:** Inj 1, 3 g **SE:** Hemorrhagic cystitis, nephrotoxicity, N/V, mild to moderate leukopenia, lethargy and confusion, alopecia, and hepatic enzyme elevations **Notes:** Administer with mesna to prevent hemorrhagic cystitis

Imatinib (Gleevec) **Uses:** **Treatment of CML, blast crisis, gastrointestinal stromal tumors (GIST)** **Action:** Inhibits BCL-ABL tyrosine kinase (signal transduction) **Dose:** *Chronic phase CML:* 400–600 mg PO qd *Accelerated/blast crisis:* 600–800 mg PO qd *GIST:* 400–600 mg qd **Caution:** [D, ?/–] Metabolized by CYP3A4 (caution with warfarin, cyclosporine, azole antifungals, erythromycin, phenytoin, rifampin, carbamazepine) **Contra:** Pregnancy **Supplied:** Caps 100 mg **SE:** GI upset, fluid retention, muscle cramps, musculoskeletal pain, arthralgia, rash, HA; neutropenia, thrombocytopenia **Notes:** Follow CBCs and LFTs at baseline and monthly; administer with large glass of water and food to ↓ GI irritation

Imipenem-Cilastatin (Primaxin) **Uses:** **Serious infections** caused by a wide variety of susceptible bacteria **Action:** Bactericidal; interferes with cell wall synthesis *Spectrum:* Gram(+) (inactive against *S aureus*, group A and B streptococci), gram(–) (not *Legionella*), anaerobes **Dose:** 250–1000 mg (imipenem) IV q6–8h; ↓ in renal disease if calculated CrCl is < 70 mL/min **Caution:** [C, +/–] Probenecid may ↑ risk for toxicity **Supplied:** Inj (imipenem/cilastatin) 250/250 mg, 500/500 mg **SE:** Seizures may occur if drug accumulates; GI upset, thrombocytopenia

Imipramine (Tofranil) **WARNING:** *Pediatric:* Antidepressants may increase risk of suicidality; consider risks and benefits of use. Patients should be closely monitored for clinical worsening, suicidality, or unusual changes in behavior **Uses: Depression, enuresis, panic attack, chronic pain** **Action:** TCA; ↑ synaptic conc of serotonin or norepinephrine in the CNS **Dose:** *Hospitalized:* Start at 100 mg/24 h PO in ÷ doses; can ↑ over several wk to max 300 mg/d *Outpatient:* Maintenance of 50–150 mg PO hs, not to exceed 200 mg/24 h **Caution:** [D, ?/–] ↑ Effects with amphetamines, anticholinergics, CNS depressants, warfarin **Contra:** Do not use with MAOIs, narrow-angle glaucoma, acute recovery phase of MI, pregnancy, CHF/angina/CVD/arrhythmias **Supplied:** Tabs 10, 25, 50 mg; caps 75, 100, 125, 150 mg **SE:** Cardiovascular symptoms, dizziness, xerostomia, discolored urine **Notes:** Less sedation than with amitriptyline

Imiquimod Cream, 5% (Aldara) **Uses: Anogenital warts, HPV, condyloma acuminata** **Action:** Unknown; may induce cytokines **Dose:** Applied 3×/wk, leave on skin for 6–10 h and wash off with soap and water, continue therapy for a max of 16 wk **Caution:** [B, ?] **Supplied:** Single-dose packets 5% (250 mg of the cream) **SE:** Local skin reactions common **Notes:** Not a cure; may weaken condoms/vaginal diaphragms, wash hands before and after application of cream

Immune Globulin, Intravenous (Gamimmune N, Sandoglobulin, Gammar IV) **Uses:** **IgG antibody deficiency disease states (e.g., congenital agammaglobulinemia, common variable hypogammaglobulinemia, and BMT), HIV, hepatitis A prophylaxis, ITP** **Action:** IgG supplementation **Dose:** *Immunodeficiency:* 100–200 mg/kg/mo IV at a rate of 0.01–0.04 mL/kg/min to a max of 400 mg/kg/dose *ITP:* 400 mg/kg/dose IV qd × 5 d *BMT:* 500 mg/kg/wk; ↓ renal insufficiency **Caution:** [C, ?] Separate administration of live vaccines by 3 mo **Contra:** Isolated immunoglobulin A deficiency with antibodies to IgA; severe thrombocytopenia or coagulation disorders **Supplied:** Inj **SE:** Adverse effects associated mostly with rate of infusion; GI upset

Inamrinone [Amrinone] (Inocor) Uses: Acute CHF, ischemic cardiomyopathy

Action: Positive inotrope with vasodilator activity **Dose:** Initial IV bolus 0.75 mg/kg over 2–3 min, then maintenance dose 5–10 mcg/kg/min; 10 mg/kg/d max; ↓ if ClCr < 10 mL/min **Caution:** [C, ?] **Contra:** Hypersensitivity to bisulfites **Supplied:** Inj 5 mg/mL **SE:** Monitor for fluid, electrolyte, and renal changes **Notes:** Incompatible with dextrose-containing solns

Indapamide (Lozol) Uses: HTN, edema, CHF **Action:** Thiazide diuretic; enhances

Na, Cl, and water excretion in the proximal segment of the distal tubule **Dose:** 1.25–5 mg/d PO **Caution:** [D, ?] ↑ Effect with loop diuretics, ACEI, cyclosporine, digoxin, lithium **Contra:** Anuria, thiazide/sulfonamide allergy, renal decompensation, pregnancy **Supplied:** Tabs 1.25, 2.5 mg **SE:** Hypotension, dizziness, photosensitivity **Notes:** Doses > 5 mg do not have additional effects on lowering BP; take early in day to avoid nocturia; use sunscreen; may take with food/milk

Indinavir (Crixivan) Uses: HIV infection **Action:** Protease inhibitor; inhibits maturation

of immature noninfectious virions to mature infectious virus **Dose:** 800 mg PO q8h; use in combination with other antiretroviral agents; take on an empty stomach; ↓ in hepatic impairment **Caution:** [C, ?] Numerous drug interactions **Contra:** Concomitant use with astemizole, cisapride, triazolam midazolam, pimozide, ergot alkaloids; not recommended to use simvastatin, lovastatin, sildenafil, St. John's wort **Supplied:** Caps 100, 200, 333, 400 mg **SE:** Nephrolithiasis, dyslipidemia, lipodystrophy, GI effects **Notes:** Drink 8-oz glasses of water/d

Indomethacin (Indocin) [See Table VII–11, pp 621–22]

Infliximab (Remicade) WARNING: Tuberculosis, invasive fungal infections, and other

opportunistic infections reported, some fatal. Tuberculin skin testing must be performed before therapy **Uses: Moderate to severe Crohn's disease; fistulizing Crohn's disease; RA (in combination with methotrexate)** **Action:** IgG1$_K$ monoclonal antibody neutralizes biologic activity of TNFα **Dose:** *Crohn's disease: Induction.* 5 mg/kg IV inf, may follow with subsequent doses given at 2 and 6 wk after initial inf Maintenance. 5 mg/kg IV inf q8wk *RA:* 3 mg/kg IV inf at 0, 2, 6 wk, followed by q8wk **Caution:** [B, ?/–] Active infection, hepatic insult **Contra:** Murine hypersensitivity, moderate/severe CHF **Supplied:** Inj **SE:** May cause hypersensitivity reaction, made up of human constant and murine variable regions; patients are predisposed to infection (especially TB); HA, fatigue, GI upset, infusion reactions; hepatotoxicity or reactivation of dormant hepatitis B may develop, monitor LFTs; pneumonia; bone marrow suppression; systemic vasculitis; pericordial effusion

Influenza Vaccine (Fluzone, FluShield, Fluvirin, FluMist) Uses: Prevent

influenza; all adults > 50 y, pregnant women (who will be in their second or third trimester during flu season), residents of nursing homes, patients with chronic diseases, health care workers, and household contacts of high-risk patients **Action:** Active immunization **Dose:** 0.5 mL/dose IM 0.5-mL IM **Caution:** [C, +] **Contra:** Egg, gentamicin, or thimerosal allergy, active infection at site; high risk of influenza complications, history of Guillain-Barré, asthma **Supplied:** Based on specific manufacturer, 0.25- and 0.5-mL pre-filled syringes **SE:** Soreness at the injection site, fever, myalgia, malaise, Guillain-Barré syndrome (controversial) **Notes:** Optimal dosing in the United States is Oct–Nov; protection begins 1–2 wk after and lasts up to 6 mo; each y, specific vaccines manufactured based on predictions of the strains to be active in flu season (December–Spring in the United States) Whole or split virus usually given to adults

Influenza virus vaccine live, intranasal (FluMist) Uses: Prevention of in-

fluenza **Action:** Live-attenuated vaccine **Dose:** *Age 9–49 y:* 1 dose (0.5 mL) per season **Caution:** [C,?/–] **Contra:** History of egg allergy, pregnancy, history of Guillain-Barré-syndrome, known or suspected immune deficiency, asthma or reactive airway disease **Supplied:** Pre-filled, single-use, intranasal sprayer **SE:** Runny nose, nasal congestion, headache, cough **Notes:** 0.25 mL administered into each nostril; do not administer concurrently with other vaccines. Avoid contact with immunocompromised individuals for 21 days

Insulin **Uses: Type 1 or type 2 DM refractory to diet change or oral hypoglycemic agents; management of acute life-threatening hyperkalemia** **Action:** Insulin supplementation **Dose:** Based on serum glucose levels; usually SC but can be given IV (only regular)/IM; typical starting dose for type 1 0.5–1 units/kg/d; type 2 0.3–0.4 units/kg/d; renal failure may ↓ insulin needs **Caution:** [B, +] **Supplied:** See Table VII–1, p 613 **SE:** Highly purified insulins ↑ free insulin; monitor patients closely for several wks when changing doses/agents

Interferon Alfa (Roferon-A, Intron A) **Uses: Hairy cell leukemia, Kaposi's sarcoma, melanoma, CML, chronic hepatitis C, follicular non-Hodgkin's lymphoma, condylomata acuminata, multiple myeloma, renal cell carcinoma, and bladder CA** **Action:** Direct antiproliferative action against tumor cells; modulation of the host immune response **Dose:** Dictated by treatment protocol *Hairy cell leukemia: Alfa-2a (Roferon-A):* 3 M units/d for 16–24 wk SC or IM *Alfa-2b (Intron A):* 2 M units/m² IM or SC 3×/wk for 2–6 mo **Contra:** Benzyl alcohol sensitivity, decompensated liver disease, autoimmune disease, rapidly progressing AIDS-related Kaposi's sarcoma **Supplied:** Injectable forms **SE:** May cause flu-like symptoms; fatigue common; anorexia in 20–30% of patients; neurotoxicity may occur at high doses; neutralizing antibodies to up to 40% of patients receiving prolonged systemic therapy

Interferon Alfa-2B and Ribavirin Combination (Rebetron) WARNING: Contraindicated in pregnant women and their male partners **Uses: Chronic hepatitis C in patients with compensated liver disease who have relapsed following α-interferon therapy** **Action:** Combination antiviral agents **Dose:** 3 M units Intron A SC 3×/wk with 1000–1200 mg of Rebetron PO ÷ bid dose for 24 wk *Patients < 75 kg:* 1000 mg of Rebetron/d **Caution:** [X, ?] **Contra:** Pregnancy, males with pregnant female partner, autoimmune hepatitis, creatinine clearance < 50 mL/min **Supplied:** *Patients < 75 kg:* Combination packs: 6 vials Intron A (3 M units/0.5 mL) with 6 syringes and alcohol swabs, 70 Rebetron caps; one 18 million-unit multidose vial of Intron A inj (22.8 M units/3.8 mL; 3 M units/0.5 mL) and 6 syringes and swabs, 70 Rebetron caps; one 18 million-unit Intron A inj multidose pen (22.5 M units/1.5 mL; 3 M units/0.2 mL) and 6 disposable needles and swabs, 70 Rebetron caps *Patients < 75 kg:* Identical except 84 Rebetron caps/pack **SE:** Flu-like syndrome, HA, anemia **Notes:** Negative pregnancy test required monthly; instruct patients in self-administration of SC Intron A

Interferon Alfacon-1 (Infergen) **Uses: Management of chronic hepatitis C** **Action:** Biologic response modifier **Dose:** 9 mcg SC 3×/wk × 24 wk **Caution:** [C, M] **Contra:** Hypersensitivity to *E coli*-derived products **Supplied:** Inj 9, 15 mcg **SE:** Flu-like syndrome, depression, blood dyscrasias **Notes:** Allow at least 48 h between inj

Interferon β-1b (Betaseron) **Uses: MS, relapsing-remitting and secondary progressive** **Action:** Biologic response modifier **Dose:** 0.25 mg SC every other day **Caution:** [C, ?] **Contra:** Hypersensitivity to human albumin products **Supplied:** Powder for inj 0.3 mg **SE:** Flu-like syndrome, depression, blood dyscrasias

Interferon γ-1b (Actimmune) **Uses: ↓ Incidence of serious infections in chronic granulomatous disease (CGD), osteopetrosis** **Action:** Biologic response modifier **Dose:** *CGD:* 50 mcg/m² SC (1.5 M units/m2) BSA > 0.5 m²; if BSA < 0.5 m², give 1.5 mcg/kg/dose; given 3×/wk **Caution:** [C, ?] **Contra:** Hypersensitivity to *E coli*-derived products **Supplied:** Inj 100 mcg (2 M units) **SE:** Flu-like syndrome, depression, blood dyscrasias

Ipecac Syrup [OTC] **Uses: Drug overdose and certain cases of poisoning** **Action:** Irritation of the GI mucosa; stimulation of the chemoreceptor trigger zone **Dose:** 15–30 mL PO, followed by 200–300 mL of water; if no emesis in 20 min, may repeat once **Caution:** [C, ?] **Contra:** Ingestion of petroleum distillates or strong acid, base, or other corrosive or caustic agents; not for use in comatose or unconscious patients **Supplied:** Syrup 15, 30 mL (OTC) **SE:** Lethargy, diarrhea, cardiotoxicity, protracted vomiting **Notes:** Caution in CNS depressant overdose; usage is falling out of favor

Ipratropium (Atrovent)   Uses: **Bronchospasm with COPD, rhinitis, and rhinorrhea**   Action: Synthetic anticholinergic agent similar to atropine   Dose: 2–4 puffs qid *Nasal:* 2 sprays/nostril bid–tid   Caution: [B, +/–]   Contra: Hypersensitivity to soya lecithin or related foods   Supplied: Met-dose inhaler 18 mcg/dose; soln for inhal 0.02%; nasal spray 0.03%, 0.06%; nasal inhaler 20 mcg/dose   SE: Nervousness, dizziness, HA, cough, bitter taste, nasal dryness   Notes: Not for acute bronchospasm

Irbesartan (Avapro) [See Table VII–4, p 615]

Irbesartan/Hydrochlorothiazide (Avalide) [See Table VII–4, p 615]

Irinotecan (Camptosar)   Uses: **Colorectal and lung CA**   Action: Topoisomerase I inhibitor; interferes with DNA synthesis   Dose: *Per protocol.* 125–350 mg/m^2 weekly to every 3 wk; ($\downarrow$ hepatic dysfunction, as tolerated per toxicities)   Caution: [D, –]   Supplied: Inj 20 mg/mL   SE: Myelosuppression, N/V/D, abdominal cramping, alopecia. Diarrhea is dose-limiting; Rx acute diarrhea with atropine; Rx subacute diarrhea with loperamide. Diarrhea correlated to levels of metabolite SN-38

Iron Dextran (Dexferrum, INFeD)   Uses: **Iron deficiency when oral supplementation not possible**   Action: Parenteral iron supplementation   Dose: Estimate iron deficiency, given IM/IV. A 0.5-mL test dose before starting iron dextran. Total replacement dose (mL) = 0.0476 × weight (kg) × [desired hemoglobin (g/dL) – measured hemoglobin (g/dL)] + 1 mL/5 kg weight (max 14 mL) *Max daily dose:* 100 mg Fe   Caution: [C, M]   Contra: Anemia without iron deficiency   Supplied: Inj 50 mg (Fe)/mL   SE: Anaphylaxis, flushing, dizziness, injection site and infusion reactions, metallic taste   Notes: Use test dose because anaphylaxis possible; give deep IM using "Z-track" technique, IV route preferred

Iron Sucrose (Venofer)   Uses: **Iron deficiency anemia in patients undergoing chronic hemodialysis who are receiving supplemental erythropoietin therapy**   Action: Iron replacement   Dose: 5 mL (100 mg) IV during dialysis, given no faster than 1 mL (20 mg) per minute   Caution: [C, M]   Contra: Anemia without iron deficiency   Supplied: 20 mg elemental iron per mL, 5-mL vials   SE: Anaphylaxis, hypotension, cramps, N/V/D, HA   Notes: Most patients require cumulative doses of 1000 mg; ensure drug administered at slow rate

Isoniazid (INH)   Uses: **Rx and prophylaxis of tuberculosis**   Action: Bactericidal; interferes with mycolic acid synthesis (disrupts cell wall)   Dose: *Active TB:* 5 mg/kg/24 h PO or IM (usually 300 mg/d) *Prophylaxis:* 300 mg/d PO for 6–12 mo $\downarrow$ in hepatic or renal dysfunction   Caution: [C, +] Acute liver disease, dialysis. Avoid alcohol   Contra: Acute liver disease, previous INH-assoc hepatitis   Supplied: Tabs 100, 300 mg; syrup 50 mg/5 mL; inj 100 mg/mL   SE: Severe hepatitis, peripheral neuropathy, GI upset, anorexia, dizziness, skin reactions   Notes: Given with 2–3 other drugs for active TB, based on INH resistance patterns where TB acquired and sensitivity results; prophylaxis generally is INH alone; IM route rarely used. To prevent peripheral neuropathy, give pyridoxine 50–100 mg/d. Check CDC guidelines (in MMWR) for specific treatment recommendations

Isoproterenol (Isuprel)   Uses: **Shock, bronchospasm, cardiac arrest, and AV nodal block**   Action: β_1- and $\beta_2$receptor stimulant   Dose: 2–10 mcg/min IV inf; titrate to effect *Inhal:* 1–2 inhal 4–6×/d   Caution: [C, ?]   Contra: Angina, tachyarrhythmias (digitalis-induced or otherwise)   Supplied: Met-inhaler; soln for neb 0.5%, 1%; inj 0.02 mg/mL, 0.2 mg/mL   SE: Insomnia, arrhythmias, HA, trembling, dizziness   Notes: Pulse > 130 BPM may induce ventricular arrhythmias

Isosorbide Dinitrate (Isordil, Sorbitrate, Dilatrate-SR)   Uses: **Rx and prevention of angina,** CHF (with hydralazine)   Action: Relaxation of vascular smooth muscle   Dose: *Acute angina:* 5–10 mg PO (chew tabs) q2–3h or 2.5–10 mg SL PRN q5–10min; > 3 doses should not be given in a 15–30 min period *Angina prophylaxis:* 5–40 mg PO q6h; do not give nitrates on a chronic q6h or qid basis > 7–10 d because tolerance may develop, provide 10–12 h drug-free intervals   Caution: [C, ?] Do not co-administer with sildenafil   Contra: Severe anemia, closed-angle glaucoma, postural hypotension, cerebral hemorrhage, head trauma (can ↑ ICP) **Supplied:** Tabs 5, 10, 20, 30, 40 mg; SR tabs 40 mg; SL tabs 2.5, 5, 10 mg; chew tabs 5, 10 mg; SR caps 40 mg **SE:** HA, ↓ BP, flushing, tachycardia, dizziness **Notes:** Higher oral dose usually needed to achieve same results as SL forms

Isosorbide Mononitrate (ISMO, Imdur)
Uses: Prevention/Treatment of angina pectoris **Action:** Relaxes vascular smooth muscle **Dose:** 20 mg PO bid, with the 2 doses 7 h apart or ER (Imdur) 30–120 mg/d PO **Caution:** [C, ?] Do not co-administer with sildenafil **Contra:** Head trauma or cerebral hemorrhage (can ↑ ICP) **Supplied:** Tabs 10, 20 mg; ER 30, 60, 120 mg **SE:** HA, dizziness, hypotension

Isotretinoin [13-*cis* Retinoic Acid] (Accutane, Amnesteem, Claravis, Sotret)
WARNING: Must not be used by pregnant women; patient must be capable of complying with mandatory contraceptive measures; must be prescribed according to product-specific risk management system **Uses: Refractory severe acne** **Action:** Retinoic acid derivative **Dose:** 0.5–2 mg/kg/d PO ÷ bid (↓ in hepatic disease, take with food) **Caution:** [X, –] Avoid tetracyclines **Contra:** Retinoid sensitivity, pregnancy **Supplied:** Caps 10, 20, 40 mg **SE:** Isolated reports of depression, psychosis, suicidal thoughts; dermatologic sensitivity, xerostomia, photosensitivity, ↑ LFTs, ↑ triglycerides **Notes:** Risk management program requires 2 negative pregnancy tests before therapy and use of 2 forms of contraception 1 mo before, during, and 1 mo after therapy; informed consent recommended; monitor LFTs and lipids

Isradipine (DynaCirc)
Uses: HTN **Action:** Ca^{2+} channel blocker **Dose:** 2.5–10 mg PO bid (do not crush or chew) **Caution:** [C, ?] Heart block, CHF **Supplied:** Caps 2.5, 5 mg; tabs CR 5, 10 mg **SE:** HA, edema, flushing, fatigue, dizziness, palpitations

Itraconazole (Sporanox)
WARNING: Potential for negative inotropic effects on the heart; if signs or symptoms of CHF occur during administration, continued use should be assessed **Uses: Fungal infections (Aspergillosis, Blastomycosis, Histoplasmosis, Candidiasis)** **Action:** Inhibits synthesis of ergosterol **Dose:** 200 mg PO or IV qd–bid (capsule with meals or cola/grapefruit juice; oral solution on empty stomach; avoid antacids) **Caution:** [C, ?] Numerous drug interactions **Contra:** CrCl < 30 mL/min, history of CHF or ventricular dysfunction, or concurrently with H_2-antagonist, omeprazole **Supplied:** Caps 100 mg; soln 10 mg/mL; inj 10 mg/mL **SE:** Nausea, rash, hepatitis, hypokalemia, CHF **Notes:** Oral solution and caps not interchangeable; often used in patients who cannot take amphotericin B. Watch for signs/symptoms of CHF with IV use

Kaolin-Pectin (Kaodene, Kao-Spen, Kapectolin, Parepectolin [OTC])
Uses: Diarrhea **Action:** Absorbent demulcent **Dose:** 60–120 mL PO after each loose stool or q3–4h PRN **Caution:** [C, +] **Contra:** Diarrhea secondary to pseuodomembranous colitis **Supplied:** Multiple OTC forms; also available with opium (Parepectolin) **SE:** Constipation, dehydration

Ketoconazole (Nizoral, Nizoral AD Shampoo [OTC])
Uses: Systemic fungal infections; topical cream for localized fungal infections due to dermatophytes and yeast; shampoo for dandruff, short term in prostate CA when rapid reduction of testosterone needed (i.e., cord compression) **Action:** Inhibits fungal cell wall synthesis **Dose:** *Oral:* 200 mg PO qd; ↑ to 400 mg PO qd for serious infections; prostate CA 400 mg PO tid (short term) *Topical:* Apply to the affected area qd (cream or shampoo) **Caution:** [C, +/–] Any agent that increases gastric pH will prevent absorption of ketoconazole; may enhance oral anticoagulants; may react with alcohol to produce a disulfiram-like reaction; numerous other drug interactions **Contra:** CNS fungal infections (poor CNS penetration), concurrent astemizole, cisapride, oral triazolam **Supplied:** Tabs 200 mg; topical cream 2%; shampoo 2% **SE:** Monitor LFTs with systemic use; can cause nausea **Notes:** Oral form multiple drug interactions

Ketoprofen (Orudis, Oruvail) [See Table VII–11, pp 621-22]

Ketorolac (Toradol) [See Table VII–11, pp 621-22]

Ketorolac Ophthalmic (Acular) [See Table VII–12, pp 621-22]

Ketotifen (Zaditor) [See Table VII–12, pp 623-25]

Labetalol (Trandate, Normodyne)　**Uses: HTN and hypertensive emergencies**　**Action:** α- and β-Adrenergic blocking agent　**Dose:** *HTN:* Initially, 100 mg PO bid, then 200–400 mg PO bid *Hypertensive emergency:* 20–80 mg IV bolus, then 2 mg/min IV infusion, titrated to effect　**Caution:** [C (D in 2nd or 3rd trimester), +]　**Contra:** Asthma/COPD, cardiogenic shock, uncompensated CHF, heart block　**Supplied:** Tabs 100, 200, 300 mg; inj 5 mg/mL　**SE:** Dizziness, nausea, ↓ BP, fatigue, cardiovascular effects

Lactic Acid and Ammonium Hydroxide [Ammonium Lactate] (Lac-Hydrin)　**Uses: Severe xerosis and ichthyosis**　**Action:** Emollient moisturizer　**Dose:** Apply bid　**Caution:** [B, ?]　**Supplied:** Lactic acid 12% with ammonium hydroxide　**SE:** Local irritation

Lactobacillus (Lactinex Granules) [OTC]　**Uses:** Control of diarrhea, especially after antibiotic therapy　**Action:** Replaces normal intestinal flora　**Dose:** 1 packet, 2 caps, or 4 tabs tid–qid (with meals or liq)　**Caution:** [A, +]　**Contra:** Milk/lactose allergy　**Supplied:** Tabs; caps; EC caps; powder in packets (all OTC)　**SE:** Flatulence

Lactulose (Chronulac, Cephulac, Enulose)　**Uses: Hepatic encephalopathy; constipation**　**Action:** Acidifies the colon, allowing ammonia to diffuse into the colon　**Dose:** *Acute hepatic encephalopathy:* 30–45 mL PO q1h until soft stools, then tid–qid *Chronic laxative therapy:* 30–45 mL PO tid–qid; adjust q1–2d to produce 2–3 soft stools/d *Rectally:* 200 g in 700 mL of water PR　**Caution:** [B, ?]　**Contra:** Galactosemia　**Supplied:** Syrup 10 g/15 mL, solution 10 g/15 mL, 10 g/packet　**SE:** Severe diarrhea, flatulence; may cause severe diarrhea and life-threatening electrolyte disturbances

Lamivudine (Epivir, Epivir-HBV)　**WARNING:** Lactic acidosis and severe hepatomegaly with steatosis reported with nucleoside analogs　**Uses: HIV infection and chronic hepatitis B**　**Action:** Inhibits HIV reverse transcriptase and hepatitis B viral polymerase, resulting in viral DNA chain termination　**Dose:** *HIV:* 150 mg PO bid *HBV:* 100 mg/d ↓ in renal impairment　**Caution:** [C, ?]　**Supplied:** Tabs 100, 150 mg (HBV); soln 5 mg/mL, 10 mg/mL　**SE:** HA, pancreatitis, anemia, GI upset, lactic acidosis

Lamotrigine (Lamictal)　**WARNING:** Serious rashes requiring hospitalization and discontinuation of treatment have been reported; rash less frequent in adults　**Uses: Partial seizures, bipolar disorder, Lennox-Gastaut**　**Action:** Phenyltriazine antiepileptic　**Dose:** *Seizures:* Initial 50 mg/d PO, then 50 mg PO bid for 2 wk, then maintenance 300–500 mg/d in 2 ÷ doses *Bipolar:* Initial 25 mg/d PO, then 50 mg PO qd for 2 wk, then 100 mg PO qd for 1 week, maintenance 200 mg/d ↓ in liver dysfunction or if with enzyme inducers or VPA　**Caution:** [C, –] Interacts with other antiepileptics　**Supplied:** Tabs 25, 100, 150, 200 mg; chew tabs 5, 25 mg　**SE:** Photosensitivity; HA, GI upset, dizziness, ataxia, rash (potentially life-threatening)　**Notes:** Value of therapeutic monitoring not established

Lansoprazole (Prevacid) [See Table VII—14, p 627]

Latanoprost (Xalatan) [See Table VII–12, pp 623–25]

Leflunomide (Arava)　**WARNING:** Pregnancy must be excluded prior to start of treatment　**Uses: Active RA**　**Action:** Inhibits pyrimidine synthesis　**Dose:** Initial 100 mg/d PO for 3 d, then 10–20 mg/d　**Caution:** [X, –]　**Contra:** Pregnancy　**Supplied:** Tabs 10, 20, 100 mg　**SE:** Monitor LFTs during initial therapy; diarrhea, infection, HTN, alopecia, rash, nausea, joint pain, hepatitis

Lepirudin (Refludan)　**Uses: Heparin-induced thrombocytopenia**　**Action:** Direct inhibitor of thrombin　**Dose:** Bolus 0.4 mg/kg IV, then 0.15 mg/kg inf; (↓ dose and infusion rate if CrCl < 60 mL/min)　**Caution:** [B, ?/–] Hemorrhagic event or severe HTN　**Contra:** Active major bleeding　**Supplied:** Inj 50 mg　**SE:** Bleeding, anemia, hematoma　**Notes:** Adjust dose based on aPTT ratio, maintain aPTT ratio of 1.5–2.0

Letrozole (Femara)　**Uses: Advanced breast CA**　**Action:** Nonsteroidal inhibitor of the aromatase enzyme system　**Dose:** 2.5 mg/d PO　**Caution:** [D, ?]　**Contra:** pregnancy

Supplied: Tabs 2.5 mg   **SE:** Requires periodic CBC, thyroid function, electrolyte, LFT, and renal monitoring; anemia, nausea, hot flashes, arthralgia

Leucovorin (Wellcovorin)   Uses: **Overdose of folic acid antagonist; augmentation of 5-FU, impaired MTX elimination**   Action: Reduced folate source; circumvents action of folate reductase inhibitors (i.e., MTX)   **Dose:** *MTX rescue:* 10 mg/m^2/dose IV or PO q6h for 72 h until MTX level < 10^{-8} *5-FU:* 200 mg/m^2/d IV 1–5 d during daily 5-FU treatment or 500 mg/m^2/wk with weekly 5-FU therapy *Adjunct to antimicrobials:* 5–15 mg/d PO   **Caution:** [C, ?/–] Should not be administered intrathecally/intraventrically   **Contra:** Pernicious anemia   **Supplied:** Tabs 5, 15, 25 mg; inj   **SE:** Allergic reaction, N/V/D, fatigue   **Notes:** Many dosing schedules for leucovorin rescue following MTX therapy

Leuprolide (Lupron, Lupron DEPOT, Lupron DEPOT-Ped, Viadur, Eligard)   Uses: **Advanced prostate CA (CAP), endometriosis, uterine fibroids, and CPP**   Action: LHRH agonist; paradoxically inhibits release of gonadotropin, resulting in decreased pituitary gonadotropins (i.e., ↓ LH); in men ↓ testosterone   **Dose:** *CAP:* 7.5 mg IM q28d or 22.5 mg IM q3mo or 30 mg IM q4mo of depot. Viadur implant (CAP only): insert in inner upper arm using local anesthesia, replace q12mo *Endometriosis (depot only):* 3.75 mg IM qmo ×6 *Fibroids:* 3.75 mg IM qmo ×3   **Caution:** [X, ?]   **Contra:** Undiagnosed vaginal bleeding, implant dosage form in women; pregnancy   **Supplied:** Lupron depot 3.75 (1 mo for fibroids, endometriosis), Lupron depot for CAP: 7.5 mg (1 mo), 22.5 (3 mo), 30 mg (4 mo); Eligard depot for CAP: 7.5 mg (1 mo); Viadur 12-mo SC implant; Lupron-PED 7.5, 11.25, 15 mg   **SE:** Hot flashes, gynecomastia, N/V, alopecia, anorexia, dizziness, HA, insomnia, paresthesias, depression exacerbation, peripheral edema, and bone pain (transient "flare reaction" at 7–14 d after the 1st dose due to LH and testosterone surge before suppression)

Levalbuterol (Xopenex)   Uses: **Asthma (Rx and prevention of bronchospasm)**   Action: Sympathomimetic bronchodilator   **Dose:** 0.63 mg neb q6–8h   **Caution:** [C, ?]   **Supplied:** Soln for inhal 0.63, 1.25 mg/3 mL   **SE:** Tachycardia, nervousness, trembling, flu syndrome   **Notes:** Therapeutically active *R*-isomer of albuterol; potential for lower incidence of cardiovascular side effects compared with albuterol—not yet proven

Levamisole (Ergamisol)   Uses: **Adjuvant therapy of Dukes C colon CA (in combination with 5-FU)**   Action: Poorly understood immunostimulatory effects   **Dose:** 50 mg PO q8h for 3 d q14d during 5-FU therapy; ↓ in hepatic dysfunction   **Caution:** [C, ?/–]   **Supplied:** Tabs 50 mg   **SE:** N/V/D, abdominal pain, taste disturbance, anorexia, hyperbilirubinemia, disulfiram-like reaction on alcohol ingestion, minimal bone marrow depression, fatigue, fever, conjunctivitis

Levetiracetam (Keppra)   Uses: **Partial onset seizures**   Action: Unknown   **Dose:** 500 mg PO bid, may ↑ to max 3000 mg/d; ↓ in renal insufficiency   **Caution:** [C, ?/–]   **Supplied:** Tabs 250, 500, 750 mg   **SE:** May cause dizziness and somnolence; may impair coordination

Levobetaxolol (Betaxon) [See Table VII–12, pp 623–25]

Levobunolol (A-K Beta, Betagan) [See Table VII–12, pp 623–25]

Levocabastine (Livostin) [See Table VII–12, pp 623–25]

Levofloxacin (Levaquin, Quixin Ophthalmic, Iquix Ophthalmic)   Uses: **Lower respiratory tract infections, sinusitis, UTI; topical for bacterial conjunctivitis, skin infections** *Spectrum:* Excellent gram(+) coverage except MRSA and *E faecium*; excellent gram(−) coverage except *S maltophilia* and *Acinetobacter* sp; poor anaerobic coverage   **Action:** Quinolone antibiotic, inhibits DNA gyrase   **Dose:** 250–500 mg/d PO or IV; ↓ in renal insufficiency, ophthal 1–2 drops in eye(s) q2h while awake for 2 d, then q4h while awake for 5 d; *Oral:* avoid antacids   **Caution:** [C, −] Interactions with cation-containing products   **Supplied:** Tabs 250, 500 mg; premixed bags 250, 500 mg; ophthal 0.5%, 1.5% sol   **SE:** N/D, dizziness, rash, GI upset, photosensitivity

Levonorgestrel (Plan B)   Uses: **Emergency contraception ("morning-after pill"); can prevent pregnancy if taken < 72 hours after unprotected sex (contraceptive fails or**

if no contraception used) Actions: progestin **Dose:** 1 pill Q12 hr × 2 **Supplied:** tab, 0.75 mg, 2 blister pack **Caution:** [X, M] **Contra:** Known/suspected pregnancy, abnormal uterine bleeding **SE:** N/V, abdominal pain, fatigue HA, menstrual changes **Notes:** Will not induce abortion; may increase risk of ectopic pregnancy

Levonorgestrel Implant (Norplant) Uses: Contraceptive Dose: Implant 6 caps in

the midforearm **Caution:** [X, +/−] **Contra:** Undiagnosed abnormal uterine bleeding, hepatic disease, thromboembolism, history of intracranial HTN, breast CA, renal impairment **Supplied:** Kits containing 6 implantable caps, each containing 36 mg **SE:** Uterine bleeding, HA, acne, nausea **Notes:** Prevents pregnancy for up to 5 y; may be removed if pregnancy desired

Levothyroxine (Synthroid, Levoxyl, others) Uses: Hypothyroidism,

myxedema coma **Action:** Supplementation of L-thyroxine **Dose:** Initially, 25–50 mcg/d PO or IV; ↑ by 25–50 mcg/d every month; usual dose 100–200 mcg/d. Titrate dosage based on clinical response and thyroid function tests; dosage can ↑ more rapidly in young to middle-aged patients **Caution:** [A, +] **Contra:** Recent MI, uncorrected adrenal insufficiency **Supplied:** Tabs 25, 50, 75, 88, 100, 112, 125, 137, 150, 175, 200, 300 mcg; inj 200, 500 mcg **SE:** Insomnia, weight loss, alopecia, arrhythmia; take with full glass of water to prevent gagging or choking

Lidocaine (Anestacon Topical, Xylocaine, others) Uses: Local anesthetic;

treatment of cardiac arrhythmias **Action:** Anesthetic; class IB antiarrhythmic **Dose:** *Antiarrhythmic, ET:* 5 mg/kg; follow with 0.5 mg/kg in 10 min if effective *IV load:* 1 mg/kg/dose bolus over 2–3 min; repeat in 5–10 min up to 200–300 mg/h; cont inf of 20–50 mcg/kg/min or 1–4 mg/min *Topical:* Apply max 3 mg/kg/dose *Local inj anesthetic:* Max 4.5 mg/kg (Table VII–17, p 000) **Caution:** [C, +] Do not use lidocaine with epinephrine on the digits, ears, or nose because vasoconstriction may cause necrosis; heart block **Supplied:** *Inj local:* 0.5, 1, 1.5, 2, 4, 10, 20% *Inj IV:* 1% (10 mg/mL), 2% 20 mg/mL); *admixture* 4, 10, 20% *IV inf:* 0.2%, 0.4%; *cream* 2%; *gel* 2, 2.5%; *oint* 2.5, 5%; *liq* 2.5%; *soln* 2, 4%; *viscous* 2% **SE:** 2nd line to amiodarone in emergency cardiac care; dilute ET dose 1–2 mL with NS; epinephrine may be added for local anesthesia to ↑ effect and ↓ bleeding; for IV forms, ↓ with liver disease or CHF; dizziness, paresthesias, and convulsions associated with toxicity; see Table VII–17 (p 000) for drug levels

Lidocaine/Prilocaine (EMLA) Uses: Topical anesthetic; adjunct to phlebotomy

or dermal procedures **Action:** Topical anesthetic **Dose:** *EMLA cream and anesthetic disc (1 g/10 cm2):* Apply thick layer 2–2.5 g to intact skin and cover with an occlusive dressing (e.g., Tegaderm) for at least 1 h *Anesthetic disc:* 1 g/10 cm² for at least 1 h **Caution:** [B, +] Methemoglobinemia **Contra:** Application on mucous membranes, broken skin, ophthalmic use; hypersensitivity to amide-type local anesthetics **Supplied:** Cream 2.5% lidocaine/2.5% prilocaine; anesthetic disc (1 g) **SE:** Burning, stinging, methemoglobinemia **Notes:** Longer contact time gives greater effect

Lindane (Kwell [OTC]) Uses: Head lice, crab lice, scabies Action: Ectoparasiti-

cide and ovicide **Dose:** *Cream or lotion:* Apply thin layer after bathing, leave on for 8–12 h, pour on laundry *Shampoo:* Apply 30 mL, develop a lather with warm water for 4 min, comb out nits **Caution:** [C, +/−] **Contra:** Open wounds, seizure disorder **Supplied:** Lotion 1%; shampoo 1% **SE:** Arrhythmias, seizures, local irritation, GI upset **Notes:** Caution with overuse; may be absorbed into blood; may repeat treatment in 7 days

Linezolid (Zyvox) Uses: Infections caused by gram(+) bacteria (including VRE),

pneumonia, skin infections **Action:** Unique action, binds ribosomal bacterial RNA; bactericidal for strep, bacteriostatic for enterococci and staph **Spectrum:** Excellent gram(+) activity including VRE and MRSA **Dose:** 400–600 mg IV or PO q12h **Caution:** [C, ?/−] Reversible MAOI, avoid foods containing tyramine and cough and cold products containing pseudoephedrine; myelosuppression **Supplied:** Inj 2 mg/mL; tabs 400, 600 mg; susp 100 mg/5 mL **SE:** HTN, N/D, HA, insomnia, GI upset **Notes:** Follow weekly CBC

Liothyronine (Cytomel) Uses: Hypothyroidism, goiter, myxedema coma, thyroid

suppression therapy **Action:** T_3 replacement **Dose:** Initial dose of 25 mcg/24 h, then titrate q1–2wk according to clinical response and TFT to maintenance of 25–100 mcg/d PO *Myxedema coma:* 25–50 mcg IV, ↓ dose in elderly **Caution:** [A, +] **Contra:** Recent MI, uncorrected adrenal insufficiency, uncontrolled HTN **Supplied:** Tabs 5, 12.5, 25, 50 mcg; inj 10 mcg/mL **SE:** Alopecia, arrhythmias, chest pain, HA, sweating **Notes:** Monitor TFT

Lisinopril (Prinivil, Zestril) [See Table VII–3, p 614]

Lithium Carbonate (Eskalith, Lithobid, others) Uses: Manic episodes of bipolar illness
Action: Effects shift toward intraneuronal metabolism of catecholamines **Dose:** *Acute mania:* 600 mg PO tid or 900 mg SR bid *Maintenance:* 300 mg PO tid–qid; follow serum levels; (↓ in renal insufficiency, elderly) **Caution:** [D, –] Many drug interactions **Contra:** Severe renal impairment or cardiovascular disease, lactation **Supplied:** Caps 150, 300, 600 mg; tabs 300 mg; SR tabs 300, 450 mg; syrup 300 mg/5 mL **SE:** Polyuria, polydipsia, nephrogenic DI, tremor; sodium retention or diuretic use may potentiate toxicity; arrhythmias, dizziness **Notes:** Table VII–17 (p 000) for drug levels.

Lodoxamide (Alomide) [See Table VII–12, pp 623–25]

Lomefloxacin (Maxaquin) Uses: UTI, acute exacerbation of chronic bronchitis; prophylaxis in transurethral procedures
Spectrum: Good gram(–) activity including *H influenzae* except *S maltophilia*, *Acinetobacter* sp, and some *P aeruginosa* **Action:** Quinolone antibiotic; inhibits DNA gyrase **Dose:** 400 mg/d PO; ↓ in renal insufficiency, avoid antacids **Caution:** [C, –] Interactions with cation-containing products **Supplied:** Tabs 400 mg **SE:** Photosensitivity, seizures, HA, dizziness

Lomustine (CCNU, CeeNU) Uses: Hodgkin's lymphoma; primary brain tumors
Actions: Nitrosourea alkylating agent **Dose:** Refer to specific protocol **Caution:** [D, ?] **Supplied:** 10, 40, 100 mg caps **SE:** Toxicity includes myelosuppression, renal injury, anorexia, nausea and vomiting, stomatitis, pulmonary fibrosis, and hepatotoxicity **Notes:** High lipid solubility translates into excellent penetration into the CNS

Loperamide (Imodium) [OTC] Uses: Diarrhea
Action: Slows intestinal motility **Dose:** Initially 4 mg PO, then 2 mg after each loose stool, up to 16 mg/d **Caution:** [B, +] Do not use in acute diarrhea caused by *Salmonella, Shigella,* or *C difficile* **Supplied:** Caps 2 mg; tabs 2 mg; liq 1 mg/5 mL (OTC) **SE:** Constipation, sedation, dizziness

Lopinavir/Ritonavir (Kaletra) Uses: HIV infection
Action: Protease inhibitor **Dose:** 3 caps or 5 mL PO bid (with food) **Caution:** [C, ?/–] Numerous drug interactions **Contra:** Concomitant drugs dependent on CYP3A or CYP2D6 **Supplied:** Caps 133.3 mg/33.3 mg (lopinavir/ritonavir), solution 400 mg/100 mg/5 mL **SE:** Solution contains alcohol, avoid disulfiram and metronidazole; GI upset, asthenia, ↑ cholesterol and triglycerides, pancreatitis; protease metabolic syndrome

Loracarbef (Lorabid) [See Table VII–9, p 619]

Loratadine (Claritin, Alavert) [OTC] Uses: Allergic rhinitis, chronic idiopathic urticaria
Action: Nonsedating antihistamine **Dose:** 10 mg/d PO (take on an empty stomach; ↓ in hepatic insufficiency) **Caution:** [B, +/–] **Supplied:** Tabs 10 mg (OTC); rapidly disintegrating Reditabs 10 mg; syrup 1 mg/mL **SE:** HA, somnolence, xerostomia

Lorazepam (Ativan, others) [C-IV] Uses: Anxiety and anxiety with depression; preop sedation; control of status epilepticus; alcohol withdrawal; antiemetic
Action: Benzodiazepine; antianxiety agent **Dose:** *Anxiety:* 1–10 mg/d PO in 2–3 ÷ doses *Preop sedation:* 0.05 mg/kg to 4 mg max IM 2 h before surgery *Insomnia:* 2–4 mg PO hs *Status epilepticus:* 4 mg/dose IV PRN q10–15 min; usual total dose 8 mg *Antiemetic:* 0.5–2 mg IV or PO q4–6h PRN. Alcohol withdrawal: 2–5 mg IV or 1–2 mg PO initially depending on severity. Subsequent dosing depends on patient (see Section 1, Chapter 16, Delirium Tremens: Major Alcohol Withdrawal) ↓ in elderly; do not administer IV > 2 mg/min or 0.05 mg/kg/min **Caution:** [D, ?/–] **Contra:** Severe pain, severe hypotension, sleep apnea, narrow-angle glaucoma, hypersensitivity to propylene glycol or benzyl alcohol **Supplied:** Tabs 0.5, 1, 2 mg; soln, oral conc 2 mg/mL; inj 2, 4 mg/mL **SE:** Sedation, ataxia, tachycardia, constipation, respiratory

depression   **Notes:** May take up to 10 min to see effect when given IV; do not administer IV faster than 2 mg/min or 0.05 mg/kg/min

Losartan (Cozaar) [See Table VII–4, p 615]

Lovastatin (Mevacor, Altocor) [See Table VII–15, p 628]

Lymphocyte Immune Globulin [Antithymocyte Globulin, ATG] (Atgam)
Uses: Allograft rejection in transplant patients; aplastic anemia if not candidates for BMT   **Action:** ↓ number of circulating, thymus-dependent lymphocytes   **Dose:** *Prevent rejection:* 15 mg/kg/day IV × 14 d, then qod × 7; initial within 24 h before/after transplant. Treat rejection: Same except use 10–15 mg/kg/day   **Caution:** [C, ?]   **Contra:** H/O reaction to other equine γ-globulin preparation, leukopenia, thrombocytopenia   **Supplied:** Inj 50 mg/mL   **SE:** Test dose 0.1 mL of a 1:1000 dilution in NS; discontinue with severe thrombocytopenia or leukopenia; rash, fever, chills, hypotension, HA, ↑ K⁺

Magaldrate (Riopan, Lowsium) [OTC]
Uses: Hyperacidity associated with peptic ulcer, gastritis, and hiatal hernia   **Action:** Low-Na antacid   **Dose:** 5–10 mL PO between meals and hs   **Caution:** [B, ?] Do not use in renal insufficiency due to Mg content   **Contra:** Ulcerative colitis, diverticulitis, ileostomy/coleostomy   **Supplied:** Susp   **SE:** GI upset   **Notes:** < 0.3 mg Na/tab or tsp

Magnesium Citrate [OTC]
Uses: Vigorous bowel preparation; constipation   **Action:** Cathartic laxative   **Dose:** 120–240 mL PO PRN (take with a beverage)   **Caution:** [B, +]   **Contra:** Severe renal disease, heart block, N/V, rectal bleeding   **Supplied:** Effervescent soln (OTC)   **SE:** Abdominal cramps, gas

Magnesium Hydroxide (Milk of Magnesia) [OTC]
Uses: Constipation   **Action:** NS laxative   **Dose:** 15–30 mL PO PRN (follow dose with 8 ounces of water)   **Caution:** [B, +]   **Contra:** Renal insufficiency or intestinal obstruction, ileostomy/colostomy   **Supplied:** Tabs 311 mg, liq 400, 800 mg/5 mL   **SE:** Diarrhea, abdominal cramps

Magnesium Oxide (Mag-Ox 400, others) [OTC]
Uses: Replacement for low plasma levels   **Action:** Mg supplementation   **Dose:** 400–800 mg/d ÷ qd–qid with full glass of water   **Caution:** [B, +]   **Contra:** Ulcerative colitis, diverticulitis, ileostomy/colostomy, heart block, renal insufficiency   **Supplied:** Caps 140 mg; tabs 400 mg (OTC)   **SE:** Diarrhea, nausea

Magnesium Sulfate
Uses: Replacement for low Mg levels; preeclampsia and premature labor; refractory hypokalemia and hypocalcemia   **Action:** Mg supplement   **Dose:** *Supplement:* 1–2 g IM or IV; repeat PRN *Preeclampsia/premature labor:* 4 g load then 1–4 g/h IV infusion; ↓ dose with low urine output or renal insufficiency   **Caution:** [B, +]   **Contra:** Heart block, renal failure   **Supplied:** Inj 100, 125, 250, 500 mg/mL; oral soln 500 mg/mL; granules 40 mEq/5 g   **SE:** CNS depression, diarrhea, flushing, heart block

Mannitol
Uses: Cerebral edema, intraocular pressure, renal impairment, poisonings   **Action:** Osmotic diuretic   **Dose:** *Diuresis:* 0.2 g/kg/dose IV over 3–5 min; if no diuresis within 2 h, discontinue *Cerebral edema:* 0.25 g/kg/dose IV push, repeated at 5-min intervals PRN; ↑ incrementally to 1 g/kg/dose PRN for increased ICP; caution with CHF or volume overload   **Caution:** [C, ?]   **Contra:** Anuria, dehydration, heart failure, PE   **Supplied:** Inj 5, 10, 15, 20, 25%   **SE:** Initial volume increase may exacerbate CHF; monitor for volume depletion, N/V/D

Mechlorethamine (Mustargen)   WARNING: Highly toxic agent, handle with care
Uses: Hodgkin's and NHL, cutaneous T-cell lymphoma (mycosis fungoides), lung CA, CML, malignant pleural effusions, and CLL   **Action:** Alkylating agent (bifunctional)   **Dose:** 0.4 mg/kg single dose or 0.1 mg/kg/d for 4 d; 6 mg/m² 1–2 ×/mo; highly volatile; must be administered within 30–60 min of preparation   **Caution:** [D, ?]   **Contra:** Presence of known infectious disease   **Supplied:** Inj 10 mg   **SE:** *Toxicity symptoms:* Myelosuppression, thrombosis, or thrombophlebitis at inj site; tissue damage with extravasation (Na thiosulfate may be used topically to treat); N/V, skin rash, amenorrhea, and sterility. High rates of sterility (especially in men) and secondary leukemia in patients treated for Hodgkin's disease

Meclizine (Antivert) **Uses:** Motion sickness; vertigo **Action:** Antiemetic, anticholinergic, and antihistaminic properties **Dose:** 25 mg PO tid–qid PRN **Caution:** [B, ?] **Contra:** N/A **Supplied:** Tabs 12.5, 25, 50 mg; chew tabs 25 mg; caps 25, 30 mg (OTC) **SE:** Drowsiness, dry mouth, and blurred vision common

Medroxyprogesterone (Provera, Depo-Provera) **WARNING:** May cause significant loss of bone density; associated with duration of use and may not be completely reversible **Uses:** Contraception; secondary amenorrhea, and abnormal uterine bleeding (AUB) caused by hormonal imbalance; endometrial CA **Action:** Progestin supplement **Dose:** *Contraception:* 150 mg IM q3mo or 450 mg IM q6mo *Secondary amenorrhea:* 5–10 mg/d PO for 5–10 d *AUB:* 5–10 mg/d PO for 5–10 d beginning on the 16th or 21st d of menstrual cycle *Endometrial CA:* 400–1000 mg/wk IM; ↓ in hepatic insufficiency **Caution:** [X, +] **Contra:** History of past thromboembolic disorders, hepatic disease, pregnancy **Supplied:** Tabs 2.5, 5, 10 mg; depot inj 100, 150, 400 mg/mL **SE:** Breakthrough bleeding, spotting, altered menstrual flow, anorexia, edema, thromboembolic complications, depression, weight gain **Notes:** Perform breast exam and Pap smear before therapy. If used as contraceptive obtain pregnancy test if last injection > 3 months earlier.

Megestrol Acetate (Megace) **Uses:** Breast and endometrial CAs; appetite stimulant in CA and HIV-related cachexia **Action:** Hormone; progesterone analogue **Dose:** *CA:* 40–320 mg/d PO in ÷ doses *Appetite:* 800 mg/d PO **Caution:** [X, –] Thromboembolism **Contra:** Pregnancy **Supplied:** Tabs 20, 40 mg; soln 40 mg/mL **SE:** May induce DVT; do not discontinue therapy abruptly; edema, menstrual bleeding; photosensitivity, insomnia, rash, myelosuppression

Meloxicam (Mobic) [See Table VII–11, pp 621–22]

Melphalan [LPAM] (Alkeran) **WARNING:** Severe bone marrow depression, leukemogenic, and mutagenic **Uses:** Multiple myeloma; ovarian, breast, and testicular CAs; melanoma; allogenic and ABMT in high doses **Action:** Alkylating agent (bifunctional) **Dose:** (Per protocol) 6 mg/d or 0.25 mg/kg/d for 4–7 d, repeated at 4- to 6-wk intervals, or 1-mg/kg single dose once q4–6wk; 0.15 mg/kg/d for 5 d q6wk *High dose for high-risk multiple myeloma:* Single dose 140 mg/m² *ABMT:* 140–240 mg/m² IV; ↓ in renal insufficiency **Caution:** [D, ?] **Supplied:** Tabs 2 mg; inj 50, 100 mg **SE:** Myelosuppression (leukopenia and thrombocytopenia), secondary leukemia, alopecia, dermatitis, stomatitis, and pulmonary fibrosis; very rare hypersensitivity reactions **Notes:** Take on empty stomach

Meningococcal Polysaccharide Vaccine (Menomune) **Uses:** Immunize against *N meningitidis* (meningococcus); recommended in certain complement deficiencies, asplenia, lab workers with exposure, recommended for college students by some professional groups **Action:** Live bacterial vaccine, active immunization **Dose:** 0.5 mL SC; do not inject intradermally or IV; epinephrine (1:1000) must be available for anaphylactic/allergic reactions **Caution:** [C, ?/–] **Contra:** Thimerosal sensitivity **Supplied:** Inj **SE:** Local injection site reactions, HA **Notes:** Active against meningococcal serotypes groups A, C, Y, and W-135 but not group B

Meperidine (Demerol) [C–II] **Uses:** Moderate to severe pain **Action:** Narcotic analgesic **Dose:** 50–150 mg PO or IM q3–4h PRN; ↓ dose in elderly and renal impairment **Caution:** [C/D (prolonged use or high doses at term, +] Do not use in renal failure **Contra:** Recent or concomitant MAOIs **Supplied:** Tabs 50, 100 mg; syrup 50 mg/mL; inj 10, 25, 50, 75, 100 mg/mL **SE:** Respiratory depression, seizures, sedation, constipation, analgesic effects potentiated with use of Vistaril **Notes:** 75 mg IM = 10 mg of morphine IM; reduces seizure threshold

Meprobamate (Equinil, Miltown) [C–IV] **Uses:** Short-term relief of anxiety **Action:** Mild tranquilizer; antianxiety **Dose:** 400 mg PO tid–qid up to 2400 mg/d; SR 400–800 mg PO bid; ↓ in renal/liver insufficiency **Caution:** [D, +/–] **Contra:** Narrow-angle glaucoma, porphyria, pregnancy **Supplied:** Tabs 200, 400, 600 mg; SR caps 200, 400 mg **SE:** May cause drowsiness, syncope, tachycardia, edema

Mercaptopurine [6-MP] (Purinethol) Uses: **Acute leukemias, 2nd-line Rx of CML and NHL, immunosuppressant therapy for autoimmune diseases (Crohn's disease)** Action: Antimetabolite; mimics hypoxanthine Dose: 80–100 mg/m^2/d or 2.5–5 mg/kg/d; maintenance 1.5–2.5 mg/kg/d; concurrent allopurinol therapy requires a 67–75% dose reduction of 6-MP because of interference with metabolism by xanthine oxidase; ↓ in renal, hepatic insufficiency Caution: [D, ?] Contra: Severe hepatic disease, bone marrow suppression, pregnancy Supplied: Tabs 50 mg SE: Mild hematologic toxicity; uncommon GI toxicity, except mucositis, stomatitis, and diarrhea; rash, fever, eosinophilia, jaundice, and hepatitis Notes: Use proper procedures for handling. Take on empty stomach; ensure adequate hydration

Meropenem (Merrem) Uses: **Intra-abdominal infections, bacterial meningitis** Action: Carbapenem; inhibits cell wall synthesis, a β-lactam. Excellent gram(+) coverage except MRSA and *E faecium* Excellent gram(–) coverage including extended-spectrum β-lactamase producers. Good anaerobic coverage Dose: 1 g IV q8h; ↓ in renal insufficiency Caution: [B, ?] Contra: β-Lactam sensitivity Supplied: Inj 1 g/30 mL, 500 mg/20 mL SE: Less seizure potential than imipenem; diarrhea, thrombocytopenia Notes: Overuse can increase bacterial resistance

Mesalamine (Rowasa, Asacol, Pentasa) Uses: **Mild to moderate distal ulcerative colitis, proctosigmoiditis, or proctitis** Action: Unknown; may topically inhibit prostaglandins Dose: *Retention enema:* qd hs or insert 1 supp bid *Oral:* 800–1000 mg PO 3–4×/d; ↓ initial dose in elderly Caution: [B, M] Contra: Salicylate sensitivity Supplied: Tabs 400 mg; caps 250 mg; supp 500 mg; rectal susp 4 g/60 mL SE: HA, malaise, abdominal pain, flatulence, rash, pancreatitis, pericarditis Notes: May discolor urine yellow-brown

Mesna (Mesnex) Uses: **↓ incidence of ifosfamide- and cyclophosphamide-induced hemorrhagic cystitis** Action: Antidote Dose: 20% of the ifosfamide dose (±) or cyclophosphamide dose IV 15 min before and 4 and 8 h after chemotherapy Caution: [B; ?/–] Contra: Thiol sensitivity Supplied: Inj 100 mg/mL, Tablet 400 mg SE: Hypotension, allergic reactions, HA, GI upset, taste perversion

Mesoridazine (Serentil) WARNING: Can prolong QT interval in a dose-related fashion; torsades de pointes reported Uses: **Schizophrenia, acute and chronic alcoholism, chronic brain syndrome** Action: Phenothiazine antipsychotic Dose: Initially, 25–50 mg PO or IV tid; ↑ to 300–400 mg/d max Caution: [C, ?/–] Contra: Phenothiazine sensitivity, co-administration with drugs that cause QTc prolongation, CNS depression Supplied: Tabs 10, 25, 50, 100 mg; oral conc 25 mg/mL; inj 25 mg/mL SE: Low incidence of extrapyramidal side effects; hypotension, xerostomia, constipation, skin discoloration, tachycardia, lowered seizure threshold, blood dyscrasias, pigmentary retinopathy at high doses

Metaproterenol (Alupent, Metaprel) Uses: **Asthma and reversible bronchospasm** Action: Sympathomimetic bronchodilator Dose: *Inhal:* 1–3 inhal q3–4h, 12 inhal max/24 h; allow at least 2 min between inhal *Oral:* 20 mg q6–8h Caution: [C, ?/–] Contra: Tachycardia or other arrhythmias Supplied: Aerosol 0.65 mg/inhal; soln for inhal 0.4, 0.6, 5%; tabs 10, 20 mg; syrup 10 mg/5 mL SE: Fewer β$_1$ effects than isoproterenol and longer acting; nervousness, tremor, tachycardia, HTN

Metaxalone (Skelaxin) Uses: **Relief of painful musculoskeletal conditions** Action: Centrally acting skeletal muscle relaxant Dose: 800 mg PO 3–4×/d Caution: [C, ?/–] Contra: Severe hepatic/renal impairment; caution in anemia Supplied: Tabs 400 mg SE: N/V, HA, drowsiness, hepatitis

Metformin (Glucophage, Glucophage XR) WARNING: Associated with lactic acidosis Uses: **Type 2 DM** Action: Decreases hepatic glucose production and intestinal absorption of glucose; improves insulin sensitivity Dose: Initial dose 500 mg PO bid; may ↑ to 2550 mg/d max; (administer with AM and PM meals; can convert total daily dose to qd dose of XR formulation) Caution: [B, +/–] Contra: Do not use if SCr > 1.4 in females or > 1.5 in males; contra in hypoxemic conditions, including acute CHF/sepsis; avoid alcohol; hold dose before and 48 h after ionic contrast   **Supplied:** Tabs 500, 850, 1000 mg; XR Tabs 500 mg   **SE:** Anorexia, N/V, rash, lactic acidosis (rare, but serious)

Methadone (Dolophine) [C-II]   Uses: Severe pain; detoxification and maintenance of narcotic addiction   Action: Narcotic analgesic   Dose: 2.5–10 mg IM q3–8h or 5–15 mg PO q8h; titrate as needed; ↑ slowly to avoid respiratory depression; (↓ in renal disease)   Caution: [B/D (prolonged use or high doses at term) + (with doses = 20 mg/24 h)] Severe liver disease   Supplied: Tabs 5, 10, 40 mg; oral soln 5, 10 mg/5 mL; oral conc 10 mg/mL; inj 10 mg/mL   SE: Respiratory depression, sedation, constipation, urinary retention, ventricular arrhythmias   Notes: Equianalgesic with parenteral morphine; longer half-life; prolongs QT interval

Methenamine (Hiprex, Urex, others)   Uses: Suppression or elimination of bacteriuria associated with chronic/ recurrent UTI   Dose: *Hippurate:* 1 g bid *Mandelate:* 1 g qid pc and hs; take with food and ascorbic acid; adequate hydration   Caution: [C, +]   Contra: Renal insufficiency, severe hepatic disease, and severe dehydration; allergy to sulfonamides   Supplied: *Methenamine hippurate (Hiprex, Urex):* 1 g tabs *Methenamine mandelate:* 500 mg, 1 g EC tabs   SE: Rash, GI upset, dysuria, increased LFTs

Methimazole (Tapazole)   Uses: Hyperthyroidism, thyrotoxicosis, and prep for thyroid surgery or radiation   Action: Blocks the formation of T_3 and T_4 Dose: *Initial:* 15–60 mg/d PO ÷ tid *Maintenance:* 5–15 mg PO qd (take with food)   Caution: [D, +/–]   Contra: Breastfeeding   Supplied: Tabs 5, 10 mg   SE: GI upset, dizziness, blood dyscrasias   Notes: Follow clinically and with TFT

Methocarbamol (Robaxin)   Uses: Relief of discomfort associated with painful musculoskeletal conditions   Action: Centrally acting skeletal muscle relaxant   Dose: 1.5 g PO qid for 2–3 d, then 1-g PO qid maintenance therapy; IV form rarely indicated   Caution: [C, +]   Contra: Myasthenia gravis, renal impairment; caution in seizure disorders   Supplied: Tabs 325, 500, 750 mg; inj 100 mg/mL   SE: Can discolor urine; drowsiness, GI upset

Methotrexate (Folex, Rheumatrex)   Uses: ALL and AML (including leukemic meningitis), trophoblastic tumors (chorioepithelioma, choriocarcinoma, chorioadenoma destruens, hydatidiform mole), breast CA, Burkitt's lymphoma, mycosis fungoides, osteosarcoma, head and neck CA, Hodgkin's and NHL, lung CA; psoriasis; and RA   Action: Inhibits dihydrofolate reductase-mediated generation of tetrahydrofolate   Dose: *CA;* Varies per protocol *RA:* 7.5 mg/wk PO as a single dose or 2.5 mg q12h PO for 3 doses/wk; "high dose" RX requires leucovorin rescue to limit hematologic and mucosal toxicity; ↓ in renal/hepatic impairment   Caution: [D, –]   Contra: Severe renal/hepatic impairment, pregnancy/lactation   Supplied: Tabs 2.5, 5, 7.5, 10, 15 mg; inj 2.5, 25 mg/mL; preservative-free inj 25 mg/mL   SE: Myelosuppression, N/V/D, anorexia, mucositis, hepatotoxicity (transient and reversible; may progress to atrophy, necrosis, fibrosis, cirrhosis), rashes, dizziness, malaise, blurred vision, alopecia, photosensitivity, renal failure, pneumonitis, and, rarely, pulmonary fibrosis. Chemical arachnoiditis and HA with IT delivery   Notes: Monitor blood counts, LFTs, renal function tests, chest x-ray, and MTX levels

Methyldopa (Aldomet)   Uses: HTN   Action: Centrally acting antihypertensive   Dose: 250–500 mg PO bid–tid (max 2–3 g/d) or 250 mg–1 g IV q6–8h; ↓ dose in renal insufficiency and in elderly   Caution: [B (oral), C (IV), +]   Contra: Liver disease; MAOIs   Supplied: Tabs 125, 250, 500 mg; oral susp 50 mg/mL; inj 50 mg/mL   SE: Can discolor urine; initial transient sedation or drowsiness frequent; edema, hemolytic anemia; hepatic disorders

Methylergonovine (Methergine)   Uses: Postpartum bleeding (uterine subinvolution)   Action: Ergotamine derivative   Dose: 0.2 mg IM after delivery of placenta, may repeat at 2–4 h intervals or 0.2–0.4 mg PO q6–12h for 2–7 d   Caution: [C, ?]   Contra: HTN, pregnancy   Supplied: Injectable forms; tabs 0.2 mg   SE: IV doses should be given over a period of > 1 min with frequent BP monitoring; HTN, N/V

Methylprednisolone (Solu-Medrol) [See Steroids, Table VII–2, p 613]

Metipranolol (Optipranolol) [See Table VII–12, pp 623–25]

Metoclopramide (Reglan, Clopra, Octamide)
Uses: Relief of diabetic gastroparesis, symptomatic GERD; chemotherapy-induced N/V, facilitate small bowel intubation and radiologic evaluation of the upper GI tract, stimulate gut in prolonged postop ileus **Action:** Stimulates motility of the upper GI tract; blocks dopamine in the chemoreceptor trigger zone **Dose:** *Diabetic gastroparesis:* 10 mg PO 30 min ac and hs for 2–8 wk PRN, or same dose given IV for 10 d, then switch to PO *Reflux:* 10–15 mg PO 30 min ac and hs *Antiemetic:* 1–3 mg/kg/dose IV 30 min before chemotherapy, then q2h for 2 doses, then q3h for 3 doses **Caution:** [B, –] Concomitant drugs with extrapyramidal ADRs **Contra:** Seizure disorders, GI obstruction **Supplied:** Tabs 5, 10 mg; syrup 5 mg/5 mL; soln 10 mg/mL; inj 5 mg/mL **SE:** Dystonic reactions common with high doses, treat with IV diphenhydramine; restlessness, drowsiness, diarrhea

Metolazone (Mykrox, Zaroxolyn)
Uses: Mild/moderate essential HTN and edema of renal disease or cardiac failure **Action:** Thiazide-like diuretic; inhibits sodium reabsorption in the distal tubules **Dose:** *HTN:* 2.5–5 mg/d PO *Edema:* 5–20 mg/d PO **Caution:** [D, +] **Contra:** Thiazide or sulfonamide sensitivity, anuria **Supplied:** Tabs Mykrox (rapid acting) 0.5 mg, Zaroxolyn 2.5, 5, 10 mg **SE:** Monitor fluid and electrolyte status during treatment; dizziness, hypotension, tachycardia, chest pain, photosensitivity; Mykrox and Zaroxolyn not bioequivalent

Metoprolol (Lopressor, Toprol XL) [See Table VII–7, pp 617–18]

Metronidazole (Flagyl, MetroGel)
Uses: Bone/joint, endocarditis, intra-abdominal, meningitis, and skin infections; amebiasis; trichomoniasis; bacterial vaginosis **Action:** Interferes with DNA synthesis *Spectrum:* Excellent coverage for anaerobic infections including *C difficile*, also *H pylori* in combination therapy **Dose:** *Anaerobic infections:* 500 mg IV q6–8h. *Amebic dysentery:* 750 mg/d PO for 5–10 d. *Trichomoniasis:* 250 mg PO tid for 7 d or 2 g PO ×1. *C difficile infection:* 500 mg PO or IV q8h for 7–10 d (PO preferred; IV only if patient NPO). *Vaginosis:* 1 applicatorful intravaginally bid or 500 mg PO bid for 7 d. *Acne rosacea/skin:* Apply bid ↓ in hepatic failure **Caution:** [B, M] Avoid alcohol **Contra:** First trimester of pregnancy **Supplied:** Tabs 250, 500 mg; ER tabs 750 mg; caps 375 mg; topical lotion and gel 0.75%; gel, vaginal 0.75% (5 g/applicator 37.5 mg in 70-g tube), cream 1% **SE:** May cause disulfiram-like reaction; dizziness, HA, GI upset, anorexia, urine discoloration **Notes:** For *Trichomonas* infections, Rx patient's partner; no aerobic bacteria activity; used in combination in serious mixed infections

Mexiletine (Mexitil)
Uses: Suppression of symptomatic ventricular arrhythmias; diabetic neuropathy **Action:** Class IB antiarrhythmic **Dose:** 200–300 mg PO q8h; 1200 mg/d max; drug interactions with hepatic enzyme inducers and suppressors requiring dosage changes (administer with food or antacids) **Caution:** [C, +] May worsen severe arrhythmias **Contra:** Cardiogenic shock or 2nd-/3rd-degree AV block without pacemaker **Supplied:** Caps 150, 200, 250 mg **SE:** Monitor LFTs; lightheadedness, dizziness, anxiety, incoordination, GI upset, ataxia, hepatic damage, blood dyscrasias

Mezlocillin (Mezlin) [See Table VII–6, p 616]

Miconazole (Monistat, others)
Uses: Candidal infections, dermatomycoses (various tinea forms) **Action:** Fungicidal; alters permeability of the fungal cell membrane **Dose:** Apply to area bid for 2–4 wk *Intravaginally:* 1 applicatorful or supp hs for 3 (4% or 200 mg) or 7 d (2% or 100 mg) **Caution:** [C, ?] Azole sensitivity **Supplied:** Topical cream 2%; lotion 2%; powder 2%; spray 2%; vaginal supp 100, 200 mg; vaginal cream 2%, 4% [OTC] **SE:** Vaginal burning, may potentiate warfarin **Notes:** Antagonistic to amphotericin B in vivo

Midazolam (Versed) [C-IV]
Uses: Preoperative sedation, conscious sedation for short procedures and mechanically ventilated patients, induction of general anesthesia **Action:** Short-acting benzodiazepine **Dose:** 1–5 mg IV or IM; titrate to effect; ↓ dose in elderly, with use of narcotics or CNS depressants **Caution:** [D, +/–] CYP3A4 substrate, several drug interactions **Contra:** Narrow-angle glaucoma; use of amprenavir, nelfinavir,

ritonavir **Supplied:** Inj 1, 5 mg/mL; syrup 2 mg/mL **SE:** Monitor for respiratory depression; hypotension in conscious sedation, nausea **Notes:** Reversal with flumazenil

Mifepristone [RU 486] (Mifeprex) **WARNING:** Patient counseling and information required, may be associated with fatal infections and bleeding **Uses:** Termination of intrauterine pregnancies of < 49 d **Action:** Antiprogestin; ↑ prostaglandins, resulting in uterine contraction **Dose:** Administered with 3 office visits: day 1, three 200-mg tablets PO; day 3 if no abortion, two 200-mg misoprostol PO; on or about day 14, verify termination of pregnancy **Caution:** [X, –] **Contra:** Anticoagulation therapy, bleeding disorders **Supplied:** Tabs 200 mg **SE:** Abdominal pain and 1–2 wk of uterine bleeding **Notes:** Must be administered under physician's supervision

Miglitol (Glyset) **Uses:** Type 2 DM **Action:** α-Glucosidase inhibitor; delays digestion of ingested carbohydrates **Dose:** Initial 25 mg PO tid; maintenance 50–100 mg tid (with 1st bite of each meal) **Caution:** [B, –] **Contra:** Obstructive or inflammatory GI disorders; avoid if SCr > 2 **Supplied:** Tabs 25, 50, 100 mg **SE:** Used alone or in combination with sulfonylureas; flatulence, diarrhea, abdominal pain

Milrinone (Primacor) **Uses:** CHF **Action:** Positive inotrope and vasodilator; little chronotropic activity **Dose:** 50 mcg/kg, then 0.375–0.75 mcg/kg/min inf; ↓ dose in renal impairment **Caution:** [C, ?] **Supplied:** Inj 1 mcg/mL **SE:** Arrhythmias, hypotension, HA **Notes:** Carefully monitor fluid/electrolyte status and BP/HR

Mineral Oil **Uses:** Constipation **Action:** Emollient laxative **Dose:** 5–45 mL PO PRN **Caution:** [C, ?] N/V, difficulty swallowing, bedridden patients **Contra:** Appendicitis, diverticulitis, ulcerative colitis **Supplied:** Liq [OTC] **SE:** Lipid pneumonia, anal incontinence, impaired vitamin absorption

Minoxidil (Loniten, Rogaine) **Uses:** Severe HTN; male and female pattern baldness **Action:** Peripheral vasodilator; stimulates vertex hair growth **Dose:** *Oral:* 2.5–10 mg PO bid–qid; ↓ oral dose in elderly *Topical:* Apply bid to affected area **Caution:** [C, +] **Supplied:** Tabs 2.5, 5, 10 mg; topical soln (Rogaine) 2% **SE:** Pericardial effusion and volume overload may occur with oral use; hypertrichosis after chronic use; edema, ECG changes, weight gain

Mirtazapine (Remeron) **WARNING:** *Pediatric:* Antidepressants may increase risk of suicidality; consider risks and benefits of use. patients should be closely monitored for clinical worsening, suicidality, or unusual changes in behavior **Uses:** Depression **Action:** Tetracyclic antidepressant **Dose:** 15 mg PO hs, up to 45 mg/d hs **Caution:** [C, ?] **Contra:** MAOIs within 14 d **Supplied:** Tabs 15, 30, 45 mg **SE:** Somnolence, increased cholesterol, constipation, xerostomia, weight gain, agranulocytosis **Notes:** Do not ↑ dose at intervals of less than 1–2 wk

Misoprostol (Cytotec) **Uses:** Prevention of NSAID-induced gastric ulcers; induction of labor, incomplete and therapeutic abortion **Action:** Prostaglandin with both antisecretory and mucosal protective properties **Dose:** Ulcer prevention: 200 mcg PO qid with meals; in females, start on 2nd or 3rd of next normal menstrual period; 25–50 mcg for induction of labor (term): 400 mcg on day 3 of mifepristone for pregnancy termination (take with food) **Caution:** [X, –] **Supplied:** Tabs 100, 200 mcg **SE:** Can cause miscarriage with potentially dangerous bleeding; HA, GI symptoms common (diarrhea, abdominal pain, constipation)

Mitomycin (Mutamycin) **Uses:** Stomach, pancreas, breast, colon cancers; squamous cell carcinoma of the anus; non–small cell lung, head, and neck, cervical, and breast cancers; bladder cancer (intravesically) **Action:** Alkylating agent; may also generate oxygen free radicals, induces DNA strand breaks **Dose:** 20 mg/m^2 q6–8wk or 10 mg/m^2 in combination with other myelosuppressive drugs; bladder CA 20–40 mg in 40 mL NS via a urethral catheter once/wk for 8 wk, followed by monthly treatments for 1 y; ↓ dose in renal/hepatic impairment **Caution:** [D, –] **Contra:** Thrombocytopenia, leukopenia, coagulation disorders, serum creatinine > 1.7 mg/dL **Supplied:** Inj **SE:** Myelosuppression (may persist up to 3–8 wk after dose and may be cumulative minimized by a lifetime dose < 50–60 mg/m^2), N/V, anorexia, stomatitis, and renal toxicity; microangiopathic hemolytic anemia (similar to he-

molytic-uremic syndrome) with progressive renal failure; venoocclusive disease of the liver, interstitial pneumonia, alopecia (rare); extravasation reactions can be severe

Mitotane (Lysodren) Uses: **Palliative treatment of inoperable adrenocortical carcinoma** Action: Unclear; induces mitochondrial injury in adrenocortical cells Dose: 8–10 g/d in 3–4 ÷ doses (begin at 2 g/d with glucocorticoid replacement); ↓ in hepatic insufficiency; adequate hydration necessary Caution: [C, ?] Supplied: Tabs 500 mg SE: Anorexia, N/V/D; acute adrenal insufficiency may be precipitated by physical stresses (shock, trauma, infection), Rx with steroids; allergic reactions (rare), visual disturbances, hemorrhagic cystitis, albuminuria, hematuria, HTN or hypotension, minor aches, fever

Mitoxantrone (Novantrone) Uses: **AML (with cytarabine), ALL, CML, prostate CA, MS, breast CA and NHL** Action: DNA-intercalating agent; inhibitor of DNA topoisomerase II Dose: Per specific protocols. ↓ dose in hepatic failure, leukopenia, thrombocytopenia; maintain hydration Caution: [D, –] Contra: Pregnancy Supplied: Inj 2 mg/mL SE: Myelosuppression, N/V, stomatitis, alopecia (infrequent), cardiotoxicity, urine discoloration

Modafinil (Provigil) Uses: **Improve wakefulness in patients with excessive daytime sleepiness associated with narcolepsy** Action: Possible mechanisms include altered dopamine and norepinephrine release, decreased GABA-mediated neurotransmission Dose: 200 mg PO Q morning Caution: [C, ?/–] Increases effects of warfarin, diazepam, phenytoin; decreases effects of oral contraceptives, cyclosporine, theophylline Supplied: Tablets 100 mg, 200 mg SE: HA, N, D, paresthesias, rhinitis, agitation Notes: Consider lower doses in elderly patients, reduce dose by 50% in patients with hepatic impairment; use with caution in patients with cardiovascular disease

Moexipril (Univasc) [See Table VII–3, p 614]

Molindone (Moban) Uses: **Psychotic disorders** Action: Piperazine phenothiazine Dose: 50–75 mg/d, ↑ to 225 mg/d if necessary Caution: [C, ?] Narrow-angle glaucoma Contra: Drug or alcohol-induced CNS depression Supplied: Tabs 5, 10, 25, 50, 100 mg; conc 20 mg/mL SE: Hypotension, tachycardia, arrhythmias, extrapyramidal symptoms, seizures, constipation, xerostomia, blurred vision

Montelukast (Singulair) Uses: **Prophylaxis and Rx of chronic asthma, seasonal allergic rhinitis** Action: Leukotriene receptor antagonist Dose: *Asthma:* 10 mg/d PO taken in PM *Rhinitis:* 10 mg qd Caution: [B, M] Supplied: Tabs 10 mg; chew tabs 4, 5 mg SE: HA, dizziness, fatigue, rash, GI upset, Churg-Strauss syndrome Notes: Not for acute asthma attacks

Morphine (Avinza ER, Duramorph, MS Contin, Kadian SR, Oramorph SR, Roxanol) [C-II] Uses: **Relief of severe pain** Action: Narcotic analgesic Dose: *Oral:* 5–30 mg q4h PRN; SR tabs 30–60 mg q8–12h (do not chew/crush) *IV/IM:* 2.5–15 mg q2–6h; supp 10–30 mg q4h Caution: [B (D if prolonged use or high doses at term) +/–] Contra: Severe asthma, respiratory depression, GI obstruction Supplied: Immediate release tabs 10, 14, 20 mg; MS Contin CR tabs 15, 30, 60, 100, 200 mg; Oramorph SR CR tabs 15, 30, 60, 100 mg; Kadian SR caps 20, 30, 50, 60, 100 mg; Avinza ER caps 30, 60, 90, 120 mg; soln 10, 20, 100 mg; supp 5, 10, 20 mg; inj 2, 4, 5, 8, 10, 15 mg/mL; Duramorph preservative-free inj 0.5, 1 mg/mL; 5, 10, 20, 30 mg suppository SE: Narcotic SE (respiratory depression, sedation, constipation, N/V, pruritus) Notes: May require scheduled dosing to relieve severe chronic pain; MS Contin commonly used SR form (do not crush)

Moxifloxacin (Avelox, Vigamox ophth) Uses: **Acute sinusitis, acute bronchitis, skin/soft tissue infections, conjunctivitis, and community-acquired pneumonia** Action: Quinolone; inhibits DNA gyrase. *Spectrum:* Excellent gram(+) coverage except MRSA and *E faecium.* Good gram(–) coverage except *P aeruginosa, S maltophilia* and *Acinetobacter* sp. Good anaerobic coverage Dose: 400 mg/d PO (avoid cation products, antacids)/IV qd; *ophthal:* 1 drop tid × 7d Caution: [C, ?/–] Quinolone sensitivity; interactions with Mg^{2+}, Ca^{2+}, Al^{2+}, and Fe^{2+}-containing products and class IA and III antiarrhythmic agents Supplied: Tabs 400 mg, inj, opthal 0.5% **SE:** Dizziness, nausea, QT prolongation, seizures, photosensitivity, tendon rupture **Notes:** Take 4 h before or 8 h after antacids

Mupirocin (Bactroban) Uses: Impetigo; eradication of MRSA in nasal carriers
Action: Inhibits bacterial protein synthesis **Dose:** *Topical:* Apply small amount to affected area *Nasal:* Apply bid in nostrils **Caution:** [B, ?] Do not use concurrently with other nasal products **Supplied:** Oint 2%; cream 2% **SE:** Local irritation, rash

Muromonab-CD3 (Orthoclone OKT3) WARNING: Can cause anaphylaxis; monitor fluid status Uses: Acute rejection following organ transplantation Action: Blocks
T-cell function **Dose:** 5 mg/d IV for 10–14 d **Caution:** [C, ?/–] Murine sensitivity, fluid overload **Contra:** Heart failure/fluid overload, history of seizures, pregnancy, uncontrolled HTN **Supplied:** Inj 5 mg/5 mL **SE:** Murine antibody; fever and chills after the 1st dose (premedicate with steroid/APAP/antihistamine); monitor closely for anaphylaxis or pulmonary edema **Notes:** Use 0.22 micron filter for administration

Mycophenolate Mofetil (CellCept) WARNING: Increased risk of infections, possible development of lymphoma Uses: Prevent organ rejection after transplant Action:
Inhibits immunologically-mediated inflammatory responses **Dose:** 1 g PO bid; used with steroids and cyclosporine; ↓ in renal insufficiency or neutropenia; *IV:* infuse over at least 2 h; *PO:* take on empty stomach, do not open capsules **Caution:** [C, ?/–] **Supplied:** Caps 250, 500 mg; inj 500 mg **SE:** N/V/D, pain, fever, HA, infection, HTN, anemia, leukopenia, edema

Nabumetone (Relafen) [See Table VII–1, p 613]

Nadolol (Corgard) [See Table VII–7, pp 617–18]

Nafcillin (Nallpen) [See Table VII–5, p 616]

Naftifine (Naftin) Uses: Tinea pedis, cruris, and tinea corporis Action: Antifungal
antibiotic **Dose:** Apply bid **Caution:** [B, ?] **Supplied:** 1% cream; gel **SE:** Local irritation

Nalbuphine (Nubain) Uses: Moderate/severe pain; preop and obstetrical analgesia Action: Narcotic agonist-antagonist; inhibits ascending pain pathways Dose: 10–20
mg IM or IV q4–6h PRN; max of 160 mg/d; single max dose, 20 mg; ↓ in hepatic insufficiency **Caution:** [B (D if prolonged or high doses at term), ?] **Contra:** Sulfite sensitivity **Supplied:** Inj 10, 20 mg/mL **SE:** Causes CNS depression and drowsiness; caution in patients receiving opiates

Naloxone (Narcan) Uses: Opioid addiction (diagnosis) and overdose Action:
Competitive narcotic antagonist **Dose:** 0.4–2.0 mg IV, IM, or SC q5min; max total dose, 10 mg **Caution:** [B, ?] May precipitate acute withdrawal in addicts **Supplied:** Inj 0.4, 1.0 mg/mL; neonatal inj 0.02 mg/mL **SE:** Hypotension, tachycardia, irritability, GI upset, pulmonary edema **Notes:** If no response after 10 mg, suspect nonnarcotic cause

Naltrexone (ReVia) Uses: Alcohol and narcotic addiction Action: Competitively
binds to opioid receptors **Dose:** 50 mg/d PO; do not give until opioid free for 7–10 d **Caution:** [C, M] **Contra:** Acute hepatitis, liver failure; opioid use **Supplied:** Tabs 50 mg **SE:** May cause hepatotoxicity; insomnia, GI upset, joint pain, HA, fatigue

Naphazoline and Antazoline (Albalon-A Ophthalmic, others) Naphazoline and Pheniramine Acetate (Naphcon A) [See Table VII—12, pp 623–25]

Naproxen (Aleve, Naprosyn, Anaprox, Naprelan) [See Table VII–11, pp 621–22]

Naratriptan (Amerge) [See Table VII–16, p 629]

Nateglinide (Starlix) Uses: Type 2 DM Action: ↑ pancreatic release of insulin
Dose: 120 mg PO tid 1–30 min pc; ↓ to 60 mg tid if near target HbA_{1c} (take 1 – 30 min before meals) **Caution:** [C, –] Caution with drugs metabolized by CYP2C9/3A4 **Contra:** Diabetic ketoacidosis, type I diabetes **Supplied:** Tabs 60, 120 mg **SE:** Hypoglycemia, URI; salicylates, nonselective β-blockers may enhance hypoglycemia

Nedocromil (Tilade)   Uses: Mild/moderate asthma   Action: Antiinflammatory agent   Dose: *Inhal:* 2 inhal 4×/d   Caution: [B, ?/–]   Supplied: Met-dose inhaler   SE: Chest pain, dizziness, dysphonia, rash, GI upset, infection   Notes: Not for acute asthma attacks

Nedocromil Sodium (Alocril) [See Table VII–12, pp 623–25]

Nefazodone   WARNING: Fatal hepatitis and liver failure possible; discontinue if LFT > 3× ULN; do not retreat *Pediatric:* Antidepressants may increase risk of suicidality; consider risks and benefits of use. Patients should be closely monitored for clinical worsening, suicidality, or unusual changes in behavior   Uses: Depression   Action: Inhibits neuronal uptake of serotonin and norepinephrine   Dose: Initially 100 mg PO bid; usual 300–600 mg/d in 2 ÷ doses   Caution: [C, ?]   Contra: MAOIs, pimozide, cisapride, CBZ   Supplied: Tabs 100, 150, 200, 250 mg   SE: Postural hypotension and allergic reactions; HA, drowsiness, xerostomia, constipation, GI upset, liver failure   Notes: Monitor LFTs, HR/BP

Nelfinavir (Viracept)   Uses: HIV infection   Action: Protease inhibitor; results in formation of immature, noninfectious virion   Dose: 750 mg PO tid or 1250 mg PO bid; take with food   Caution: [B, ?] Many significant drug interactions   Contra: Phenylketonuria, triazolam/midazolam use or any other drug highly dependent on CYP3A4   Supplied: Tabs 250 mg; oral powder   SE: Food increases absorption; interacts with St. John's wort; dyslipidemia, lipodystrophy, diarrhea, rash

Neomycin, Bacitracin, and Polymyxin B (Neosporin Ointment) [See Bacitracin, Neomycin, and Polymyxin, p 000]

Neomycin, Colistin, and Hydrocortisone (Cortisporin-TC Otic Drops)

Neomycin, Colistin, Hydrocortisone, and Thonzonium (Cortisporin-TC Otic Suspension)   Uses: External otitis, infections of mastoidectomy and fenestration cavities   Action: Antibiotic and anti-inflammatory   Dose: 4–5 drops in ear(s) tid–qid   Caution: [C, ?]   Contra: Supplied: Otic drops and susp   SE: Local irritation

Neomycin and Dexamethasone (AK-Neo-Dex Ophthalmic, NeoDecadron Ophthalmic [See Table VII–12, pp 623–25]

Neomycin and Polymyxin B (Neosporin Cream [OTC])   Uses: Infection in minor cuts, scrapes, and burns   Action: Bactericidal antibiotic   Dose: Apply bid–qid   Caution: [C, ?]   Supplied: Cream neomycin 3.5 mg/polymyxin B 10,000 units/g   SE: Local irritation   Notes: Different from Neosporin oint

Neomycin, Polymyxin B, and Dexamethasone (Maxitrol) [See Table VII–12, pp 623–25]

Neomycin-Polymyxin Bladder Irrigant [Neosporin GU Irrigant]   Uses: Continuous irrigant for prophylaxis against bacteriuria and gram(–) bacteremia associated with indwelling catheter use   Action: Bactericidal antibiotic   Dose: 1 mL irrigant added to 1 L of 0.9% NaCl; continuous bladder irrigation with 1L of soln/24 h   Caution: [D, ?]   Supplied: Soln Neomycin sulfate 40 mg and polymixin B 200,000 units/mL; Ampules 1, 20 mL   SE: Slight possibility for neomycin-induced ototoxicity or nephrotoxicity   Notes: Potential for bacterial or fungal superinfection; not for injection

Neomycin, Polymyxin, and Hydrocortisone (Cortisporin Ophthalmic and Otic) [Also see Table VII–12, pp 623–25]   Uses: Ocular and otic bacterial infections   Action: Antibiotic and anti-inflammatory   Dose: *Otic:* 3–4 drops in the ear(s) 3–4 times/d *Ophth:* Apply a thin layer to the eye(s) or 1 drops 1–4 ×/d   Caution: [C, ?]   Supplied: Otic susp; ophth soln; ophth oint   SE: Local irritation

Neomycin, Polymyxin-B, and Prednisolone (Poly-Pred Ophthalmic) [See Table VII–12, pp 623–25]

Neomycin Sulfate (Myciguent [OTC])   Uses: Hepatic coma and preoperative bowel preparation   Action: Aminoglycoside, poorly absorbed orally; suppresses GI bacterial flora   Dose: 3–12 g/24 h PO in 3–4 ÷ doses   Caution: [C, ?/–] Caution in renal failure, neuromuscular disorders, hearing impairment   Contra: Intestinal obstruction   Supplied:

Tabs 500 mg; oral soln 125 mg/5 mL **SE:** Hearing loss with long-term use; rash, N/V **Notes:** Do not use parenterally due to ↑ toxicity. Part of the Condon bowel prep

Nesiritide (Natrecor) **Uses: Acutely decompensated CHF** **Action:** Human B-type natriuretic peptide **Dose:** 2 mcg/kg IV bolus, then 0.01 mcg/kg/min IV **Caution:** [C, ?/–] Patients in whom vasodilators are not appropriate **Contra:** SBP < 90, cardiogenic shock **Supplied:** Vials 1.5 mg **SE:** Hypotension, HA, GI upset, arrhythmias, ↑ Cr **Notes:** Requires continuous BP monitoring

Nevirapine (Viramune) **WARNING:** Reports of fatal hepatotoxicity even after short-term use; severe life-threatening skin reactions (Stevens-Johnson, toxic epidermal necrolysis, and hypersensitivity reactions); monitor closely during 1st 8 wk of treatment **Uses: HIV infection** **Action:** Nonnucleoside reverse transcriptase inhibitor **Dose:** Initially 200 mg/d for 14 d, then 200 mg bid **Caution:** [C, +/–] Oral contraceptive use **Supplied:** Tabs 200 mg; susp 50 mg/5 mL **SE:** May cause life-threatening rash; HA, fever, diarrhea, neutropenia, hepatitis **Notes:** Give without regard to food; not recommended to initiate in women if CD4 > 250 or men > 400 unless benefit outweighs risk of potential hepatotoxicity

Niacin (Niaspan) **Uses: Adjunctive therapy in patients with significant hyperlipidemia** **Action:** Inhibits lipolysis; decreases esterification of triglycerides; increases lipoprotein lipase activity **Dose:** 1–6 g PO in divided doses tid; max of 9 g/d **Caution:** [A (C if doses > RDA), +] **Contra:** Liver disease, peptic ulcer, arterial hemorrhage **Supplied:** SR caps 125, 250, 300, 400, 500 mg; tabs 25, 50, 100, 250, 500 mg; SR tabs 150, 250, 500, 750 mg; elixir 50 mg/5 mL **SE:** Upper body and facial flushing and warmth following dose; may cause GI upset; HA, flatulence, paresthesias, liver damage, may exacerbate peptic ulcer, gout; may worsen glucose control in DM **Notes:** Administer with food; flushing may be ↓ by taking an aspirin or NSAID 30–60 min before dose

Nicardipine (Cardene) **Uses: Chronic stable angina and HTN; prophylaxis of migraine** **Action:** Ca channel blocker **Dose:** *Oral:* 20–40 mg PO tid *SR:* 30–60 mg PO bid *IV:* 5 mg/h IV cont inf; ↑ by 2.5 mg/h q15min to max 15 mg/h; ↓ dose in renal/hepatic impairment **Caution:** [C, ?/–] Heart block, CAD **Contra:** Cardiogenic shock **Supplied:** Caps 20, 30 mg; SR caps 30, 45, 60 mg; inj 2.5 mg/mL **SE:** Flushing, tachycardia, hypotension, edema, HA **Notes:** *Oral-to-IV conversion:* 20 mg tid = 0.5 mg/h, 30 mg tid = 1.2 mg/h, 40 mg tid = 2.2 mg/h; take with food (not high fat)

Nicotine Gum (Nicorette [OTC]) **Uses: Aid to smoking cessation for the relief of nicotine withdrawal** **Action:** Provides systemic delivery of nicotine **Dose:** Chew 9–12 pieces/d PRN; max 30 pieces/d **Caution:** [C, ?] **Contra:** Life-threatening arrhythmias, unstable angina **Supplied:** 2 mg, 4 mg/piece; mint, orange, original flavors **SE:** Tachycardia, HA, GI upset, hiccups **Notes:** Patients must stop smoking and perform behavior modification for max effect

Nicotine Nasal Spray (Nicotrol NS) **Uses: Aid to smoking cessation for the relief of nicotine withdrawal** **Action:** Provides systemic delivery of nicotine **Dose:** 0.5 mg/actuation; 1–2 sprays/h, not to exceed 10 sprays/h **Caution:** [D, M] **Contra:** Life-threatening arrhythmias, unstable angina **Supplied:** Nasal inhaler 10 mg/mL **SE:** Local irritation, tachycardia, HA, taste perversion **Notes:** Patients must stop smoking and perform behavior modification for max effect

Nicotine Transdermal (Habitrol, Nicoderm CQ [OTC], Nicotrol [OTC]) **Uses: Aid to smoking cessation for the relief of nicotine withdrawal** **Action:** Provides systemic delivery of nicotine **Dose:** Individualized to the patient's needs; apply 1 patch (14–22 mg/d), and taper over 6 wk **Caution:** [D, M] **Contra:** Life-threatening arrhythmias, unstable angina **Supplied:** Habitrol and Nicoderm CQ 7, 14, 21 mg of nicotine/24 h; Nicotrol 5, 10, 15 mg/24 h; **SE:** Insomnia, pruritus, erythema, local site reaction, tachycardia **Notes:** Nicotrol to be worn for 16 h to mimic smoking patterns; others worn for 24 h; patients must stop smoking and perform behavior modification for max effect

Nifedipine (Procardia, Procardia XL, Adalat, Adalat CC) **Uses: Vasospastic or chronic stable angina and HTN; tocolytic** **Action:** Ca channel blocker **Dose:** SR

tabs 30–90 mg/d *Tocolysis:* 10–20 mg PO q4–6h   **Caution:** [C, +] Heart block, aortic stenosis   **Contra:** Immediate-release preparation for urgent or emergent HTN; acute MI   **Supplied:** Caps 10, 20 mg; SR tabs 30, 60, 90 mg   **SE:** HA common on initial treatment; reflex tachycardia may occur with regular release dosage forms; peripheral edema, hypotension, flushing, dizziness   **Notes:** Adalat CC and Procardia XL not interchangeable; sublingual administration is neither safe nor effective and should be abandoned

Nilutamide (Nilandron)   WARNING: Interstitial pneumonitis possible; most cases in 1st 3 mo; follow chest x-ray before treatment   Uses: Combination with surgical castration for metastatic prostate CA   Action: Nonsteroidal antiandrogen   Dose: 300 mg/d PO in ÷ doses for 30 d, then 150 mg/d   Caution: [C, ?]   Contra: Severe hepatic impairment or respiratory insufficiency   Supplied: Tabs 150 mg   SE: Hot flashes, loss of libido, impotence, N/V/D, gynecomastia, hepatic dysfunction (follow LFTs), interstitial pneumonitis   Notes: May cause a severe reaction when taken with alcohol

Nimodipine (Nimotop)   Uses: Prevent vasospasm after subarachnoid hemorrhage   Action: Ca channel blocker   Dose: 60 mg PO q4h for 21 d; ↓ dose in hepatic failure   Caution: [C, ?]   Supplied: Caps 30 mg   SE: Hypotension, HA, constipation   Notes: Contents of caps may be administered via NG tube if caps cannot be swallowed whole

Nisoldipine (Sular)   Uses: HTN   Action: Ca channel blocker   Dose: 10–60 mg/d PO; do not take with grapefruit juice or high-fat meal; ↓ starting doses in elderly or hepatic impairment   Caution: [C, ?]   Contra: N/A   Supplied: ER tabs 10, 20, 30, 40 mg   SE: Edema, HA, flushing

Nitrofurantoin (Macrodantin, Furadantin, Macrobid)   WARNING: Pulmonary reactions possible   Uses: Prevention and treatment of UTI   Action: Bacteriostatic; interferes with carbohydrate metabolism   *Spectrum:* Susceptible gram(−) and some gram(+) bacteria; *Pseudomonas, Serratia,* and most *Proteus* sp. generally resistant   Dose: *Suppression:* 50–100 mg/d PO *Treatment:* 50–100 mg PO qid. Take with food, milk, or antacid   Caution: [B, +] Avoid if CrCl < 50 mL/min, pregnant at term   Supplied: Caps and tabs 50, 100 mg; SR caps 100 mg; susp 25 mg/5 mL   SE: GI side effects common; dyspnea and a variety of acute and chronic pulmonary reactions, peripheral neuropathy   Notes: Macrocrystals (Macrodantin) cause less nausea than other forms of the drug

Nitroglycerin (Nitrostat, Nitrolingual, Nitro-Bid Ointment, Nitro-Bid IV, Nitrodisc, Transderm-Nitro, Others)   Uses: Angina pectoris, acute and prophylactic therapy, CHF, BP control   Action: Relaxation of vascular smooth muscle, dilates coronary arteries   Dose *Sublingual:* 1 tab q5min SL PRN for 3 doses *Translingual:* 1–2 metdoses sprayed onto oral mucosa q3–5min, max 3 doses *Oral:* 2.5–9 mg tid *IV:* 5–20 mcg/min, titrated to effect *Topical:* Apply ½ in. of oint to the chest wall tid, wipe off at night *TD:* 0.2–0.4 mg/h/patch qd   Caution: [B, ?] Restrictive cardiomyopathy   Contra: IV: Pericardial tamponade, constrictive pericarditis PO: Concurrent use with sildenafil, tadalafil, vardenafil, head trauma, closed-angle glaucoma   Supplied: SL tabs 0.3, 0.4, 0.6 mg; translingual spray 0.4 mg/dose; SR caps 2.5, 6.5, 9, 13 mg; SR tabs 2.6, 6.5, 9.0 mg; inj 0.5, 5, 10 mg/mL; oint 2%; TD patches 0.1, 0.2, 0.4, 0.6 mg/hr; buccal CR 2, 3 mg   SE: HA, hypotension, lightheadedness, GI upset   Notes: Tolerance to nitrates develops with chronic use after 1–2 wk; can be avoided by providing a nitrate-free period each day, using shorter-acting nitrates tid, and removing long-acting patches and oint before hs to prevent tolerance

Nitroprusside (Nipride, Nitropress)   Uses: Hypertensive crisis, CHF, controlled hypotension periop (↓ bleeding), aortic dissection, pulmonary edema   Action: ↓ SVR   Dose: 0.5–10 mcg/kg/min IV inf, titrated to effect; usual dose 3 mcg/kg/min   Caution: [C, ?] Decreased cerebral perfusion   Contra: High output failure, compensatory HTN   Supplied: Inj 25 mg/mL   SE: Excessive hypotensive effects, palpitations, HA   Notes: Thiocyanate, the metabolite, excreted by the kidney; thiocyanate toxicity at levels of 5–10 mg/dL, more likely when used for > 2–3 d; if used to treat aortic dissection, use β-blocker concomitantly

Nizatidine (Axid)   Uses: Duodenal ulcers, GERD, heartburn   Action: H$_2$-receptor antagonist   Dose: *Active ulcer:* 150 mg PO bid or 300 mg PO hs; maint 150 mg PO hs

GERD: 300 mg PO bid; maint PO bid *Heartburn:* 75 mg PO bid. ↓ dose in renal impairment **Caution:** [B, +] **Supplied:** Caps 75, 150, 300 mg **SE:** Dizziness, HA, constipation, diarrhea; 75 mg tabs available OTC

Norepinephrine (Levophed) **Uses: Acute hypotension, cardiac arrest (adjunct)**
Action: Peripheral vasoconstrictor acting on both the arterial and venous beds **Dose:** 8–12 mcg/min IV, titrate to effect **Caution:** [C, ?] **Contra:** Hypotension due to hypovolemia **Supplied:** Inj 1 mg/mL **SE:** Bradycardia, arrhythmia **Notes:** Correct blood volume depletion as much as possible prior to vasopressor therapy; interaction with TCAs leads to severe HTN; infuse into large vein to avoid extravasation; phentolamine 5–10 mg/10 mL NS injected locally for extravasation

Norethindrone Acetate/Ethinyl Estradiol (FemHRT) **Uses: Treatment of moderate to severe vasomotor symptoms associated with menopause; prevention of osteoporosis** **Action:** Hormone replacement **Dose:** 1 tab qd **Caution** [X, –] **Supplied:** 1 mg norethindrone/5 mcg ethinyl estradiol tabs **SE:** Thrombosis, dizziness, HA, libido changes **Notes:** Use in women with intact uterus.

Norfloxacin (Noroxin, Chibroxin Ophth) **Uses: Complicated and uncomplicated UTI due to gram(–) bacteria, prostatitis, gonorrhea and infectious diarrhea** **Action:** Quinolone, inhibits DNA gyrase *Spectrum:* Susceptible infections due to *E faecalis, E coli, K pneumoniae, P mirabilis, P aeruginosa, S epidermidis, S saprophyticus* **Dose:** 400 mg PO bid *Gonorrhea:* 800 mg single dose *Prostatitis:* 400 mg PO bid **Caution:** [C, –] Tendinitis/tendon rupture, quinolone sensitivity, dose ↓ in renal impairment **Contra:** History of hypersensitivity or tendinitis with fluoroquinolones **Supplied:** Tabs 400 mg **SE:** Photosensitivity, HA, GI **Notes:** Drug interactions with antacids, theophylline, and caffeine; good concentrations in the kidney and urine, poor blood levels; do not use for urosepsis

Norgestrel (Ovrette) **Uses: Contraceptive** **Action:** Prevent follicular maturation and ovulation **Dose:** 1 tab/d PO; begin day 1 of menses **Caution:** [X, ?] **Contra:** Thromboembolic disorders, breast CA, pregnancy, severe hepatic disease **Supplied:** Tabs 0.075 mg **SE:** Edema, breakthrough bleeding, thromboembolism **Notes:** Progestin-only products have higher rate of failure in prevention of pregnancy

Nortriptyline (Aventyl, Pamelor) **WARNING:** *Pediatric:* Antidepressants increase risk of suicidality; consider risks and benefits of use. Patients should be closely monitored for clinical worsening, suicidality, or unusual changes in behavior **Uses: Endogenous depression** **Action:** TCA; increases the synaptic CNS concentrations of serotonin and/or norepinephrine **Dose:** 25 mg PO tid–qid; doses > 150 mg/d not recommended *Elderly:* 10–25 mg hs; ↓ dose with hepatic insufficiency **Caution:** [D, +/–] Narrow-angle glaucoma, CV disease **Contra:** TCA hypersensitivity, concomitant use of MAOI **Supplied:** Caps 10, 25, 50, 75 mg; soln 10 mg/5 mL **SE:** Many anticholinergic side effects (blurred vision, urinary retention, dry mouth) **Notes:** Max effect seen after 2 wk of therapy

Nystatin (Mycostatin) **Uses: Mucocutaneous *Candida* infections (oral, skin, vaginal)** **Action:** Alters membrane permeability *Spectrum:* Susceptible *Candida* sp. **Dose:** *Oral:* 400,000–600,000 units PO "swish and swallow" qid *Vaginal:* 1 tab vaginally hs for 2 wk *Topical:* Apply bid–tid to affected area **Caution:** [B (C oral), +] **Contra:** N/A **Supplied:** Oral susp 100,000 units/mL; oral tabs 500,000 units; troches 200,000 units; vaginal tabs 100,000 units; topical cream and oint 100,000 units/g **SE:** GI upset, Stevens-Johnson syndrome **Notes:** Not absorbed orally; not effective for systemic infections

Octreotide (Sandostatin, Sandostatin LAR) **Uses: Suppresses/inhibits severe diarrhea associated with carcinoid and neuroendocrine GI tumors (i.e., VIPoma, ZE syndrome); bleeding esophageal varices** **Action:** Long-acting peptide; mimics natural hormone somatostatin **Dose:** 100–600 mcg/d SC/IV in 2–4 ÷ doses; initiate at 50 mcg qd–bid *Sandostatin LAR (depot):* 10–30 mg IM q4wk **Caution:** [B, +] Hepatic/renal impairment **Supplied:** Inj 0.05, 0.1, 0.2, 0.5, 1 mg/mL; 10, 20, 30 mg/5 mL depot **SE:** N/V, abdominal discomfort, flushing, edema, fatigue, cholelithiasis, hyper-/hypoglycemia, hepatitis

Ofloxacin (Floxin, Ocuflox Ophthalmic)   Uses: **Lower respiratory tract, skin and skin structure, and urinary tract infections, prostatitis, uncomplicated gonorrhea, and** *Chlamydia* **infections; topical for bacterial conjunctivitis; otitis externa, if perforated eardrum > 12 y**   Action: Bactericidal; inhibits DNA gyrase *Spectrum:* Susceptible infection due to *S pneumoniae, S aureus, S pyogenes, H influenzae, P mirabilis, N gonorrhoeae, C trachomatis, E coli* Dose: 200–400 mg PO bid or IV q12h. Ophth 1–2 drops in eye(s) q2–4h for 2 d, then qid for 5 more d. Otic 10 drops in ear(s) bid for 10 d; ↓ dose in renal impairment; take on empty stomach   Caution: [C, –] Drug interactions with antacids, sucralfate, and Al⁺², Ca⁺², Mg⁺², Fe⁺², or Zn⁺²-containing products, which ↓ absorption   Contra: Quinolone hypersensitivity   Supplied: Tabs 200, 300, 400 mg; inj 20, 40 mg/mL; ophth and otic 0.3%   SE: N/V/D, photosensitivity, insomnia, and HA   Notes: Ophth form can be used in ears

Olanzapine (Zyprexa, Zyprexa Zydis)   WARNING: May increase risk of hyperglycemia and diabetes   Uses: **Bipolar mania, schizophrenia, acute agitation in schizophrenia, psychotic disorders**   Action: Dopamine and serotonin antagonist   Dose: *Bipolar/schizophrenia:* 5–10 mg/d, ↑ weekly PRN to 20 mg/d max   *Agitation:* 10–20 mg IM q2–4 hr PRN up to 40 mg daily max   Caution: [C, –]   Contra: N/A   Supplied: Tabs 2.5, 5, 7.5, 10, 15, 20 mg; oral disintegrating tabs 5, 10, 15, 20 mg   SE: HA, somnolence, orthostatic hypotension, tachycardia, dystonia, xerostomia, constipation   Notes: Takes weeks to titrate to therapeutic dose; cigarette smoking decreases levels; brand name may be confused with Zyrtec (cetirizine)

Olmesartan (Benicar) [See Table VII–4, p 615]

Olopatadine (Patanol) [See Table VII–12, pp 623–25]

Olsalazine (Dipentum)   Uses: **Maintenance of remission of ulcerative colitis**   Action: Topical anti-inflammatory activity   Dose: 500 mg PO bid; take with food   Caution: [C, M] Salicylate sensitivity   Contra: N/A   Supplied: Caps 250 mg   SE: Diarrhea, HA, blood dyscrasias, hepatitis   Notes: N/A

Omalizumab (Xolair)   Uses: **Treatment of moderate to severe asthma in patients 12 years of age and above, who have shown reactivity to an allergen and whose symptoms are inadequately controlled with inhaled corticosteroids**   Action: Anti-IgE antibody   Dose: 150–375 mg SC every 2–4 wk (dosage and dosing frequency determined by total serum IgE level and body weight—see package labeling for dose determination charts)   Caution: [B, ?/–]   Supplied: 150 mg in single-use 5-mL vial   SE: Injection site reaction, sinusitis, headache, anaphylaxis reported within 2 h of administration in 3 patients   Notes: Continue other asthma medications as indicated

Omeprazole (Prilosec, Zegerid) [See Table VII–14, p 627]

Ondansetron (Zofran)   Uses: **Prevent chemotherapy-associated and postoperative N/V**   Action: Serotonin receptor antagonist   Dose: *Chemotherapy:* 0.15 mg/kg/dose IV before chemotherapy, then repeat 4 and 8 h after 1st dose or 4–8 mg PO tid; give 1st dose 30 min before chemotherapy. For chemotherapy, administer on a schedule, not PRN *Postop:* 4 mg IV immediately before induction of anesthesia or postop. ↓ Dose with hepatic impairment;   Caution: [B, +/–]   Contra: N/A   Supplied: Tabs 4, 8 mg; inj 2 mg/mL   SE: Diarrhea, HA, constipation, dizziness

Oprelvekin (Neumega)   Uses: **Prevent severe thrombocytopenia due to chemotherapy**   Action: Promotes proliferation and maturation of megakaryocytes (interleukin-11)   Dose: 50 mcg/kg/d SC for 10–21 d   Caution: [C, ?/–]   Contra: N/A   Supplied: 5 mg powder for inj   SE: Tachycardia, palpitations, arrhythmias, edema, HA, dizziness, insomnia, fatigue, fever, nausea, anemia, dyspnea

Oral Contraceptives, Biphasic, Monophasic, Triphasic, Progestin Only   Uses: **Birth control and regulation of anovulatory bleeding**   Action: *Birth control:* Suppresses LH surge, prevents ovulation; progestins thicken cervical mucus; inhibits fallopian tubule cilia, ↓ endometrial thickness to ↓ chances of fertilization *Anovulatory bleeding:* Cyclic hormones mimic body's natural cycle and help regulate endometrial lining, resulting in regular bleeding q28d; may also reduce uterine bleeding and dysmenorrhea **Dose:** 28-d cycle pills taken qd; 21-d cycle pills taken qd, no pills taken during the last 7 d of the cycle (during menses); some products now available as transdermal patch **Caution:** [X, +] Migraine, HTN, diabetes, sickle cell disease, gallbladder disease **Contra**: Undiagnosed abnormal vaginal bleeding, pregnancy, estrogen-dependent malignancy, hypercoagulation disorders, liver disease, hemiplegic migraine, and smokers > 35 y **Supplied:** 28-d cycle pills (21 hormonally active pills + 7 placebo/Fe supplementation); 21-d cycle pills (21 hormonally active pills). **SE:** Intramenstrual bleeding, oligomenorrhea, amenorrhea, increased appetite/weight gain, loss of libido, fatigue, depression, mood swings, mastalgia, HAs, melasma, ↑ vaginal discharge, acne/greasy skin, corneal edema, nausea **Notes:** Taken correctly, 99.9% effective for preventing pregnancy; not protective against STDs; encourage additional barrier contraceptive. Long term, can ↓ risk of ectopic pregnancy, benign breast disease, ovarian and uterine CA *Treatment for menstrual cycle control:* Start with a monophasic pill. Pill must be taken for 3 mo before switching to another brand. If abnormal bleeding continues, change to pill with higher estrogen dose *Treatment for birth control:* Choose pill with most beneficial side effect profile for particular patient. Side effects numerous and due to symptoms of estrogen excess or progesterone deficiency. Each pill's side effect profile is unique (found in package insert); tailor treatment to specific patient

Orlistat (Xenical)
Uses: Management of obesity in patients with BMI ≥ 30 kg/m² or ≥ 27 kg/m² in presence of other risk factors; type 2 DM, dyslipidemia **Action:** Reversible inhibitor of gastric and pancreatic lipases **Dose:** 120 mg PO tid with a fat-containing meal **Caution:** [B, ?] May lower cyclosporine levels and lessen daily dose requirements for warfarin **Contra:** Cholestasis, chronic malabsorption **Supplied:** Capsules 120 mg **SE:** abdominal pain/discomfort, fatty/oily stools, fecal urgency **Notes:** Do not administer if meal contains no fat. GI effects increase with higher-fat meals. Supplement with fat-soluble vitamins

Orphenadrine (Norflex)
Uses: Muscle spasms **Action:** Central atropine-like effects cause indirect skeletal muscle relaxation, euphoria, and analgesia **Dose:** 100 mg PO bid, 60 mg IM/IV q12h **Caution:** [C, +] **Contra:** Glaucoma, GI obstruction, cardiospasm, myasthenia gravis **Supplied:** Tabs 100 mg; SR tabs 100 mg; inj 30 mg/mL **SE:** Drowsiness, dizziness, blurred vision, flushing, tachycardia, constipation

Oseltamivir (Tamiflu)
Uses: Prevention and treatment of influenza A and B **Action:** Inhibits viral neuraminidase **Dose:** 75 mg PO bid for 5 d; ↓ dose in renal impairment **Caution:** [C, ?/–] **Supplied:** Caps 75 mg, powder 12 mg/mL **SE:** N/V, insomnia **Notes:** Initiate within 48 h of symptom onset or exposure

Oxacillin (Bactocill, Prostaphlin) [See Table VII–5, p 616]

Oxaprozin (Daypro) [See Table VII–11, pp 621–22]

Oxazepam (Serax) [C-IV]
Uses: Anxiety, acute alcohol withdrawal, anxiety with depressive symptoms **Action:** Benzodiazepine **Dose:** 10–15 mg PO tid–qid; severe anxiety and alcohol withdrawal may require up to 30 mg qid; avoid abrupt discontinuation **Caution:** [D, ?] **Contra:** N/A **Supplied:** Caps 10, 15, 30 mg; tabs 15 mg **SE:** Sedation, ataxia, dizziness, rash, blood dyscrasias, dependence **Notes:** Metabolite of diazepam (Valium)

Oxcarbazepine (Trileptal)
Uses: Partial seizures **Action:** Blocks voltage-sensitive Na+ channels, resulting in stabilization of hyperexcited neural membranes **Dose:** 300 mg PO bid, ↑ dose weekly to target maintenance dose of 1200–2400 mg/d. ↓ dose in renal insufficiency **Caution:** [C, –] Possible cross-sensitivity to carbamazepine **Supplied:** Tabs 150, 300, 600 mg **SE:** Hyponatremia, HA, dizziness, fatigue, somnolence, GI upset, diplopia, mental concentration difficulties **Notes:** Do not abruptly discontinue

Oxiconazole (Oxistat)
Uses: Tinea pedis, tinea cruris, and tinea corporis **Action:** Antifungal antibiotic **Dose:** Apply bid *Spectrum:* Effective against most strains of *Epidermophyton floccosum, Trichophyton mentagrophytes, Trichophyton rubrum, Malassezia furfur* **Caution:** [B, M] **Supplied:** Cream 1%; lotion **SE:** Local irritation

Oxybutynin (Ditropan, Ditropan XL)   Uses: Symptomatic relief of urgency, nocturia, and incontinence associated with neurogenic or reflex neurogenic bladder   **Action:** Direct smooth muscle antispasmodic; ↑ bladder capacity   **Dose:** 5 mg PO tid–qid. XL 5 mg PO qd; ↑ to 30 mg/d PO (5 and 10 mg/tab); ↓ dose in elderly; periodic drug holidays recommended   **Caution:** [B, ? (use with caution)]   **Contra:** Glaucoma, myasthenia gravis, GI or GU obstruction, ulcerative colitis, megacolon   **Supplied:** Tabs 5 mg; XL tabs 5, 10, 15 mg; syrup 5 mg/5 mL   **SE:** Anticholinergic side effects; drowsiness, xerostomia, constipation, tachycardia

Oxybutynin transdermal system (Oxytrol)   Uses: Treatment of overactive bladder   **Action:** Direct smooth-muscle antispasmodic; increase bladder capacity   **Dose:** One 3.9 mg/d system applied twice weekly to abdomen, hip, or buttock   **Caution:** [B, ?/–]   **Contra:** Urinary retention, gastric retention, or uncontrolled narrow-angle glaucoma   **Supplied:** 3.9 mg/d transdermal system   **SE:** Anticholinergic effects, itching/redness at application site   **Notes:** Avoid re-application to the same site within 7 d

Oxycodone [Dihydrohydroxycodeinone] (OxyContin, OxyIR, Roxicodone) [C-II]   WARNING: Swallow whole, do not crush; high abuse potential   Uses: Moderate/severe pain, normally used in combination with nonnarcotic analgesics   **Action:** Narcotic analgesic   **Dose:** 5 mg PO q6h PRN; ↓ in severe liver disease   **Caution:** [B (D if prolonged use or near term), M]   **Contra:** Hypersensitivity, respiratory depression   **Supplied:** Immediate-release caps (OxyIR) 5 mg; tabs (Percolone) 5 mg; CR (OxyContin) 10, 20, 40, 80 mg; liq 5 mg/5 mL; soln conc 20 mg/mL   **SE:** Hypotension, sedation, dizziness, GI upset, constipation, risk of abuse   **Notes:** Usually prescribed in combination with APAP or ASA; OxyContin used for chronic CA pain; may be sought after as drug of abuse

Oxycodone and Acetaminophen (Percocet, Tylox) [C-II]   Uses: Moderate to severe pain   **Action:** Narcotic analgesic   **Dose:** 1–2 tabs/caps PO q4–6h PRN (acetaminophen max dose 4 g/d)   **Caution:** [B (D if prolonged use or near term), M]   **Contra:** Hypersensitivity, respiratory depression   **Supplied:** Percocet tabs, mg oxycodone/mg APAP: 2.5/325, 5/325, 7.5/325, 10/325, 7.5/500, 10/650; Tylox caps 5 mg of oxycodone, 500 mg of APAP; soln 5 mg of oxycodone and 325 mg of APAP/5 mL   **SE:** Hypotension, sedation, dizziness, GI upset, constipation

Oxycodone and Aspirin (Percodan, Percodan-Demi) [C-II]   Uses: Moderate/moderately severe pain   **Action:** Narcotic analgesic with NSAID   **Dose:** 1–2 tabs/caps PO q4–6h PRN; ↓ dose in severe hepatic failure   **Caution:** [B (D if prolonged use or near term), M]   Peptic ulcer   **Supplied:** Percodan 4.5 mg oxycodone hydrochloride, 0.38 mg oxycodone terephthalate, 325 mg ASA; Percodan-Demi 2.25 mg oxycodone hydrochloride, 0.19 mg oxycodone terephthalate, 325 mg ASA   **SE:** Sedation, dizziness, GI upset, constipation

Oxymorphone (Numorphan) [C-II]   Uses: Moderate to severe pain, sedative   **Action:** Narcotic analgesic   **Dose:** 0.5 mg IM, SC, IV initially, 1–1.5 mg q4–6h PRN *PR:* 5 mg q4–6h PRN   **Caution:** [B, ?]   **Supplied:** Inj 1, 1.5 mg/mL; supp 5 mg   **SE:** Hypotension, sedation, GI upset, constipation, histamine release   **Notes:** Chemically related to hydromorphone

Oxytocin (Pitocin)   Uses: Induction of labor and control of postpartum hemorrhage; promotion of milk letdown in lactating women   **Action:** Stimulates muscular contractions of the uterus, stimulates milk flow during nursing   **Dose:** 0.001–0.002 units/min IV inf; titrate to desired effect to a max of 0.02 units/min *Breastfeeding:* 1 spray in both nostrils 2–3 min before feeding   **Caution:** [Uncategorized, no anomalies expected, +/–]   **Contra:** Where vaginal delivery is not favorable, fetal distress   **Supplied:** Inj 10 units/mL; nasal soln 40 units/mL   **SE:** Uterine rupture and fetal death; arrhythmias, anaphylaxis, water intoxication   **Notes:** Monitor vital signs closely; nasal form for breast-feeding only

Paclitaxel (Taxol, Abraxane)   Uses: Ovarian and breast CA   **Action:** Mitotic spindle poison promotes microtubule assembly and stabilization against depolymerization   **Dose:** Refer to specific protocol; glass or polyolefin containers using polyethylene-lined nitroglycerin tubing sets; PVC inf sets result in leaching of plasticizer; ↓ dose in hepatic failure; maintain adequate hydration   **Caution:** [D, ?/–]   **Contra:** Neutropenia less than 1500 cells/mm,^{3} solid tumors **Supplied:** Inj 6 mg/mL, Abraxane - 5 mg/mL albumin-bound drug **SE:** Myelosuppression, peripheral neuropathy, transient ileus, myalgia, bradycardia, hypotension, mucositis, N/V/D, fever, rash, HA, and phlebitis; hematologic toxicity schedule-dependent; leukopenia dose-limiting by 24-h inf; neurotoxicity dose-limiting by short (1–3 h) inf **Notes:** Hypersensitivity reactions (dyspnea, hypotension, urticaria, rash) usually within 10 min of starting inf; minimize with corticosteroid, antihistamine (H₁- and H₂-antagonist) pretreatment

Palonosetron (Aloxi) **WARNING: May prolong QTc interval** **Uses: Prevention of acute and delayed nausea and vomiting with moderately and highly emetogenic cancer chemotherapy** **Action:** 5HT₃ serotonin receptor antagonist **Dose:** 0.25 mg IV 30 min before chemotherapy; do not repeat within 7 d **Caution:** [B, ?] **Supplied:** 0.25 mg/5 mL vial **SE:** Headache, constipation, dizziness, abdominal pain, and anxiety

Pamidronate (Aredia) **Uses: Hypercalcemia of malignancy and Paget's disease; palliation of symptomatic bone metastases** **Action:** Inhibition of normal and abnormal bone resorption **Dose:** *Hypercalcemia:* 60 mg IV over 4 h or 90 mg IV over 24 h *Paget's disease:* 30 mg/d IV for 3 d; slow inf rate necessary **Caution:** [D, ?/–] **Contra:** Pregnancy **Supplied:** Powder for inj 30, 60, 90 mg **SE:** Fever, tissue irritation at inj site, uveitis, fluid overload, HTN, abdominal pain, N/V, constipation, UTI, bone pain, hypokalemia, hypocalcemia, hypomagnesemia, and hypophosphatemia **Notes:** Slow infusion rate necessary

Pancrelipase (Pancrease, Cotazym, Creon, Ultrase) **Uses: Exocrine pancreatic secretion deficiency (CF, chronic pancreatitis, other pancreatic insufficiency) and for steatorrhea of malabsorption syndrome** **Action:** Pancreatic enzyme supplementation **Dose:** 1–3 caps (tabs) with meals and snacks; dosage ↑ to 8 caps (tabs); do not crush or chew enteric-coated products; dosage is dependent on digestive requirements of patient; avoid antacids **Caution:** [C, ?/–] **Contra:** Hypersensitivity to pork products **Supplied:** Caps, tabs **SE:** N/V, abdominal cramps **Notes:** Each patient requiring pancreatic supplementation should receive individualized enzymatic therapy

Pancuronium (Pavulon) **Uses: Treatment of patients on mechanical ventilation** **Action:** Nondepolarizing neuromuscular blocker **Dose:** 2–4 mg IV q2–4h PRN; ↓ dose for renal/hepatic impairment; intubate patient and keep on controlled ventilation; use an adequate amount of sedation or analgesia **Caution:** [C, ?/–] **Supplied:** Inj; 1, 2 mg/mL **SE:** Tachycardia, HTN, pruritus, other histamine reactions

Pantoprazole (Protonix) [See Table VII–14, p 627]

Paregoric (Camphorated Tincture of Opium) [C-III] **Uses: Diarrhea, pain, and neonatal opiate withdrawal syndrome** **Action:** Narcotic **Dose:** 5–10 mL PO qd–qid PRN **Caution:** [B (D if prolonged use or high dose near term, +] **Contra:** Convulsive disorder **Supplied:** Liq 2 mg morphine = 20 mg opium/5 mL **SE:** Hypotension, sedation, constipation **Notes:** Contains anhydrous morphine from opium; short-term use only

Paroxetine (Paxil, Paxil CR) **WARNING: *Pediatric:* Antidepressants may increase risk of suicidality; consider risks and benefits of use. Patients should be closely monitored for clinical worsening, suicidality, or unusual changes in behavior** **Uses: Depression, OCD, panic disorder, social anxiety disorder, PMDD** **Action:** Serotonin reuptake inhibitor **Dose:** 10–60 mg PO single daily dose in AM; CR 25 mg/d PO; ↑ 12.5 mg/wk (max range 26–62.5 mg/d) **Caution:** [B ?/–] **Contra:** MAOI **Supplied:** Tabs 10, 20, 30, 40 mg; susp 10 mg/5 mL; CR 12.5, 25 mg **SE:** Sexual dysfunction, HA, somnolence, dizziness, GI upset, diarrhea, xerostomia, tachycardia

Pegfilgrastim (Neulasta) **Uses: ↓ The frequency of infection in patients with nonmyeloid malignancies receiving myelosuppressive anticancer drugs that cause febrile neutropenia** **Actions:** Colony-stimulating factor **Dose:** 6 mg SC × 1 per chemo cycle; never give between 14 d before and 24 h after dose of cytotoxic chemotherapy **Caution:** [C, M] Caution in sickle cell **Contra:** Hypersensitivity to drugs used to treat *E coli* or to filgrastim **Supplied:** Syringes: 6 mg/0.6 mL **SE:** HA, fever, weakness, fatigue, dizziness, insomnia, edema, N/V/D, stomatitis, anorexia, constipation, taste perversion, dyspepsia, abdominal pain, granulocytopenia, neutropenic fever, ↑ LFT, uric acid, arthralgia, myalgia, bone pain, ARDS, alopecia, splenic rupture, aggravation of sickle cell disease

Peg interferon alfa 2a (Pegasys) **Uses:** Chronic hepatitis C with compensated liver disease **Action:** Biologic response modifier **Dose:** 180 mcg (1 mL) SC once weekly × 48 wk; ↓ dose in renal impairment **Caution:** [C, ?/–] **Contra:** Autoimmune hepatitis, decompensated liver disease **Supplied:** 180 mcg/mL inj **SE:** **Notes:** May aggravate neuropsychiatric, autoimmune, ischemic, and infectious disorders

Peg interferon alfa 2b (PEG-Intron) **Uses:** Treatment of hepatitis C **Action:** Immune modulation **Dose:** 1 mcg/kg/wk SC; 1.5 mcg/kg/wk combined with ribavirin **Caution:** [C, ?/–] Caution in patients with psychiatric history **Contra:** Autoimmune hepatitis, decompensated liver disease, hemoglobinopathy **Supplied:** Vials 50, 80, 120, 150 mcg/0.5 mL **SE:** Depression, insomnia, suicidal behavior, GI upset, alopecia, pruritus **Notes:** ↓ Flu-like symptoms by giving at bedtime or with APAP; neutropenia and thrombocytopenia may require discontinuation; follow CBC and platelets

Pemirolast (Alamast) [See Table VII–12, pp 623–25]

Penbutolol (Levatol) [See Table VII–7, pp 617–18]

Penciclovir (Denavir) **Uses:** Herpes simplex (herpes labialis/cold sores) **Action:** Competitive inhibitor of DNA polymerase **Dose:** Apply topically at 1st sign of lesions, then q2h for 4 d **Caution:** [B, ?/–] **Contra:** Hypersensitivity **Supplied:** Cream 1% [OTC] **SE:** Erythema, HA **Notes:** Do not apply to mucous membranes

Penicillin G, Aqueous (Potassium or Sodium) (Pfizerpen, Pentids) **Uses:** Bacteremia, endocarditis, pericarditis, respiratory tract infections, meningitis, neurosyphilis, skin/skin structure infections **Action:** Bactericidal; inhibits cell wall synthesis *Spectrum:* Most gram(+) infections (except staphylococci), including streptococci; *N meningitidis,* syphilis, clostridia, and anaerobes (except *Bacteroides*) **Dose:** 400,000–800,000 units PO qid; IV doses vary greatly depending on indications; range 0.6–24 M units/d in ÷ doses q4h; ↓ in renal impairment **Caution:** [B, M] **Contra:** Hypersensitivity **Supplied:** Tabs 200,000, 250,000, 400,000, 800,000 units; susp 200,000, 400,000 units/5 mL; powder for inj **SE:** Beware of hypersensitivity reactions; interstitial nephritis, diarrhea, hypersensitivity, seizures **Notes:** Contains 1.7 mEq of potassium per million units

Penicillin G Benzathine (Bicillin) **Uses:** Single-dose treatment regimen for streptococcal pharyngitis, rheumatic fever, glomerulonephritis prophylaxis, and syphilis **Action:** Bactericidal; inhibits cell wall synthesis *Spectrum:* Same as Penicillin G above **Dose:** 1.2–2.4 M units deep IM inj q2–4wk **Caution:** [B, M] **Contra:** Hypersensitivity **Supplied:** Inj 300,000, 600,000 units/mL **SE:** Pain at injection site, acute interstitial nephritis, anaphylaxis **Notes:** Sustained action with detectable levels up to 4 wk; considered drug of choice for treatment of noncongenital syphilis; Bicillin L-A contains the benzathine salt only; Bicillin C-R contains a combination of benzathine and procaine (300,000 units procaine with 300,000 units benzathine/mL or 900,000 units benzathine with 300,000 units procaine/2 mL)

Penicillin G Procaine (Wycillin, Others) **Uses:** Respiratory tract infections, scarlet fever, skin and soft tissue infections, syphilis **Action:** Bactericidal; inhibits cell wall synthesis *Spectrum:* Moderately severe infections caused by penicillin G-sensitive organisms that respond to low, persistent serum levels **Dose:** 0.6–4.8 M units/d in ÷ doses q12–24h; give probenecid at least 30 min before penicillin to prolong action **Caution:** [B, M] **Contra:** Hypersensitivity **Supplied:** Inj 300,000, 500,000, 600,000 units/mL **SE:** Pain at injection site, interstitial nephritis, anaphylaxis **Notes:** Long-acting parenteral penicillin; blood levels up to 15 h

Penicillin V (Pen-Vee K, Veetids, Others) **Uses:** Susceptible streptococci infections, otitis media, URIs, skin/soft tissue infections (PCN-sens staph) **Action:** Bactericidal; inhibits cell wall synthesis *Spectrum:* Most gram(+) infections, including streptococci **Dose:** 250–500 mg PO q6h, q8h, q12h; ↓ in severe renal disease; take on empty stomach **Caution:** [B, M] **Contra:** Hypersensitivity **Supplied:** Tabs 125, 250, 500 mg; susp 125, 250 mg/5 mL **SE:** GI upset, interstitial nephritis, anaphylaxis, convulsions **Notes:** Well-tolerated oral penicillin; 250 mg = 400,000 units penicillin G

Pentamidine (Pentam 300, NebuPent) Uses: **Treatment and prevention of PCP** Action: Inhibits DNA, RNA, phospholipid, and protein synthesis Dose: 4 mg/kg/24 h IV qd for 14–21 d *Prevention:* 300 mg once q4wk, administered via Respigard II neb; IV requires ↓ dose in renal impairment Caution: [C, ?] Supplied: Inj 300 mg/vial; aerosol 300 mg SE: Associated with pancreatic islet cell necrosis leading to hyperglycemia; chest pain, fatigue, dizziness, rash, GI upset, pancreatitis, renal impairment, blood dyscrasias Notes: Follow CBC (leukopenia and thrombocytopenia); monitor glucose and pancreatic function monthly for the 1st 3 mo; monitor for hypotension after IV administration

Pentazocine (Talwin) [C-IV] Uses: **Moderate to severe pain** Action: Partial narcotic agonist-antagonist Dose: 30 mg IM or IV; 50–100 mg PO q3–4h PRN; ↓ dose in renal/hepatic impairment Caution: [C (1st trimester, D if prolonged use or high doses near term), +/–] Contra: Hypersensitivity Supplied: Tabs 50 mg (+ naloxone 0.5 mg); inj 30 mg/mL SE: Associated with considerable dysphoria; drowsiness, GI upset, xerostomia, seizures Notes: 30–60 mg IM equianalgesic to 10 mg of morphine IM

Pentobarbital (Nembutal, Others) [C-II] Uses: **Insomnia, convulsions, and induced coma after severe head injury** Action: Barbiturate Dose: *Sedative:* 20–40 mg PO or PR q6–12h *Hypnotic:* 100–200 mg PO or PR hs PRN *Induced coma:* Load 5–10 mg/kg IV, then maintenance 1–3 mg/kg/h IV cont inf to keep the serum level between 20 and 50 mg/mL Caution: [D, +/–] Significant hepatic impairment Contra: Hypersensitivity Supplied: Caps 50, 100 mg; elixir 18.2 mg/5 mL (= 20 mg pentobarbital); supp 30, 60, 120, 200 mg; inj 50 mg/mL SE: Can cause respiratory depression, hypotension when used aggressively IV for cerebral edema; bradycardia, hypotension, sedation, lethargy, hangover, rash, Stevens-Johnson syndrome, blood dyscrasias, respiratory depression Notes: Tolerance to sedative-hypnotic effect acquired within 1–2 wk

Pentosan Polysulfate Sodium (Elmiron) Uses: **Relief of pain/discomfort associated with interstitial cystitis** Action: Acts as buffer on bladder wall Dose: 100 mg PO tid on empty stomach with water 1 h ac or 2 h pc Caution: [B, ?/–] Contra: Hypersensitivity Supplied: Caps 100 mg SE: Alopecia, diarrhea, nausea, HAs, ↑ LFTs, anticoagulant effects, thrombocytopenia Notes: Patients should be reassessed after 3 mo

Pentoxifylline (Trental) Uses: **Symptomatic management of peripheral vascular disease** Action: Lowers blood cell viscosity by restoring erythrocyte flexibility Dose: 400 mg PO tid pc; treat for at least 8 wk to see full effect; decrease to bid if GI or CNS effects occur Caution: [C, +/–] Contra: Cerebral or retinal hemorrhage Supplied: Tabs 400 mg SE: Dizziness, HA, GI upset

Pergolide (Permax) Uses: **Parkinson's disease** Action: Centrally active dopamine receptor agonist Dose: Initially, 0.05 mg PO tid, titrated q2–3d to desired effect; usual maintenance 2–3 mg/d in ÷ doses Caution: [B, ?/–] Contra: Ergot sensitivity Supplied: Tabs 0.05, 0.25, 1.0 mg SE: Dizziness, somnolence, confusion, nausea, constipation, dyskinesia, rhinitis, MI Notes: May cause hypotension during initiation of therapy

Perindopril Erbumine (Aceon) [See Table VII–3, p 614]

Permethrin (Nix [OTC], Elimite) Uses: **Eradication of lice and scabies** Action: Pediculicide Dose: Saturate hair and scalp; allow 10 min before rinsing Caution: [B, ?/–] Contra: Hypersensitivity Supplied: Topical liq 1%; cream 5% SE: Local irritation Notes: Disinfect clothing, bedding, combs/brushes

Perphenazine (Trilafon) Uses: **Psychotic disorders, severe nausea, intractable hiccups** Action: Phenothiazine; blocks dopaminergic receptors in the brain Dose: *Antipsychotic:* 4–16 mg PO tid; max 64 mg/d *Hiccups:* 5 mg IM q6h PRN or 1 mg IV at intervals not < 1–2 mg/min to a max of 5 mg; ↓ dose in hepatic insufficiency Caution: [C, ?/–] Narrow-angle glaucoma, severe hyper-/hypotension Contra: Phenothiazine sensitivity, bone marrow depression, severe liver or cardiac disease Supplied: Tabs 2, 4, 8, 16 mg; oral conc 16 mg/5 mL; inj 5 mg/mL SE: Hypotension, tachycardia, bradycardia, extrapyramidal symptoms, drowsiness, seizures, photosensitivity, skin discoloration, blood dyscrasias, constipation

Phenazopyridine (Pyridium, Others)   Uses: **Lower urinary tract irritation**   Action: Local anesthetic on urinary tract mucosa   Dose: 100–200 mg PO tid; ↓ in renal insufficiency   Caution: [B, ?] Hepatic disease   Contra: Renal insufficiency   Supplied: Tabs 100, 200 mg   SE: GI disturbances; causes red-orange urine color, which can stain clothing; HA, dizziness, acute renal failure, methemoglobinemia; some products available OTC

Phenelzine (Nardil)   WARNING: *Pediatric: Antidepressants may increase risk of suicidality; consider risks and benefits of use. Patients should be closely monitored for clinical worsening, suicidality, or unusual changes in behavior*   Uses: **Depression**   Action: MAOI   Dose: 15 mg tid *Elderly:* 15–60 mg/d in ÷ doses   Caution: [C, –]   Contra: Interactions with SSRI, ergots, triptans, CHF, h/o liver disease   Supplied: Tabs 15 mg   SE: May cause postural hypotension; edema, dizziness, sedation, rash, sexual dysfunction, xerostomia, constipation, urinary retention   Notes: May take 2–4 wk to see therapeutic effect; avoid tyramine-containing foods

Phenobarbital [C-IV]   Uses: **Seizure disorders, insomnia, and anxiety**   Action: Barbiturate   Dose: *Sedative-hypnotic:* 30–120 mg/d PO or IM PRN *Anticonvulsant:* Loading dose of 10–12 mg/kg in 3 ÷ doses, then 1–3 mg/kg/24 h PO, IM, or IV   Caution: [D, M]   Contra: Porphyria, liver dysfunction   Supplied: Tabs 8, 15, 16, 30, 32, 60, 65, 100 mg; elixir 15, 20 mg/5 mL; inj 30, 60, 65, 130 mg/mL   SE: Bradycardia, hypotension, hangover, Stevens-Johnson syndrome, blood dyscrasias, respiratory depression   Notes: Tolerance develops to sedation; paradox hyperactivity seen in pediatric patients; long half-life allows single daily dosing (Table VII–17, p 630)

Phenylephrine (Neo-Synephrine)   Uses: **Vascular failure in shock, hypersensitivity, or drug-induced hypotension; nasal congestion; mydriatic**   Action: α-Adrenergic agonist   Dose: *Mild/moderate hypotension:* 2–5 mg IM or SC elevates BP for 2 h; 0.1–0.5 mg IV elevates BP for 15 min *Severe hypotension/shock:* Initiate cont inf at 100–180 mg/min; after BP is stabilized, maintenance rate of 40–60 mg/min *Nasal congestion:* 1–2 Sprays/nostril PRN *Ophth:* 1 Drop 15–30 min before exam   Caution: [C, +/–] HTN, acute pancreatitis, hepatitis, coronary disease, narrow-angle glaucoma, hyperthyroidism   Contra: Bradycardia, arrhythmias   Supplied: Inj 10 mg/mL; nasal soln 0.125, 0.16, 0.25, 0.5, 1%; ophth soln 0.12, 2.5, 10%   SE: Arrhythmias, HTN, peripheral vasoconstriction activity potentiated by oxytocin, MAOIs, and TCAs; HA, weakness, necrosis, decreased renal perfusion   Notes: Promptly restore blood volume if loss has occurred; use large veins for inf to avoid extravasation; phentolamine 10 mg in 10–15 mL of NS for local inj as antidote for extravasation

Phenytoin (Dilantin)   Uses: **Seizure disorders**   Action: Inhibits seizure spread in the motor cortex   Dose: *Load:* 15–20 mg/kg IV, max inf rate 25 mg/min or PO in 400-mg doses at 4-h intervals *Maintenance:* Initially, 200 mg PO or IV bid or 300 mg hs; then follow serum concentrations; avoid oral susp if possible due to erratic absorption   Caution: [D, +]   Contra: Heart block, sinus bradycardia   Supplied: Caps 30, 100 mg; chew tabs 50 mg; oral susp 30, 125 mg/5 mL; inj 50 mg/mL   SE: Nystagmus and ataxia early signs of toxicity; gum hyperplasia with long-term use *IV:* Hypotension, bradycardia, arrhythmias, phlebitis; peripheral neuropathy, rash, blood dyscrasias, Stevens-Johnson syndrome   Notes: Follow levels (Table VII–17, p 630); phenytoin is bound to albumin, and levels reflect both bound and free phenytoin; in the presence of ↓ albumin and azotemia, low phenytoin levels may be therapeutic (normal free levels); changes in dosage (increase or decrease) should not be carried out at intervals shorter than 7–10 d

Physostigmine (Antilirium)   Uses: **Antidote for TCA, atropine, and scopolamine overdose; glaucoma**   Action: Reversible cholinesterase inhibitor   Dose: 2 mg IV or IM q20min   Caution: [C, ?]   Contra: GI or GU obstruction, CV disease   Supplied: Inj 1 mg/mL; ophth oint 0.25%   SE: Rapid IV administration associated with convulsions; cholinergic side effects; may cause asystole, sweating, salivation, lacrimation, GI upset, changes in heart rate   Notes: Excessive readministration of physostigmine can result in cholinergic crisis; all symptoms of cholinergic crisis can be reversed with atropine

Phytonadione [Vitamin K] (AquaMEPHYTON, Others)   Uses: **Coagulation disorders caused by faulty formation of factors II, VII, IX, and X; hyperalimentation** Action: Needed for the production of factors II, VII, IX, and X   Dose: *Anticoagulant-induced prothrombin deficiency:* 1–10 mg PO or IV slowly *Hyperalimentation:* 10 mg IM or IV qwk   Caution: [C, +]   Contra: Hypersensitivity   Supplied: Tabs 5 mg; inj 2, 10 mg/mL   SE: Anaphylaxis can result from IV dosage; administer IV slowly; GI upset (oral), inj site reactions   Notes: With parenteral treatment, the 1st change in prothrombin usually seen in 12–24 h

Pilocarpine (Isopto Carpine, Pilocar, Pilopine HS gel) [See Table VII–12, pp 623–25]

Pimecrolimus (Elidel)   Uses: **Atopic dermatitis**   Action: T-lymphocyte inhibition   Dose: Apply bid for at least 1 wk after resolution; apply to dry skin only; wash hands after use   Caution: [C, ?/–] Caution with local infection, lymphadenopathy   Contra: Hypersensitivity   Supplied: Ointment 0.03%, 0.1%: 30-g, 60-g tubes   SE: Phototoxicity, local irritation/burning, flu-like symptoms

Pindolol (Visken) [See Table VII–7, pp 617–18]

Pioglitazone (Actos)   Uses: **Type 2 DM**   Action: Increases insulin sensitivity   Dose: 15–45 mg/d PO   Caution: [C, –]   Contra: Hepatic impairment   Supplied: Tabs 15, 30, 45 mg   SE: Weight gain, upper respiratory infection, HA, hypoglycemia, edema

Piperacillin (Pipracil) [See Table VII–6, p 616]

Piperacillin-Tazobactam (Zosyn) See Table VII–6, p 616]

Pirbuterol (Maxair)   Uses: **Prevention and treatment of reversible bronchospasm** Action: β_2-Adrenergic agonist   Dose: 2 inhal q4–6h; max 12 inhal/d   Caution: [C, ?/–]   Supplied: Aerosol 0.2 mg/actuation; Autohaler dry powder 0.2 mg/actuation   SE: Nervousness, restlessness, trembling, HA, taste changes, tachycardia

Piroxicam (Feldene) [See Table VII–11, pp 621–22]

Plasma Protein Fraction (Plasmanate, Others)   Uses: **Shock and hypotension**   Action: Plasma volume expansion   Dose: Initially, 250–500 mL IV (not > 10 mL/min); subsequent inf depends on clinical response   Caution: [C, +]   Contra: Renal insufficiency, CHF   Supplied: Inj 5%   SE: Hypotension associated with rapid infusion; hypocoagulability, metabolic acidosis, PE   Notes: 130–160 mEq Na/L; not substitute for RBC

Pneumococcal 7–Valent Conjugate Vaccine (Prevnar)   Uses: **Immunization against pneumococcal infections in infants and children**   Action: Active immunization   Dose: 0.5 mL IM/dose; series of 3 doses; 1st dose at 2 mo of age with subsequent doses q2mo   Caution: [C, +] Thrombocytopenia   Contra: Diphtheria toxoid sensitivity, febrile illness   Supplied: Inj   SE: Local reactions, arthralgia, fever, myalgia

Pneumococcal Vaccine Polyvalent (Pneumovax-23)   Uses: **Immunization against pneumococcal infections in patients predisposed to or at high risk of acquiring these infections; all people ≥65 y**   Action: Active immunization   Dose: 0.5 mL IM   Caution: [C, ?]   Contra: *Do not* vaccinate during immunosuppressive therapy   Supplied: Injection 25 mg each of polysaccharide isolates per 0.5-mL dose   SE: Fever, inj site reaction, hemolytic anemia, thrombocytopenia, anaphylaxis

Podophyllin (Podocon-25, Condylox Gel 0.5%, Condylox)   Uses: **Topical therapy of benign growths (genital and perianal warts [condylomata acuminata], papillomas, fibroids)**   Action: Direct antimitotic effect; exact mechanism unknown   Dose: Condylox gel and Condylox: Apply 3 consecutive d/wk for 4 wk. Use Podocon-25 sparingly on the lesion, leave on for 1–4 h, then thoroughly wash off   Caution: [C, ?] Immunocompromise   Contra: DM, bleeding lesions,   Supplied: Podocon-25 (with benzoin) 15-mL bottles; Condylox gel 0.5% 35 g clear gel; Condylox soln 0.5% 35 g   SE: Local reactions, significant absorption; anemias, tachycardia, paresthesias, GI upset, renal/hepatic damage   Notes: Podocon-25 applied only by the clinician; do not dispense

Polyethylene Glycol [PEG]-Electrolyte Solution (GoLYTELY, CoLyte)

Uses: Bowel prep prior to examination or surgery **Action:** Osmotic cathartic **Dose:** After 3- to 4-h fast, drink 240 mL of soln q10min until 4 L is consumed **Caution:** [C, ?] **Contra:** GI obstruction, bowel perforation, megacolon, ulcerative colitis **Supplied:** Powder for reconstitution to 4 L in container **SE:** 1st BM should occur in approximately 1 h; cramping or nausea, bloating

Polymyxin B and Hydrocortisone (Otobiotic Otic)

Uses: Superficial bacterial infections of external ear canal **Action:** Antibiotic anti-inflammatory combination **Dose:** 4 drops in ear(s) tid–qid **Caution:** [B, ?] **Contra:** N/A **Supplied:** Soln polymyxin B 10,000 units/hydrocortisone 0.5%/mL **SE:** Useful in neomycin allergy, local irritation

Potassium Citrate (Urocit-K)

Uses: Alkalinize urine, prevention of urinary stones (uric acid, calcium stones if hypocitraturic) **Action:** Urinary alkalinizer **Dose:** 10–20 mEq PO tid with meals, max 100 mEq/d **Caution:** [A, +] **Contra:** Severe renal impairment, dehydration, hyperkalemia, peptic ulcer; use of potassium-sparing diuretics or salt substitutes **Supplied:** **SE:** GI upset, hypocalcemia, hyperkalemia, metabolic alkalosis **Notes:** Tabs 540 mg = 5 mEq, 1080 mg = 10 mEq

Potassium Citrate and Citric Acid (Polycitra-K)

Uses: Alkalinize urine, prevention of urinary stones (uric acid, calcium stones if hypocitraturic) **Action:** Urinary alkalinizer **Dose:** 10–20 mEq PO tid with meals, max 100 mEq/d **Caution:** [A, +] **Contra:** Severe renal impairment, dehydration, hyperkalemia, peptic ulcer; use of potassium-sparing diuretics or salt substitutes **Supplied:** Soln 10 mEq/5 mL; powder 30 mEq/packet **SE:** GI upset, hypocalcemia, hyperkalemia, metabolic alkalosis

Potassium Iodide [Lugol's Solution] (SSKI, Thyro-Block)

Uses: Thyroid storm, reduction of vascularity before thyroid surgery, block thyroid uptake of radioactive isotopes of iodine, thin bronchial secretions **Action:** Iodine supplement **Dose:** *Preop thyroidectomy:* 50–250 mg PO tid (2–6 drops strong iodine soln); administer 10 d preop **Caution:** [D, +] Hyperkalemia, tuberculosis, PE, bronchitis, renal impairment **Contra:** Iodine sensitivity **Supplied:** Tabs 130 mg; soln (SSKI) 1 g/mL; Lugol's soln, strong iodine 100 mg/mL; syrup 325 mg/5 mL **SE:** Fever, HA, urticaria, angioedema, goiter, GI upset, eosinophilia

Potassium Supplements (Kaon, Kaochlor, K-Lor, Slow-K, Micro-K, Klorvess, Others)

Uses: Prevention or treatment of hypokalemia (often related to diuretic use) **Action:** Supplementation of potassium **Dose:** 20–100 mEq/d PO ÷ qd–bid; IV 10–20 mEq/h, max 40 mEq/h and 150 mEq/d (monitor frequent potassium levels when using high-dose IV infusions) **Caution:** [A, +] Use cautiously in renal insufficiency as well as with NSAIDs and ACE inhibitors **Contra:** Hyperkalemia **Supplied:** Oral forms; injectable forms **SE:** Can cause GI irritation; bradycardia, hyperkalemia, heart block **Notes:** Mix powder and liquid with beverage (unsalted tomato juice, etc); follow serum K⁺; Cl⁻ salt recommended in coexisting alkalosis; for coexisting acidosis use acetate, bicarbonate, citrate, or gluconate salt

Pramipexole (Mirapex)

Uses: Parkinson's disease **Action:** Dopamine agonist **Dose:** 1.5–4.5 mg/d PO, beginning with 0.375 mg/d in 3 ÷ doses; titrate dosage slowly **Caution:** [C, ?/–] **Supplied:** Tabs 0.125, 0.25, 1, 1.5 mg **SE:** Postural hypotension, asthenia, somnolence, abnormal dreams, GI upset, Epstein-Barr syndrome

Pramoxine (Anusol Ointment, Proctofoam-NS, Others)

Uses: Relief of pain and itching from external and internal hemorrhoids and anorectal surgery; topical for burns and dermatosis **Action:** Topical anesthetic **Dose:** Apply cream, oint, gel, or spray freely to anal area q3h **Caution:** [C, ?] **Contra:** N/A **Supplied:** [OTC] All 1%; foam (Proctofoam NS), cream, oint, lotion, gel, pads, spray **SE:** Contact dermatitis

Pramoxine + Hydrocortisone (Enzone, Proctofoam-HC)

Uses: Relief of pain and itching from hemorrhoids **Action:** Topical anesthetic, anti-inflammatory **Dose:** Apply freely to anal area tid–qid **Caution:** [C, ?/–] **Contra:** N/A **Supplied:** Cream pramoxine 1% acetate 0.5/1%; foam pramoxine 1% hydrocortisone 1%; lotion pramoxine 1% hydrocortisone 0.25/1/2.5%, pramoxine 2.5% and hydrocortisone 1%   **SE:** Contact dermatitis

Pravastatin (Pravachol) [See Table VII–15, p 628]

Prazosin (Minipress)   **Uses:** HTN   **Action:** Peripherally acting α-adrenergic blocker   **Dose:** 1 mg PO tid; can ↑ to max daily dose of up to 20 mg/d   **Caution:** [C, ?]   **Contra:**   **Supplied:** Caps 1, 2, 5 mg   **SE:** Dizziness, edema, palpitations, fatigue, GI upset   **Notes:** Can cause orthostatic hypotension, take the 1st dose hs; tolerance develops to this effect; tachyphylaxis may result

Prednisolone [See Table VII–2, p 613]

Prednisone [See Table VII–2, p 613]

Probenecid (Benemid, Others)   **Uses:** Prevention of gout and hyperuricemia; prolongs serum levels of penicillins or cephalosporins   **Action:** Renal tubular blocking agent   **Dose:** *Gout:* 250 mg bid for 1 wk, then 0.5 g PO bid; can ↑ by 500 mg/mo up to 2–3 g/d *Antibiotic effect:* 1–2 g PO 30 min before antibiotic dose   **Caution:** [B, ?]   **Contra:** High-dose ASA, moderate/severe renal impairment   **Supplied:** Tabs 500 mg   **SE:** HA, GI upset, rash, pruritus, dizziness, blood dyscrasias   **Notes:** Do not use during acute gout attack

Procainamide (Pronestyl, Procan)   **Uses:** Supraventricular and ventricular arrhythmias   **Action:** Class 1A antiarrhythmic; depresses the excitability of cardiac muscle to electrical stimulation and slows conduction in the atrium, the bundle of His and the ventricle   **Dose:** *Recurrent VF/VT:* 20 mg/min IV (max total 17 mg/kg) *Maintenance:* 1–4 mg/min *Stable wide-complex tachycardia of unknown origin, AF with rapid rate in WPW:* 20 mg/min IV until arrhythmia suppression, hypotension, QRS widens > 50%, then 1–4 mg/min *Chronic dosing:* 50 mg/kg/d PO in ÷ doses q4–6h; ↓ dose in renal/hepatic impairment   **Caution:** [C, +]   **Contra:** CHB, 2nd- or 3rd-degree heart block without pacemaker, torsades de pointes, SLE   **Supplied:** Tabs and caps 250, 375, 500 mg; SR tabs 250, 500, 750, 1000 mg; inj 100, 500 mg/mL   **SE:** Can cause hypotension and a lupus-like syndrome; GI upset, taste perversion, arrhythmias, tachycardia, heart block, angioneurotic edema   **Notes:** Follow levels (Table VII–17, p 000)

Procarbazine (Matulane)   **WARNING:** Highly toxic; handle with care   **Uses:** Hodgkin's disease, NHL, brain tumors   **Action:** Alkylating agent; inhibits DNA and RNA synthesis   **Dose:** Refer to specific protocol   **Caution:** [D, ?] Alcohol ingestion   **Contra:** Inadequate bone marrow reserve   **Supplied:** Caps 50 mg   **SE:** Myelosuppression, hemolytic reactions (with G6PD deficiency), N/V/D; disulfiram-like reaction; cutaneous reactions; constitutional symptoms, myalgia, and arthralgia; CNS effects, azoospermia, and cessation of menses   **Notes:** N/A

Prochlorperazine (Compazine)   **Uses:** N/V, agitation, and psychotic disorders   **Action:** Phenothiazine; blocks postsynaptic dopaminergic CNS receptors   **Dose:** *Antiemetic:* 5–10 mg PO tid–qid or 25 mg PR bid or 5–10 mg deep IM q4–6h *Antipsychotic:* 10–20 mg IM acutely or 5–10 mg PO tid–qid for maintenance; ↑ doses may be required for antipsychotic effect   **Caution:** [C, +/–] Narrow-angle glaucoma, severe liver/cardiac disease   **Contra:** Phenothiazine sensitivity, bone marrow suppression   **Supplied:** Tabs 5, 10, 25 mg; SR caps 10, 15, 30 mg; syrup 5 mg/5 mL; supp 2.5, 5, 25 mg; inj 5 mg/mL   **SE:** Extrapyramidal side effects common; treat with diphenhydramine

Promethazine (Phenergan)   **Uses:** N/V, motion sickness   **Action:** Phenothiazine; blocks postsynaptic mesolimbic dopaminergic receptors in the brain   **Dose:** 12.5–50 mg PO, PR, or IM bid–qid PRN   **Caution:** [C, +/–]   **Supplied:** Tabs 12.5, 25, 50 mg; syrup 6.25 mg/5 mL, 25 mg/5 mL; supp 12.5, 25, 50 mg; inj 25, 50 mg/mL   **SE:** Drowsiness, tardive dyskinesia, EPS, lowered seizure threshold, hypotension, GI upset, blood dyscrasias, photosensitivity

Propafenone (Rythmol)   **Uses:** Life-threatening ventricular arrhythmias and AF   **Action:** Class IC antiarrhythmic; blocks the fast inward sodium current in heart muscle and Purkinje fibers, and slows the rate of increase of phase 0 of the action potential   **Dose:**

150–300 mg PO q8h **Caution:** [C, ?] Amprenavir or ritonavir use **Contra:** Uncontrolled CHF, bronchospasm, cardiogenic shock, conduction disorders **Supplied:** Tabs 150, 225, 300 mg **SE:** Dizziness, unusual taste, 1st-degree heart block, arrhythmias, prolongation of QRS and QT intervals; fatigue, GI upset, blood dyscrasias

Propantheline (Pro-Banthine) Uses: PUD, Symptomatic treatment of small intestine hypermotility, spastic colon, ureteral spasm, bladder spasm, pylorospasm **Action:** Antimuscarinic agent **Dose:** 15 mg PO ac and 30 mg PO hs; ↓ dose in elderly **Caution:** [C, ?] **Contra:** Narrow-angle glaucoma, ulcerative colitis, toxic megacolon, GI or GU obstruction **Supplied:** Tabs 7.5, 15 mg **SE:** Anticholinergic side effects (dry mouth and blurred vision common)

Propofol (Diprivan) Uses: Induction or maintenance of anesthesia; continuous sedation in intubated patients **Action:** Sedative hypnotic; mechanism unknown **Dose:** *Anesthesia:* 2–2.5 mg/kg induction, then 0.1–0.2 mg/kg/min inf *ICU sedation:* 5–50 mcg/kg/min cont inf; ↓ dose in elderly, debilitated, or ASA II or IV patients **Caution:** [B, +] **Contra:** When general anesthesia is CI **Supplied:** Inj 10 mg/mL **SE:** May ↑ triglycerides with extended dosing; hypotension, pain at injection site, apnea, anaphylaxis **Notes:** 1 mL of propofol contains 0.1 g fat

Propoxyphene (Darvon), Propoxyphene and Acetaminophen (Darvocet), and Propoxyphene and Aspirin (Darvon Compound-65, Darvon-N + Aspirin) [C-IV] Uses: Mild/moderate pain **Action:** Narcotic analgesic **Dose:** 1–2 PO q4h PRN; ↓ dose in hepatic impairment, elderly **Caution:** [C (D if prolonged use), M] Hepatic impairment (APAP), peptic ulcer (ASA); severe renal impairment **Contra:** Hypersensitivity **Supplied:** *Darvon:* Propoxyphene HCl caps 65 mg *Darvon-N:* Propoxyphene napsylate 100-mg tabs *Darvocet-N:* Propoxyphene napsylate 50 mg/APAP 325 mg *Darvocet-N 100:* Propoxyphene napsylate 100 mg/APAP 650 mg *Darvon Compound-65:* Propoxyphene HCl 65-mg/ASA 389-mg/caffeine 32-mg caps *Darvon-N with ASA:* Propoxyphene napsylate 100 mg/ASA 325 mg **SE:** Overdose can be lethal; hypotension, dizziness, sedation, GI upset, ↑ levels on LFTs

Propranolol (Inderal) [Also see Table VII–7, pp 617–18] Uses: HTN, angina, MI, hyperthyroidism; prevents migraines and atrial arrhythmias **Action:** Competitively blocks β-adrenergic receptors, β_1, β_2; only β-blocker to block conversion of T4 to T3 **Dose:** *Angina:* 80–320 mg/d PO ÷ bid–qid or 80–160 mg/d SR *Arrhythmia:* 10–80 mg PO tid–qid or 1 mg IV slowly, repeat q5min up to 5 mg *HTN:* 40 mg PO bid or 60–80 mg/d SR, ↑ weekly to max 640 mg/d *Hypertrophic subaortic stenosis:* 20–40 mg PO tid–qid *MI:* 180–240 mg PO ÷ tid–qid *Migraine prophylaxis:* 80 mg/d ÷ qid–tid, ↑ weekly to max 160–240 mg/d ÷ tid–qid; wean off if no response in 6 wk *Pheochromocytoma:* 30–60 mg/d ÷ tid–qid *Thyrotoxicosis:* 1–3 mg IV single dose; 10–40 mg PO q6h *Tremor:* 40 mg PO bid, ↑ as needed to max 320 mg/d; ↓ dose in renal impairment **Caution:** [C (1st trimester, D if 2nd or 3rd trimester), +] **Contra:** Uncompensated CHF, cardiogenic shock, bradycardia, heart block, PE, severe respiratory disease **Supplied:** Tabs 10, 20, 40, 60, 80 mg; SR caps 60, 80, 120, 160 mg; oral soln 4, 8 mg/mL; 80 mg/mL; inj 1 mg/mL **SE:** Bradycardia, hypotension, fatigue, GI upset, erectile dysfunction, hypoglycemia

Propylthiouracil [PTU] Uses: Hyperthyroidism **Action:** Inhibits production of T3 and T4 and conversion of T4 to T3 **Dose:** *Initial:* 100 mg PO q8h (may need up to 1200 mg/d); after patient is euthyroid (6–8 wk), taper dose by ⅓ q4–6wk to maintenance: 50–150 mg/24 h; can usually be discontinued in 2–3 y; ↓ dose in elderly **Caution:** [D, –] **Contra:** Hypersensitivity **Supplied:** Tabs 50 mg **SE:** Monitor patient clinically; monitor thyroid function tests, fever, rash, leukopenia, dizziness, GI upset, taste perversion, SLE-like syndrome

Protamine (Generic) Uses: Reversal of heparin effect **Action:** Neutralizes heparin by forming a stable complex **Dose:** Based on amount of heparin reversal desired; give IV slowly; 1 mg reverses approximately 100 units of heparin given in the preceding 3–4 h, 50 mg max dose **Caution:** [C, ?] **Contra:** Hypersensitivity **Supplied:** Inj 10 mg/mL **SE:** Follow coagulation studies; may have anticoagulant effect if given without heparin; hypotension, bradycardia, dyspnea, hemorrhage

Pseudoephedrine (Sudafed, Novafed, Afrinol, Others) [OTC-must be dispensed by pharmacist in some states]
Uses: Decongestant **Action:** Stimulates α-adrenergic receptors, resulting in vasoconstriction **Dose:** 30–60 mg PO q6–8h; SR caps 120 mg PO q12h; decrease dose in renal insufficiency **Caution:** [C, +] **Contra:** Poorly controlled HTN or CAD disease and in MAOIs **Supplied:** Tabs 30, 60 mg; caps 60 mg; SR tabs 120, 240 mg; SR caps 120 mg; liq 7.5 mg/0.8 mL, 15, 30 mg/5 mL **SE:** HTN, insomnia, tachycardia, arrhythmias, nervousness, tremor **Notes:** Ingredient in many cough and cold preparations

Psyllium (Metamucil, Serutan, Effer-Syllium) [OTC]
Uses: Constipation and diverticular disease of the colon **Action:** Bulk laxative **Dose:** 1 tsp (7 g) in a glass of water PO qd–tid **Caution:** [B, ?] Psyllium in effervescent (Effer-Syllium) form usually contains K^+; use caution in patients with renal failure; phenylketonuria (in products with aspartame) **Contra:** Do not use if suspected bowel obstruction **Supplied:** Granules 4, 25 g/tsp; powder 3.5 g/packet **SE:** Diarrhea, abdominal cramps, bowel obstruction, constipation, bronchospasm

Pyrazinamide (Generic)
Uses: Active TB in combination with other agents **Action:** Bacteriostatic; mechanism unknown **Dose:** 15–30 mg/kg/24 h PO ÷ tid–qid; max 2 g/d; ↓ dose for renal/hepatic impairment **Caution:** [C, +/–] **Contra:** Severe hepatic damage, acute gout **Supplied:** Tabs 500 mg **SE:** Hepatotoxicity, malaise, GI upset, arthralgia, myalgia, gout, photosensitivity **Notes:** Use in combination with other anti-TB drugs; consult *MMWR* for the latest TB recommendations; dosage regimen differs for directly observed therapy

Pyridoxine (Vitamin B$_6$)
Uses: Treatment and prevention of vitamin B$_6$ deficiency **Action:** Supplementation of vitamin B$_6$ **Dose:** *Deficiency:* 10–20 mg/d PO *Drug-induced neuritis:* 100–200 mg/d; 25–100 mg/d prophylaxis **Caution:** [A (C if doses exceed RDA), +] **Supplied:** Tabs 25, 50, 100 mg; inj 100 mg/mL **SE:** Allergic reactions, HA, nausea

Quazepam (Doral) [C-IV]
Uses: Insomnia **Action:** Benzodiazepine **Dose:** 7.5–15 mg PO hs PRN; ↓ dose in the elderly, hepatic failure **Caution:** [X, ?/–] Narrow-angle glaucoma **Contra:** Pregnancy, sleep apnea **Supplied:** Tabs 7.5, 15 mg **SE:** Sedation, hangover, somnolence, respiratory depression **Notes:** Do not discontinue abruptly

Quetiapine (Seroquel)
WARNING: May increase risk of hyperglycemia and diabetes **Uses:** Acute exacerbations of schizophrenia **Action:** Serotonin and dopamine antagonism **Dose:** 150–750 mg/d; initiate at 25–100 mg bid–tid; slowly ↑ dose; ↓ dose for hepatic and geriatric patients **Caution:** [C, –] **Supplied:** Tabs 25, 100, 200 mg **SE:** Multiple reports of confusion with Serzone (former branded nefazodone product); HA, somnolence, weight gain, orthostatic hypotension, dizziness, cataracts, neuroleptic malignant syndrome, tardive dyskinesia, QT prolongation

Quinapril (Accupril) [See Table VII–3, p 614]

Quinidine (Quinidex, Quinaglute)
Uses: Prevention of tachydysrhythmias, malaria **Action:** Class 1A antiarrhythmic; increases the refractory period in atrial and ventricular muscle, in SA and AV conduction systems, and the Purkinje fibers **Dose:** *Conversion of AF or flutter:* Use after digitalization, 200 mg q2–3h for 8 doses; then ↑ daily dose to a max of 3–4 g or until normal rhythm; ↓ dose in renal impairment **Caution:** [C, +] Ritonavir use **Contra:** Digitalis toxicity and AV block; conduction disorders **Supplied:** *Sulfate:* Tabs 200, 300 mg; SR tabs 300 mg *Gluconate:* SR tabs 324 mg; inj 80 mg/mL **SE:** Extreme hypotension may be seen with IV administration. Syncope, QT prolongation, GI upset, arrhythmias, fatigue, cinchonism (tinnitus, hearing loss, delirium, visual changes), fever, hemolytic anemia, thrombocytopenia, rash **Notes:** Follow serum levels (Table VII–17, p 000; sulfate salt is 83% quinidine; gluconate salt is 62% quinidine. Must use in combination with drug that slows AV conduction (e.g., digoxin, diltiazem, β-blocker)

Quinupristin-Dalfopristin (Synercid)
Uses: Infections caused by vancomycin-resistant *E faecium* and other gram(+) organisms **Action:** Inhibits both the early and late

phases of protein synthesis at the ribosomes **Spectrum:** Susceptible infections due to van-comycin-resistant *Enterococcus faecium*, methicillin-susceptible *S aureus*, and *S pyogenes*; NOT active against *E faecalis* **Dose:** 7.5 mg/kg IV q8–12h (use central line if possible); not compatible with NS or heparin; therefore, flush IV lines with dextrose; ↓ in hepatic failure **Caution:** [B, M] **Contra:** Hypersensitivity **Supplied:** Inj 500 mg (150 mg quinupristin/350 mg dalfopristin) **SE:** Hyperbilirubinemia, inf site reactions and pain, arthralgia, myalgia **Notes:** Multiple drug interactions (e.g., cyclosporine)

Rabeprazole (Aciphex) [See Table VII–14, p 627]

Raloxifene (Evista)   Uses: Prevention of osteoporosis   Action: Partial antagonist of estrogen that behaves like estrogen   **Dose:** 60 mg/d   **Caution:** [X, –]   **Contra:** Throm-boembolism, pregnancy   **Supplied:** Tabs 60 mg   **SE:** Chest pain, insomnia, rash, hot flashes, GI upset, hepatic dysfunction

Ramipril (Altace) [See Table VII–3, p 614]

Ranitidine (Zantac)   Uses: Duodenal ulcer, active benign ulcers, hypersecretory conditions, and GERD   Action: H_2-receptor antagonist   **Dose:** *Ulcer:* 150 mg PO bid, 300 mg PO hs, or 50 mg IV q6–8h; or 400 mg IV/d cont inf, then maintenance of 150 mg PO hs *Hypersecretion:* 150 mg PO bid, up to 600 mg/d *GERD:* 300 mg PO bid; maintenance 300 mg PO hs; ↓ dose in renal failure   **Caution:** [B, +]   **Supplied:** Tabs 75, 150, 300 mg; syrup 15 mg/mL; inj 25 mg/mL   **SE:** Dizziness, sedation, rash, GI upset   **Notes:** Oral and parenteral doses differ; available OTC in 75 mg and 150 mg tabs

Repaglinide (Prandin)   Uses: Type 2 DM   Action: Stimulates insulin release from pancreas   **Dose:** 0.5–4 mg PO ac, start 1–2 mg, ↑ to 16 mg/d max; take pc   **Caution:** [C, ?/–]   **Contra:** DKA, type 1 DM   **Supplied:** Tabs 0.5, 1, 2 mg   **SE:** HA, hyper-/hypo-glycemia, GI upset

Reteplase (Retavase)   Uses: Post-AMI   Action: Thrombolytic agent   **Dose:** 10 units IV over 2 min, 2nd dose in 30 min 10 units IV over 2 min   **Caution:** [C, ?/–]   **Contra:** Internal bleeding, spinal surgery or trauma, history of CVA vascular malformations, uncon-trolled hypotension, sensitivity to thrombolytics   **Supplied:** Inj 10.8 units/2 mL   **SE:** Bleed-ing, allergic reactions

Ribavirin (Virazole)   Uses: RSV infection in infants and hepatitis C (in combina-tion with interferon alfa-2b)   Action: Unknown   **Dose:** *RSV:* 6 g in 300 mL sterile water inhaled over 12–18 h *Hep C:* 600 mg PO bid in combination with interferon alfa-2b (see Rebe-tron, p 000)   **Caution:** [X, ?]   **Contra:** Pregnancy, autoimmune hepatitis, CrCl < 50 mL/min **Supplied:** Powder for aerosol 6 g; caps 200 mg   **SE:** May accumulate on soft contact lenses; fatigue, HA, GI upset, anemia, myalgia, alopecia, bronchospasm   **Notes:** Aerosolized by a SPAG; monitor Hgb/Hct frequently; PRG test monthly

Rifabutin (Mycobutin)   Uses: Prevention of *M avium* complex infection in AIDS patients with a CD4 count < 100   Action: Inhibits DNA-dependent RNA polymerase activity **Dose:** 150–300 mg/d PO   **Caution:** [B; ?/–] WBC < 1000/mm³ or platelets < 50,000/mm³; ri-tonavir   **Contra:** Hypersensitivity   **Supplied:** Caps 150 mg   **SE:** Discolored urine, rash, neutropenia, leukopenia, myalgia, ↑ LFTs   **Notes:** Adverse effects/drug interactions similar to rifampin

Rifampin (Rifadin)   Uses: TB and treatment and prophylaxis of *N meningitidis, H influenzae,* and *S aureus* carriers; adjunct for severe *S aureus*   Action: Inhibits DNA-de-pendent RNA polymerase activity   **Dose:** *N meningitidis and H influenzae:* Carrier 600 mg/d PO for 4 d *TB:* 600 mg PO or IV qd or 2×/wk with combination therapy regimen; ↓ dose in he-patic failure   **Caution:** [C, +] Amprenavir, multiple drug interactions   **Contra:** Hypersensitiv-ity, presence of active *N meningitidis* infection   **Supplied:** Caps 150, 300 mg; inj 600 mg **SE:** Orange-red discoloration of bodily fluids, increased LFTs, flushing, HA   **Notes:** Never use as single agent for active TB; multiple drug interactions; concomitant use with saquinavir/ritonavir may cause hepatitis

Rifapentine (Priftin)   Uses: Pulmonary TB   Action: Inhibits DNA-dependent RNA polymerase activity **Spectrum:** *Mycobacterium* tuberculosis   **Dose:** *Intensive phase:* 600 mg

PO 2×/wk for 2 mo; separate doses by 3 or more days *Continuation phase:* 600 mg/wk PO for 4 mo; should be part of 3–4 drug regimen **Caution:** [C, red/orange breast milk] *Drug Interactions:* ↓ Efficacy of protease inhibitors, antiepileptics, β-blockers, calcium channel blockers **Contra:** Hypersensitivity to rifamycins **Supplied:** 150 mg tablets **SE:** Neutropenia, hyperuricemia, HTN, HA, dizziness, rash, GI upset, blood dyscrasias, increased LFTs, hematuria, discolored secretions **Notes:** Monitor LFTs if history of liver dysfunction

Rimantadine (Flumadine) Uses: Prophylaxis and treatment of influenza A viral infections **Action:** Antiviral agent **Dose:** 100 mg PO bid; change to qd in severe renal/hepatic impairment and elderly; initiate within 48 h of symptom onset **Caution:** [C, breastfeeding unsafe] *Drug Interactions:* Cimetidine **Supplied:** Tabs 100 mg; syrup 50 mg/5 mL (raspberry) **SE:** Orthostatic hypotension, edema, dizziness, GI upset, lowered seizure threshold **Notes:** Avoid in pregnancy or breastfeeding

Rimexolone (Vexol Ophthalmic) [See Table VII–12, pp 623–25]

Risedronate (Actonel) Uses: Paget's disease; treat/prevent glucocorticoid-induced osteoporosis or postmenopausal osteoporosis **Action:** Bisphosphonate; inhibits osteoclast-mediated bone resorption **Dose:** *Paget's:* 30 mg/d PO for 2 mo *Osteoporosis treatment/prevention:* 5 mg PO qd or 35 mg PO qwk; take 30 min before 1st food/drink of the day, and maintain upright position for at least 30 min after administration. Not recommended in CrCl < 30 mL/min **Caution:** [C, ?/–] Calcium supplements and antacids decrease absorption **Contra:** Hypersensitivity, hypocalcemia, esophageal abnormalities, unable to stand/sit for 30 min **Supplied:** Tabs 5, 30 mg, and 35 mg **SE:** HA, diarrhea, abdominal pain, arthralgia; flu-like symptoms, rash, esophagitis, bone pain **Notes:** Monitor alkaline phosphatase, Ca^{2+}, Phos, K^+ periodically

Risperidone (Risperdal) WARNING: May increase risk of hyperglycemia and diabetes **Uses: Psychotic disorders (schizophrenia), dementia of the elderly, bipolar disorder, mania, Tourette's disorder, autism** **Action:** Benzisoxazole antipsychotic agent **Dose:** 0.5–6 mg PO bid; ↓ starting doses in elderly, renal/hepatic impairment **Caution:** [C, –] ↑ hypotension with antihypertensives, clozapine **Supplied:** Tabs 0.25, 0.5, 1, 2, 3, 4 mg; soln 1 mg/mL **SE:** Orthostatic hypotension, extrapyramidal reactions with higher doses, tachycardia, arrhythmias, sedation, dystonias, neuroleptic malignant syndrome, sexual dysfunction, constipation, xerostomia, blood dyscrasias, cholestatic jaundice, weight gain **Notes:** May take several weeks to see effect

Ritonavir (Norvir) Uses: HIV infection **Actions:** Protease inhibitor; inhibits maturation of immature noninfectious virions to mature infectious virus **Dose:** Start at 300 mg PO bid and titrate over 1 week to 600 mg PO bid (titration ↓ GI SE); dose adjustments required with amprenavir, indinavir, nelfinavir and saquinavir; take with food **Caution:** [B, +] *Drug Interactions:* ergotamine, amiodarone, bepridil, flecainide, propafenone, quinidine, pimozide, midazolam, triazolam **Supplied:** Caps 100 mg; soln 80 mg/mL **SE:** ↑ triglycerides, ↑ LFTs, N/V/D/C, abdominal pain, taste perversion, anemia, weakness, HA, fever, malaise, rash, paresthesias **Notes:** Store in refrigerator

Rivastigmine (Exelon) Uses: Mild/moderate dementia associated with Alzheimer's disease **Action:** Enhances cholinergic activity **Dose:** 1.5 mg PO bid; ↑ to 6 mg bid, with increases at 2-wk intervals (take with food) **Caution:** [B, ?] β-Blockers, CA^+ channel blockers, smoking, neuromuscular blockade, digoxin **Contra:** Hypersensitivity to rivastigmine or carbamates **Supplied:** Caps 1.5, 3, 4.5, 6 mg; soln 2 mg/mL **SE:** Dose-related GI adverse effects (A/N/V/D); dizziness, insomnia, fatigue, tremor, diaphoresis, HA **Notes:** Swallow capsules whole, do not break, chew, or crush; avoid concurrent ethanol use

Rizatriptan (Maxalt, Maxalt MLT) [See Table VII–16, p. 629]

Rocuronium (Zemuron) Uses: Skeletal muscle relaxation during rapid-sequence intubation, surgery, or mechanical ventilation. **Action:** Nondepolarizing neuromuscular blockade **Dose:** *Rapid sequence intubation:* 0.6–1.2 mg/kg IV. *Continuous infusion* 4–16 mcg/kg/min IV; reduce dose in patients with hepatic impairment **Caution:** [C, ?] Aminoglycosides, vancomycin, tetracycline, polymyxins enhance blockade **Supplied:** 10 mg/mL 5-, 10-mL vials **SE:** BP changes, tachycardia

Ropinirole (Requip)   Uses: **Treatment of Parkinson's disease**   Action: Dopamine agonist   Dose: Initial dose 0.25 mg PO tid, with weekly dosage increases of 0.25 mg per dose, up to total daily dose of 3 mg   Caution: [C, ?/–] Severe cardiovascular disease, severe renal or hepatic impairment   Supplied: Tablets 0.25 mg, 0.5 mg, 1 mg, 2 mg, 5 mg   SE: Syncope, postural hypotension, N/V, HA, somnolence, hallucinations, dyskinesias   Notes: Discontinuation requires a 7-d taper

Rosiglitazone (Avandia)   Uses: **Type 2 DM**   Action: ↑ Insulin sensitivity   Dose: 4–8 mg/d PO or in 2 ÷ (with or without meals)   Caution: [C, –] Not for DKA   Contra: Active liver disease, use with caution in ESRD (renal elimination)   Supplied: Tabs 2, 4, 8 mg   SE: Weight gain, hyperlipidemia, HA, edema, fluid retention, exacerbate CHF, hyper-/hypoglycemia, hepatic damage   Notes: Take with or without meals

Rosuvastatin (Crestor) [See Table VII–15, p 628]

Salmeterol (Serevent)   Uses: **Asthma, exercise-induced asthma, COPD**   Action: Sympathomimetic bronchodilator, β_2-agonist   Dose: 1 diskus-dose inhaled bid   Caution: [C, ?/–]   Contra: Need for acute bronchodilation; within 14 d of MAOI use   Supplied: Dry powder diskus   SE: HA, pharyngitis, tachycardia, arrhythmias, nervousness, GI upset, tremors   Notes: Not for acute attacks; should also prescribe short-acting β-agonist

Saquinavir (Fortovase)   Uses: **HIV infection**   Action: HIV protease inhibitor   Dose: 1200 mg PO tid within 2 h pc (dose adjust with ritonavir, delavirdine, lopinavir, and nelfinavir)   Caution: [B, +] Drug interactions: rifampin, ketoconazole, statins, sildenafil, triazolam, midazolam, ergots   Contra: Hypersensitivity, sun exposure without sunscreen/clothing, triazolam, midazolam, ergots   Supplied: Caps 200 mg   SE: Dyslipidemia, lipodystrophy, rash, hyperglycemia, GI upset, weakness, hepatic dysfunction   Notes: Take 2 h after meal; avoid direct sunlight

Sargramostim [GM-CSF] (Prokine, Leukine)   Uses: **Myeloid recovery after BMT or CA chemotherapy**   Action: Activates mature granulocytes and macrophages   Dose: 250 mcg/m^2/d IV for 21 d (BMT)   Caution: [C, ?/–] Lithium, corticosteroids   Contra: > 10% blasts, hypersensitivity to yeast, concurrent chemo/radiation   Supplied: Inj 250 mcg, 500 mcg   SE: Bone pain, fever, hypotension, tachycardia, flushing, GI upset, myalgia   Notes: Rotate SC inj sites; use APAP for pain

Scopolamine, Scopolamine Transdermal (Scopace, Transderm-Scop)   Uses: **Prevention of N/V associated with motion sickness, anesthesia, and opiates; mydriatic, cycloplegic, treatment of iridiocyclitis**   Action: Anticholinergic, antiemetic   Dose: Apply 1 TD patch behind the ear q3d; 0.4–0.8 PO, repeat PRN q4–6h; apply at least 4 h before exposure; ↓ dose in elderly   Caution: [C, +] APAP, levodopa, ketoconazole, digitalis, KCL   Contra: Narrow-angle glaucoma, GI or GU obstruction, thyrotoxicosis, paralytic ileus   Supplied: Patch 1.5 mg, tabs 0.4 mg, ophthalmic 0.25%   SE: Dry mouth, drowsiness, blurred vision, tachycardia, constipation   Notes: Do not blink excessively after eye drops; wait 5 min to use other eye drops; activity with patch requires several hours

Secobarbital (Seconal) [C-II]   Uses: **Insomnia, preanesthetic agent**   Action: Rapid-acting barbiturate   Dose: 100–200 mg PO, 100–300 mg PO pre-op; ↓ dose in elderly   Caution: [D, +] CYP2C9, 3A3/4, 3A5-7 inducer; ↑ toxicity with other CNS depressants   Contra: Porphyria, pregnancy   Supplied: Caps 100 mg   SE: Tolerance acquired in 1–2 wk; respiratory depression, CNS depression, porphyria, photosensitivity

Selegiline (Eldepryl)   Uses: **Parkinson's disease**   Action: Inhibits MAO activity   Dose: 5 mg PO bid; ↓ dose in elderly   Caution: [C, ?] Meperidine, SSRI, and TCAs   Contra: Concurrent meperidine   Supplied: Tabs/caps 5 mg   SE: Nausea, dizziness, orthostatic hypotension, arrhythmias, tachycardia, edema, confusion, xerostomia   Notes: ↓ Carbidopa/levodopa when used in combo

Selenium Sulfide (Exsel Shampoo, Selsun Blue Shampoo, Selsun Shampoo)   Uses: **Scalp seborrheic dermatitis, itching and flaking of the scalp due to dandruff; tinea versicolor**   Action: Antiseborrheic   Dose: *Dandruff, seborrhea:* Massage 5–10 mL into wet scalp, leave on 2–3 min, rinse, and repeat; use 2×/wk, then once q1–4wk PRN *Tinea versicolor:* Apply 2.5% qd for 7 d on area and lather with small amounts of water; leave on skin for 10 min, then rinse **Caution:** [C, ?] **Contra:** Open wounds **Supplied:** Shampoo 1% [OTC], 2.5% **SE:** Dry or oily scalp, lethargy, hair discoloration, local irritation **Notes:** Do not use more than 2×/wk

Sertraline (Zoloft)

WARNING: *Pediatric:* Antidepressants may increase risk of suicidality; consider risks and benefits of use. Patients should be closely monitored for clinical worsening, suicidality, or unusual changes in behavior **Uses: Depression, panic disorders, obsessive–compulsive disorder (OCD), post-traumatic stress disorders (PTSD), social anxiety disorder, eating disorders, premenstrual disorders** **Action:** Inhibits neuronal uptake of serotonin **Dose:** *Depression:* 50–200 mg/d PO *PTSD:* 25 mg PO qd×1 wk, then 50 mg PO qd, max 200 mg/d **Caution:** [C, ?/–] Haloperidol (serotonin syndrome), sumatriptan, linezolid **Contra:** MAOI use within 14 d; caution in hepatic impairment, concomitant pimozide **Supplied:** Tabs 25, 50, 100 mg **SE:** Can activate manic/hypomanic state; weight loss; insomnia, somnolence, fatigue, tremor, xerostomia, nausea, dyspepsia, diarrhea, ejaculatory dysfunction, ↓ libido, hepatotoxicity

Sevelamer (Renagel)

Uses: Reduction of serum phosphorus in end-stage renal disease **Action:** Binds phosphate within intestinal lumen **Dose:** 2–4 capsules PO tid with meals, with subsequent adjustment based on serum phosphorus **Caution:** [C, ?] **Contra:** Bowel obstruction **Supplied:** Capsules 403 mg **SE:** BP changes, N/V/D, dyspepsia, thrombosis **Notes:** Instruct patient not to open or chew capsules; may reduce fat-soluble vitamin absorption; 800 mg sevelamer = 667 mg calcium acetate

Sibutramine (Meridia) [C-IV]

Uses: Obesity **Action:** Blocks uptake of norepinephrine, serotonin, and dopamine **Dose:** 10 mg/d PO, may ↓ to 5 mg after 4 wk **Caution:** [C, –] SSRIs, lithium, dextromethorphan, opioids **Contra:** MAOI use within 14 d, uncontrolled HTN, arrhythmias **Supplied:** Caps 5, 10, 15 mg **SE:** HA, insomnia, xerostomia, constipation, rhinitis, tachycardia, HTN **Notes:** Use with low-calorie diet, monitor BP and heart rate

Sildenafil (Viagra)

Uses: Erectile dysfunction **Action:** Smooth muscle relaxation and increased inflow of blood to the corpus cavernosum; inhibits phosphodiesterase type 5 responsible for cGMP breakdown; ↑ cGMP activity **Dose:** 25–100 mg PO 1 h before sexual activity, max dosing is once daily; ↓ dose if > 65 y (avoid fatty foods with dose) **Caution:** [B, ?] Potent CYP3A4 inhibitors (e.g., protease inhibitors) **Contra:** Nitrates; retinitis pigmentosa; hepatic/severe renal impairment **Supplied:** Tabs 25, 50, 100 mg **SE:** HA; flushing; dizziness; blue haze visual disturbance, usually reversible; cardiac events in absence of nitrates debatable **Notes:** Caution in patients with CAD

Silver Nitrate (Dey-Drop, others)

Uses: Removal of granulation tissue and warts; prophylaxis in burns **Action:** Caustic antiseptic and astringent **Dose:** Apply to moist surface 2–3×/wk for several wk or until effect **Caution:** [C, ?] **Contra:** Do not use on broken skin **Supplied:** Topical impregnated applicator sticks, oint 10%, soln 10, 25, 50%; ophth 1% ampule **SE:** May stain tissue black, usually resolves; local irritation, methemoglobinemia **Notes:** Discontinue if redness or irritation develops

Silver Sulfadiazine (Silvadene)

Uses: Prevention and treatment of infection in 2nd- and 3rd-degree burns **Action:** Bactericidal **Dose:** Aseptically cover the affected area with ⅟₁₆-in. coating bid **Caution:** [B, ?/–] **Supplied:** Cream 1% **SE:** Itching, rash, skin discoloration, blood dyscrasias, hepatitis, allergy **Notes:** Can have systemic absorption with extensive application

Simethicone (Mylicon) [OTC]

Uses: Flatulence **Action:** Defoaming action **Dose:** 40–125 mg PO pc and hs PRN **Caution:** [C, ?] **Contra:** Intestinal perforation or obstruction **Supplied:** Tabs 80, 125 mg; caps 125 mg; drops 40 mg/0.6 mL **SE:** Diarrhea, nausea

Simvastatin (Zocor) [See Table VII–15, p 628]

Sirolimus [Rapamycin] (Rapamune)   WARNING: Can cause immunosuppression and infections   Uses: **Prophylaxis of organ rejection**   Action: Inhibits T-lymphocyte activation   Dose: *> 40 kg.* 6 mg PO on day 1, then 2 mg/d PO; *< 40 kg.* 3 mg/m^2 load, then 1 mg/m^2/d (dilute in water or orange juice; do not drink grapefruit juice while on sirolimus); take 4 h after cyclosporine; ↓ dose in hepatic impairment   Caution: [C, ?/–] Grapefruit juice, ketoconazole   Supplied: Soln 1 mg/mL, tabs 1 mg   SE: HTN, edema, chest pain, fever, HA, insomnia, acne, rash, hypercholesterolemia, hyper-/hypokalemia, GI upset, infections, blood dyscrasias, arthralgia, tachycardia, renal impairment, hepatic artery thrombosis, graft loss and death in de novo liver transplantation   Notes: Routine blood levels not needed except in liver failure (trough 9–17 ng/mL)

Smallpox vaccine (Dryvax)   Uses: **Immunization against smallpox (variola virus)**   Actions: Active immunization (live attenuated vaccinia virus)   Dose: 2–3 punctures of bifurcated needle dipped in vaccine into deltoid, posterior triceps muscle; check site for reaction in 6–8 d; if major reaction, the site will scab and heal, leaving a scar; if mild/equivocal reaction, repeat using 15 punctures   Caution: [X, –]   Contra: *Nonemergency use:* Febrile illness, immunosuppression, history of eczema and their household contacts. *Emergency use.* No absolute contraindications   Supplied: Vial for reconstitution; ~100 million pock-forming units/mL   SE: Malaise, fever, regional lymphadenopathy, encephalopathy, rashes, spread of inoculation to other sites administered; Stevens-Johnson syndrome, eczema vaccinatum with severe disability

Sodium Bicarbonate (NaHCO$_3$)   Uses: **Alkalinization of urine, RTA, metabolic acidosis, hyperkalemia, TCA overdose**   Dose: *Cardiac arrest:* Initiate adequate ventilation, 1 mEq/kg/dose IV; can repeat 0.5 mEq/kg in 10 min once or based on acid–base status *Metabolic acidosis:* 2–5 mEq/kg IV over 8 h and PRN based on acid–base status *Alkalinize urine:* 4 g (48 mEq) PO, then 1–2 g (48 mEq) q4h; adjust based on urine pH; 2 ampules in 1 L D$_5$W at 100–250 mL/h IV, monitor urine pH and serum bicarbonate *Chronic renal failure:* 1–3 mEq/kg/d PO. *Distal RTA:* 1 mEq/kg/d PO   Caution: [C, ?]   Contra: Alkalosis, hypernatremia, severe pulmonary edema, hypocalcemia   Supplied: Powder, tabs; 300 mg = 3.6 mEq; 325 mg = 3.8 mEq; 520 mg = 6.3 mEq; 600 mg = 7.3 mEq; 650 mg = 7.6 mEq; injection 1 mEq/1 mL vial or ampules   SE: Belching, edema, flatulence, hypernatremia, metabolic alkalosis   Notes: 1 g neutralizes 12 mEq of acid; 50 mEq bicarb = 50 mEq Na—can make 3 ampules in 1 L D$_5$W to = D$_5$NS w/150 mEq bicarb

Sodium Citrate (Bicitra)   Uses: **Alkalinize urine; dissolve uric acid and cysteine stones**   Action: Urinary alkalinizer, metabolic acidosis   Dose: 2–6 tsp (10–30 mL) diluted in 1–3 oz water PO pc and hs; best after meals   Caution: [C, +]   Contra: Aluminum-based antacids; severe renal impairment or sodium-restricted diets   Supplied: 15- or 30-mL unit dose: 16 (473 mL) or 4 (118 mL) fl oz   SE: Tetany, metabolic alkalosis, hyperkalemia, GI upset; avoid use of multiple 50-mL ampules; can cause hypernatremia/hyperosmolality   Notes: 1 mL = 1 mEq Na and 1 mEq bicarb

Sodium Oxybate (Xyrem) [C-III]   Uses: **Narcolepsy-associated cataplexy**   Action: Inhibitory neurotransmitter   Dose: 2.25 g PO qhs, second dose 2.5–4 h later; may increase to max of 9 g/d   Caution: [B, ?/–]   Contra: Succinic semialdehyde dehydrogenase deficiency; potentiates ethanol   Supplied: 500 mg/mL 180 mL oral soln   SE: Confusion, depression, diminished level of consciousness, incontinence, significant vomiting, respiratory depression, psychiatric symptoms   Notes: May lead to dependence; synonym for gammahydroxybutyrate (GHB), a substance abused recreationally and as a "date rape" drug; controlled distribution requires prescriber and patient registration; must be administered when patient is in bed

Sodium Phosphate (Visicol)   Uses: **Bowel evacuation before colonoscopy**   Action: Hyperosmotic   Dose: 3 tabs with at least 8 oz clear liquid every 15 min for a total of 20 tabs the night before the procedure; 3–5 h before the colonoscopy, repeat the process   Caution: [C, ?] Renal impairment, electrolyte disturbances   Contra: Megacolon, bowel obstruction, CHF, ascites, unstable angina, gastric retention, bowel perforation, colitis, hypomotility   Supplied: Tabs 2 g   SE: QT prolongation, diarrhea, hypernatremia, flatulence, cramps

Sodium Polystyrene Sulfonate (Kayexalate) Uses: Hyperkalemia Action:
Sodium and potassium ion-exchange resin **Dose:** 15–60 g PO or 30–60 g PR q6h based on serum K^+ (given with an agent, e.g., sorbitol, to promote movement through the bowel) **Caution:** [C, M] **Contra:** Hypernatremia **Supplied:** Powder; susp 15 g/60 mL sorbitol **SE:** Can cause hypernatremia, hypokalemia, sodium retention, GI upset, fecal impaction; enema acts more quickly than PO **Notes:** Oral route is most effective

Sorbitol (generic) Uses: Constipation Action: Laxative Dose: 30–60 mL of a
20–70% soln PO PRN **Caution:** [B, +] **Contra:** Anuria **Supplied:** Liq 70% **SE:** Edema, electrolyte losses, lactic acidosis, GI upset, xerostomia **Notes:** May be vehicle for many liquid formulations (e.g., zinc, Kayexalate)

Sotalol (Betapace) WARNING: Monitor patients for first 3 days of therapy to reduce
risks of induced arrhythmia **Uses: Ventricular arrhythmias, AF** **Action:** β-Adrenergic-blocking agent **Dose:** 80 mg PO bid; may be ↑ to 240–320 mg/d; ↓ dose in renal failure **Caution:** [B (1st trimester) (D if 2nd or 3rd trimester), +] **Contra:** Asthma, bradycardia, prolonged QT interval, 2nd- or 3rd-degree heart block without pacemaker, cardiogenic shock, uncontrolled CHF, CrCl < 40 mL/min **Supplied:** Tabs 80, 120, 160, 240 mg **SE:** Bradycardia, chest pain, palpitations, fatigue, dizziness, weakness, dyspnea **Notes:** BETAPACE should not be substituted for BETAPACE AF because of significant differences in labeling

Sotalol (Betapace AF) WARNING: To minimize risk of induced arrhythmia, patients
initiated/reinitiated on BETAPACE AF should be placed for a minimum of 3 d (on their maintenance dose) in a facility that can provide cardiac resuscitation, continuous ECG monitoring, and calculations of CrCl; BETAPACE should not be substituted for BETAPACE AF because of differences in labeling **Uses: Maintain sinus rhythm for symptomatic A fib/flutter** **Action:** β-Adrenergic-blocking agent **Dose:** *Initial ClCr > 60 mL/min:* 80 mg PO q12h. *ClCr 40–60 mL/min:* 80 mg PO q2h; ↑ to 120 mg during hospitalization; monitor QT interval 2–4 h after each dose, with dose reduction or discontinuation if QT interval > 500 ms **Caution:** [B (1st trimester; D if 2nd or 3rd trimester), +] **Contra:** Asthma, bradycardia, prolonged QT interval, 2nd- or 3rd-degree heart block without pacemaker, cardiogenic shock, uncontrolled CHF, CrCl < 40 mL/min; caution if converting from previous antiarrhythmic therapy **Supplied:** Tabs 80, 120, 160 mg **SE:** Bradycardia, chest pain, palpitations, fatigue, dizziness, weakness, dyspnea **Notes:** Routinely evaluate renal function and QT interval

Sparfloxacin (Zagam) Uses: Community-acquired pneumonia, acute exacerba-
tions of chronic bronchitis **Action:** Quinolone antibiotic; inhibits DNA gyrase **Dose:** 400 mg PO on day 1, then 200 mg q24h for 10 d; ↓ dose in renal dysfunction **Caution:** [C, ?/–] Interactions with theophylline, caffeine, sucralfate, warfarin, and antacids **Contra:** QT prolongation; do not administer with drugs that prolong QT interval **Supplied:** Tabs 200 mg **SE:** Significant phototoxicity (even from daylight through windows); restlessness, N/V/D, rash, ruptured tendons, ↑ LFTs, sleep disorders, confusion, convulsions **Notes:** MUST protect from sunlight up to 5 d after last dose

Spironolactone (Aldactone) Uses: Hyperaldosteronism, ascites from CHF or
cirrhosis **Action:** Aldosterone antagonist; K-sparing diuretic **Dose:** 25–100 mg PO qid; CHF (NYHA class III–IV) 25–50 mg/d; take with food **Caution:** [D, +] **Contra:** Hyperkalemia, renal failure, anuria **Supplied:** Tabs 25, 50, 100 mg **SE:** Hyperkalemia and gynecomastia, arrhythmia, sexual dysfunction, confusion, dizziness

Stavudine (Zerit) WARNING: Lactic acidosis and severe hepatomegaly with steatosis
and pancreatitis reported **Uses: Advanced HIV disease** **Action:** Reverse-transcriptase inhibitor **Dose:** *> 60 kg:* 40 mg bid *< 60 kg:* 30 mg bid; ↓ dose in renal failure **Caution:** [C, +] **Contra:** Hypersensitivity **Supplied:** Caps 15, 20, 30, 40 mg; soln 1 mg/mL **SE:** Peripheral neuropathy, HA, chills, fever, malaise, rash, GI upset, anemias, lactic acidosis, ↑ LFTs, pancreatitis **Notes:** Take with plenty of water

Steroids, Systemic (see also Table VII–2, p 613) The following relates
only to the commonly used systemic glucocorticoids Uses: Endocrine
disorders (adrenal insufficiency), rheumatoid disorders, collagen-vascular diseases,

dermatologic diseases, allergic states, cerebral edema, nephritis, nephrotic syndrome, immunosuppression for transplantation, hypercalcemia, malignancies (breast, lymphomas), preoperatively (in any patient who has been on steroids in the previous year, known hypoadrenalism, preop for adrenalectomy); injection into joints/tissue **Action:** Glucocorticoid **Dose:** Varies with use and institutional protocols

- *Adrenal insufficiency, acute:* Hydrocortisone 100 mg IV; then 300 mg/d ÷ q6h; convert to 50 mg PO q8h×6 doses, taper to 30–50 mg/d ÷ bid
- *Adrenal insufficiency, chronic (physiologic replacement):* May need mineralocorticoid supplementation such as Florinef. Hydrocortisone 20 mg PO qAM, 10 mg PO qPM; cortisone 0.5–0.75 mg/kg/d ÷ bid; cortisone 0.25–0.35 mg/kg/d IM; dexamethasone 0.03–0.15 mg/kg/d or 0.6–0.75 mg/msp]2/d ÷ q6–12h PO, IM, IV
- *Asthma, acute:* Methylprednisolone 60 mg PO/IV q6h or dexamethasone 12 mg IV q6h
- *Extubation/airway edema:* Dexamethasone 0.5–1 mg/kg/d IM/IV ÷ q6h (start beginning 24 h before extubation; continue for 4 additional doses)
- *Immunosuppressive/anti-inflammatory:* Hydrocortisone 15–240 mg PO, IM, IV q12h; methylprednisolone: 4–48 mg/d PO, taper to lowest effective dose; methylprednisolone sodium succinate 10–80 mg/d IM; prednisone or prednisolone 5–60 mg/d PO ÷ qd–qid
- *Septic shock* (controversial): Hydrocortisone 500 mg–1 g IM/IV q2–6h
- *Status asthmaticus:* Hydrocortisone 1–2 mg/kg/dose IV q6h; then decrease by 0.5–1 mg/kg q6h
- *Rheumatic disease:*

Intra-articular: Hydrocortisone acetate 25–37.5 mg large joint, 10–25 mg small joint; methylprednisolone acetate 20–80 mg large joint, 4–10 mg small joint
Intrabursal: Hydrocortisone acetate 25–37.5 mg
Intraganglial: Hydrocortisone acetate 25–37.5 mg
Tendon sheath: Hydrocortisone acetate 5–12.5 mg

- *Perioperative steroid coverage:* Hydrocortisone 100 mg IV night before surgery, 1 h preop, intraop, and 4, 8, and 12 h postop; pod #1 100 mg IV q6h; pod #2 100 mg IV q8h; pod #3 100 mg IV q12h; pod #4 50 mg IV q12h; pod #5 25 mg IV q12h; then resume prior oral dosing if chronic use or discontinue if only perioperative coverage required
- *Cerebral edema:* Dexamethasone 10 mg IV; then 4 mg IV q4–6h

Caution: [C, ?/–] **Contra:** Active varicella infection, serious infection except TB, fungal infections **Supplied:** Table VII–2, p 613 **Notes/SE:** Hydrocortisone succinate administered systemically, acetate form intra-articular; all can cause increased appetite, hyperglycemia, hypokalemia, osteoporosis, nervousness, insomnia, "steroid psychosis," adrenal suppression; never abruptly stop steroids, especially in chronic treatment; taper dose

Streptokinase (Streptase, Kabikinase)
Uses: Coronary artery thrombosis, acute massive PE, DVT, and some occluded vascular grafts **Action:** Activates plasminogen to plasmin that degrades fibrin **Dose:** *PE:* Loading dose of 250,000 units IV through a peripheral vein over 30 min, then 100,000 units/h IV for 24–72 h *Coronary artery thrombosis:* 1.5 million units IV over 60 min *DVT or arterial embolism:* Load as with PE, then 100,000 units/h for 72 h *Occluded catheter* (not recommended): 10,000–25,000 units in NS to final volume of catheter (leave in place for 1 h, aspirate and flush catheter with NS) **Caution:** [C, +] **Contra:** Streptococcal infection or streptokinase use in last 6 mo, active bleeding, CVA, TIA, spinal surgery, or trauma in last month, vascular anomalies, severe hepatic or renal disease, endocarditis, pericarditis, severe uncontrolled HTN **Supplied:** Powder for inj 250,000, 600,000, 750,000, 1,500,000 units **SE:** Bleeding, hypotension, fever, bruising, rash, GI upset, hemorrhage, anaphylaxis **Notes:** If maintenance inf inadequate to maintain thrombin clotting time 2–5× control, refer to the package insert for adjustments. Antibodies remain 3–6 mo following dose

Streptomycin Uses: **TB, streptococcal or enterococcal endocarditis** Action: Aminoglycoside; interferes with protein synthesis Dose: *Endocarditis:* 1 g q12h 1–2wk, then 500 mg q12h 1–4wk; *TB:* 15 mg/kg/d (up to 1 g), directly observed therapy (DOT) 2×wk–20–30 mg/kg/dose (max 1.5 g), DOT 3×wk to 25—30 mg/kg/dose (max 1 g); ↓ dose in renal failure, either IM or IV over 30–60 min Caution: [D, +] Contra: Pregnancy Supplied: Inj 400 mg/mL (1-g vial) SE: Increased incidence of vestibular and auditory toxicity, neurotoxicity, nephrotoxicity—pk 20–30 mcg/mL, tr < 5 mcg/mL; toxic pk > 50, tr > 10

Streptozocin (Zanosar) Uses: **Pancreatic islet cell tumors and carcinoid tumors** Action: DNA-DNA (interstrand) cross-linking; DNA, RNA, and protein synthesis inhibitor Dose: Refer to specific protocol; decrease dose in renal failure Caution: [D, ?/–] Contra: Caution in renal failure, pregnancy Supplied: Inj 1 g SE: N/V, duodenal ulcers; myelosuppression rare (20%) and mild; nephrotoxicity (proteinuria and azotemia often heralded by hypophosphatemia) dose-limiting. Hypo-/hyperglycemia may occur; phlebitis and pain at inj site Notes: Monitor renal function

Succimer (Chemet) Uses: **Lead poisoning (lead levels > 45 mcg/mL)** Action: Heavy-metal chelating agent Dose: 10 mg/kg/dose q8h × 5 d then 10 mg/kg/dose q12h for 14 d; ↓ dose in renal dysfunction Caution: [C, ?] Contra: Hypersensitivity Supplied: Caps 100 mg SE: Rash, fever, GI upset, hemorrhoids, metallic taste, drowsiness, ↑ LFTs Notes: Monitor lead levels, maintain adequate hydration, may open capsules

Succinylcholine (Anectine, Quelicin, Sucostrin) Uses: **Adjunct to general anesthesia to facilitate ET intubation and to induce skeletal muscle relaxation during surgery or mechanically supported ventilation** Action: Depolarizing neuromuscular blocking agent Dose: 1–1.5 mg/kg IV over 10–30 s, followed by 0.04–0.07 mg/kg PRN or 10–100 mcg/kg/min infusion; ↓ in severe liver disease Caution: [C, M] Contra: At risk for malignant hyperthermia; myopathy; recent major burn, multiple trauma, extensive skeletal muscle denervation Supplied: Inj 20, 50, 100 mg/mL; powder for inj 500 mg, 1 g/vial SE: May precipitate malignant hyperthermia, respiratory depression, or prolonged apnea; multiple drugs potentiate succinylcholine; observe for cardiovascular effects (arrhythmias, hypotension, brady-tachycardia); increased intraocular pressure, postoperative stiffness, salivation, myoglobinuria Notes: May be given IVP or infusion or IM in the deltoid

Sucralfate (Carafate) Uses: **Duodenal ulcers, gastric ulcers, stomatitis, GERD, preventing stress ulcers, esophagitis** Action: Forms ulcer-adherent complex that protects against acid, pepsin, and bile acid Dose: 1 g PO qid, 1 h before meals and hs; continue 4–8 wk unless healing demonstrated by x-ray or endoscopy; separate from other drugs by 2 h; take on empty stomach—before meals Caution: [B, +] Supplied: Tabs 1 g; susp 1 g/10 mL SE: Constipation frequent; diarrhea, dizziness, xerostomia Notes: Aluminum may accumulate in renal failure

Sulfacetamide (Bleph-10, Cetamide, Sodium Sulamyd) [See Table VII–12, pp 623–25]

Sulfacetamide and Prednisolone (Blephamide, others) [See Table VII–12, pp 623–25]

Sulfasalazine (Azulfidine, Azulfidine EN) Uses: **Ulcerative colitis, RA, juvenile RA, active Crohn's, ankylosing spondylitis, psoriasis** Action: Sulfonamide; actions not clear Dose: Initially, 1 g PO tid–qid; ↑ to a max of 8 g/d in 3–4 ÷ doses; maintenance 500 mg PO qid; ↓ dose in renal failure Caution: [B (D if near term), M] Contra: Sulfonamide or salicylate sensitivity, porphyria, GI or GU obstruction; avoid in hepatic impairment Supplied: Tabs 500 mg; EC tabs 500 mg; oral susp 250 mg/5 mL SE: Can cause severe GI upset; discolors urine; dizziness, HA, photosensitivity, oligospermia, anemias, Stevens-Johnson syndrome Notes: May cause yellow-orange skin discoloration or stain contact lenses; avoid long sunlight exposure

Sulfinpyrazone (Anturane) Uses: **Acute and chronic gout** Action: Inhibits renal tubular absorption of uric acid Dose: 100–200 mg PO bid for 1 wk, then ↑ as needed to maintenance of 200–400 mg bid (max 800 mg/d, take with food or antacids, and plenty of fluids; avoid salicylates) **Caution:** [C (D if near term), ?/–] **Contra:** Avoid in renal impairment, avoid salicylates; peptic ulcer; blood dyscrasias, near term pregnancy, hypersensitivity **Supplied:** Tabs 100 mg; caps 200 mg **SE:** N/V, stomach pain, urolithiasis, leukopenia **Notes:** Take with plenty of water

Sulindac (Clinoril) [See Table VII–11, pp 621–22]

Sumatriptan (Imitrex) [See Table VII–16, p 629])

Tacrine (Cognex) Uses: Mild/moderate Alzheimer's dementia **Action:** Cholinesterase inhibitor **Dose:** 10–40 mg PO qid to 160 mg/d; separate doses from food **Caution:** [C, ?] **Contra:** Previous tacrine-induced jaundice **Supplied:** Caps 10, 20, 30, 40 mg **SE:** ↑ LFT, HA, dizziness, GI upset, flushing, confusion, ataxia, myalgia, bradycardia **Notes:** Serum conc > 20ng/mL assoc with more SE, monitor LFTs

Tacrolimus [FK 506] (Prograf, Protopic) Uses: Prophylaxis of organ rejection, eczema **Action:** Macrolide immunosuppressant **Dose:** *IV:* 0.05–0.1 mg/kg/d as cont inf *PO:* 0.15–0.3 mg/kg/d ÷ into 2 doses *Eczema:* Apply bid, continue 1 wk after clearing; decrease dose in hepatic/renal impairment **Caution:** [C, –] Do not use with cyclosporine **Supplied:** Caps 1, 5 mg; inj 5 mg/mL; ointment 0.03, 0.1% **SE:** Neurotoxicity and nephrotoxicity, HTN, edema, HA, insomnia, fever, pruritus, hypo-/hyperkalemia, hyperglycemia, GI upset, anemia, leukocytosis, tremors, paresthesias, pleural effusion, seizures, lymphoma **Notes:** Monitor serum drug levels; Serum conc > 20 see Table VII–17, p 630

Tamoxifen (Nolvadex) Uses: Breast CA (postmenopausal, estrogen receptor positive), reduction of breast CA in high-risk women, metastatic male breast CA, mastalgia, pancreatic CA, gynecomastia, ovulation induction **Action:** Nonsteroidal antiestrogen; mixed agonist-antagonist effect **Dose:** 20–40 mg/d PO (typically 10 mg bid or 20 mg/d) **Caution:** [D, –] **Contra:** Caution in leukopenia, thrombocytopenia, hyperlipidemia **Supplied:** Tabs 10, 20 mg **SE:** Uterine malignancy and thrombotic events in breast CA prevention trials; menopausal symptoms (hot flashes, N/V) in premenopausal patients; vaginal bleeding and menstrual irregularities; skin rash, pruritus vulvae, dizziness, HA, peripheral edema; acute flare of bone metastasis pain and hypercalcemia; retinopathy reported (high dose) **Notes:** ↑ Risk of pregnancy in premenopausal women by inducing ovulation

Tamsulosin (Flomax) Uses: BPH **Action:** Antagonist of prostatic α-receptors **Dose:** 0.4 mg/d PO; do not crush, chew, or open caps **Caution:** [B, ?] **Contra:** Female gender **Supplied:** Caps 0.4, 0.8 mg **SE:** HA, dizziness, syncope, somnolence, decreased libido, GI upset, retrograde ejaculation, rhinitis, rash, angioedema **Notes:** Not for use as antihypertensive

Tazarotene (Tazorac) Uses: Facial acne vulgaris; stable plaque psoriasis up to 20% body surface area **Action:** Keratolytic **Dose:** *Acne:* Cleanse face, dry, and apply thin film q hs on acne lesions *Psoriasis:* Apply hs **Caution:** [X, ?/–] **Contra:** Retinoid sensitivity **Supplied:** Gel 0.05, 0.1% **SE:** Burning, erythema, irritation, rash, photosensitivity, desquamation, bleeding, skin discoloration **Notes:** Discontinue if excessive pruritus, burning, skin redness or peeling until symptoms resolve

Tegaserod maleate (Zelnorm) WARNING: Rare reports of ischemic colitis **Uses:** Short-term treatment of constipation-predominant IBS in women, chronic idiopathic constipation in pts < 65 y **Action:** 5HT₄ serotonin agonist **Dose:** 6 mg PO bid pc for 4–6 wk; may continue for 2nd course **Caution:** [B, ?/–] **Contra:** Severe renal, moderate-severe hepatic impairment, history of bowel obstruction, gallbladder disease, sphincter of Oddi dysfunction, abdominal adhesions **Supplied:** Tabs 2, 6 mg **SE:** Do not administer if diarrhea is present because drug increases GI motility; discontinue if abdominal pain worsens **Notes:** Maintain adequate hydration

Telmisartan (Micardis) [See Table VII–4, p 615]

Temazepam (Restoril) [C-IV] Uses: Insomnia, anxiety, depression, panic attacks **Action:** Benzodiazepine **Dose:** 15–30 mg PO hs PRN; ↓ dose in elderly **Caution:** [X; ?/–] potentiates CNS depressive effects of opioids, barbiturates, alcohol, antihistamines, MAOIs, TCAs **Contra:** Narrow-angle glaucoma **Supplied:** Caps 7.5, 15, 30 mg **SE:**

Confusion, dizziness, drowsiness, hangover **Notes:** Abrupt discontinuation after > 10 days of use may cause withdrawal

Tenecteplase (TNKase) Uses: **Restore perfusion and reduce mortality with acute MI** Action: Thrombolytic; TPA Dose: 30–50 mg; see following table:

Weight (kg)	TNKase (mg)	Volume TNKase*(mL)
< 60	30	6
≥ 60 to < 70	35	7
≥ 70 to < 80	40	8
≥ 80 to < 90	45	9
≥ 90	50	10

*From one vial of reconstituted TNKase.

Caution: [C, ?] ↑ bleeding with concurrent NSAIDs, ticlodipine, clopidogrel, GPIIb/IIIa antagonists **Contra:** Bleeding, CVA, major surgery (intracranial, intraspinal) or trauma within 2 mo **Supplied:** Inj 50 mg, reconstitute with 10 mL sterile water **SE:** Bleeding, hypersensitivity **Notes:** Do not shake when reconstituting; do NOT use D₅W either in the IV line or to reconstitute

Teniposide (VM-26, Vumon) Uses: **Small cell lung cancer, Kaposi's sarcoma, non-Hodgkin's lymphoma** Action: Topoisomerase II inhibitor, interfering with strand passage and DNA ligase activities of topoisomerase II. Cell cycle-specific activity at S, early G_2 phase Dose: Refer to specific protocol.↓ dose in Down's syndrome, leukemia, renal failure; consider adjustment in hepatic impairment Caution: [D, ?] Supplied: 10 mg/mL 5 mL ampule SE: Toxicity includes myelosuppression (especially leukopenia and thrombocytopenia), hypotension, chemical phlebitis, skin rashes, hypertension, hypersensitivity reactions (urticaria, flushing, rashes, or hypotension), and secondary leukemia

Tenofovir (Viread) Uses: **HIV infection** Action: Nucleotide reverse transcriptase inhibitor Dose: 300 mg po qd with a meal Caution: [B, ?/–] Didanosine (separate admin times), lopinavir, ritonavir Contra: CrCl < 60 mL/min; caution with known risk factors for liver disease Supplied: Tabs 300 mg SE: GI upset, metabolic syndrome, hepatotoxicity; separate didanosine doses by 2 h Notes: Take with fatty meal; available in combination with emtricitabine, known as Truvada

Terazosin (Hytrin) Uses: **BPH and HTN** Action: α_1-Blocker (blood vessel and bladder neck/prostate) Dose: Initially, 1 mg PO hs; ↑ 20 mg/d max Caution: [C, ?] ↑ Hypotension with β-blocker, calcium channel blocker, ACEI Contra: α-Antagonist sensitivity Supplied: Tabs 1, 2, 5, 10 mg; caps 1, 2, 5, 10 mg SE: Hypotension and syncope after 1st dose; dizziness, weakness, nasal congestion, peripheral edema common; palpitations, GI upset Notes: Caution with 1st dose syncope. If for HTN, combine with thiazide diuretic

Terbinafine (Lamisil) Uses: **Onychomycosis, athlete's foot, jock itch, ringworm, cutaneous candidiasis, pityriasis versicolor** Action: Inhibits squalene epoxidase resulting in fungal death Dose: Oral: 250 mg/d PO for 6–12 wk Topical: Apply to affected area; ↓ dose in renal/hepatic impairment Caution: [B, –] May ↑ effects of drugs metab by CYP2D6 Contra: Liver disease or kidney impairment Supplied: Tabs 250 mg; cream 1% SE: HA, dizziness, rash, pruritus, alopecia, GI upset, taste perversion, neutropenia, retinal damage, Stevens-Johnson syndrome Notes: Effect may take months due to need for new nail growth; do not use occlusive dressings

Terbutaline (Brethine, Bricanyl) Uses: **Reversible bronchospasm (asthma, COPD); inhibition of labor (tocolytic)** Action: Sympathomimetic Dose: Bronchodilator: 2.5–5 mg PO qid or 0.25 mg SC; may repeat in 15 min (max 0.5 mg in 4 h) Met-dose inhaler: 2 inhal q4–6h Premature labor: Acutely 2.5–10 mg/min/IV, gradually ↑ as tolerated q10–20min; maintenance 2.5–5 mg PO q4–6h until term; ↓ dose in renal failure Caution: [B, +] ↑ Toxicity with MAOIs, TCAs; diabetes, HTN, hyperthyroidism; tachycardia Supplied: Tabs 2.5, 5 mg; inj 1 mg/mL; met-dose inhaler SE: HTN, hyperthyroidism; high doses may precipitate β_1-adrenergic effects; nervousness, trembling, tachycardia, HTN, dizziness Notes: Caution with diabetes

Terconazole (Terazol 7)   Uses: **Vaginal fungal infections**   Action: Topical antifungal   Dose: 1 applicatorful or 1 supp intravaginally hs for 3–7 d   Caution: [C, ?]   Supplied: Vaginal cream 0.4%, vaginal supp 80 mg   SE: Vulvar or vaginal burning   Notes: Insert high into vagina

Teriparatide (Forteo)   Uses: **Severe/refractory osteoporosis**   Action: PTH (recombinant)   Dose: 20 mcg SC qd in thigh or abdomen   Caution: [C, ?/–]   Contra: Osteosarcoma in animals—do not administer if Paget's disease, prior radiation, bone metastases, hypercalcemia; caution in urolithiasis   Supplied: 3-mL prefilled device (discard after 28 d)   SE: Symptomatic orthostatic hypotension upon administration, N/D, ↑ Ca, leg cramps   Notes: Not recommended for use > 2 y

Tetanus Immune Globulin   Uses: **Passive immunization against tetanus for a suspected contaminated wound and unknown immunization status**   Action: Passive immunization   Dose: 250–500 units IM (higher doses if delayed therapy)   Caution: [C, ?]   Contra: Thimerosal sensitivity   Supplied: Inj 250-unit vial or syringe   SE: Pain, tenderness, erythema at injection site; fever, angioedema, muscle stiffness, anaphylaxis   Notes: May begin active immunization series at different inj site if required

Tetanus Toxoid   Uses: **Tetanus prophylaxis**   Action: Active immunization   Dose: Based on previous immunization status   Caution: [C, ?]   Contra: Chloramphenicol use, neurologic symptoms with previous use, active infection (for routine primary immunization)   Supplied: Inj tetanus toxoid, fluid, 4–5 Lf units/0.5 mL; tetanus toxoid, adsorbed, 5, 10 Lf units/0.5 mL   SE: Local erythema, induration, sterile abscess; chills, fever, neurologic disturbances

Tetracycline (Achromycin V, Sumycin)   Uses: **Broad-spectrum antibiotic**   Spectrum: *Gram(+) positive: Staphylococcus, Streptococcus Gram(–): H pylori.* Atypicals: *Chlamydia, Rickettsia,* and *Mycoplasma*   Action: Bacteriostatic; inhibits protein synthesis   Dose: 250–500 mg PO bid–qid; ↓ dose in renal/hepatic impairment   Caution: [D, +]   Contra: *Pregnancy,* antacids, dairy products   Supplied: Caps 100, 250, 500 mg; tabs 250, 500 mg; oral susp 250 mg/5 mL   SE: Photosensitivity, GI upset, renal failure, pseudotumor cerebri, hepatic impairment

Thalidomide (Thalomid)   Uses: **Erythema nodosum leprosum, graft-versus-host disease, aphthous ulceration in HIV-positive patients**   Action: Inhibits neutrophil chemotaxis, decreases monocyte phagocytosis   Dose: *GVHD:* 1000–1600 mg PO qd *Stomatitis:* 200 mg bid for 5 d, then 200 mg qd for up to 8 wk *ENL:* 100–300 mg PO qhs   Caution: [X, –] May increase HIV viral load; use caution if history of seizures   Contra: *Pregnancy:* Sexually active males not using latex condoms, or females not using 2 forms of contraception   SE: Dizziness, drowsiness, rash, fever, orthostasis, Stevens-Johnson syndrome, peripheral neuropathy, seizures   Supplied: 50-mg cap   Notes: MD must register with STEPS risk management program; informed consent necessary; immediately discontinue if skin rash develops

Theophylline (Theo-24, Theochron, Others)   Uses: **Asthma, bronchospasm**   Action: Relaxes smooth muscle of the bronchi and pulmonary blood vessels   Dose: 900 mg PO ÷ q6h; SR products may be ÷ q8–12h (maintenance); ↓ dose in hepatic failure   Caution: [C, +] Multiple interactions, including caffeine, smoking, carbamazepine, barbs, β-blockers, ciprofloxacin, E-mycin, INH, loop diuretics   Contra: Arrhythmia, hyperthyroidism, uncontrolled seizures   Supplied: Elixir 80, 150 mg/15 mL; liq 80, 160 mg/15 mL; caps 100, 200, 250 mg; tabs 100, 125, 200, 225, 250, 300 mg; SR caps 50, 75, 100, 125, 200, 250, 260, 300 mg; SR tabs 100, 200, 250, 300, 400, 450, 500 mg   SE: N/V, tachycardia, and seizures; nervousness, arrhythmias   Notes: See drug levels in Table VII–17 (p 000); many drug interactions

Thiamine [Vitamin B₁]   Uses: **Thiamine deficiency (beriberi), alcoholic neuritis, Wernicke's encephalopathy**   Action: Dietary supplementation   Dose: *Deficiency:* 100 mg/d IM for 2 wk, then 5–10 mg/d PO for 1 mo *Wernicke's encephalopathy:* 100 mg IV in single dose, then 100 mg/d IM for 2 wk   Caution: [A (C if doses exceed RDA), +]   Supplied:

Tabs 5, 10, 25, 50, 100, 500 mg; inj 100, 200 mg/mL **SE:** Angioedema, paresthesias, rash, anaphylaxis with rapid IV administration **Notes:** IV thiamine use associated with anaphylactic reaction; must give IV slowly

Thiethylperazine (Torecan) Uses: N/V Action: Antidopaminergic antiemetic
Dose: 10 mg PO, PR, or IM qd–tid; ↓ dose in hepatic failure **Caution:** [X, ?] **Contra:** Phenothiazine and sulfite sensitivity, pregnancy **Supplied:** Tabs 10 mg; supp 10 mg; inj 5 mg/mL **SE:** Extrapyramidal reactions may occur; xerostomia, drowsiness, orthostatic hypotension, tachycardia, confusion

6-Thioguanine [6-TG] (Tabloid) Uses: AML, ALL, CML Action: Purine-based
antimetabolite (substitutes for natural purines interfering with nucleotide synthesis) **Dose:** 2–3 mg/kg/d PO; ↓ dose in severe renal/hepatic impairment **Caution:** [D, –] **Contra:** Resistance to mercaptopurine **Supplied:** Tabs 40 mg **SE:** Myelosuppression (especially leukopenia and thrombocytopenia), N/V/D, anorexia, stomatitis, rash, hyperuricemia; hepatotoxicity occurs rarely

Thioridazine (Mellaril) WARNING: Dose-related QT prolongation Uses: Schizophrenia, psychosis Action: Phenothiazine antipsychotic Dose: Initially, 50–100 mg PO
tid; maintenance 200–800 mg/24 h PO in 2–4 ÷ doses. **Caution:** [C, ?] ↑ Phenothiazines, QTc prolonging agents, aluminum (↓) **Contra:** Phenothiazine sensitivity **Supplied:** Tabs 10, 15, 25, 50, 100, 150, 200 mg; oral conc 30, 100 mg/mL; oral susp 25, 100 mg/5 mL **SE:** Low incidence of extrapyramidal effects; ventricular arrhythmias; hypotension, dizziness, drowsiness, neuroleptic malignant syndrome, seizures, skin discoloration, photosensitivity, constipation, sexual dysfunction, blood dyscrasias, pigmentary retinopathy, hepatic impairment **Notes:** Avoid alcohol, must dilute oral conc in 2–4 oz liquid

Thiotepa (see Triethylene-Triphosphamide)

Thiothixene (Navane) Uses: Psychotic disorders Action: Antipsychotic Dose:
Mild to moderate psychosis: 2 mg PO tid, up to 20–30 mg/d *Severe psychosis:* 5 mg PO bid; ↑ to a max of 60 mg/24 h PRN *IM use:* 16–20 mg/24 h ÷ bid–qid; max 30 mg/d **Caution:** [C, ?] **Contra:** Phenothiazine sensitivity **Supplied:** Caps 1, 2, 5, 10, 20 mg; oral conc 5 mg/mL; inj 2, 5 mg/mL **SE:** Drowsiness and extrapyramidal side effects most common; hypotension, dizziness, drowsiness, neuroleptic malignant syndrome, seizures, skin discoloration, photosensitivity, constipation, sexual dysfunction, blood dyscrasias, pigmentary retinopathy, hepatic impairment **Notes:** Dilute oral conc immediately before administration

Tiagabine (Gabitril) Uses: Adjunctive therapy in treatment of partial seizures,
bipolar disorder **Action:** Inhibition of GABA **Dose:** Initially 4 mg/d PO, ↑ by 4 mg during 2nd wk; ↑ PRN by 4–8 mg/d based on response, 56 mg/d/max **Caution:** [C, M] **Supplied:** Tabs 4, 12, 16, 20 mg **SE:** Dizziness, HA, somnolence, memory impairment, tremors **Notes:** Use gradual withdrawal; used in combination with other anticonvulsants

Ticarcillin (Ticar) [See Table VII–6, p 616]

Ticarcillin/Potassium Clavulanate (Timentin) [See Table VII–6, p 616]

Ticlopidine (Ticlid) WARNING: Neutropenia/agranulocytosis, TTP, and aplastic anemia reported Uses: ↓ Risk of thrombotic stroke, protect grafts post-CABG, diabetic mi-
croangiopathy, ischemic heart disease, DVT prophylaxis, graft prophylaxis after renal transplantation **Action:** Platelet aggregation inhibitor **Dose:** 250 mg PO bid with food **Caution:** [B, ?/–] ↑ Toxicity of ASA, anticoagulants, NSAIDs, theophylline **Contra:** Bleeding, hepatic impairment, neutropenia, thrombocytopenia **Supplied:** Tabs 250 mg **SE:** Bleeding, GI upset, rash, ↑ on LFTs **Notes:** monitor hematologic status 1st 3 mo

Timolol (Blocadren) [See Table VII–7, pp 617–18]

Timolol, Ophthalmic (Timoptic) [See Table VII–12, pp 623–25]

Tinzaparin (Innohep) Uses: Treatment of DVT with or without PE Action: Low-
molecular-weight heparin **Dose:** 175 units/kg SC qd at least 6 d until warfarin dose stabilized **Caution:** [B, ?] Pork hypersensitivity, active bleeding; caution in mild to moderate renal

dysfunction **Contra:** Hypersensitivity to sulfites, heparin, benzyl alcohol; heparin-induced thrombocytopenia **Supplied:** 20,000 units/mL in 2 mL MDV **SE:** Bleeding, bruising, thrombocytopenia, pain at injection site, ↑ LFTs **Notes:** Anti-Xa levels monitoring tool; no effect on bleeding time, platelet function, PT, or aPTT

Tioconazole (Vagistat) **Uses:** Vaginal fungal infections **Action:** Topical antifungal **Dose:** 1 applicatorful intravaginally hs (single dose) **Caution:** [C, ?] **Supplied:** Vaginal oint 6.5% **SE:** Local burning, itching, soreness, polyuria **Notes:** Insert high into vagina

Tirofiban (Aggrastat) **Uses:** Acute coronary syndrome **Action:** Glycoprotein IIB/IIIa inhibitor **Dose:** Initially 0.4 mcg/kg/min for 30 min, followed by 0.1 mcg/kg/min; use in combination with heparin; ↓ dose in renal insufficiency **Caution:** [B, ?/–] **Contra:** Bleeding, intracranial neoplasm, vascular malformation, stroke/surgery/trauma within last 30 d, severe HTN **Supplied:** Inj 50, 250 mcg/mL **SE:** Bleeding, bradycardia, coronary dissection, pelvic pain, rash

Tobramycin (Nebcin) **Uses:** Serious gram(–) infections **Action:** Aminoglycoside; inhibits protein synthesis *Spectrum:* Gram(–) bacteria (including *Pseudomonas*) **Dose:** 1–2.5 mg/kg/dose IV q8–24h; ↓ with renal insufficiency **Caution:** [C, M] **Contra:** Aminoglycoside sensitivity **Supplied:** Inj 10, 40 mg/mL **SE:** Nephrotoxic and ototoxic **Notes:** Monitor CrCl and serum concentrations for dosage adjustments (Tables VII–18, VII–19, VII–20, and VII–21, pp 630-34)

Tobramycin Ophthalmic (AK-Tob, Tobrex) [See Table VII–12, pp 623-25]

Tobramycin and Dexamethasone Ophthalmic (TobraDex) [See Table VII–12, pp 623-25]

Tolazamide (Tolinase) [See Table VII–13, p 626]

Tolazoline (Priscoline) **Uses:** Peripheral vasospastic disorders **Action:** Competitively blocks α-adrenergic receptors **Dose:** 10–50 mg IM/IV/SC qid (adjust with ↓ renal function) **Caution:** [C, ?] **Contra:** CAD **Supplied:** Inj 25 mg/mL **SE:** Hypotension, peripheral vasodilation, tachycardia, arrhythmias, GI upset, blood dyscrasias, renal failure, GI bleeding

Tolbutamide (Orinase) [See Table VII–13, p 626]

Tolcapone (Tasmar) **Uses:** Adjunct to carbidopa/levodopa in Parkinson's disease **Action:** Catechol-O-methyltransferase inhibitor slows metabolism of levodopa **Dose:** 100 mg PO with first daily dose of levodopa/carbidopa, followed by doses 6 and 12 hours later. Reduce dose in renal impairment **Caution:** [C, ?] **Contra:** Hepatic impairment; nonselective MAO inhibitors **Supplied:** Tabs 100 mg, 200 mg **SE:** Constipation, xerostomia, vivid dreams, hallucinations, anorexia, N/D, orthostasis, liver failure **Notes:** Do not abruptly discontinue or ↓ dose; requires LFT monitoring

Tolmetin (Tolectin) [See Table VII–11, pp 621–22]

Tolnaftate (Tinactin) [OTC] **Uses:** Tinea pedis, tinea cruris, tinea corporis, tinea manus, tinea versicolor **Action:** Topical antifungal **Dose:** Apply to area bid for 2–4 wk **Caution:** [C, ?] **Contra:** Nail and scalp infections **Supplied:** OTC 1% liq; gel; powder; cream; soln **SE:** Local irritation **Notes:** Avoid ocular contact, infection should improve in 7–10 d

Tolterodine (Detrol, Detrol LA) **Uses:** Overactive bladder (frequency, urgency, incontinence) **Action:** Anticholinergic **Dose:** Detrol 1–2 mg PO bid; Detrol LA 2–4 mg/d **Caution:** [C, ?/–] ↑ toxicity with CYP2D6 and 3A3/4 inhibitors **Contra:** Urinary retention, gastric retention, or uncontrolled narrow-angle glaucoma **Supplied:** Tabs 1, 2 mg; Detrol LA tabs 2, 4 mg **SE:** Dry mouth, blurred vision **Notes:** Significant drug interactions with CYP2D6, CYP3A3/4 substrates

Topiramate (Topamax) **Uses:** Adjunctive treatment for complex partial seizures and tonic-clonic seizures, bipolar disorder, neuropathic pain, migraine prophylaxis **Action:** Anticonvulsant **Dose:** Seizures: Total dose 400 mg/d PO. Migraine prophylaxis:

Total dose 100 mg/d PO. See product information for 8-wk titration schedule; ↓ dose in renal failure **Caution:** [C, ?/–] May cause metabolic acidosis, thus requiring monitoring **Supplied:** Tabs 25, 100, 200 mg; caps sprinkles 15, 25, 50 mg **SE:** May precipitate kidney stones; fatigue, dizziness, psychomotor slowing, memory impairment, GI upset, tremor, nystagmus; acute secondary angle closure glaucoma requiring drug discontinuation **Notes:** May be associated with weight loss; metabolic acidosis generally responsive to dose reduction or discontinue; discontinuation requires taper

Topotecan (Hycamtin) **WARNING:** Chemotherapy precautions, bone marrow suppression possible **Uses:** Ovarian CA (cisplatin-refractory), small cell lung CA, sarcoma **Action:** Topoisomerase I inhibitor; interferes with DNA synthesis **Dose:** 1.5 mg/m²/d as a 1-h IV inf for 5 consecutive d, repeated q3wk; ↓ dose in renal failure **Caution:** [D, –] **Supplied:** 4 mg vials **SE:** Myelosuppression, N/V/D, drug fever, skin rash

Torsemide (Demadex) **Uses:** Edema, HTN, CHF, and hepatic cirrhosis **Action:** Loop diuretic; inhibits reabsorption of sodium and chloride in ascending loop of Henle and distal tubule **Dose:** 5–20 mg/d PO or IV **Caution:** [B, ?] **Contra:** Sulfonylurea sensitivity **Supplied:** Tabs 5, 10, 20, 100 mg; inj 10 mg/mL **SE:** Orthostatic hypotension, HA, dizziness, photosensitivity, electrolyte imbalance, blurred vision, renal impairment **Notes:** 20 mg torsemide equivalent to 40 mg furosemide

Tramadol (Ultram) **Uses:** Moderate/severe pain **Action:** Centrally acting analgesic **Dose:** 50–100 mg PO q4–6h PRN, not to exceed 400 mg/d **Caution:** [C, ?/–] **Contra:** Opioid dependency; MAOIs **Supplied:** Tabs 50 mg **SE:** Dizziness, HA, somnolence, GI upset, respiratory depression, anaphylaxis (sensitivity to codeine) **Notes:** Lowers seizure threshold, tolerance or dependence may develop

Tramadol/Acetaminophen (Ultracet) **Uses:** Short-term management of acute pain (< 5 d) **Action:** Centrally acting analgesic; nonnarcotic analgesic **Dose:** 2 tab PO q4–6h PRN; 8 tab/d max; *Elderly/renal impairment:* Use lowest possible dose; 2 tab q12h max if CrCl < 30 **Caution:** [C, –] Seizures, hepatic/renal impairment, or history of addictive tendencies **Contra:** Acute intoxication **Supplied:** Tabs 37.5 mg tramadol/325 mg APAP **SE:** SSRIs, TCAs, opioids, MAOIs increase risk of seizures; dizziness, somnolence, tremor, headache, N/V/D, constipation, dry mouth, liver toxicity, rash, pruritus, increased sweating, physical dependence **Notes:** Avoid alcohol use

Trandolapril (Mavik) [See Table VII–3, p 614]

Trastuzumab (Herceptin) **Uses:** Treatment of metastatic breast cancer tumors that overexpress the HER2/neu protein **Actions:** Monoclonal antibody binds to the human epidermal growth factor receptor 2 protein (HER2); mediates cellular cytotoxicity **Dose:** Refer to specific protocol **Caution:** [B, ?] CV dysfunction, hypersensitivity/infusion reactions **Supplied** 440-mg vial **SE:** Anemia, cardiomyopathy, nephrotic syndrome, pneumonitis **Notes:** Infusion-related reactions should be minimized with acetaminophen, diphenhydramine, and meperidine

Trazodone (Desyrel) **WARNING:** *Pediatric:* Antidepressants may increase risk of suicidality; consider risks and benefits of use. Patients should be closely monitored for clinical worsening, suicidality, or unusual changes in behavior **Uses:** Depression, hypnotic, augment other antidepressants **Action:** Antidepressant; inhibits reuptake of serotonin and norepinephrine **Dose:** 50–150 mg PO qd–qid; max 600 mg/d *Sleep:* 50 mg PO, qhs, PRN **Caution:** [C, ?/–] **Supplied:** Tabs 50, 100, 150, 300 mg **SE:** Dizziness, HA, sedation, nausea, xerostomia, syncope, confusion, tremor, hepatitis, extrapyramidal reactions **Notes:** May take 1–2 wk for symptomatic improvement; may interact with CYP3A4 inhibitors to increase conc, carbamazepine to decrease trazodone conc

Treprostinil Sodium (Remodulin) **Uses:** NYHA Class II-IV pulmonary arterial hypertension **Action:** Vasodilation, inhibition of platelet aggregation **Dose:** 0.625-1.25 ng/kg/min continuous infusion **Caution:** [B, ?/–] **Supplied:** 1, 2.5, 5, 10 mg/mL injection **SE:** Additive effects with anticoagulants, antihypertensives; infusion site reactions **Notes:** Initiate in monitored setting; do not discontinue or reduce dose abruptly

Tretinoin, Topical [Retinoic Acid] (Retin-A, Avita, Renova)
Uses: Acne vulgaris, sun-damaged skin, wrinkles (photo aging), some skin CAs **Action:** Exfoliant retinoic acid derivative **Dose:** Apply qd hs (if irritation develops, ↓ frequency) *Photoaging:* Start with 0.025%, increase to 0.1% over several months (apply only every 3 d if on neck area; dark skin may require bid application) **Caution:** [C, ?] **Contra:** Retinoid sensitivity **Supplied:** Cream 0.025, 0.05, 0.1%; gel 0.01, 0.025, 0.1%; microformulation gel 0.1%; liq 0.05% **SE:** Avoid sunlight; edema; skin dryness, erythema, scaling, changes in pigmentation, stinging, photosensitivity

Triamcinolone (Azmacort)
Uses: Chronic treatment of asthma **Actions:** Topical steroid **Dose:** Two inhalations tid–qid or 4 inhalations bid **Caution:** [C, ?] **SE:** Cough, oral candidiasis **Supplied:** *Inhaler:* 100 mcg/metered spray **Notes:** Instruct patients to rinse mouth after use; not for acute asthma

Triamcinolone and Nystatin (Mycolog-II)
Uses: Cutaneous candidiasis **Action:** Antifungal and anti-inflammatory **Dose:** Apply lightly to area bid; max 25 d **Caution:** [C, ?] **Contra:** Varicella; systemic fungal infections **Supplied:** Cream and oint 15, 30, 60, 120 mg **SE:** Local irritation, hypertrichosis, changes in pigmentation **Notes:** For short-term use (< 7 d)

Triamterene (Dyrenium)
Uses: Edema associated with CHF, cirrhosis **Action:** Potassium-sparing diuretic **Dose:** 100–300 mg/24 h PO ÷ qd–bid; ↓ dose in renal/hepatic impairment **Caution:** [B (manufacturer; D expert opinion), ?/–] **Contra:** Hyperkalemia, renal impairment, diabetes; caution with other potassium-sparing diuretics **Supplied:** Caps 50, 100 mg **SE:** Hyperkalemia, blood dyscrasias, liver damage, and other reactions

Triazolam (Halcion) [C-IV]
Uses: Short-term management of insomnia **Action:** Benzodiazepine **Dose:** 0.125–0.25 mg/d PO hs PRN; ↓ dose in elderly **Caution:** [X, ?/–] **Contra:** Narrow-angle glaucoma; cirrhosis; concurrent amprenavir, ritonavir, or nelfinavir **Supplied:** Tabs 0.125, 0.25 mg **SE:** Tachycardia, chest pain, drowsiness, fatigue, memory impairment, GI upset **Notes:** Additive CNS depression with alcohol and other CNS depressants

Triethanolamine (Cerumenex) [OTC]
Uses: Cerumen (ear wax) removal **Action:** Ceruminolytic agent **Dose:** Fill the ear canal and insert the cotton plug; irrigate with water after 15 min; repeat PRN **Caution:** [C, ?] **Contra:** Perforated tympanic membrane, otitis media **Supplied:** Soln 6, 12 mL **SE:** Local dermatitis, pain, erythema, pruritus

Triethylene-Triphosphamide (Thio-Tepa, Tespa, TSPA)
Uses: Hodgkin's lymphoma and NHL; leukemia; breast, ovarian, and bladder CAs (IV and intravesical therapy), preparative regimens for allogeneic and autologous BMT in high doses **Action:** Polyfunctional alkylating agent **Dose:** 0.5 mg/kg q1–4wk, 6 mg/m² IM or IV×4 d q2–4wk, 15–35 mg/m² by cont IV inf over 48 h; 60 mg into the bladder and retained 2 h q1–4wk; 900–125 mg/m² in ABMT regimens (the highest dose that can be administered without ABMT is 180 mg/m²); 1–10 mg/m² (typically 15 mg) intravesically once or twice a wk; 0.8 mg/kg in 1–2 L of soln may be instilled intraperitoneally; ↓ dose in renal failure **Caution:** [D, –] **Supplied:** Inj 15 mg **SE:** Myelosuppression, N/V, dizziness, HA, allergy, paresthesias, alopecia

Trifluoperazine (Stelazine)
Uses: Psychotic disorders **Action:** Phenothiazine; blocks postsynaptic CNS dopaminergic receptors in the brain **Dose:** 2–10 mg PO bid; ↓ dose in elderly/debilitated patients **Caution:** [C, ?/–] **Contra:** History of blood dyscrasias; phenothiazine sensitivity **Supplied:** Tabs 1, 2, 5, 10 mg; oral conc 10 mg/mL; inj 2 mg/mL **SE:** Orthostatic hypotension, EPS, dizziness, neuroleptic malignant syndrome, skin discoloration, lowered seizure threshold, photosensitivity, blood dyscrasias **Notes:** Oral conc must be diluted to 60 mL or more before administration; requires several weeks for onset of effects

Trifluridine (Viroptic)
Uses: Herpes simplex keratitis and conjunctivitis **Action:** Antiviral **Dose:** 1 drops q2h (max 9 drops/d); ↓ to 1 drop q4h after healing begins; treat up to 14 d **Caution:** [C, M] **Supplied:** Soln 1% **SE:** Local burning, stinging

Trihexyphenidyl (Artane) Uses: **Parkinson's disease** Action: Blocks excess acetylcholine at cerebral synapses Dose: 2–5 mg PO qd–qid Caution: [C, +] Contra: Narrow-angle glaucoma, GI obstruction, myasthenia gravis, bladder obstructions Supplied: Tabs 2, 5 mg; SR caps 5 mg; elixir 2 mg/5 mL SE: Dry skin, constipation, xerostomia, photosensitivity, tachycardia, arrhythmias

Trimethobenzamide (Tigan) Uses: **N/V** Action: Inhibits medullary chemoreceptor trigger zone Dose: 250 mg PO or 200 mg PR or IM tid–qid PRN Caution: [C, ?] Contra: Benzocaine sensitivity Supplied: Caps 100, 250 mg; supp 100, 200 mg; inj 100 mg/mL SE: Drowsiness, hypotension, dizziness; hepatic impairment, blood dyscrasias, seizures Notes: In the presence of viral infections, may mask emesis or mimic CNS effects of Reye syndrome; may cause parkinsonian-like syndrome

Trimethoprim (Trimpex, Proloprim) Uses: **UTI due to susceptible gram(+) and gram(−) organisms; suppression of UTI** Action: Inhibits dihydrofolate reductase Dose: 100 mg/d PO bid or 200 mg/d PO; ↓ dose in renal failure Caution: [C, +] Contra: Megaloblastic anemia due to folate deficiency Supplied: Tabs 100, 200 mg; oral soln 50 mg/5 mL SE: Rash, pruritus, megaloblastic anemia, hepatic impairment, blood dyscrasias Notes: Take with plenty of water

Trimethoprim (TMP)–Sulfamethoxazole (SMX) [Co-Trimoxazole] (Bactrim, Septra) Uses: **UTI treatment and prophylaxis, otitis media, sinusitis, bronchitis** Action: SMX-inhibiting synthesis of dihydrofolic acid; TMP-inhibiting dihydrofolate reductase to impair protein synthesis *Spectrum:* includes *Shigella*, *P carinii*, and *Nocardia* infections, *Mycoplasma, Enterobacter sp, Staphylococcus, Streptococcus,* and more Dose: 1 DS tab PO bid or 5–20 mg/kg/24 h (based on TMP) IV in 3–4 ÷ doses *P carinii:* 15–20 mg/kg/d IV or PO (TMP) in 4 ÷ doses *Nocardia:* 10–15 mg/kg/d IV or PO (TMP) in 4 ÷ doses *UTI prophylaxis:* 1 PO qd; ↓ dose in renal failure; maintain hydration Caution: [B (D if near term), +] Contra: Sulfonamide sensitivity, porphyria, megaloblastic anemia with folate deficiency, significant hepatic impairment Supplied: Regular tabs 80 mg TMP/400 mg SMX; DS tabs 160 mg TMP/800 mg SMX; oral susp 40 mg TMP/200 mg SMX/5 mL; inj 80 mg TMP/ 400 mg SMX/5 mL SE: Allergic skin reactions, photosensitivity, GI upset, Stevens-Johnson syndrome, blood dyscrasias, hepatitis Notes: Synergistic combination, interacts with warfarin

Trimetrexate (Neutrexin) WARNING: Must be used with leucovorin to avoid toxicity Uses: **Moderate to severe PCP** Action: Inhibits dihydrofolate reductase Dose: 45 mg/m^2 IV q24h for 21 d; ↓ in hepatic impairment Caution: [D, ?/−] Contra: Methotrexate sensitivity Supplied: Inj SE: Use cytotoxic cautions; infuse over 60 min; seizure, fever, rash, GI upset, anemias, and ↑ LFTs, peripheral neuropathy, renal impairment Notes: Administer with leucovorin 20 mg/m^2 IV q6h for 24 d

Triptorelin (Trelstar Depot, Trelstar LA) Uses: **Palliation of advanced prostate CA** Action: ↓ Gonadotropin secretion when given continuously; following 1st administration, there is a transient surge in LH, FSH, testosterone, and estradiol. After chronic/continuous administration (usually 2–4 wk), a sustained decrease in LH and FSH secretion and marked reduction of testicular and ovarian steroidogenesis are observed. A reduction of serum testosterone similar to surgical castration Dose: 3.75 mg IM monthly or 11.25 mg IM q3mo Caution: [X, NA] Contra: Not indicated in females Supplied: Injection depot 3.75 mg; long-acting 11.25 mg SE: Dizziness, emotional lability, fatigue, headache, insomnia HTN, diarrhea, vomiting, impotence, urinary retention, urinary tract infection, pruritus, anemia, injection site pain, musculoskeletal pain, allergic reactions

Trovafloxacin (Trovan) Uses: **Life-threatening infections including pneumonia, complicated intra-abdominal, gynecologic/pelvic, or skin infections** Action: Fluoroquinolone antibiotic inhibits DNA gyrase Dose: 200 mg/d; dosage reduction in hepatic impairment Caution: [C, −] Use with caution in children Contra: Hepatic impairment Supplied: Injection 5 mg/mL in 40 and 60 mL; tablets 100, 200 mg SE: Liver failure, dizziness, HA, N, rash Notes: Use restricted to hospitals; hepatotoxicity led to restricted availability

Urokinase (Abbokinase)   Uses: PE, DVT, restore patency to IV catheters   Action: Converts plasminogen to plasmin that causes clot lysis   Dose: *Systemic effect:* 4400 units/kg IV over 10 min, followed by 4400–6000 units/kg/h for 12 h *Restore catheter patency:* Inject 5000 units into catheter and gently aspirate   Caution: [B, +]   Contra: Do not use within 10 d of surgery, delivery, or organ biopsy; bleeding, CVA, vascular malformation   Supplied: Powder for inj 5000 units/mL, 250,000 units vial   SE: Bleeding, hypotension, dyspnea, bronchospasm, anaphylaxis, cholesterol embolism

Valacyclovir (Valtrex)   Uses: Herpes zoster; genital herpes   Action: Prodrug of acyclovir, inhibits viral DNA replication *Spectrum:* Herpes simplex I and II   Dose: 1 g PO tid *Genital herpes:* 500 mg bid × 7 d *Herpes prophylaxis:* 500–1000 mg/d; ↓ dose in renal failure   Caution: [B, +]   Supplied: Caps 500 mg   SE: HA, GI upset, dizziness, pruritus, photophobia

Valdecoxib (Bextra) [See Table VII–11, pp 621–22]

Valganciclovir (Valcyte)   Uses: Treatment of CMV   Action: Ganciclovir prodrug, inhibits viral DNA synthesis   Dose: Induction, 900 mg PO bid with food × 21 d, then 900 mg PO qd; dose adjustment in renal dysfunction   Caution: [C, ?/–] Use with imipenem/cilastatin, nephrotoxic drugs   Contra: Hypersensitivity to acyclovir, ganciclovir, valganciclovir; ANC < 500/m^2; platelets < 25,000; Hgb < 8 g/dL   Supplied: Tabs 450 mg   SE: Bone marrow suppression   Notes: Requires frequent CBCs; renal function monitoring required

Valproic Acid (Depakene, Depakote)   Uses: Treatment of epilepsy, mania; prophylaxis of migraines, Alzheimer's behavior disorder   Action: Anticonvulsant; increases the availability of GABA   Dose: *Seizures:* 30–60 mg/kg/24 h PO ÷ tid (after initiation of 10–15 mg/kg/24 h) *Mania:* 750 mg in 3 ÷ doses, ↑ 60 mg/kg/d max *Migraines:* 250 mg bid, ↑ 1000 mg/d max; ↓ dose in hepatic impairment   Caution: [D, +]   Contra: Hepatic impairment   Supplied: Caps 250 mg; syrup 250 mg/5 mL   SE: Monitor LFTs and serum levels (Table VII–17, p 000); phenobarbital and phenytoin may alter levels; somnolence, dizziness, GI upset, diplopia, ataxia, rash, thrombocytopenia, hepatitis, pancreatitis, prolonged bleeding times, alopecia, weight gain, hyperammonemic encephalopathy reported in patients with urea cycle disorders

Valrubicin (Valstar)   Uses: Intravesical treatment of BCG-refractory bladder carcinoma-in-situ when immediate cystectomy would be associated with unacceptable morbidity or mortality   Action: Semisynthetic doxorubicin analogue; cytotoxic   Doses: Refer to specific protocol   Caution: [C,?/–]   Contra: Bladder capacity of < 75 mL or active UTI; Do *not* use within 1–2 weeks of biopsy as systemic absorption can cause myelosuppression   Supplied: 40 mg/mL 5-mL vial   SE: Local bladder symptoms; neutropenia, GI effects, fever more common with intraperitoneal use   Notes: Dilute 800 mg in approximately 75 mL normal saline. Minimal systemic absorption with intact bladder

Valsartan (Diovan) [See Table VII–4, p 615]

Valsartan/Hydochlorothiazide(Diovan HCT) [See Table VII–4, p 615]

Vancomycin (Vancocin, Vancoled)   Uses: Serious MRSA infections; enterococcal infections; oral treatment of *C difficile* pseudomembranous colitis   Action: Inhibits cell wall synthesis *Spectrum:* Gram(+) bacteria and some anaerobes (includes MRSA, *Staphylococcus* sp, *Enterococcus* sp, *Streptococcus* sp, *C difficile*)   Dose: 1 g IV q12h; for colitis 125–500 mg PO q6h; ↓ in renal insufficiency   Caution: [C, M]   Supplied: Caps 125, 250 mg; powder for oral soln; powder for inj 500 mg, 1000 mg, 10 g/vial   SE: ↓ in renal insufficiency (for drug levels, Table VII–18, p 000). Ototoxic and nephrotoxic; GI upset (oral), neutropenia   Notes: Not absorbed PO, local effect in gut only; give IV dose slowly (over 1–3 h) to prevent "red-man syndrome" (a red flushing of the head, neck and upper torso); IV product may be given PO for colitis

Vardenafil (Levitra)   WARNING: May prolong QTc interval   Uses: Erectile dysfunction   Action: Phosphodiesterase 5 inhibitor   Dose: 10 mg PO 60 min before sexual activity; 2.5 mg if administered with CYP3A4 inhibitors; administer no more than once daily or in doses greater than 20 mg **Caution:** [B, –] **Contra:** Nitrates **Supplied:** 2.5-mg, 5-mg, 10-mg, 20-mg tabs **SE:** Hypotension, headache, dyspepsia, priapism **Notes:** Concomitant α-blockers may cause hypotension; caution in patients with cardiovascular, hepatic or renal disease

Varicella Virus Vaccine (Varivax)

Uses: Prevention of varicella (chickenpox) infection **Action:** Active immunization **Dose:** 0.5 mL SC, repeated in 4–8 wk **Caution:** [C, M] **Contra:** Immunocompromise; neomycin-anaphylactoid reaction, blood dyscrasias; immunosuppressive drugs; avoid pregnancy for 3 mo after injection **Supplied:** Powder for inj **SE:** Live attenuated virus; may cause mild varicella infection; fever, local reactions, irritability, GI upset **Notes:** Recommended for all patients who have not had chickenpox

Vasopressin [Antidiuretic Hormone, ADH] (Pitressin)

Uses: Diabetes insipidus; postop treatment of abdominal distention; adjunct treatment of GI bleeding and esophageal varices; pulseless VT and VF, adjunct systemic vasopressor (IV drip) **Action:** Posterior pituitary hormone, potent GI vasoconstrictor, potent peripheral vasoconstrictor **Dose:** *Diabetes insipidus:* 2.5–10 units SC or IM tid–qid *GI hemorrhage:* 0.2–0.4 units/min; ↓ dose in cirrhosis; caution in vascular disease *VT/VF:* 40 units IVP× 1 *Vasopressor:* 0.01–0.1 units/kg/min **Caution:** [B, +] **Contra:** hypersensitivity **Supplied:** Inj 20 units/mL **SE:** HTN, arrhythmias, fever, vertigo, GI upset, tremor **Notes:** Addition of vasopressor to concurrent norepinephrine or epinephrine infusions

Vecuronium (Norcuron)

Uses: Skeletal muscle relaxation during surgery or mechanical ventilation **Action:** Nondepolarizing neuromuscular blocker **Dose:** 0.08–0.1 mg/kg IV bolus; maint 0.010–0.015 mg/kg after 25–40 min; additional doses q12–15min PRN; ↓ dose in severe renal/hepatic impairment **Caution:** [C, ?] Drug interactions causing ↑ effect of vecuronium (e.g., aminoglycosides, tetracycline, succinylcholine) **Supplied:** Powder for inj 10 mg **SE:** Bradycardia, hypotension, itching, rash, tachycardia, CV collapse **Notes:** Fewer cardiac effects than with pancuronium

Venlafaxine (Effexor)

WARNING: *Pediatric:* Antidepressants may increase risk of suicidality; consider risks and benefits of use. Patients should be closely monitored for clinical worsening, suicidality, or unusual changes in behavior **Uses:** Depression, generalized anxiety, social anxiety disorder; OCD, chronic fatigue syndrome, ADHD, autism **Action:** Potentiation of CNS neurotransmitter activity **Dose:** 75–375 mg/d PO ÷ into 2–3 equal doses; ↓ dose in renal/hepatic impairment **Caution:** [C, ?/–] **Contra:** MAOIs **Supplied:** Tabs 25, 37.5, 50, 75, 100 mg; ER caps 37.5, 75, 150 mg **SE:** HTN, HA, somnolence, GI upset, sexual dysfunction; actuates mania or seizures **Notes:** Avoid alcohol, can ↑ mean heart rate

Verapamil (Calan, Isoptin)

Uses: Angina, HTN, PSVT, AF, atrial flutter, migraine prophylaxis, hypertrophic cardiomyopathy, bipolar disorder **Action:** Ca^{2+} channel blocker **Dose:** *Arrhythmias:* 2nd line for PSVT with narrow QRS complex and adequate BP 2.5–5 mg IV over 1–2 min; repeat 5–10 mg in 15–30 min PRN (30 mg max) *Angina:* 80–120 mg PO tid, ↑ 480 mg/24 h max *HTN:* 80–180 mg PO tid or SR tabs 120–240 mg PO qd to 240 mg bid; ↓ dose in renal/hepatic impairment **Caution:** [C, +] Amiodarone/β-blockers/flecainide can cause bradycardia; statins, midazolam, tacrolimus, theophylline levels may be increased **Contra:** Conduction disorders, cardiogenic shock; caution with elderly patients **Supplied:** Tabs 40, 80, 120 mg; SR tabs 120, 180, 240 mg; SR caps 120, 180, 240, 360 mg; inj 5 mg/2 mL **SE:** Gingival hyperplasia, constipation, hypotension, bronchospasm, heart rate or conduction disturbances

Vinblastine (Velban, Velbe)

WARNING: Chemotherapeutic agent; handle with caution **Uses:** Hodgkin's and NHLs, mycosis fungoides, CAs (testis, renal cell, breast, non–small cell lung, AIDS-related Kaposi's sarcoma, choriocarcinoma), histiocytosis **Action:** Inhibits microtubule assembly through binding to tubulin **Dose:** 0.1–0.5 mg/kg/wk (4–20 mg/m²); ↓ dose in hepatic failure **Caution:** [D, ?] **Contra:** Intrathecal use **Supplied:** Inj 1 mg/mL **SE:** Myelosuppression (especially leukopenia), N/V (rare), constipation, neurotoxicity (like vincristine but less frequent), alopecia, rash; myalgia, tumor pain

Vincristine (Oncovin, Vincasar PFS) WARNING: Chemotherapeutic agent; handle with caution ***Fatal if administered intrathecally*** Uses: **ALL, breast and small cell lung carcinoma, sarcoma (e.g., Ewing's, rhabdomyosarcoma), Wilms' tumor, Hodgkin's lymphoma and NHL, neuroblastoma, multiple myeloma** Action: Promotes disassembly of mitotic spindle, causing metaphase arrest Dose: $0.4–1.4$ mg/m^2 (single doses 2 mg/max); ↓ dose in hepatic failure Caution: [D, ?] Contra: Intrathecal use Supplied: Inj 1 mg/mL SE: Neurotoxicity commonly dose limiting, jaw pain (trigeminal neuralgia), fever, fatigue, anorexia, constipation and paralytic ileus, bladder atony; no significant myelosuppression with standard doses; soft tissue necrosis possible with extravasation

Vinorelbine (Navelbine) WARNING: Chemotherapeutic agent; handle with caution Uses: **Breast and non–small cell lung CA** (alone or with cisplatin) Action: Inhibits polymerization of microtubules, impairing mitotic spindle formation; semisynthetic vinca alkaloid Dose: 30 mg/m^2/wk; ↓ dose in hepatic failure Caution: [D, ?] Contra: Intrathecal use Supplied: Inj 10 mg SE: Myelosuppression (especially leukopenia), mild GI effects, and infrequent neurotoxicity (6–29%); constipation and paresthesias (rare); tissue damage can result from extravasation

Vitamin B$_1$ [See Thiamine, p 596]

Vitamin B$_6$ [See Pyridoxine, p 585]

Vitamin B$_{12}$ [See Cyanocobalamin, p 524]

Vitamin K [See Phytonadione, p 581]

Voriconazole (VFEND) Uses: **Invasive aspergillosis, serious fungal infections** Action: Inhibits ergosterol synthesis Spectrum: Several types of fungus including *Aspergillus, Scedosporium* sp, *Fusarium* sp Dose: IV: 6 mg/kg q12h × 2, then 4 mg/kg bid; may reduce to 3 mg/kg per dose PO: < 40 kg: 100 mg q 12h, up to 150 mg; > 40 kg: 200 mg q 12 h, up to 300 mg; ↓ dose in mild/moderate hepatic impairment; IV only one dose in renal impairment/ESRD Caution: [D, ?/–] Contra: Severe hepatic impairment Supplied: Tabs 50, 200 mg; 200 mg inj SE: Visual changes, fever, rash, GI upset, ↑ LFTs Notes: Must screen for multiple drug interactions (e.g., increase dose when given with phenytoin); administer oral doses on empty stomach

Warfarin (Coumadin) Uses: **Prophylaxis and treatment of PE and DVT, AF with embolization, other postoperative indications** Action: Inhibits vitamin K-dependent production of clotting factors in the order VII-IX-X-II Dose: Adjust to keep INR 2.0–3.0 for most; mechanical valves INR is 2.5–3.5 *ACCP guidelines:* 5–7.5 mg initially (unless rapid therapeutic INR needed); use ≤ 5 mg if patient is elderly or has other bleeding risk factors ↓. *Alternate:* 10–15 mg PO, IM, or IV qd for 1–3 d; maintenance 2–10 mg/d PO, IV, or IM; follow daily INR initially to adjust dosage; monitor vitamin K intake; consider ↓ doses in hepatic impairment or elderly Caution: [X, +] Contra: Severe hepatic or renal disease, bleeding, peptic ulcer, pregnancy Supplied: Tabs 1, 2, 2.5, 3, 4, 5, 6, 7.5, 10 mg; inj SE: Bleeding caused by overanticoagulation (PT > 3 control or INR > 5.0–6.0) or injury and INR within therapeutic range Notes: INR preferred test; to rapidly correct overcoumadinization, use vitamin K, FFP or both; highly teratogenic; do not use in pregnancy. Caution patient on taking warfarin with other meds, especially ASA *Common warfarin interactions:* Potentiated by APAP, alcohol (with liver disease), amiodarone, cimetidine, ciprofloxacin, cotrimoxazole, erythromycin, fluconazole, flu vaccine, isoniazid, itraconazole, metronidazole, omeprazole, phenytoin, propranolol, quinidine, tetracycline. Inhibited by barbiturates, carbamazepine, chlordiazepoxide, cholestyramine, dicloxacillin, nafcillin, rifampin, sucralfate, high vitamin K foods; bleeding, alopecia, skin necrosis, purple toe syndrome

Zafirlukast (Accolate) Uses: **Adjunctive treatment of asthma** Action: Selective and competitive inhibitor of leukotrienes Dose: 20 mg bid (empty stomach) Caution: [B, –] Interacts with warfarin to ↑ INR Supplied: Tabs 20 mg SE: Hepatic dysfunction, usually reversible on discontinuation; HA, dizziness, GI upset; Churg-Strauss syndrome Notes: Not for acute asthma; take on empty stomach

Zalcitabine (Hivid) WARNING: Use with caution in patients with neuropathy, pancreatitis, lactic acidosis, hepatitis Uses: **HIV** Action: Antiretroviral agent Dose: 0.75 mg PO tid; ↓ dose in renal failure Caution: [C, +] Supplied: Tabs 0.375, 0.75 mg SE: Peripheral neuropathy, pancreatitis, fever, malaise, anemia, hypo-/hyperglycemia, hepatic impairment Notes: May be used in combination with zidovudine

Zaleplon (Sonata) Uses: **Insomnia** Action: A nonbenzodiazepine sedative hypnotic, a pyrazolopyrimidine Dose: 5–20 mg hs PO PRN; ↓ dose in renal/hepatic insufficiency, elderly Caution: [C, ?/–] Caution in mental/psychological conditions Supplied: Caps 5, 10 mg SE: HA, edema, amnesia, somnolence, photosensitivity Notes: Take immediately before desired onset

Zanamivir (Relenza) Uses: **Influenza A and B** Action: Inhibits viral neuraminidase Dose: 2 inhal (10 mg) bid for 5 d; initiate within 48 h of symptoms Caution: [C, M] Contra: Pulmonary disease Supplied: Powder for inhal 5 mg SE: Bronchospasm, HA, GI upset Notes: Uses a Diskhaler for administration

Zidovudine (Retrovir) WARNING: Neutropenia, anemia, lactic acidosis, and hepatomegaly with steatosis Uses: **HIV infection, prevention of maternal transmission of HIV** Action: Inhibits reverse transcriptase Dose: 200 mg PO tid or 300 mg PO bid or 1–2 mg/kg/dose IV q4h *Pregnancy:* 100 mg PO 5×/d until the start of labor, then during labor 2 mg/kg over 1 h followed by 1 mg/kg/h until clamping of the umbilical cord; ↓ dose in renal failure Caution: [C, ?/–] Contra: Life-threatening hypersensitivity Supplied: Caps 100 mg; tabs 300 mg; syrup 50 mg/5 mL; inj 10 mg/mL SE: Hematologic toxicity, HA, fever, rash, GI upset, malaise

Zidovudine and Lamivudine (Combivir) WARNING: Neutropenia, anemia, lactic acidosis, and hepatomegaly with steatosis Uses: **HIV infection** Action: Combination of reverse transcriptase inhibitors Dose: 1 tab bid; ↓ dose in renal failure Caution: [C, ?/–] Supplied: Caps zidovudine 300 mg/lamivudine 150 mg SE: Hematologic toxicity, HA, fever, rash, GI upset, malaise, pancreatitis Notes: Combination product decreases daily pill burden

Zileuton (Zyflo) Uses: **Chronic treatment of asthma** Action: Inhibitor of 5-lipoxygenase Dose: 600 mg PO qid Caution: [C, ?/–] Contra: Hepatic impairment Supplied: Tabs 600 mg SE: Hepatic damage, HA, GI upset, leukopenia Notes: Monitor LFTs every month × 3, then q2–3 mo; must take on a regular basis; not for acute asthma

Ziprasidone (Geodon) WARNING: A typical antipsychotics may increase risk of hyperglycemia and diabetes Uses: **Schizophrenia, acute agitation** Action: Atypical antipsychotic Dose: 20 mg PO bid with food, may increase in 2-d intervals up to 80 mg bid; agitation 10–20 mg IM PRN up to 40 mg/d. Separate 10-mg doses by 2h and 20-mg doses by 4 h Caution: [C, –] Contra: QT prolongation, recent MI, uncompensated heart failure, meds that prolong QT interval Supplied: Caps 20, 40, 60, 80 mg; Inj 20 mg/mL SE: Bradycardia; monitor electrolytes; rash, somnolence, respiratory disorder, Epstein-Barr syndrome, weight gain, orthostatic hypotension Notes: Caution in hypokalemia/hypomagnesemia

Zoledronic Acid (Zometa) Uses: **Hypercalcemia of malignancy (HCM),** ↓ skeletal-related events in prostate CA, multiple myeloma, and metastatic bone lesions Action: Bisphosphonate; inhibits osteoclastic bone resorption Dose: *HCM:* 4 mg IV over at least 15 min; may retreat in 7 d if adequate renal function *Bone lesions/myeloma:* 4 mg IV over at least 15 min repeat q3–4wk PRN; prolonged with Cr ↑ Caution: [C, ?/–] Loop diuretics, aminoglycosides; ASA-sensitive asthmatics Contra: Bisphosphonate hypersensitivity Supplied: Vial 4 mg SE: Adverse effects ↑ with renal dysfunction; fever, flu-like syndrome, GI upset, insomnia, anemia; electrolyte abnormalities; osteonecrosis of jaw Notes: Requires vigorous prehydration; do not exceed recommended doses/infusion duration to minimize dose-related renal dysfunction; follow Cr; conduct dental exam prior to initiation

Zolmitriptan (Zomig, Zomig ZMT) [see Table VII–16, p 629]

Zolpidem (Ambien) [C-IV] Uses: **Short-term treatment of insomnia** Action: Hypnotic agent Dose: 5–10 mg PO hs PRN; ↓ dose in elderly, hepatic insufficiency Cau-

tion: [B, +] **Supplied:** Tabs 5, 10 mg **SE:** HA, dizziness, drowsiness, nausea, myalgia
Notes: May be habit forming

Zonisamide (Zonegran)   Uses: **Adjunct treatment complex-partial seizures**   Ac-
tion: Anticonvulsant   **Dose:** Initial 100 mg/d PO; may ↑ to 400 mg/d   **Caution:** [C, −] ↑ Toxicity with CYP3A4 inhib; ↓ levels with concurrent carbamazepine, phenytoin, phenobarbital,
VPA   **Contra:** Hypersensitivity to sulfonamides   **Supplied:** Caps 100 mg   **SE:** Dizziness,
drowsiness, confusion, ataxia, memory impairment, paresthesias, psychosis, nystagmus,
diplopia, tremor; anemia, leukopenia; GI upset, nephrolithiasis, Stevens-Johnson syndrome;
monitor for ↓ sweating and ↑ body temperature   **Notes:** Swallow capsules whole

3. MINERALS: INDICATIONS/EFFECTS, RDA/DOSAGE, SIGNS/SYMPTOMS OF DEFICIENCY AND TOXICITY, AND OTHER

Calcium [See also p 516]   **Indications/Effects:** Strengthens bones and teeth, used
as adjunct with osteoporosis medications to promote bone rebuilding. May decrease blood
pressure, aids premenstrual symptoms (pain, cramping, mood swings)   **RDA/Dosage:** *Age
50 & under:* 1000 mg daily *Age > 50:* 1200 mg. *Postmenopausal women not taking estrogen
and men > 65 y:* 1500 mg daily. *Men and postmenopausal women taking estrogen (50–65 y):*
1000 mg daily.   **Signs/Symptoms of Deficiency:** Osteoporosis (over time) leading to increased risk of fractures.   **Signs/Symptoms of Toxicity: (> 2500 mg/d):** Constipation,
anorexia, dry mouth, nausea, polyuria, renal calculi   **Other:** Avoid calcium sources from
dolomite, oyster shell, and bone meal because they may contain heavy metal contamination
(lead, arsenic). Caffeine and cigarette smoking may reduce calcium absorption. Hyperthyroidism, diabetes mellitus, use of corticosteroids, and use of loop diuretics all either reduce
calcium absorption or increase excretion; calcium supplementation should be strongly considered in these cases. Vitamin D/calcium combination decreases fracture rate and increases absorption in elderly

Chromium   **Indications/Effects:** Required for normal glucose metabolism (trace element)   **RDA/Dosage:** 50–200 mcg   **Signs/Symptoms of Deficiency:** Rare; may cause
development of adult diabetes mellitus and atherosclerosis, peripheral neuropathy
Signs/Symptoms of Toxicity: Irritation of GI tract (nausea, vomiting, ulcers), renal damage
and eczema/dermatitis from occupational exposure   **Other:** Balanced diet fulfills RDA. Supplements may cause hypoglycemia in type I diabetics

Copper   **Indications/Effects:** Bone formation, hematopoiesis, enzyme component
RDA/Dosage: Balanced diet meets daily requirements   **Signs/Symptoms of Deficiency:**
Anemia in malnourished children.   **Signs/Symptoms of Toxicity:** Self-limiting nausea, vom-
iting, diarrhea (usually caused by occupational exposure)

Iron [See also p 556]   **Indications/Effects:** Energy transfer and carrying oxygen, prevention of microcytic anemia   **RDA/Dosage:** Adult females 10–15 mg daily (30 mg if pregnant), males 10 mg daily   **Signs/Symptoms of Deficiency:** Microcytic, hypochromic
anemia; fatigue, breathlessness, pallor, dizziness, headache   **Signs/Symptoms of Toxicity
(> 75 mg/d):** Nausea, diarrhea, abdominal pain, anorexia   **Other:** Iron may decrease the absorption of other minerals when given concomitantly. In addition, it has numerous drug interactions and should not be given at the same time as other prescribed medications (e.g.,
antacids, tetracycline). Concern exists in males of the risk of hemochromatosis when supple-
menting iron; in middle-aged men this can increase the risk of heart disease and hepatic disease. Iron is the most common cause of pediatric poisonings in the home. It is available in
numerous salt forms with differing elemental iron content

Iron Salt	Elemental Iron
Fumarate	33%
Gluconate	12%
Sulfate	20–30%

Magnesium [See also p 562] Indications/Effects: Strengthens bones and teeth, reduces neurologic irritability in patients at risk for seizures (e.g., eclampsia), may reduce premenstrual symptoms (headache, fluid retention, mood changes), maintains normal sinus rhythm **RDA/Dosage:** 200–400 mg (1 g = 82.3 mEq) **Signs/Symptoms of Deficiency:** Weakness, confusion, tingling, muscle contractions, cramps **Signs/Symptoms of Toxicity (> 350 mg/d):** Diarrhea, nausea, drowsiness, lethargy, sweating, slurred speech

Selenium Indications/Effects: Decreases risk of heart disease (antioxidant), essential for normal function of immune system and thyroid gland **RDA/Dosage:** *Women:* 55 mcg *Men:* 70 mcg **Signs/Symptoms of Deficiency:** Rare, due to TPN or GI malabsorptive diseases; can cause cardiomyopathy ("Keshan disease") **Signs/Symptoms of Toxicity (> 400 mg/d):** *Selenosis:* GI upset, hair loss, white-blotchy nails, mild nerve damage **Other:** Balanced diet meets RDA requirements (dietary source: plant foods)

Zinc Indications/Effects: Supplementation strengthens immune system if patient is zinc deficient; may prevent macular degeneration; may improve cognition. Zinc supports normal growth and development during pregnancy, childhood, and adolescence **RDA/Dosage:** *Females:* 12 mg *Males:* 10 mg **Signs/Symptoms of Deficiency:** Impaired night vision, immune function, taste; also poor appetite, poor growth, delayed wound healing, anemia, hyperplasia, hepatosplenomegaly. **Signs/Symptoms of Toxicity (> 100–450 mg/d):** Altered iron function, reduced immune function, lowered HDL levels, GI intolerance, anemia, copper deficiency **Other:** High calcium intake (> 1400 mg/d) reduces zinc absorption, requiring increased zinc intake of 18 mg/d

4. NATURAL PRODUCTS: USES, EFFICACY, DOSE, CAUTION, ADVERSE EFFECTS, AND DRUG INTERACTIONS

Black Cohosh Uses: Symptoms of menopause (especially hot flashes) as well as premenstrual syndrome, hypercholesterolemia, and peripheral arterial disease; has anti-inflammatory and sedative effects **Efficacy:** May have short-term benefit on menopausal symptoms **Dose:** 40—160 mg daily **Caution:** Overdose can cause nausea, vomiting, dizziness, nervous system and visual disturbances, bradycardia, and (possibly) seizures. Contraindicated in pregnancy (associated with miscarriage, premature birth) **Adverse Effects:** Nausea, dizziness, visual changes, migraine, increased sweating, hypotension **Drug Interactions:** May further reduce lipids and/or blood pressure when used with prescription medications

Chamomile Uses: Antispasmodic, sedative, anti-inflammatory, astringent, antibacterial **Dose:** 10—15 g daily (taken as 3 g dried flower heads tid–qid between meals; can steep in 250 mL hot water) **Caution:** Avoid use if allergic to chrysanthemums, ragweed, asters (family *Compositae*) **Adverse Effects:** Contact dermatitis, hypersensitivity reaction (allergy, anaphylaxis) if allergic to ragweed **Drug Interactions:** Monitor anticoagulant levels due to additive anticoagulant effects. Additive with other medications that cause sedation (benzodiazepines). Chamomile can cause delayed gastric absorption of medications if concomitantly administered, owing to altered GI motility

Cranberry (*Vaccinium macrocarpon*) Uses: Prevention and treatment of urinary tract infections **Efficacy:** Possibly effective **Dose:** 150 mg/d **Caution:** May increase risk of kidney stones in susceptible individuals **Adverse Effects:** None known **Drug Interactions:** May increase risk of bleeding when used with warfarin

Dong Quai (*Angelica polymorpha, sinensis*) Uses: Uterine stimulant; menstrual cramps, irregular menses, and menopausal symptoms; an anti-inflammatory, vasodilator, CNS stimulant, immunosuppressant, analgesic, antipyretic, antiasthmatic **Efficacy:** Does not appear to be effective for menopausal symptoms **Dose:** Average daily dose of 4.5 g PO **Caution:** Avoid in pregnancy and lactation **Adverse Effects:** Diarrhea, photosensitivity, skin cancer **Drug Interactions:** Blood-thinning agents (increases INR in patients on warfarin)

Echinacea (*Echinacea purpurea*)   **Uses:** Immune system stimulant; prevention/treatment of colds, flu; as supportive therapy for colds and chronic infections of the respiratory tract and lower urinary tract   **Efficacy:** Not well established; may reduce severity and duration of upper respiratory infections   **Dose:** 6–9 mL expressed juice or 2–5 g dried root   **Caution:** Should not be used in progressive systemic or immune diseases, such as tuberculosis, collagen-vascular disorders, and multiple sclerosis. May interfere with immunosuppressive therapy. Echinacea is not recommended for use during pregnancy; should not be used for longer than 8 consecutive weeks because of possible immunosuppression   **Adverse Effects:** Nausea; rash   **Drug Interactions:** Avoid use with anabolic steroids, amiodarone, methotrexate, corticosteroids, cyclosporine

Ephedra/Ma Huang   **Uses:** Stimulant, aid in weight loss, aid in bronchial dilation   **Dose:** USE NOT RECOMMENDED DUE TO REPORTED DEATHS (> 100 mg/d can be life-threatening). US SALES BANNED BY FDA IN 2004   **Caution:** Adverse cardiac events, seizures, strokes, and death   **Adverse Effects:** Nervousness, headache, insomnia, palpitations, vomiting, hyperglycemia   **Drug Interactions:** Interacts with digoxin, antihypertensives, antidepressants, diabetic medications

Evening Primrose Oil   **Uses:** Premenstrual syndrome, diabetic neuropathy, attention deficit/hyperactivity disorder   **Efficacy:** Possibly beneficial for PMS, but not effective for menopausal symptoms   **Dose:** 2–4 g/d   **Adverse Effects:** Indigestion, nausea, soft stools, headache   **Drug Interactions:** Induces metabolism of phenobarbital, lowering seizure threshold

Feverfew (*Tanacetum parthenium*)   **Uses:** Prophylaxis and treatment of migraine; fever; menstrual disorders; arthritis; toothache; insect bites   **Efficacy:** Weak evidence for migraine prevention   **Dose:** 125 mg of dried leaf (containing at least 0.2% of parthenolide)   **Caution:** Not recommended during pregnancy   **Adverse Effects:** Occasional mouth ulceration or gastric disturbance, swollen lips, abdominal pain; long-term adverse effects are unknown   **Drug Interactions:** Aspirin and warfarin (possible increased bleeding risk)

Garlic (*Allium sativum*)   **Uses:** Antioxidant; used for hyperlipidemia and hypertension; used as anti-infective (antibacterial, antifungal); tick repellent (orally)   **Efficacy:** Lowers cholesterol by only 4–6%; modest reduction in blood pressure; possibly reduces risk of GI and prostate cancers   **Dose:** 400–1200 mg dried garlic powder (2–5 mg of allicin)   **Caution:** Do *not* use in pregnancy because of its abortifacient properties; should be discontinued at least 7 d before surgery (bleeding risk)   **Adverse Effects:** Increased serum insulin levels, decreased serum lipid and cholesterol levels, anemia, burning sensation in mouth, nausea/vomiting, diarrhea   **Drug Interactions:** Warfarin and aspirin (inhibits platelet aggregation). Additive effect with antidiabetic agents may lead to hypoglycemia. CYP4503A4 inducer (may decrease cyclosporine, HIV/AIDS antivirals, oral contraceptives)

Ginger (*Zingiber officinale*)   **Uses:** Prevention of motion sickness, morning sickness, and nausea and vomiting due to anesthesia.   **Efficacy:** Demonstrated benefit in reduction of N/V from motion or pregnancy; weaker evidence for benefit postoperatively or with cancer chemotherapy   **Dose:** 1–4 g rhizome or 0.5–2 g of powdered drug daily   **Caution:** Ginger is to be used only after consultation with a physician in a patient with gallstones; excessive amounts may cause CNS depression and may interfere with cardiac function or anticoagulant activity   **Adverse Effects:** Heartburn   **Drug Interactions:** Excessive consumption of ginger (dosage not stated) may interfere with cardiac, antidiabetic, or anticoagulant therapy (inhibits platelet aggregation)

Ginkgo Biloba   **Uses:** Memory deficits, dementia, anxiety, improvement of distance and pain-free walking in peripheral occlusive vessel disease, vertigo, tinnitus, asthma/bronchospasm, antioxidant uses, premenstrual symptoms (especially breast tenderness), impotence, SSRI-induced sexual dysfunction   **Dose:** 60–80 mg standardized dry extract bid–tid   **Efficacy:** Small benefit on cognition in dementia; no demonstrated benefit in healthy adults   **Caution:** Risk of bleeding due to antagonism of platelet activating factor is a concern, especially if patient is on concomitant antiplatelet agents (discontinue 3 d before surgery); new re-

ports of possible increased risk of seizures   **Adverse Effects:** GI upset, headaches, dizziness, heart palpitations, rash   **Drug Interactions:** Aspirin, other salicylates, warfarin

Ginseng   **Uses:** "Energy booster," stress reduction, enhancement of brain activity and physical endurance (adaptogenic), antioxidant, aid in glucose control   **Efficacy:** Not well established   **Dose:** 1–2 g of root or 100–300 mg of extract (standardized to contain 7% ginsenosides) tid   **Caution:** Use with caution in patients with cardiac disorders, diabetes, hypotension, hypertension, mania, and schizophrenia, and in patients receiving corticosteroids. Avoid during pregnancy. Discontinue at least 7 d before surgery (bleeding risk)   **Adverse Effects:** Controversial "ginseng abuse syndrome" (nervousness, excitation, headache, insomnia) reported in high doses; palpitations, vaginal bleeding, breast nodules, hypoglycemia   **Drug Interactions:** Warfarin, antidepressants (augmented stimulant effect), caffeine (augmented stimulant effect), antidiabetic agents (additive hypoglycemic effect)

Glucosamine Sulfate (also called Chitosamine) and Chondroitin Sulfate
Uses: Osteoarthritis (glucosamine is the rate-limiting step in glycosaminoglycan biosynthesis and promotes cartilage rebuilding; chondroitin is a biologic polymer that acts as the flexible connecting matrix between protein filaments in cartilage and draws fluid and nutrients into joint, creating "shock absorption")   **Efficacy:** Controversial   **Dose:** Glucosamine 500 PO tid; chondroitin 400 mg tid   **Caution:** None known   **Adverse Effects:** Glucosamine may increase insulin resistance in diabetics; because these agents are concentrated in cartilage, the theory is that they are unlikely to produce severely toxic or teratogenic effects   **Drug Interactions:** Glucosamine–none known, chondroitin–monitor anticoagulant therapy

Kava Kava (Kava Kava Root Extract, *Piper methysticum*)   **Uses:** Anxiety, stress, restlessness, and insomnia   **Efficacy:** May have mild anxiolytic benefit   **Dose:** Standardized extract (70% kavalactones) 100 mg 2–3 × daily   **Caution:** Growing evidence of hepatotoxicity risk has resulted in bans in Europe and Canada. Not recommended during pregnancy and lactation. Discontinue at least 24 h before surgery (may increase sedative effect of anesthetics)   **Adverse Effects:** Mild gastrointestinal disturbances; in rare cases, allergic skin reactions can occur; may increase cholesterol; elevation of liver enzymes/jaundice; may cause rash and/or vision changes, red eyes, puffy face, muscle weakness   **Drug Interactions:** Avoid using with other sedatives, alcohol, or stimulants. Potentiation of effectiveness is possible for substances acting on the CNS, such as alcohol, barbiturates, and other psychopharmacologic agents

Melatonin   **Uses:** Insomnia, jet lag; use as antioxidant, use as immunostimulant   **Efficacy:** Sedative effects most pronounced in elderly patients with decreased endogenous melatonin levels; some evidence of benefit for jet lag   **Dose:** 1–3 mg 20 minutes before bedtime (controlled-release: administer 2 h before bedtime)   **Caution:** Use synthetic rather than product derived from animal pineal gland; avoid if patient has autoimmune disease, AIDS/HIV, or is trying to get pregnant   **Adverse Effects:** "Heavy head," headache, depression, daytime sedation, dizziness   **Drug Interactions:** β-Blockers, corticosteroids, NSAIDs, benzodiazepines

Milk Thistle *(Silybum marianum)*   **Uses:** Prophylaxis and treatment of liver damage from alcohol, toxins, cirrhosis, chronic hepatitis, fatty liver, cholestasis, and cholangitis; includes preventive use in individuals with chronic exposure to toxins (painters, farmers, chemical workers, etc)   **Efficacy:** Administration before exposure has been reported to be more effective than use after damage has occurred   **Dose:** 70–200 mg tid   **Adverse Effects:** Possible GI intolerance   **Drug Interactions:** None known

Saw Palmetto (*Serenoa repens*)   **Uses:** Treatment of benign prostatic hypertrophy (BPH) stages 1 and 2 (inhibits testosterone-5-alpha-reductase)   **Efficacy:** Small to significant benefit for prostatic symptoms (urinary flow, prostate size, sexual function)   **Dose:** 320 mg qd   **Caution:** Because of its hormonal effects, should be avoided in pregnancy, during lactation, and in women of childbearing years   **Adverse Effects:** Mild GI upset, mild headache. Large amounts may cause diarrhea   **Drug Interactions:** May increase iron absorption; may increase effects of estrogen replacement

St. John's Wort (*Hypericum perforatum*)

Uses: Mild to moderate depression and anxiety, gastritis, insomnia, vitiligo; use as anti-inflammatory; use as immune stimulant/anti-HIV/antiviral **Efficacy:** Variable; demonstrated benefit for mild/moderate depression in several well-controlled clinical trials, but not always seen in clinical practice **Dose:** 2–4 g of herb or 0.2–1.0 mg of total hypericin in standardized extract preparations daily. Commonly available preparations: 300 mg PO tid (0.3% hypericin) **Caution:** Excessive doses may potentiate existing MAOI therapy and may cause an allergic reaction. Not recommended during pregnancy **Adverse Effects:** Photosensitivity, dry mouth, dizziness, constipation, confusion **Drug Interactions:** Should not be used at the same time as prescription antidepressants, especially MAOIs. Serious drug interactions include decrease in efficacy of cyclosporine (with resultant organ rejection), digoxin (with congestive heart failure exacerbation), protease inhibitors, theophylline, and oral contraceptives. Potent cytochrome P450 3A4 enzyme inducer **Other:** Potency of St. John's wort can vary widely from one product and batch to another based on harvesting and extraction techniques. St. John's wort may result in fluctuating mood when taken chronically

Valerian (*Valeriana officinalis*)

Note: Combined with hops in commercial OTC sleep product Alluna **Uses:** Anxiolytic, sedative, restlessness, dysmenorrhea **Efficacy:** Probably effective as a sedative (shown to reduce sleep latency) **Dose:** 2–3 g extract qd–bid **Caution:** None known **Adverse Effects:** Sedation, hangover effect, headache, cardiac disturbances, and GI upset **Drug Interactions:** Use with caution when taking other sedating agents; alcohol or prescription sedatives may cause drowsiness that could impair function

Yohimbine (*Pausinystalia yohimbe*)

Uses: To improve sexual vigor (impotence) **Efficacy:** Variable **Dose:** 5 mg tid (should only be used under direction of physician) **Cautions:** May exacerbate schizophrenia or mania (if patient is predisposed). α_2-Adrenergic antagonism causes hypotension, abdominal distress, and weakness at high doses (overdose can be fatal); salivation, dilated pupils, irregular heartbeat **Adverse Effects:** Anxiety, tremors, dizziness, high blood pressure, increased heart rate. Do not use in patients with renal/hepatic diseases **Drug Interactions:** Do not combine with antidepressants, especially MAOIs or similar agents

5. UNSAFE HERBS: TOXICITY

Agent	Toxicities
Aconite	Salivation, nausea/vomiting, blurred vision, cardiac arrhythmias
Calamus	Possible carcinogenicity
Chaparral	Hepatotoxicity, possible carcinogenicity
Chinese herbal mixtures	May contain Ma huang or other dangerous herbs
Coltsfoot	Hepatotoxicity, possible carcinogenicity
Comfrey	Hepatotoxicity, carcinogenicity
Juniper	High allergy potential, diarrhea, seizures, nephrotoxicity
Licorice	Large daily amounts (> 30 g) over months can result in hypokalemia, sodium/fluid retention with resultant hypertension, myoglobinuria, and hyporeflexia
Life root	Hepatotoxicity, liver cancer
Ma-huang/ephedra	Elevated BP, MI, stroke, psychosis
Pokeweed	Severe GI cramping, nausea, diarrhea, vomiting, labored breathing, hypotension, seizures
Sassafras	Vomiting, stupor, hallucinations, dermatitis, abortion, hypothermia, liver cancer
Yohimbine	Hypotension, abdominal distress, CNS stimulation (including mania and psychosis in predisposed individuals)

6. VITAMINS: INDICATIONS/EFFECTS, RDA/DOSAGE, SIGNS/SYMPTOMS OF DEFICIENCY AND TOXICITY, AND OTHER

Vitamin A **Indications/Effects:** *General:* Healthy skin and vision, resistance to infection, bone and sperm development *Pregnancy:* Maintains healthy fetus and prevents neural tube defects, may decrease maternal transmission of AIDS to fetus **RDA/Dosage:** *Males:* 1000 mcg/d (5000 units) (900 mcg/d per IOM report*). *Females:* 800 mcg/d (4000 units) (700 mcg/d*) *Food and Nutrition Board, Institute of Medicine, the National Academies, 2001. www.iom.edu **Signs/Symptoms of Deficiency:** (Vitamin A deficiency is rare) Anemia, night blindness, diarrhea, renal calculi, tooth decay, flaking skin **Signs/Symptoms of Toxicity:** > 3000 mcg/d (= 10,000 units) can result in fatigue, night sweats, GI upset, headache, dry skin, alopecia, pruritus, and hepatotoxicity; in pregnancy can result in birth defects (head, heart, brain, spinal column); chronic, high doses may lead to bone mineral loss with subsequent osteoporotic hip fractures **Other:** Should avoid vitamin A supplements if patient smokes or drinks > 2 drinks/d

Folate (Folic Acid, Pteroylglutamic Acid) [See also p 545] Indications/Effects: *General:* Prevention of stroke, heart disease (via decreased homocysteine levels), dementia, cancer (antioxidant effect) *Pregnancy:* Prevention of neural tube defects **RDA/Dosage:** *To prevent deficiency:* Males: 200 mcg. Females: 180 mcg. *To promote health and prevent chronic disease:* 400 mcg daily. *Women of childbearing age:* 800 mcg daily to reduce the risk of spina bifida and other neural tube defects to the fetus **Signs/Symptoms of Deficiency:** Megaloblastic and macrocytic anemia, glossitis; risk of deficiency increased on methotrexate **Signs/Symptoms of Toxicity:** Few (irritability, nausea), but doses of > 1000 mcg/d can mask B_{12} deficiency **Other:** Enhances the metabolism of phenytoin

Thiamine (Vitamin B₁) [See also p 596] Indications/Effects: Carbohydrate metabolism, myocardial function **RDA/Dosage:** *Males:* 1.5 mg *Females:* 1.1 mg **Signs/Symptoms of Deficiency:** Most likely to occur in chronic alcoholics and/or those with poor nutritional intake (e.g., cachectic elderly in nursing home); peripheral neuropathy, nystagmus, confusion, ataxia, high-output heart failure. Early stages of deficiency known as Wernicke's encephalopathy, which is reversible, may progress to Korsakoff's psychosis, which is not. Dose to treat encephalopathy: 100 mg IV, then 50–100 mg IM/IV qd until normal diet resumed **Signs/Symptoms of Toxicity:** Unknown

Vitamin B₆ (Pyridoxine) [See also p 585] Indications/Effects: Reduces the severity/risk of depression, PMS, hypertension, carpal tunnel syndrome, morning sickness. May help reduce cardiovascular disease by effects on homocysteine levels **RDA/Dosage:** *Under age 50:* 1.3 mg *Age > 50:* Males 1.7 mg, females 1.5 mg **Signs/Symptoms of Deficiency:** Microcytic anemia, glossitis, cheilosis, irritability, muscle fasciculations, dermatitis, neuritis, seizures, renal calculi **Signs/Symptoms of Toxicity:** (> 2 g/d) Ataxia, distal paresthesias, muscle weakness, nerve damage **Other:** May reduce the effect of levodopa in Parkinson's disease; avoid use in these patients. Often prescribed concomitantly with isoniazid, cycloserine, or penicillamine to prevent CNS adverse effects (pyridoxine dose 10–50 mg/d)

Vitamin B₁₂ (Cyanocobalamin) [See also p 524] Indications/Effects: Prevents anemia, promotes healthy nerve conduction, decreases homocysteine accumulation, delays progression from HIV-positive status to AIDS **RDA/Dosage:** 2.4 mcg (patients > age 50 may not absorb B_{12} well when given PO so should take 100 mcg/d PO or 100–1000 mcg/mo IM if > 50 and also taking folate) **Signs/Symptoms of Deficiency:** Fatigue, nerve damage/neuropathy, dementia, depression, confusion, pernicious anemia (lack of intrinsic factor), megaloblastic anemia, glossitis, paralysis **Signs/Symptoms of Toxicity:** (> 100 mg/d) Diarrhea **Other:** Avoid megadoses of vitamin C due to destruction of vitamin B_{12}. Contraindicated in hereditary optic nerve atrophy; potassium levels may fall rapidly when replacing B_{12} at high doses. *Increased B_{12} requirements:* Pregnancy, hyperthyroidism. *Increased B_{12} excre-

tion: Alcoholics. Strict vegans (no egg/milk intake) need B_{12} supplement if not eating fortified cereals

Vitamin C (Ascorbic Acid) **Indications/Effects:** Antioxidant, healthy gums, assists in collagen formation, improves iron absorption, may improve wound healing, may shorten duration of a viral upper respiratory infection **RDA/Dosage*:** *Males:* 90 mg *Females:* 75 mg *Smokers:* Add 35 mg. *Food and Nutrition Board, Institute of Medicine, the National Academies, 2000. www.iom.edu **Signs/Symptoms of Deficiency:** Anemia, hemorrhage, muscle weakness, gum disease (scurvy), delayed wound healing, skin changes including perifollicular hyperkeratotic papules and hemorrhage and purpura **Signs/Symptoms of Toxicity (> 2000 mg/d):** Abdominal cramps, nausea, diarrhea, nosebleeds. May increase risk of renal calculi and exacerbate hemochromatosis; interferes with absorption of vitamin B_{12}

Vitamin D **Indications/Effects:** Assists in calcium and phosphorus absorption; may reduce risks of colon and breast cancer **RDA/Dosage:** Under age 50, 200 units. Age 50–70, 400 units. Over age 70, 600 units (may have difficulty with absorption) **Signs/Symptoms of Deficiency:** Osteomalacia, increased risk of fractures (especially in postmenopausal women), muscle spasms **Signs/Symptoms of Toxicity (> 1000 units/d):** Nausea, headache, fatigue, heart irregularities, anorexia, metallic taste, increased calcium levels with subsequent renal disease **Other:** Requires UV light to convert to active forms (sufficient amount of sun exposure: 5–15 minutes, 2–3 ×/wk)

Vitamin E **Indications/Effects:** Cardioprotective (decreases LDL oxidation, anticoagulant, 40% reduction in CHD on 100 units qd × 2 y), immunostimulant, protects against cataracts, slows progression of Alzheimer's disease, reduces premenstrual symptoms **RDA/Dosage:** 15 mg/33 units (although many studies use 100–400 units qd–qid for prevention of CV/CNS disease) **Signs/Symptoms of Deficiency:** Deficiency more likely on low-fat diet; may need to supplement; erythrocyte hemolysis, peripheral neuropathy **Signs/Symptoms of Toxicity (> 1000 units/d):** Can result in bleeding (inhibits platelet aggregation); this effect may occur at lower doses on warfarin. Also fatigue, headache, nausea, diarrhea, flatulence, blurred vision, dermatitis **Other:** Discontinue use before surgery because of its effects on platelet aggregation and tendon healing

Vitamin K [See also p 581] **Indications/Effects:** Enhances production of clotting factors, healthy bone formation **RDA/Dosage:** 65—80 mcg (1 mcg/kg) **Signs/Symptoms of Deficiency:** Rare, but more likely to occur in hospitalized patients, newborn infants, those on tube feedings, and/or those on antibiotics, especially sulfas; bruising, bleeding **Signs/Symptoms of Toxicity:** Usually not toxic in older children/adults **Other:** Blocks pharmacologic effects of warfarin (as a supplement and in dietary intake)

REFERENCES

Anonymous: *Dietary Reference Intakes: Applications in Dietary Assessment.* National Academy Press;2000.

Anonymous: *Review of Natural Products,* Facts & Comparisons, Inc.;2001.

Dasgupta A. Review of abnormal laboratory test results and toxic effects due to use of herbal medicines. *Am J Clin Pathol* 2003;120(1):127.

Fowler JB, German TC: The essence of herbal products for the hospital pharmacist. *Pharmacy Practice News* 2001;1:28.

Jellin J, Gregory P, Batz F (eds). Natural Medicines Comprehensive Database. Therapeutic Research Faculty; Stockton, CA (www.naturaldatabase.com). Accessed January 30, 2004.

Internet Sites: Food and Drug Administration: www.fda.gov

Medical Sites: www.drkoop.com, www.webmd.com, www.medscape.com

TABLES

TABLE VII–1. INSULINS.

Type of Insulin	Onset (hr)	Peak (hr)	Duration (hr)	Compatible to Mix With
■ **Rapid-acting**				
Aspart (Novolog)	0.25	0.5–1.5	3–5	All
Glulisine (Apidra)	0.25	0.5–1.5	3–4	All
Lispro (Humalog)	0.25	0.5–1.5	3–4	All
Regular Iletin II	0.5–1	5–10	6–8	All
Humulin R	0.5–1	5–10	6–8	All
Novolin R	0.5–1	5–10	6–8	All
■ **Intermediate-acting**				
NPH Iletin II	1–1.5	4–6	24	Regular
Humulin N	1–1.5	4–6	24	Regular
Novolin N	1–1.5	4–6	24	Regular
Lente Iletin II	1–2.5	7.5	24	Regular, Semilente
■ **Long-acting**				
Humulin U	4–8	10–30	36	Regular
Ultralente	4–8	10–30	36	Regular
Insulin Glargine (Lantus)	1–1.5	Peakless	24	Do not mix with other insulins
■ **Combinations**				
Humulin 70/30	0.5	4–8	24	
Novolin 70/30	0.5	4–8	24	

TABLE VII–2. COMPARISON OF GLUCOCORTICOIDS (also see Steroids, Systemic).

Drug (Trade)	Equivalent Dose (mg)	Anti-inflammatory Potency	Mineralocorticoid Potency
■ **Short-acting**			
Cortisone (Cortone)	25	0.8	2
Hydrocortisone (Cortef)	20	1	2
■ **Intermediate-acting**			
Methylprednisolone (Medrol)	4	5	0
Prednisone (Deltasone)	5	4	1
Prednisolone (Delta-Cortef)	5	4	1
Triamcinolone	4	5	0
■ **Long-acting**			
Betamethasone (Celestone)	0.6–0.75	20–30	0
Dexamethasone (Decadron)	0.75	20–30	0

TABLE VII–3. ANGIOTENSIN-CONVERTING ENZYME INHIBITORS.[1]

Drug (Trade)	Hypertension	Heart Failure	Left Ventricular Dysfunction
Benazepril (Lotensin)	10–40 mg/d divided q day–bid		
Captopril (Capoten)	25–50 mg bid–tid	6.25–25 mg tid	Titrate to 50 mg tid
Enalapril (Vasotec)	5–40 mg/d divided q day–bid	2.5–10 mg bid	Titrate to 10 mg bid
Fosinopril (Monopril)	10–40 mg q day	10–40 mg q day	
Lisinopril (Prinivil, Zestril)	10–40 mg q day	5–20 mg q day	
Moexipril (Univasc)	7.5–30 mg/d divided q day–bid		
Perindopril (Aceon)	4–16 mg/d	4 mg/d	
Quinapril (Accupril)	10–80 mg q day	5–20 mg bid	
Ramipril (Altace)	2.5–20 mg/d divided q day–bid	1.25–5 mg bid	
Trandolapril (Mavik)	2–8 mg/d	1 mg/d	

[1]*Notes:*
1. Pro-drugs (metabolized to active agent): Benazepril, Enalapril, Fosinopril, Moexipril, Perindopril, Quinapril, Ramipril, Trandolapril.
2. Persistent, nonproductive cough has occurred with the use of *all* ACE inhibitors. Cough typically resolves within 1–4 days after therapy is discontinued. Angiotensin-II receptor antagonists (see Table 7–4) are less frequently associated with cough.
3. Co-administration of ACE inhibitors with potassium preparations may result in elevated serum potassium concentrations.
4. Strictly contraindicated in pregnancy. Women of child-bearing age should be warned regarding risk of teratogenicity and use of ACE inhibitors.

TABLE VII–4. ANGIOTENSIN RECEPTOR ANTAGONISTS.

Drug (Trade)	Daily Dosage Range	Renal Dysfunction	Product Availability (mg)
Candesartan (Atacand)	8–32 mg q day	No adjustment necessary	Tablets 4, 8, 16, 32
Eprosartan (Teveten)	400–800 mg q day	No adjustment necessary	Tablets 400, 600
Irbesartan (Avapro)	140–300 mg q day	No adjustment necessary	Tablets 75, 150, 300
Irbesartan/ Hydrochlorothiazide (Avalide)	1–2 tablets q day	HCTZ not recommended in severe impairment	Tablets Irbesartan 150/HCTZ 12.5 Irbesartan 300/HCTZ 12.5
Losartan (Cozaar)	25–100 mg q day or bid	No adjustment necessary	Tablets 25, 50
Losartan/ Hydrochlorothiazide (Hyzaar)	50/12.5 mg 1–2 q day 100 mg/25 mg q day	HCTZ not recommended in severe impairment	Tablets Losartan 50/HCTZ 12.5 Losartan 100/HCTZ 25
Olmesartan (Benicar)	20–40 mg per day	No adjustment necessary	Tablets 5,20,40
Telmisartan (Micardis)	20–80 mg q day	No adjustment necessary	Tablets 40, 80
Valsartan (Diovan)	80–320 mg q day	Decrease dose if $Cl_{cr} < 10$ mL/min	Capsules 80, 160
Valsartan/ Hydrochlorothiazide (Diovan HCT)	1–2 capsules q day	HCTZ not recommended in severe impairment	Tablets Valsartan 80/HCTZ 12.5 Valsartan 160/HCTZ 12.5

TABLE VII–5. ANTISTAPHYLOCCOCCAL PENICILLINS.[1, 2]

Drug (Brand)	Dosage	Dosing Interval	Suplied	Notes
Oxacillin (Bactocill)	1–2 g	4–6 hr	Injection	
Nafcillin (Nafcil, Unipen)	1–2 g	4–6 hr	Injection	No dosage adjustments for renal function
Cloxacillin (Cloxapen, Tegopen)	250–500 mg	6 hr	Oral	Administer on an empty stomach
Dicloxacillin (Dynapen, Dycill)	250–500 mg	6 hr	Oral	Administer on an empty stomach

[1] **Indications:** Treatment of infections caused by susceptible strains of *Staphylococcus* and *Streptococcus*.
[2] **Actions:** Bactericidal: Inhibit cell wall synthesis.

TABLE VII–6. EXTENDED-SPECTRUM PENICILLINS.[1–3]

Drug (Brand)	Dose	Dosing Interval	mEq Na$^+$ Per Gram	Notes
Ticarcillin (Ticar)	3 g	4–6 hr	5.2	May cause hypokalemia/ sodium overload, acquired platelet dysfunction with the potential for bleeding to occur
Ticarcillin-clavulanate (Timentin)	3.1 g	4–6 hr	4.75	Clavulanate is a beta-lactamase inhibitor
Mezlocillin (Mezlin)	3 g	4–6 hr	1.85	Activity against *Entero-bacteriaceae*
Piperacillin (Pipracil)	3 g	4–6 hr	1.85	Best activity against *Pseudomonas*
Piperacillin-tazobactam (Zosyn)	3.375 g	6 hr		Tazobactam is a beta-lactamase inhibitor (Does not improve activity against *Pseudomonas* when compared to pipera-cillin without tazobactam)

[1] **Indications:** Treatment of infections caused by susceptible gram-negative bacteria (including *Klebsiella, Proteus, E coli, Enterobacter, P aeruginosa, Serratia*) involving the skin, bone and joints, respiratory tract, urinary tract, abdomen, and vascular system.
[2] **Actions:** Bactericidal, inhibits cell wall synthesis.
[3] **Notes:** These agents are often used in combination with an aminoglycoside to treat *P aeruginosa* and in neuropenic patients with a fever. Dosage adjustment necessary in renal impairment.

TABLE VII–7. BETA-ADRENERGIC BLOCKING AGENTS.[1-4]

Drug (Trade)	Receptor	Angina	Hypertension	Myocardial Infarction	Congestive Heart Failure
Acebutolol (Sectral)	B₁, ISA		200–400 mg bid		
Atenolol (Tenormin)	B₁	50–100 mg q day	50–100 mg q day	5 mg IV × 2 doses, then 50 mg PO bid	
Betaxolol (Kerlone)	B₁		10–20 mg q day		
Bisoprolol (Zebeta)	B₁		5–10 mg q day		
Carteolol (Cartrol)	B₁, B₂, ISA		2.5–5 mg q day		
Carvedilol (Coreg)	B₁, B₂, α		6.25–25 mg bid		3.125–25 bid
Esmolol (Brevibloc)	(See p 511)				
Labetalol (Trandate, Normodyne)	B₁, B₂, α₁		100–400 mg bid		
Metoprolol (Lopressor, Toprol XL)	B₁	50–100 mg bid	100–450 mg q day	5 mg IV × 3 doses, then 50 mg PO Q 6 hr × 48 hr, then 100 mg PO bid	6.25–50 mg bid **or** 12.5–200 mg XL q day
Nadolol (Corgard)	B₁, B₂	40–80 mg q day	40–80 mg q day		
Penbutolol (Levatol)	B₁, B₂, ISA		20–40 mg q day		
Pindolol (Visken)	B₁, B₂, ISA		5–10 mg bid		

(continued)

TABLE VII–7. BETA-ADRENERGIC BLOCKING AGENTS (continued).

Drug (Trade)	Receptor	Angina	Hypertension	Myocardial Infarction	Congestive Heart Failure
Propranolol (Inderal)	B_1, B_2	160 mg SR q day	120–160 mg SR q day	60 mg tid–qid	
Sotalol (Betapace)	(See p 000)				
Timolol (Blocadren)	B_1, B_2		10–20 mg bid	10 mg bid	

Notes: ISA = intrinsic sympathomimetic activity.

Other Uses:

Cardiac Arrhythmias:	Various agents and doses
Migraine Prophylaxis:	Atenolol 50–100 mg/d **or**
	Nadolol 40–80 mg/d **or**
	[1]Propranolol 80–240 mg/d
Essential Tremor:	Propranolol 40 mg bid; maximal dose 320 mg/d
Adjunctive Therapy:	Pheochromocytoma (after alpha-adrenergic drugs are added)
	Hyperthyroidism (propranolol)
	Rebleeding of esophageal varices in cirrhotic patients and alcohol withdrawal (atenolol)

[1]FDA-approved indication.

Precautions:

1 Use with caution in diabetic patients. May blunt symptoms/signs of acute hypoglycemia; nonselective agents may potentiate insulin-induced hypoglycemia. Beta-blockade also reduces the release of insulin in response to hyperglycemia.

2 May increase serum lipid concentrations. May not be as pronounced with agents having intrinsic sympathomimetic activity.

3 Use with caution in patients with congestive heart failure (decreased myocardial contractility) and chronic obstructive pulmonary diseases (potential blockade of B_2 receptors).

4 When discontinuing chronically administered beta-blockers, particularly in patients with ischemic heart disease, reduce dose gradually, especially with agents with a short half-life (propranolol, metoprolol).

TABLE VII–8. FIRST-GENERATION CEPHALOSPORINS.[1–3]

Drug (Brand)	Dose	Dosing Interval	Supplied	Notes
Cefadroxil (Duricef, Ultracef)	500 mg–1 g	12–24 hr	Capsules, tablets	
Cefazolin (Ancef, Kefzol)	1–2 g	8 hr	Injection	For surgical prophylaxis most widely used antibiotic
Cephalexin (Keflex)	250–500 mg	qid	Capsules, tablets	
Cephradine (Velosef)	250–500 mg 1 g	qid 6 hr	Capsules Injection	

[1]**Indications:** Treatment of infections caused by susceptible strains of *Streptococcus, Staphylococcus, E coli, Proteus, and Klebsiella* involving the skin, bone and joints, upper and lower respiratory tract, and urinary tract.
[2]**Actions:** Bactericidal; inhibits cell wall synthesis.
[3]**Dosage adjustments:** Necessary in renal impairment.

TABLE VII–9. SECOND-GENERATION CEPHALOSPORINS.[1–3]

Drug (Brand)	Dose	Dosing Interval	Supplied	Notes
Cefaclor (Ceclor)	250–500 mg	8 hr	Capsules Tablets	
Cefotetan (Cefotan)	1–2 g	12 hr	Injection	Activity against anaerobes
Cefoxitin (Mefoxin)	1–2 g	6 hr	Injection	Best activity against anaerobes
Cefprozil (Cefzil)	250–500 mg	q day–bid	Tablets	Use higher doses for otitis and pneumonia
Cefuroxime (Zinacef, Ceftin)	750 mg–1.5 g 250–500 mg	8 hr bid	Injection Tablets	Ceftin should be taken with food
Loracarbef (Lorabid)	200–400 mg	bid	Capsules	Similar to cefaclor

[1]**Indications:** Treatment of infections caused by susceptible bacteria involving the upper and lower respiratory tract, skin, bone, urinary tract, abdomen, and female reproductive system.
[2]**Actions:** Bactericidal; inhibits cell wall synthesis.
[3]**Notes:** More active than 1st-generation agents against *H influenzae, E coli, Klebsiella* species, and *P mirabilis*. Risk of hypoprothrombinemia or bleeding has been associated with cephalosporins containing a N-methylthiotetrazole (NMTT) side chain. These agents include cefotetan, cefmetazole, and cefoperazone (3rd-generation). Administration of vitamin K will prevent clinical bleeding associated with these drugs for patients with vitamin K deficiency.
  Dosage adjustment necessary in renal impairment.

TABLE VII–10. THIRD- AND FOURTH-GENERATION CEPHALOSPORINS.[1-3]

Drug (Brand)	Dose	Interval	Supplied	Notes
Cefdinir (Omnicef)	300–600 mg	12–24 hr	Capsules	
Cefditoren	200–400	12 hr	Tablets	200 mg skin, 400 mg bronchitis and pharyngitis
Cefepime[4] (Maxipime)	1–2 g	12 hr	Injection	
Cefixime (Suprax)	200–400 mg	12–24 hr	Tablets, suspension	Use suspension for otitis media
Cefoperazone (Cefobid)	1–2 g	12 hr	Injection	See Footnote 3, Table 7–9
Cefotaxime (Claforan)	1–2 g	4–8 hr	Injection	Crosses the blood-brain barrier
Cefpodoxime (Vantin)	200–400 mg	12 hr	Tablets	Drug interations with agents increasing the gastric pH
Ceftazidime (Fortaz, Ceptaz) Tazidime, Tazicef)	1–2 g	8 hr	Injection	Best activity against *Pseudomonas.* Crosses the blood-brain barrier.
Ceftibuten (Cedax)	400 mg	12 hr	Capsule	Take on an empty stomach
Ceftizoxime (Cefizox)	1–2 g	8–12 hr	Injection	
Ceftriaxone (Rocephin)	1–2 g	12–24 hr	Injection	Treatment of choice for gonorrhea. Crosses the blood-brain barrier.

[1]*Indications:* Treatment of infections caused by susceptible bacteria involving the respiratory tract, skin, bone and joints, and urinary tract; treatment of meningitis, febrile neutropenia, and septicemia.
[2]*Actions:* Bactericidal; inhibits cell wall synthesis.
[3]*Notes:* Less active against gram-positive cocci than 1st- and 2nd-generation agents. Increased activity against gram-negative aerobes (*Enterobacteriaceae* including *Enterobacter* and *Serratia*) due to increased stability to beta-lactamases. May be used in combination with an aminoglycoside. Dosage adjustment necessary in renal impairment.
[4]*Notes:* 4th-generation cephalosporin.

TABLE VII–11. NONSTEROIDAL ANTI-INFLAMMATORY DRUGS.[1]

Drug (Trade)	Arthritis	Analgesia	Dysmenorrhea	Maximum Daily Dose (MG)
■ **Salicylates[2]**				
Diflunisal[3] (Dolobid)	500 mg bid–tid	500 mg bid–tid		1500
■ **Acetic acids[2]**				
Diclofenac (Cataflam, Voltaren)	50–75 mg bid–tid	50 mg tid	50 mg tid	200
Etodolac (Lodine)	200–400 mg bid–tid	200–400 mg q 6–8 hr		1200
Indomethacin (Indocin)	25–50 mg bid–tid			200 **or** SR 150
Ketorolac (Toradol)		IV/IM 15–30 mg q 6 hr; PO 10 mg q 6 hr		IV: 120; PO: 40; do not use for more than 5 days
Nabumetone (Relafen)	1000–2000 mg/d divided q day–bid			2000
Sulindac (Clinoril)	150–200 mg bid			400
Tolmetin (Tolectin)	200–600 mg tid			2000
■ **Oxicams[2]**				
Piroxicam (Feldene)	10–20 mg q day			20

(continued)

TABLE VII–11. NONSTEROIDAL ANTI-INFLAMMATORY DRUGS (continued).

Drug (Trade)	Arthritis	Analgesia	Dysmenorrhea	Maximum Daily Dose (MG)
■ Propionic acids[2]				
Fenoprofen (Nalfon)	300–600 mg tid–qid	200 mg q 4–6 hr		3200
Flurbiprofen (Ansaid)	50–100 mg bid–qid			300
Ibuprofen (Advil, Motrin)	400–800 mg tid–qid	400 mg q 4–6 hr	400 mg q 4 hr	3200
Ketoprofen (Orudis)	50–75 mg tid–qid	25–50 mg q 6–8 hr		300
Meloxicam[4, 6] (Mobic)	7.5–15 mg q day			
Naproxen (Naprosyn)	250–500 mg bid	250 mg q 6–8 hr	250 mg q 6–8 hr	1500
Naproxen sodium (Aleve, Anaprox)	275–550 mg bid	275 mg q 6–8 hr	275 mg q 6–8 hr	1375
Oxaprozin (Daypro)	600–1200 mg q day			1200
■ Selective COX-2 Inhibitors				
Celecoxib[5–7] (Celebrex)	100 mg bid or 200 mg q day (osteoarthritis) 100–200 mg bid (rheumatoid arthritis)			400
Valdecoxib[6–8] (Bextra)	10 mg q day		20 mg q 1–2 hr	40

Notes:

[1] Can cause renal insufficiency/failure, especially in the elderly. **Do not take** in the third trimester of pregnancy. Information regarding CV risks of long term use is emerging.

[2] Chronic **use can cause gastrointestinal bleeding from gastroduodenal ulceration.** Inhibits platelet **aggregation except for meloxicam.**

[3] First dose 1000 mg, then 500 mg bid-tid.

[4] Inhibits COX-2 more than COX-1.

[5] Dosage for familial adenomatous polyposis is 400 mg bid. Doses greater than 200 mg/day may not be associated with CV risks.

[6] Does not inhibit platelet aggregation.

[7] Avoid with sulfa allergy.

[8] Associated **with** Stevens-Johnsons syndrome and toxic epidermal necrolysis. Use contraindicated in patients immediately following CABG.

TABLE VII–12. OPHTHALMIC AGENTS.

Drug (Trade)	Strength (%)	Dosing Schedule
AGENTS FOR GLAUCOMA		
Alpha-$_2$ adrenergic agonists		
Brimonidine (Alphagan)	0.2	1 gtt tid
Apraclonidine (Iopidine)	0.5, 1.0	1–2 gtts tid (0.5%), 1 gtt 1 hr prior to surgery (1.0%)
Dipivefrin (Propine)	0.1	1 gtt q 12 hr
Beta-blockers		
Betaxolol (Betoptic-S, Betoptic)	0.25, 05	1 gtt bid
Levobunolol (Betagan Liquifilm)	0.25, 0.5	1 gtt q day–bid
Metipranolol (OptiPranolol)	0.3	1 gtt bid
Timolol[1] (Timoptic)	0.25, 0.5	1 gtt q day–bid
Carteolol (Ocupress)	1.0	1 gtt bid
Levobetaxolol (Betaxon)	0.5	1 gtt bid
Carbonic anhydrase inhibitors		
Brinzolamide (Azopt)	1.0	1 gtt tid
Dorzolamide (Trusopt)	2.0	1 gtt tid
Miotics, cholinesterase inhibitors		
Carbachol (Isopto Carbachol)	0.75–3	1–2 gtts tid
Physostigmine (Isopto Eserine)	0.25–0.5	2 gtts up to qid
Demecarium (Humorsol)	0.125, 0.25	1–2 gtts twice weekly, up to 1–2 gtts bid
Echothiophate iodine (Phospholine iodide)	0.03, 0.06, 0.125, 0.25	1 gtt bid
Pilocarpine (Isopto Carpine, Pilocar)	0.25–10	1–2 gtts up to 6 × per day
(Pilopine HS gel)	4.0	0.5 inch q HS

(continued)

TABLE VII–12. OPHTHALMIC AGENTS *(continued)*.

Drug (Trade)	Strength (%)	Dosing Schedule
Prostaglandin agonists		
Latanoprost[2] (Xalatan)	0.005	1 drop q HS
Combination agents		
Dorzolamide and Timolol (Cosopt)	2/0.5	1 drop bid
ANTIBIOTICS		
Bacitracin (See p 000)		
Chloramphenicol (AK-Chlor)	oint/sol	1–2 drops or 0.5 inch q3–4 hr
Ciprofloxacin (Ciloxan)	solution	1–2 drops 4–6 × per day
Erythromycin (AK-Mycin, Ilotycin)	ointment	0.5 inch 2–8 × per day
Gatifloxacin (Zymar)	solution	Days 1 & 2: 1 drop q 2 hr up to 8 times
		Days 3–7: 1 drop qid
Gentamicin (Garamycin)	oint/sol	1–2 drops or 0.5 inch 2–3 × per day, up to q 3–4 hr
Levofloxacin (Quixin, Iquix)	solution	Days 1 & 2: 1–2 drops q 2 hr up to 8 times/day
		Days 3–7: 1–2 drops q 4 hr up to 4 times/day
Moxifloxacin (Vigamox)	solution	1 drop tid
Neomycin, Polymyxin B,	sus	1–2 drops q 3–4
Hydrocortisone 1% (Cortisporin)		
Norfloxacin (Chibroxin)	solution	1–2 drops qid
Ofloxacin (Ocuflox)	solution	Days 1 & 2: 1–2 drops q 2–4 hr
		Days 3–7: 1–2 drops qid
Sulfacetamide Sodium	10–30% oint/sol	1–2 drops q 1–3 hr or 0.5 inch q day–qid
(Sodium Sulamyd, Bleph 10)		
Tobramycin (Tobrex)	oint/sol	1–2 drops or 0.5 inch 2–3 × per day, up to q 3–4 hr
ANTI-INFLAMMATORY		
NSAIDs		
Diclofenac (Voltaren)	0.1	1 drop qid (post-op inflammation following cataract surgery)
Flurbiprofen (Ocufen)	0.03	1 drop q 4 hr × 3 days (ocular inflammation)
Ketorolac (Acular)	0.5	1 drop qid (relieves itching due to seasonal allergic conjunctivitis)

Corticosteroids

Dexamethasone (AK-Dex, others)	0.05 (oint), 0.1 (sol)	1–2 drops or 0.5 inch tid–qid
Fluorometholone (FML, Flarex)	0.1	1–2 drops bid–qid
Prednisolone (AK-Pred, Pred Forte)	0.12, 0.125, 1.0	1–2 drops q 1 hr day, q 2 night until response, then 1 drop q 4 hr
Rimexolone (Vexol)	1	1–2 drops q 1 hr to qid

Antihistamine

Olopatadine (Patanol)	0.1	1–2 drops qbid

Decongestant/anti-allergy

Ketotifen[3] (Zaditor)	0.025	1 drop bid–tid
Levocabastine (Livostin)	0.05	1 drop qid
Naphazoline and Antazoline (Albalon-A)	0.05/0.5	1–2 drops tid–qid
Naphazoline and Pheniramine Acetate (Naphcon A)	0.025/0.3	1–2 drops tid–qid

Mast cell stabilizers

Lodoxamide (Alomide)	0.1	1–2 drops qid
Nedocromil sodium (Alocril)	2	1–2 drops bid
Pemirolast potassium (Alamast)	0.1	1–2 drops qid

COMBINATION AGENTS (also see Glaucoma)

Gentamicin and Prednisolone (Pred-G)	Oint/sol	0.5 inch bid–tid (oint), 1–2 drops q 2–4 hr up to q 2 hr (sol)
Neomycin & Dexamethasone (Dex-Neo-Dex)	Oint/sol	0.5 inch tid–qid (oint), 1–2 drops q 3–4 hr (sol)
Neomycin, Polymyxin, Hydrocortisone (Cortisporin)	Oint/sol	0.5 inch q day–qid (oint), 1–2 drops bid–qid
Neomycin, Polymyxin, & Dexamethasone (Maxitrol)	Oint/sol	0.5 inch tid–qid (oint), 1–2 drops q 4–6 hr (sol)
Neomycin, Polymyxin, & Prednisolone (Poly-Pred)	Oint/sol	0.5 inch tid–qid (oint), 1–2 drops q 4–6 hr (sol)
Sulfacetamide & Prednisolone (Blephamide)	Oint/sol	0.5 inch q day—qid (oint), 1–3 drops q 2–3 hr

Notes:
1 Systemic absorption may cause bradycardia.
2 May darken light irides.
3 Wait at least 10 minutes before putting in contact lens.

TABLE VII–13. SULFONYLUREA AGENTS.[1, 2]

Drug (Trade)	Duration of Activity (hr)	Equivalent Dose (mg)	Dosing Schedule
■ First-generation			
Acetohexamide (Dymelor)	24	500	250–1500 mg q day
Chlorpropamide (Diabinese)	≥ 60	250	100–500 mg q day
Tolazamide (Tolinase)	12–24	250	100–500 mg q day
Tolbutamide (Orinase)	6–12	1000	500–1000 mg bid
■ Second-generation			
Glipizide[3] (Glucotrol, Glucotrol-XL)	10–16	10	5–15 mg q day–bid
Glyburide non-micronized[4] (DiaBeta, Micronase)	24	5	1.25–10 mg q day–bid
Glyburide micronized[4] (Glynase)	24	3	1.5–6 mg q day–bid
Glimepiride (Amaryl)	24	2	1–4 mg q day 8 mg q day[5]

[1]*Indications:* Management of non-insulin-dependent diabetes mellitus (NIDDM).
[2]*Actions:* Stimulates the release of insulin from the pancreas; increases insulin sensitivity at peripheral sites; reduces glucose output from the liver.
[3]*Glipizide:* Give approximately 30 minutes before a meal. Divide total daily doses when doses exceed 15 mg. Maximum daily recommended daily dose is 40 mg.
[4]*Glyburide:* Administer with first main meal. Maximum recommended daily dose non-micronized, 20 mg; micronized, 12 mg.
[5]Given with the first main meal in patients receiving low-dose insulin.

TABLE VII-14. PROTON PUMP INHIBITORS.[1-3]

	Duodenal Ulcer	Gastric Ulcer	Hypersecretory Conditions	GERD Healing	GERD Maintenance	H pylori Eradication
Esomeprazole (Nexium)[2] –Delayed-release capsules: 20, 40 mg				20–40 mg q day × 4–8 wk	20 mg q day	40 mg q day, & Amoxicillin 1 g bid, & Clarithromycin 500 mg bid × 10 days
Lansoprazole (Prevacid)[3] –Delayed-release capsules: 15, 30 mg –Orally disintegrating delayed release tablets: 15, 30 mg –Granules for oral suspension, delayed release: 15, 30 mg	15 mg q day × 4 wk	30 mg q day × 8 wk	60 mg q day up to 90 mg bid (divide doses > 120 mg/d)	15–30 mg q day × 8 wk	15 mg q day	30 mg bid; Amoxicillin 1 g bid; & Clarithromycin 500 mg bid × 14 days
Omeprazole (Prilosec) –Delayed-release tablets (OTC): 20 mg –Delayed-release capsules: 10, 20, 40 mg –Powder for suspension: 20 mg (Zegerid)	20 mg q day × 4–8 wk	40 mg q day × 4–8 wk	60 mg q day up to 120 mg tid (divide doses > 80 mg/d)	20–40 mg q day × 4–8 wk	20 mg q day	20 mg q day, & Amoxicillin 1 g bid & Clarithromycin 500 mg bid × 10 days **OR** 40 mg q day & Clarithromycin 500 mg tid × 14 days
Pantoprazole (Protonix)[3] –Delayed-release tablet: 20, 40 mg			80 mg q day up to 240 mg (in 2 divided doses)	40 mg × 8 wk	40 mg × 12 mo	
Rabeprazole (Aciphex) –Delayed-release tablet: 20 mg	20 mg q day × 4 wk	60 mg q day	20 mg × 4–8 wk	20 mg q day		

Notes:

[1] All products are delayed-release formulations. Swallow whole—do not crush or chew.

[2] If patient has difficulty swallowing the capsule, open delayed-release capsule and mix the pellets inside the capsule in 1 tablespoon of applesauce. Swallow immediately—do not chew or crush pellets.

[3] Available in an IV formulation.

TABLE VII-15. HMG-CoA REDUCTASE INHIBITORS. [1-3]

	Dose	Comparative Dosages	Hydrophilic/ Lipophilic	Metabolism	LFT Monitoring
Atorvastatin (Lipitor) Tablet: 10, 20, 40, 80 mg	10–80 mg q day	10 mg	Lipophilic	P450 3A4	Baseline or elevation of dose, 12 wk, semiannually
Fluvastatin (Lescol) Capsule: 20, 40 mg Tablet, extended release: 80 mg	20–80 mg q day	40 mg	Lipophilic	P450 2C9	Baseline or elevation of dose, 12 wk, semiannually
Lovastatin (Mevacor, Altocor) Tablet: 10, 20, 40 mg	10–80 mg q day	40 mg	Lipophilic	P450 3A4	Baseline or elevation of Dose, 6 wk, 12 wk, semiannually
Pravastatin (Pravachol) Tablet: 10, 20, 40, 80 mg	10–40 mg q day	40 mg	Hydrophilic	Not extensively metabolized	Baseline or elevation of dose, 12 wk
Rosuvastatin (Crestor) Tablet: 5, 10, 20, 40 mg	5–40 mg q day	5 mg	Hydrophilic	P450 2C9/2C19 (not extensively metabolized	Baseline or elevation of dose, 12 wk, semiannually
Simvastatin (Zocor) [5] Tablet: 10, 20, 40, 80 mg	10–80 mg q day	20 mg	Lipophilic	P450 3A4	Baseline or elevation of dose, semiannually

Notes:
1. Pregnancy category X.
2. Maximum response occurs in 4–6 weeks.
3. Counsel patients to report unexplained muscle pain, tenderness or weakness due to risk of myopathy, or jaundice and abdominal pain due to risk of hepatic injury.
4. Do not exceed 5 mg q day with cyclosporin or 10 mg q day with gemfibrozil or CrCl < 30 mL/min.
5. Available in combination with cholesterol absorption inhibitor ezetimibe. Vytorin tablets available as 10 mg ezetimibe with 10, 20, 40 or 80 mg simvastatin.

TABLE VII–16. 5-HT$_3$ RECEPTOR AGONISTS

Drug	Initial Dose	Repeat Dose	Max Dose/24 h	Supplied
Almotriptan (Axert)	6.25 or 12.5 mg PO	×1 in 2 hr	25 mg	Tabs 6.25, 12.5 mg
Eletriptan[a] (Relpax)	20 or 40 mg	×1 in 2 hr	80 mg	Tabs 20, 40 mg
Frovatriptan (Frova)	2.5 mg PO	in 2 hr	7.5 mg	Tabs 2.5 mg
Naratriptan (Amerge)	1 or 2.5 mg PO[b]	in 4 hr	5 mg	Tabs 1, 2.5 mg
Rizatriptan (Maxalt, Maxalt-MLT	5 or 10 mg PO[c]	in 2 hr	30 mg	Tabs 5, 10 mg; Disintegrating tabs, 5, 10 mg
Sumatriptan (Imitrex)	25, 50, or 100 mg PO	in 2 hr	200 mg	Tabs 25, 50, 100 mg
	5–20 mg intranasally	in 2 hr	40 mg	Nasal spray 5, 20 mg
	6 mg SC	in 1 hr	12 mg	Inj 12 mg/mL
Zolmitriptan (Zomig, Zomig ZMT)	2.5 or 5 mg PO	in 2 hr	10 mg	Tabs 2.5, 5 mg; Disintegrating tabs 2.5 mg

Precautions/contraindications: (C, M) ischemic heart disease, coronary artery vasospasm, Prinzmetal's angina, uncontrolled HTN, hemiplegic or basilar migraine, ergots, use of another serotonin agonist within 24 hr use with MAOI. Side effects: dizziness, somnolence, paresthesias, nausea, flushing, dry mouth, coronary vasospasm, chest tightness, HTN, GI upset.
[a]Do not use within 72 hours of drugs that are potent CYP3A4 inhibitors.
[b]Reduce dose in mild renal and hepatic insufficiency (2.5 mg/d MAX); contraindicated with severe renal (CrCl < 15 mL/min) or hepatic impairment.
[c]Initiate therapy at 5 mg PO (15 mg/d max) in patients receiving propranolol.

TABLE VII–17. NON-ANTIBIOTIC DRUG LEVELS.

Drug	Therapeutic Level	Toxic Level
Carbamazepine	8.0–12.0 mcg/mL	> 15.0 mcg/mL
Digoxin	0.8–2.0 ng/mL	> 2.0 ng/mL
Ethanol		> 80–100 mg/100 mL (legally intoxicated) 100–200 mg/100 mL (labile) 150–300 mg/100 mL (confusion) 250–400 mg/100 mL (stupor) 350–500 mg/100 mL (coma) > 450 mg/100 mL (death)
Ethosuximide	40–100 mcg/mL	> 150 mcg/mL
Lidocaine	1.5–6.5 mcg/mL	> 6.5 mcg/mL
Lithium	0.6–1.2 mmol/L	> 2.0 mmol/L
Phenobarbital	15.0–40.0 mcg/mL	> 45.0 mcg/mL
Phenytoin (total)	10.0–20.0 mcg/mL	> 20.0 mcg/mL
Phenytoin (free)	1–2 mcg/mL	> 2.0 mcg/mL
Procainamide	4.0–10.0 mcg/mL	> 16.0 mcg/mL
N-acetylprocainamide (NAPA-active metabolite of procainamide)	5.0–30.0 mcg/mL	> 40.0 mcg/mL
Quinidine	3.0–5.0 mcg/mL	> 7 mcg/mL
Salicylate	20–30 mcg/mL	40–50 mcg/mL
Tacrolimus	5–15 ng/mL	
Theophylline	5–15 mcg/mL	> 20.0 mcg/mL
Valproic acid	50–100 mcg/mL	> 150 mcg/mL

Note: Each lab may have its own set of values that vary slightly from those given.
Modified and reproduced with permission from Gomella LG, ed. Clinician's Pocket Reference. *10th ed.* McGraw-Hill; 2004.

TABLE VII–18. THERAPEUTIC DRUG LEVELS: ANTIBIOTICS.

Antibiotic	Trough (mcg/mL) Maintain Below Upper Limit	Peak (mcg/mL)
Amikacin	5.0–7.5	25–35
Gentamicin	1.0–2.0	5–8
Gentamicin (24-hour dosing with normal renal function)	1.0–2.0	> 10
Tobramycin	1.0–2.0	5–8
Tobramycin (24-hour dosing with normal renal function)	1.0–2.0	> 10
Vancomycin	5.0–10.0	20–40

[1]*Modified and reproduced with permission from Gomella LG, ed.* Clinician's Pocket Reference. *10th ed.* McGraw-Hill; 2004.

TABLE VII–19. AMINOGLYCOSIDE DOSING IN ADULTS: EVERY 8- OR 12-HOUR DOSING (FOR Q DAY DOSING OF GENTAMICIN AND TOBRAMYCIN SEE PAGES 000 AND 000, RESPECTIVELY).

1. Select the loading dose:
   Gentamicin   1.5–2.0 mg/kg
   Tobramycin   1.5–2.0 mg/kg
   Amikacin   5.0–7.5 mg/kg

2. Calculate the estimated creatinine clearance (CrCl) based on serum creatinine (SCr), age, and weight (kg); OR order a formal creatinine clearance, if time permits.

$$\text{CrCl for male} = \frac{\left(140 - \text{age} \times \text{ weight in kg}\right)}{\left(\text{ScCr} \times 72\right)} \times 100$$

   CrCl for female = 0.85 × (CrCl male)

3. By using Table VII–20, p XXX, you can now select the maintenance dose (as a percentage of the chosen loading dose) most appropriate for the patient's renal function based on CrCl and dosing interval. Shaded areas are the percentages and intervals suggested for any given creatinine clearance. For patients over 60 years old, it is recommended to give the dose no more frequently than every 12 hours.

4. Empiric dosing, as above, is used to begin therapy. Serum levels (see Table VII–18, p 630) should be monitored and adjustments made in the dosing based on the drug levels for optimal therapy.

Note: See Table VII–18, p 000, for the trough and peak levels of the aminoglycosides gentamicin, tobramycin, and amikacin. Peak levels should be drawn 30 minutes after the dose is completely infused; trough levels should be drawn 30 minutes prior to dose. As a general rule, draw the peak and trough around the fourth maintenance dose. Therapy can be initiated with the recommended guidelines. **These calculations are not valid for netilmicin.**
[1]*Modified and reproduced with permission from Gomella LG, ed.* Clinician's Pocket Reference. *10th ed. McGraw-Hill; 2004.*

TABLE VII–20. AMINOGLYCOSIDE DOSING: PERCENTAGE OF LOADING DOSE REQUIRED FOR DOSAGE INTERVAL SELECTED.

Creatinine Clearance (mL/min)	Dosing Interval (hr)		
	8	12	24
90	90%	—	—
80	88	—	—
70	84	—	—
60	79	91%	—
50	74	87	—
40	66	80	—
30	57	72	92%
25	51	66	88
20	45	59	83
15	37	50	75
10	29	40	64
7	24	33	55
5	20	28	48
2	14	20	35
0	9	13	25

Note: Shaded areas indicate suggested dosage intervals.
Reproduced with permission from Hull JH, Sarubbi FA: Gentamicin serum concentrations: Pharmacokinetic predictions. Ann Intern Med 1976;85:183–189.

TABLE VII–21. AMINOGLYCOSIDE DOSING: ONCE-DAILY DOSING OF GENTAMICIN AND TOBRAMYCIN (*NOT* AMIKACIN).

Several studies suggest that larger doses of aminoglycosides given once daily are just as effective, and less toxic, than conventional dosing given three times a day. Once-daily dosing of gentamicin and tobramycin regimens takes advantage of concentration-dependent killing through the optimization of peak concentration/MIC ratio. In addition, there are potential cost savings for nursing, pharmacy, and laboratory personnel.

Inclusion Criteria: All patients ordered aminoglycosides for prophylaxis, empiric therapy, or documented infection. (Aminoglycosides are usually indicated as synergistic or adjunctive therapy with other antibiotics as double coverage for gram-negative infections.)

Exclusion Criteria:
1. Patients with ascites
2. Patients with burns on > 20% of body surface
3. Pregnant patients
4. Patients receiving dialysis
5. Patients with gram-positive bacterial endocarditis
6. Pediatric patients

Initial Dose: Doses will be based on __DOSING BODY WEIGHT__, ideal body weight plus 40% of estimated adipose tissue mass (*see Dosing Guidelines*). Patients with estimated $Cl_{cr} \geq 40$ mL/min/1.73 m^2 will receive initial gentamicin dose of 7 mg/kg-DBW, infused over 30 minutes. Patients with estimated creatinine clearances < 40 mL/min/1.73 m^2 will receive an initial gentamicin dose of 3 mg/kg, infused over 30 minutes.

Monitoring: Two random concentrations will be obtained to monitor. Once-daily dosing of gentamicin and tobramycin:

The *1st random* concentration will be drawn *4 hours** after completion of the *1st* dose. The average 4-hour random sample, with a 7 mg/kg dose will be ~ 13–15 mg/L 4 hours after a 30-minute infusion. *Note:* The Therapeutic Drug Monitoring Lab should be notified that the expected gentamicin/tobramycin level will be greater than 10 mg/L.

The *2nd random* concentration will be drawn *12 hours* after completion of the *1st* dose.

> **The rationale for the 4-hour sample versus a "peak" is to determine the serum concentration after the distribution phase. A study (Jennings HJ, Davis GA, June 2000) was conducted at the University of Kentucky Medical Center that demonstrated a prolonged distribution phase following a 7 mg/kg dose in trauma surgery patients.*

Subsequent Doses: Scr/BUN should be measured at baseline and 2 times per week thereafter. Subsequent doses will be the same as the initial dose, but the dosing intervals will be adjusted to achieve troughs *less than or equal to 1 mg/L.* Appropriate dosing intervals include every 24, 36, or 48 hours.

> *If the serum concentration following a 7 mg/kg dose requires > 48 hours to decline to 1 mg/L, then 3 mg/kg or conventional dosing may be warranted. Some patients may have a prolonged "drug-free" period that may warrant conventional dosing to maintain concentrations. Patients should not receive a single dose of 7 mg/kg more frequently than every 24 hours until more studies are available.*

(*continued*)

TABLE VII–21. AMINOGLYCOSIDE DOSING: ONCE-DAILY DOSING OF GENTAMICIN AND TOBRAMYCIN (*NOT* AMIKACIN) (*continued*).

INITIAL DOSING GUIDELINES FOR ADULTS:

1. Estimate Creatinine Clearance (Cl_{cr}) using <u>Actual Body Weight</u> (ABW) for nonobese patients; in obese patients (> *125% IBW*) use <u>Dosing Body Weight</u> (see below for equation).

$$\text{Males} \quad Cl_{cr} = \frac{(140 - \text{Age}) \times \text{ABW}}{72 \times \text{Scr}} \qquad \text{Females} \quad Cl_{cr} = Cl_{cr} \times 0.85$$

2. Estimate Body Surface Area (BSA) using the Mosteller equation:

$$\text{BSA (m}^2) = \frac{\sqrt{\text{Ht(cm)} \times \text{Wt (kg)}}}{60} \quad \text{(Mosteller; } N \text{ } Engl \text{ } J \text{ } Med \text{ 1987;317:1098)}$$

3. Calculate Standardized Creatinine Clearance:

$$Cl_{cr(Std)} = Cl_{cr} \times \frac{1.73\text{m}^2}{\text{BSA}}$$

4. Determine <u>Ideal Body Weight</u> (IBW).

$$\begin{aligned} \text{IBW (kg)} &= \textbf{50 (kg) + (2.3 (kg)} \times \textbf{ea. inch over 5 ft) \quad male} \\ &= \textbf{45 (kg) + (2.3 (kg)} \times \textbf{ea. inch over 5 ft) \quad female} \end{aligned}$$

5. Calculate <u>Dosing Body Weight</u> (DBW):

$$\text{DBW} = \text{IBW} + 0.4 \text{ (ABW} - \text{IBW)}$$

(*If ABW* < *IBW, then DBW* = *ABW*)

6. Calculate the patient's dose based on Dosing Body Weight:
   a) **If Cl_{cr}(std) $\geq$ 40 mL/min/1.73 m², then give 7 mg/kg − DBW.**
   b) **If Cl_{cr}(std) < 40 mL/min/1.73 m², then give 3 mg/kg − DBW.**

Dilute dose in 100 mL of either 5% Dextrose or Normal Saline and infuse over 30 minutes.

Order two random concentrations at **4 and 12 hours** after the end of 1st dose. *Notify lab of the patient's name to allow for proper dilution of sample.*

Modified and reproduced with permission from Davis GA: Clinical Pharmacokinetics Service Policy and Procedural Manual. 23rd ed. *University of Kentucky Medical Center; 2000.*

Appendix

CONTENTS

TABLE A–1. FAHRENHEIT/CENTIGRADE TEMPERATURE CONVERSION.

°F	°C	°C	°F
95.0	35.0	35.0	95.0
96.0	35.5	35.5	95.9
97.0	36.1	36.0	95.8
98.0	36.6	36.5	97.7
98.6	37.0	37.0	98.6
99.0	37.2	37.5	99.5
100.0	37.7	38.0	100.4
101.0	38.3	38.5	101.3
102.0	38.8	39.0	102.2
103.0	39.4	39.5	103.1
104.0	40.0	40.0	104.0
105.0	40.5	40.5	104.9
106.0	41.1	41.0	105.8
	$°C = (°F - 32) \times 5/9$		$°F = (°C \times 95) \div 32$

Modified and Reproduced with permission from Gomella LG, ed. Clinician's Pocket Reference. 10th ed. McGraw-Hill; 2004.

TABLE A–2. POUNDS/KILOGRAMS WEIGHT CONVERSION.

lb	kg	kg	lb
1	0.5	1	2.2
2	0.9	2	4.4
4	1.8	3	6.6
6	2.7	4	8.8
8	3.6	5	11.0
10	4.5	6	13.2
20	9.1	8	17.6
30	13.6	10	22.0
40	18.2	20	44.0
50	22.7	30	66.0
60	27.3	40	88.0
70	31.8	50	110.0
80	36.4	60	132.0
90	40.9	70	154.0
100	45.4	80	176.0
150	68.2	90	198.0
200	90.8	100	220.0
$kg = lb \times 0.454$			$lb = kg \times 2.2$

[1] *Reproduced with permission from Gomella LG, ed.* Clinician's Pocket Reference. *10th ed. McGraw-Hill; 2004.*

TABLE A–3. GLASGOW COMA SCALE.

Parameter	Response		Score
Eyes	Open	Spontaneously	4
		To verbal command	3
		To pain	2
		No response	1
Best motor response	To verbal command	Obeys	6
	To painful stimulus	Localizes pain	5
		Flexion-withdrawal	4
		Decorticate (flex)	3
		Decerebrate (extend)	2
		No response	1
Best verbal response		Oriented, converses	5
		Disoriented, converses	4
		Inappropriate responses	3
		Incomprehensible sounds	2
		No response	1

Note: The Glasgow Coma Scale (EMV Scale) is a fairly reliable and objective way to monitor changes in levels of consciousness. It is based on eye opening, motor responses, and verbal responses (EMV). A person's EMV score is based on the total of the three different responses. The score ranges from 3 (lowest) to 15 (highest). *Modifided and reproduced with permission from Gomella LG, ed.* Clinician's Pocket Reference. *10th ed. McGraw-Hill; 2004.*

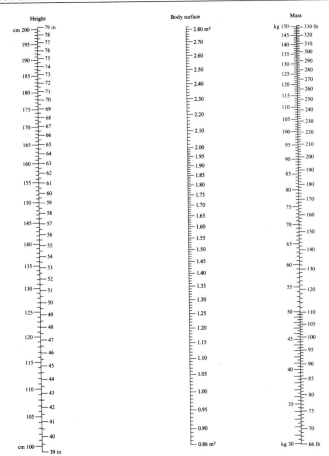

Figure A–1. Calculating body surface area. To determine the body surface of an adult, use a straightedge to connect height and mass. The point of intersection in the body surface line gives the body surface area in meters squared (m^2). (Reproduced with permission from Lentner C, ed. *Geigy Scientific Tables*. Vol 1. 8th ed. Basel: CIBA-Geigy;1981:227.

TABLE A–4. ENDOCARDITIS PROPHYLAXIS.[1, 2]

■ **Dental and upper respiratory procedures[2]**

Oral

Amoxicillin[3]	2 g PO 1 hr before procedure
Penicillin allergy:	
Clindamycin	600 mg PO 1 hr before procedure
OR	
Cephalexin[4] OR	2 g PO 1 hr before procedure
Cefadroxil[4]	
OR	
Azithromycin or Clarithromycin	500 mg PO 1 hr before procedure

Parenteral

Ampicillin	2 g IV or IM 30 min before procedure
Penicillin allergy:	
Clindamycin	600 mg IV within 30 min before procedure
OR	
Cefazolin[4]	1 g IV or IM within 30 min before procedure

■ **Gastrointestinal and genitourinary procedures[2]**

Oral

Amoxicillin[3]	2 g PO 1 hr before procedure

Parenteral[4]

Ampicillin	2 g IV or 1 M within 30 min before procedure
plus/minus	
Gentamicin	1.5 mg/kg (120 mg maximum dose) IV or IM 30 min before procedure
Penicillin allergy:[5]	
Vancomycin	1 g IV infused *slowly over 1 hr* beginning 1 hr before procedure
plus/minus	
Gentamicin	1.5 mg/kg (120 maximum dose) IV or IM 30 min before procedure

Modified and reproduced with permission from Med Lett *1999;41:80.*

[1] For patients with previous endocarditis, valvular heart disease, prosthetic heart valves, or complex cyanotic congenital heart disease (eg, tetralogy of Fallot), the risk is considered high. The risk is also considered high enough to treat in patients with other forms of congenital heart disease (but not uncomplicated secundum atrial septal defect), acquired valvular disease (eg, rheumatic heart disease), hypertrophic cardiomyopathy, and mitral valve prolapse with regurgitation or thickened valve leaflets. Viridans streptococci are the most likely cause of bacterial endocarditis after dental or upper respiratory procedures; enterococci are the most common cause of endocarditis after gastrointestinal or genitourinary procedures.

[2] For a review of the risk of bacteremia and endocarditis with various procedures, see Dajani AS, Taubert KA, Wilson W et al: Prevention of bacterial endocarditis: Recommendations by the American Heart Association. *JAMA* 1997;277:1794; and Durack DT: Prophylaxis of infective endocarditis. In: Mandell GL, Bennet JE, Dolin R, eds. *Principles and Practice of Infectious Diseases.* 5th ed. Churchill Livingstone; 2000:917. Among dental procedures, tooth extraction and gingival surgery (including implant placement) are thought to have the highest risk for bacterial endocarditis (Durack DT: Antibiotics for prevention of endocarditis during dentistry: Time to scale back? *Ann Intern Med* 1998;129:829.

[3] Amoxicillin is recommended because of its excellent bioavailability and good activity against streptococci and enterococci.

[4] Not recommended for patients with a history of immediate-type allergic reaction to penicillin (eg, urticaria, angioedema, anaphylaxis).

[5] Gentamicin should be added for patients with a high risk for bacterial endocarditis (see footnote 1). High-risk patients given parenteral ampicillin before the procedure should receive a dose of ampicillin 1 g IV or IM or a dose of amoxicillin 1 g PO 6 hours after the first dose.

TABLE A–5. SPECIMEN TUBES FOR VENIPUNCTURE.

Tube Color	Additives	General Use
Red	None	Clot tube to collect serum for chemistry, cross-matching, serology
Red and black (hot pink)	Silicone gel for rapid clot	As above, but not for osmolality or blood bank work
Blue	Sodium citrate (binds calcium)	Coagulation studies (best kept on ice, not for fibrin split products)
Blue/yellow label		Fibrin split products
Royal blue		Heavy metals, arsenic
Purple	Disodium EDTA (binds calcium)	Hematology, not for lipid profiles
Green	Sodium heparin	Ammonia, cortisol, ionized calcium (best kept on ice)
Green/glass beads		LE prep
Gray	Sodium fluoride	Lactic acid
Yellow	Transport medium	Blood cultures

Note: Individual labs may vary slightly from these listings.
Reproduced with permission from Gomella LG, Lefor AT: Surgery On Call. 3rd ed. McGraw-Hill; 2001.

Subject Index

NOTE: Page numbers in **boldface** type indicate a major discussion. A *t* following a page number indicates tabular material, and an *f* following a page number indicates a figure. Drugs are listed under their generic names. When a drug trade name is listed, the reader is referred to under their generic name.